OSTEOPOROSIS
Etiology, Diagnosis, and Management

Osteoporosis
Etiology, Diagnosis, and Management

Editors

B. Lawrence Riggs, M.D.
Consultant, Division of Endocrinology,
Metabolism and Internal Medicine
Mayo Clinic and Mayo Foundation
Professor of Medicine
Mayo Medical School
Rochester, Minnesota

L. Joseph Melton III, M.D.
Consultant, Section of Clinical Epidemiology
Mayo Clinic and Mayo Foundation
Professor of Epidemiology
Mayo Medical School
Rochester, Minnesota

Raven Press   New York

Raven Press, 1185 Avenue of the Americas, New York, New York 10036

Made in the United States of America

International Standard Book Number 0-88167-350-1

The material contained in this volume was submitted as previously unpublished material, except in the instances in which credit has been given to the source from which some of the illustrative material was derived.

Great care has been taken to maintain the accuracy of the information contained in the volume. However, neither Raven Press nor the editors can be held responsible for errors or for any consequences arising from the use of the information contained herein.

Materials appearing in this book prepared by individuals as part of their official duties as U.S. Government employees are not covered by the above-mentioned copyright.

9 8 7 6 5 4 3 2 1

Library of Congress Cataloging-in-Publication Data

Osteoporosis : etiology, diagnosis, and management.

Includes bibliographies and index.
1. Osteoporosis. I. Riggs, B. Lawrence (Byron Lawrence), 1931–   II. Melton, L. Joseph.
RC931.O730774   1988   616.7′16   85-43142
ISBN 0-88167-350-1

To our wives, Janet and Jane, for their support and forbearance

Preface

Osteoporosis is a disease whose time has come. Not long ago there was little interest in osteoporosis. Most physicians thought that it was a boring disease, and many believed it to be untreatable and the inevitable consequence of old age. Treatment of osteoporosis, when it occurred, was largely confined to patients with the vertebral fracture syndrome. Hip and Colles' fractures were usually ignored. Diagnosis of osteoporosis was limited to patients with nontraumatic vertebral fractures because there was no effective way to measure bone density.

All this has now changed. Largely as a consequence of the NIH Consensus Development Conference in 1984, the magnitude of the problem has been recognized. It has become clear to physicians that there are effective strategies for treatment and prevention. There has been wide media coverage. A recent national television poll showed that awareness among the lay public of the existence of osteoporosis as a disease has increased from 15 percent to 85 percent. All health care providers dealing with middle-aged women are being besieged with questions about it. The National Osteoporosis Foundation (1625 Eye Street, N.W., Suite 1011, Washington, D. C. 20006) has recently been established, and plans are underway to develop regional and local chapters for enhancing public awareness, increasing patient education and encouraging adoption of general preventive measures. Three of the National Institutes of Health (NIAMS, NIA, and NIDDK) have developed an initiative to increase funding for research on osteoporosis.

There are major new findings regarding the ontogeny, regulation and the function of bone cells. A relationship between the immune system and cells of the osteoclast's lineage has been discovered. The bone cell remodeling cycle has been defined and its kinetics measured. Bone cells have been shown to respond not only to systemic factors but to a myriad of local regulators and growth factors.

There is an emerging consensus that osteoporosis is a heterogeneous disorder with multiple causes. Many of the causes and risk factors for bone loss have been identified by physiologic and epidemiologic studies, and their relative importance is being quantified. Additionally, the recent development of methods to culture human bone cells from biopsy samples should lead to a definition of the role of intrinsic abnormalities of bone cell function in pathogenesis.

Diagnostic methods have improved dramatically. Bone density at the site of fractures can now be measured with $< 3\%$ precision, and bone turnover can be assessed conveniently by measuring an ever-growing number of newly discovered circulating bone-related proteins.

Using methods to quantify bone turnover and bone density, it has been established which forms of treatment are effective and which are not. Three antiresorptive regimens are currently approved by the Food and Drug Administration for the treatment of osteoporosis—calcium, estrogen, and calcitonin—and drugs of this class, such as the second generation diphosphonates, are under development. It has been documented that estrogen is effective in retarding postmenopausal bone loss, and new treatment approaches are being developed to minimize its side effects. For established osteoporosis, there is increasing interest in using formation-stimulating regimens that have the potential to restore bone mass above the fracture threshold, thereby effecting a "clinical cure." Among these, therapy with sodium fluoride is being intensively studied and results are being evaluated for relatively new regimens, such as the 1-34 synthetic fragment of parathyroid hormone in low dosage, combined therapy with calcitonin and oral phosphate and coherence therapy utilizing sequential activating and depressing agents. Stimulating bone formation using growth factors produced by recombinant-DNA technology is an exciting prospect. In such a favorable setting, it is reasonable to hope that this enormous public health problem can be brought under control within the coming decade.

The amount of relevant information required for a full understanding of etiology, diagnosis, and treatment far exceeds that covered in existing chapters of medical and subspecialty textbooks, review articles, and simple primers containing general principles for care. The time seemed right for a comprehensive textbook that would give an indepth coverage to the major aspects of the disease. We have attempted to meet this need with a multi-authored textbook by leading experts in their respective areas. We hope that the book will be valuable for practitioners of many disciplines, for residents in training, and for research scientists working in this field.

B. Lawrence Riggs
L. Joseph Melton III

Contents

I. Basic Science

II.   Clinical Aspects

III. Pathophysiology

IV. Management

Contributors

Jon E. Block, Ph.D.
Department of Radiology
University of California
School of Medicine
San Francisco, California 94143

Edmund Y. S. Chao, Ph.D.
Section of Biomechanical Research
Mayo Clinic and Mayo Foundation
200 First Street S.W.
Rochester, Minnesota 55905

Charles H. Chesnut III, M.D.
Division of Nuclear Medicine RC-70
University Hospital
University of Washington
Seattle, Washington 98195

Charles N. Cornell, M.D.
Orthopaedic Surgery
Cornell University Medical College
The Hospital for Special Surgery
535 East 70th Street
New York, New York 10021

Pierre Delmas, M.D., Ph.D.
Hôpital E. Herriot
Place d'Arsonval
69003 Lyon, France

Richard Eastell, M.D.
Endocrine Research Unit
Mayo Clinic and Mayo Foundation
200 First Street S.W.
Rochester, Minnesota 55905

Erik Fink Eriksen, M.D.
Endocrine Research Unit
Mayo Clinic and Mayo Foundation
200 First Street S.W.
Rochester, Minnesota 55905

Bruce Ettinger, M.D.
Department of Internal Medicine
Kaiser Permanente Medical Group
2200 O'Farrel Street
San Francisco, California 94115

Larry W. Fisher, Ph.D.
National Institute of Dental Research
National Institutes of Health
Laboratory Biological Structure
Building 30, Room 106
9000 Rockville Park
Bethesda, Maryland 20892

J. C. Gallagher, M.D.
Department of Medicine
Creighton University
601 North 30th
Omaha, Nebraska 68132

Harry K. Genant, M.D.
Department of Radiology
University of California
Moffit Hospital
San Francisco, California 94143

Steven T. Harris, M.D.
Department of Medicine
University of California
San Francisco, California 94143

John H. Healey, M.D.
Department of Orthopaedic Surgery
Cornell University Medical College
Metabolic Bone Disease
The Hospital for Special Surgery
Division Orthopaedic Surgery
Memorial Sloan-Kettering Cancer Center
535 East 70th Street
New York, New York 10021

Robert P. Heaney, M.D.
Department of Internal Medicine
The Creighton University
  School of Medicine
2500 California Street
Omaha, Nebraska 68178

Hunter Heath III, M.D.
Division of Endocrinology, Metabolism, and
  Internal Medicine
Mayo Clinic and Mayo Foundation
200 First Street S.W.
Rochester, Minnesota 55905

Stephen F. Hodgson, M.D.
Division of Endocrinology, Metabolism, and
*   Internal Medicine*
Mayo Clinic and Mayo Foundation
200 First Street S.W.
Rochester, Minnesota 55905

Rajiv Kumar, M.D.
Divison of Nephrology and Internal Medicine
Mayo Clinic and Mayo Foundation
200 First Street S.W.
Rochester, Minnesota 55905

Joseph M. Lane, M.D.
Division of Metabolic Bone Disease
The Hospital for Special Surgery
535 East 70th Street
New York, New York 10021

Robert Lindsay, M.B., Ch.B., Ph.D.
Regional Bone Center
Department of Clinical Medicine
Helen Hayes Hospital
Route 9W
West Haverstraw, New York 10993

Richard B. Mazess, Ph.D.
Department of Medical Physics
University of Wisconsin
1530 Medical Sciences Center
1300 University Avenue
Madison, Wisconsin 53706

L. Joseph Melton III, M.D.
Section of Clinical Epidemiology
Mayo Clinic and Mayo Foundation
200 First Street S.W.
Rochester, Minnesota 55905

Pierre J. Meunier, M.D.
Hospices Civils De Lyon
Hopital Edouard-Herriot
Place d'Arsonval 69374
Lyon Cedex 2, France

Michael A. Parfitt, M.D.
Mineral Metabolism Research Laboratory
Henry Ford Hospital
2799 West Grand Boulevard
Detroit, Michigan 48202

William A. Peck, M.D.
The Jewish Hospital of St. Louis
216 South Kingshighway
St. Louis, Missouri 63110

B. Lawrence Riggs, M.D.
Division of Endocrinology, Metabolism, and
*   Internal Medicine*
Mayo Clinic and Mayo Foundation
200 First Street S.W.
Rochester, Minnesota 55905

Pamela Gehron Robey, Ph.D.
National Institute of Dental Research
National Institutes of Health
Laboratory Biological Structure
Building 30, Room 106
9000 Rockville Park
Bethesda, Maryland 20892

Mehrsheed Sinaki, M.D.
Department of Physical Medicine and
*   Rehabilitation*
Mayo Clinic and Mayo Foundation
200 First Street S.W.
Rochester, Minnesota 55905

Peter Steiger, Ph.D.
Department of Radiology
University of California
San Francisco, California 94143

John D. Termine, Ph.D.
Bone Research Branch
National Institute of Dental Research
National Institutes of Health
Building 30, Room 216
Bethesda, Maryland 20205

James B. Vogler, M.D.
Department of Radiology
Duke University
Durham, North Carolina 27710

Heinz W. Wahner, M.D.
Section of Nuclear Medicine
Mayo Clinic and Mayo Foundation
200 First Street S.W.
Rochester, Minnesota 55905

William Woods, M.D.
The Jewish Hospital of St. Louis
216 South Kingshighway
St. Louis, Missouri 63110

Marian F. Young, Ph.D.
National Institute of Dental Research
National Institutes of Health
Laboratory Biological Structure
Building 30, Room 106
9000 Rockville Park
Bethesda, Maryland 20892

OSTEOPOROSIS
Etiology, Diagnosis, and Management

Osteoporosis: Etiology, Diagnosis, and Management, edited by B. Lawrence Riggs and L. Joseph Melton, III. Raven Press, New York © 1988.

1

The Cells of Bone

William A. Peck and William L. Woods

Department of Medicine, Jewish Hospital at Washington University Medical Center, St. Louis, Missouri 63110

Over 20 years have passed since Frost's pioneering biological and histomorphometric observations elaborated our modern concept of local skeletal remodeling (135,136). Most subsequently developed theories only modify the original. That is to say, skeletal tissue is renewed when a local group of diverse cells, comprising the basic multicellular unit (BMU), remodel a microscopic quantum of bone. Remodeling is an orderly cascade involving: (1) *initiation,* the generation of an impulse that alters the status of a resting bone surface (trabecular, cortical endosteal or haversian), lowering its threshold for activation; (2) *activation,* the provocation of the earliest preresorptive cellular responses to the initiating stimulus; (3) *resorption,* the removal of mineral and organic matrix; (4) *reversal,* the termination of resorptive processes and the priming of the osteoblast system; (5) *formation,* the osteoblastic repair of the resorption cavity (see 23,200,313 for reviews) (Fig. 1). The operational elements of this system, the cells of bone, include osteoclasts and osteoblasts, which subserve the sequential processes of resorption and formation at each remodeling locus, and the precursors of these highly specialized cells. Exciting recent research has added more participants to this fundamental cellular gestalt: cells of the bone

marrow compartment and immune regulatory system, which may act not only as bone cell progenitors but also as regulators of the remodeling process.

The complex cellular systems that comprise the BMU *tend* to preserve bone mass in the short term. This stems from the temporal and spatial orderliness of the remodeling sequence and the approximate quantitative and qualitative balance of resorption and formation. "Coupling" is the term often applied to this balance. In the long term, however, bone mass is not preserved. In fact, the gradual, progressive decline in bone mass which typifies the adult human skeleton is merely the summation of slight short-term losses at many remodeling loci. As Jaworski has recently pointed out (190), virtually lifelong erosion of trabecular and paramedullary cortical bone as the marrow cavity expands is evidence of physiological imbalance. Furthermore, there is no "balance" possible when thin trabecular plates are completely eroded, thus eliminating the scaffold for bone formation.

Yet the achievement of short-term "near balance" or "approximate coupling" points to the close regulation of individual remodeling events and coordination among them; the efficiency of the BMU is impressive. Not surpris-

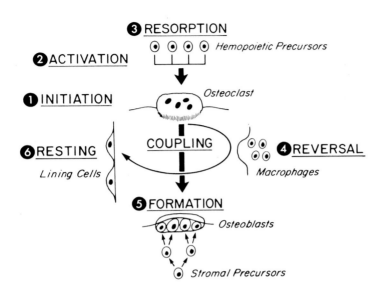

❸ RESORPTION
❷ ACTIVATION
❶ INITIATION
❻ RESTING
Lining Cells
COUPLING
❹ REVERSAL
❺ FORMATION

Hemopoietic Precursors
Osteoclast
Macrophages
Osteoblasts
Stromal Precursors

FIG. 1. The remodeling cycle. In this schema, a combination of local and systemic influences are envisaged as preparing specific regions or domains for remodeling by lowering the lining cell threshold for activation. Theoretically, threshold reduction may be reversible. Osteocytes may be involved in determining the activation threshold by transducing physical impulses and conducting the transduced signal to the bone surface. Activation involves contraction (shape change) and collagenase release, which combine to expose chemotactically active sites on the underlying surface for osteoclast attraction. PGE may facilitate the osteoclast response and may act as an autocrine/paracrine stimulus to activation.

ingly, therefore, new advances in knowledge have moved us far beyond the traditional triad of systemic regulators: PTH as the resorption stimulator, calcitonin as the inhibitor, and vitamin D, via its active metabolite, as a resorption promoter and provider of mineral. These systemic regulators, responsive to homeostatic demands, would not in themselves suffice to coordinate the phases of remodeling. One can now identify multiple locally posited and elaborated agents which control and integrate bone cell growth, specialization and function. Not only do the cells of bone emerge as local generators of regulatory agents *de novo*, but also as transducers or converters of local and systemic messages into new chemical messages.

In this chapter, we will first describe the principal cells of bone and their origins: the osteoclast, the osteoblast and the bone lining cell-osteocyte complex. Reference is made to relationships with mast cells, cells of the marrow compartment and of the immune regulatory system. We will then consider the physiological regulators of these cells, local and systemic, as part of the remodeling scenario. Finally, areas for further research will be set forth.

We have elected to emphasize the cells associated with skeletal remodeling and to exclude from detailed consideration a number of potentially relevant topics: the cellular aspects of endochondral ossification and epiphyseal function, skeletal embryogenesis, fracture healing, the biology of the periosteum, and the secondary level of bone organization (supracellular level of bone biology), each of which could warrant an individual tome. Furthermore, constraints of space and time preclude an extensive consideration of the impact of many pharmacological agents on bone cells. We stress one additional caveat: many recent observations have stemmed from *in vitro* studies, often using embryonic or transformed cell systems. We do not repeatedly mention, though often tempted to do so, the importance of caution in interpreting these data and in extrapolating them to *in vivo* physiology. Let this one preemptive statement suffice.

THE CELLS OF BONE

The Osteoclast

Multinucleated osteoclasts have been established as the principal agencies of bone resorption. We have accumulated considerable information about the nature, lineage and regulation of osteoclasts, and the ways in which osteoclast activity is linked to other events in the remodeling scenario (see 31,83,255,431 for recent reviews). Other cell types in bone, such as macrophages, osteocytes, and perhaps even osteoblasts, may be capable of bone dissolution under highly selective circumstances, but probably are not responsible for bulk removal of structurally intact bone under physiological conditions. These and other cell types may well participate in regulating osteoclast activity and a subset of the macrophage population may serve as osteoclast precursors.

The Nature of the Osteoclast

Osteoclasts are large, usually multinucleated cells attached to bony surfaces. The morphological *sine qua non* of the active osteoclast is the functionally specialized region of attachment, including the characteristic ruffled border surrounded by an organelle-free, actin-containing clear zone (202,209,241,245,375). Ruffled border-free osteoclasts are believed to be the mobile form of the cell. Osteoclasts are enriched in mitochondria and lysosomes, and appear to contain cytoplasmic electron-dense organelles reminiscent of the coated pits which are involved with the internalization of receptor-bound ligands (202) (Fig. 2). Tartrate-inhibitable acid phosphatase (273,275), among other lysosomal enzymes and carbonic anhydrase (11,138,452), are characteristic of the osteoclast. The ruffled border, in intimate contact with the bone surface, is the site of resorption. Its projections are intertwined with disaggregating bone mineral; both mineral crystals and collagen fibrils are identifiable at that interface. It is likely that crystals are phagocytosed and divided in cytoplasmic vacuoles. By contrast, collagen fragments have not been demonstrated within active osteoclasts.

Mechanism of Osteoclast-mediated Resorption

Recent studies have disclosed exciting new information about the cellular mechanism of osteoclast-mediated resorption. Novel lines of in-

vestigation include: the role of carbonic anhydrase in osteoclast activity and the involvement of osteoclast-derived cathepsins in bone dissolution. Extending the classical view of osteoclast-mediated bone resorption, which depicted the secretion of lysosomal enzymes and hydrogen ion secreted at the ruffled border-bone surface interface (the acid theory of bone solubilization), Waite and Kenny postulated that carbonic anhydrase might facilitate hydroxyapatite dissolution (462). Substantial experimental evidence supports this theory. A variety of resorption stimulators increase skeletal carbonic anhydrase activity and their resorptive effects are inhibited by acetazolamide and other carbonic anhydrase inhibitors (156–159,276,328,461,463). PTH-mediated increases in skeletal carbonic anhydrase have been localized to osteoclasts (8). Acetazolamide has also been found to block partially the development of disuse atrophy in rat bone (208). Recently, osteopetrosis, suggestive of osteoclast inactivity, has been reported in association with a genetic deficiency in a carbonic anhydrase isoenzyme (carbonic anhydrase II) (402). The osteoclast is the only cell type at the remodeling locus that is enriched in carbonic anhydrase (11). Although carbonic anhydrase is associated with several cellular structures, its distribution on the plasma membrane is conducive to hydrogen ion excretion.

From the foregoing observations, carbonic anhydrase would appear to participate in bone resorption. Accordingly, carbonic anhydrase catalyzes the conversion of metabolically produced carbon dioxide to carbonic acid, which yields hydrogen ion upon dissociation. Hydrogen is then pumped into the resorbing space, providing an appropriate milieu for the action of lysosomal acid hydrolases (453,454).

In addition to possible H^+ secretion, other ionic shifts may promote the resorption-associated movement of Ca^{2+} from bone into the extracellular spaces. Kreiger and Tashjian have obtained evidence that stimulated release of Ca^{2+} requires a Na^+ exchange mechanism. Three strategies, all designed to increase the "effective" intracellular Na^+ concentration, inhibited hormone-mediated resorption in or-

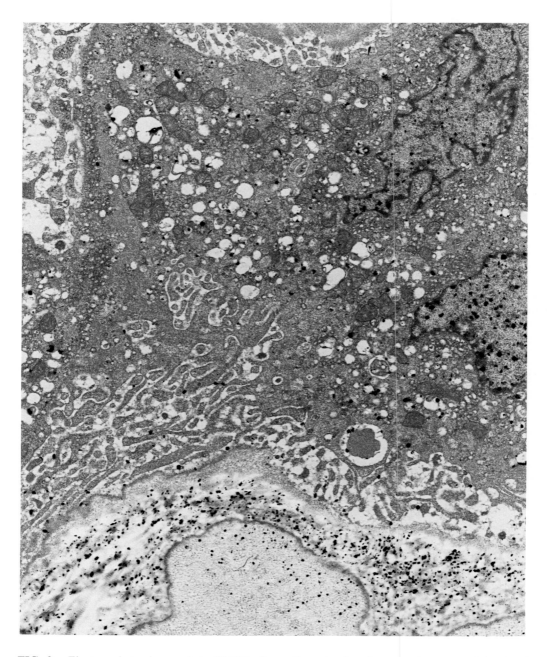

FIG. 2. Electron photomicrograph (x 12,000) of an active osteoclast demonstrating two nuclei and a characteristic ruffled membrane. Black particles represent acid phosphatase reaction product; note that acid phosphatase is found within the resorbing bone tissue. Acid phosphatase was localized by the Gomori technique using β-glycerol phosphate as substrate.

gan-cultured bones: blockade of Na^+-K^+ ATP-ase (ouabain, vanadate), exposure to monovalent cation inophores, and incubation at lowered extracellular Na^+ concentrations (221–223).

The osteoclast is highly enriched in lysosomes and elaborates a variety of lysosomal enzymes upon exposure to stimulators of bone resorption. A major question has arisen, however, concerning the mechanism whereby the organic matrix is resorbed during osteoclast activity. Whereas it had long been assumed that osteoclasts might elaborate a collagenolytic enzyme, mammalian neutral collagenase, found in many tissues, is not a lysosomal enzyme. In fact, the skeletal form of this collagenase resides in and is elaborated by osteoblasts (167,307,308,339,379,380). Osteoblasts also elaborate a peptide inhibitor of collagenase (289,308).

Osteoclasts do appear to participate in collagen dissolution, but not by producing mammalian collagenase. They have been shown to release proteases which are capable of degrading bone collagen. For example, osteoclasts produce a lysomal cysteine protease, cathepsin B, which may actually be collagenolytic or may have the capacity to activate mammalian collagenase previously incorporated into the extracellular matrix by osteoblasts (96). Cathepsin inhibitors have been found to inhibit PTH-induced bone resorption *in vitro* and to blunt certain indices of bone resorption *in vivo* (95).

The Lineage of Osteoclasts

It is now recognized that osteoclasts arise by fusion rather than by mitosis, and derive from a stem cell that is found in the circulation and, ultimately, in hematopoietic tissue. Particularly pivotal among a pioneering series of experiments using radiographic, chimeric, and parabiotic techniques (see 23,31,200,254 for reviews) were the observations of Walker and colleagues in animals with hereditary osteopetrosis, a disease characterized by failure of osteoclastic modeling of bone. Infusion of spleen cells from normal animals or cross-circulatory perfusion with blood from normal littermates cured the osteopetrosis, whereas in normal animals cross-circulatory perfusion with blood from diseased animals created the defect (464–466). Since these results were reported, considerable effort has been expended in order to identify the nature and lineage of the "preosteoclast."

The possibility that cells of the monocyte-macrophage series are preosteoclasts has considerable appeal. Macrophages are enormously versatile cells of the hematopoietic series (see 293 for review). There are functional and morphological similarities between macrophages and osteoclasts (38,182,306,487), and macrophages are chemotactically attracted to bone surfaces (246,277,283,286). Cells with the morphological traits of mononuclear phagocytes are found in remodeling loci (444). Furthermore, they release radioactively labeled Ca^{2+} from devitalized bone *in vitro* (201,261, 282,433). Cells of the monocyte-macrophage series have high-affinity receptors for the bone-resorbing hormone $1\alpha,25$–$(OH)_2D_3$ (26,266). $1\alpha,25$–$(OH)_2D_3$ enhances their maturation and perhaps their fusion (1,2,5,21). Multinucleated, mineral-resorbing osteoclast-like cells have been shown to develop *in vitro* in bone marrow preparations from several animal species (36,186,417,440). Co-culture of embryonic mouse long bones with proliferating bone marrow mononuclear phagocytes results in the development of multinucleated, mineral-resorbing osteoclasts (36,37). Although osteoclast-specific antigens have been identified, osteoclasts have also been found to share common determinants with cultured monocytes and inflammatory polykaryons (310). In addition, defective macrophage function accompanies the osteoclast defects in certain forms of osteopetrosis (84,253,254,441).

An impressive body of data, however, suggests that the lineage of osteoclasts excludes mature mononuclear phagocytes or macrophages. First, multinucleated cells derived from osteoclastomas (giant cell tumors of bone) fail to cross-react with all but several of many antigranulocyte-monocyte antibodies.

Osteoclasts lack Fc receptors, which are found in monocytes, tissue macrophages, and inflammatory polykaryons (38,198). Second, osteoclasts isolated from newborn rodents do not express markers characteristic of mononuclear phagocytes, including T-200, the hematopoietic tissue-restricted surface determinant (183). Third, multinucleated cells formed from mononuclear phagocytes differ structurally from osteoclasts (182). Fourth, osteoclasts isolated from rabbit, rat, mouse and human bone can resorb slices of human cortical bone, whereas monocytes, peritoneal macrophages, inflammatory polykaryons, and a variety of myeloid cell lines fail to do so (61,64,68). That $1\alpha,25$–$(OH)_2D_3$ promotes macrophage differentiation cannot be used as an argument in favor of the macrophagic lineage of osteoclasts, since this hormone can promote the differentiation of many cell types, and, indeed, can induce monocytes to differentiate and acquire antigens which are not found on osteoclasts *(vide infra)*.

Subsequent studies have examined the lineage of the osteoclast in greater detail, and point to a mononuclear cell within the hematopoietic system as the osteoclast progenitor. Phenotypic osteoclasts emerge from the nonadherent cell population derived from cultures of bone marrow (186). Resorption-stimulating hormones (e.g., PTH, $1\alpha,25$–$(OH)_2D_3$ and PGE_2) facilitate the development of these osteoclast-like cells (186). By contrast, convincing modulation of phagocytic macrophages into osteoclasts has not been demonstrated. Burger et al. demonstrated that proliferating cells of the marrow mononuclear phagocyte series formed mineral-resorbing osteoclasts (36). In subsequent studies, Burger, Van der Meer and Nijweide showed that osteoclasts could develop from mouse peritoneal exudate cells elicited by calf serum injection, though osteoclast development was slower and more erratic than with bone marrow mononuclear phagocytes (37). This suggests that the exudate, enriched in mature macrophages, also contained a small number of osteoclast precursors which may have proliferated before their fusion to form osteoclasts. Hence, fully differentiated cells of

the monocyte/macrophage series do not seem to be osteoclast progenitors. Any large population of mature macrophages, however, may contain a small number of such progenitors.

From these observations and others, therefore, it appears that a "preosteoclast" does exist in bone marrow, presumably in the circulation and in distant reticuloendothelial repositories as well. Since osteoclasts represent a small minority of all skeletal cells, it would not be surprising if the number of osteoclast precursors in hematopoietic tissue was diminutive.

Two caveats must be added to the foregoing discussion. Under certain circumstances, mononuclear phagocytes may assist osteoclasts in the resorption process and, indeed, may fuse with existing osteoclasts derived from a separate lineage (484,485). Furthermore, it is conceivable that the osteoclast lineage may exhibit developmental or ontological variations. Bone-resorbing cells in the early fetus may originate from different precursors than those of the adult.

Following their development, mature osteoclasts migrate to bone surfaces where they attach and resorb a quantum of bone. The process of attraction of osteoclasts to bone surfaces has been examined recently. Several matrix components, including type I collagen and osteocalcin (bone gla protein) have been shown to be chemotactic for macrophages, and these same agencies may attract osteoclasts as well (246,277,283,286). Virtually nothing is known about the termination of osteoclast activity, nor the fate of osteoclasts upon completion of their resorptive task. A chemical signal within the matrix may dictate the end of the resorptive phase, and it has been suggested that osteoclasts then undergo scission, perhaps into mononuclear phagocytes (see 23).

The Osteoblast

Osteoblasts (see 370 for review) *in situ* occur as a contiguous layer of cells which, in their active state, are cuboidal (15–30 μ), asymmetric, and contain intracellular organelles typical of cells vigorously engaged in protein synthesis (177). They form functional gap junctions with their neighbors and with subjacent osteocyte processes (105,191). They contain numerous microtubules and bundles of actin filaments along the inner surfaces of their plasma membranes (209). The osteoblasts are oriented in bone according to underlying matrix fibers (197). Resting bone surfaces are lined by flattened cells that are believed to be inactive osteoblasts (bone lining cells).

The Lineage of Osteoblasts

Osteoblasts emerge from the complex microenvironment of the marrow cavity via a lineage which is separate from that of the osteoclast (see 312 for review). That microenvironment contains not only the hematopoietic system, believed to yield the osteoclast, but also the stromal system, which includes osteoblast ancestors. Among the differentiated progeny of the stromal cell system are the fibroblast, the adipocyte, the reticular cell and the osteogenic cell. It is held that mature osteoblasts specialize nonmitotically (i.e., modulate) from their immediate precursors (preosteoblasts), which themselves derive ultimately from mitotically competent stem cells (see 311,370 for reviews). Therefore, the availability of mature osteoblasts is a function of the stem cell mass and its mitotic activity.

Synthetic Functions of the Osteoblast

The principal protein elaborated by osteoblasts is Type 1 collagen, almost the exclusive collagen of bone matrix. Elegant studies have aided in uncovering the steps in the transcription and translation of bone procollagen, its posttranslational modifications, and its elaboration into the extracellular spaces (304, 460,473,479). Enrichment in alkaline phosphatase is a hallmark of the active osteoblast. Skeletal alkaline phosphatase is of the bone–liver–intestine type, and is expressed principally on the plasma membrane, where it appears to act as an ectoenzyme (106,144,401). The osteobast synthesizes, in addition to collagen, a variety of matrix components, including osteocalcin (bone gla protein) (203,299,400) and osteonectin (309,365,439,472) (vide infra). Osteoblasts may well be the source of chondro (osteo) inductive factor(s), which has (have) been extracted from bone matrix (384,451). Osteoblasts are also capable of synthesizing prostaglandins of the E series and other prostanoids (139,300,371,482), mammalian collagenase in response to stimulators of bone resorption (167,307,308,339,379,380), a collagenase inhibitor (289,308) and plasminogen activator (160).

Osteocalcin is a 5800-dalton protein easily purified from bone that contains three γ-carboxyglutamic acid residues (see 333 for review). These residues are responsible for its binding to bone, since uncarboxylated osteocalcin is not bound. The γ-carboxylation process is vitamin K-dependent in this protein, as it is for other γ-carboxyglutamic acid-containing proteins, such as certain clotting factors. Rat osteosarcoma cells and cells derived from human bone segments, but not untransformed rodent or avian bone cells, elaborate osteocalcin in vitro (24,203,231,298). Interestingly, $1\alpha,25-(OH)_2D_3$ markedly enhances the synthesis and secretion of osteocalcin in bone and the effect of the D metabolite is inhibited by glucocorticoids and by PTH (24,231,334,400). Although its physiological role is unknown, osteocalcin is a chemotactically active matrix protein (246,286). Furthermore, the possibility that it may serve to prevent excess mineralization has been suggested (336).

Price, Urist, and Otowara have identified a second γ-carboxyglutamic acid-containing protein in bone (335). Unlike osteocalcin, so-called matrix gla protein was isolated only from demineralized bone matrix under denaturing conditions. It is strongly associated with the collagenous matrix which remains after demineralization.

Osteonectin is a phosphoserine-containing glycoprotein with a molecular weight of 32 Kd (as determined by guanidine HCl gel filtration) which exhibits saturable, exchangeable, and simultaneous binding to collagen and hydroxyapatite (372,437,439). The osteonectin-collagen complex potentiates calcium-phosphate deposition. Osteonectin is secreted by osteoblastic cells (365), but cells from other connective tissues can produce an osteonectin-like material, which, however, does not accumulate in those tissues. It is likely that osteonectin is involved in hydroxyapatite nucleation, stabilization, and organization (97,438).

Additional proteins of possible osteoblast origin include bone characteristic sialoproteins, proteoglycans, and phosphoproteins (119,120, 130,131,397,405). Each of these proteins may play crucial roles in the elaboration, mineralization, and perhaps resorption of matrix. For example, it has been suggested that the small proteoglycans may alter the kinetics of fibril formation by osteoblasts.

Osteoblasts and Matrix Mineralization

Clearly, osteoblasts manufacture a variety of proteins found in the organic matrix of bone. With the recognition that the specific function of osteoblasts *in vivo* is to produce calcified matrix, the role of osteoblasts in the mineralization process has received considerable attention. There are three requirements for physiologic mineralization (see 436 for review): (1) a structurally normal and appropriately positioned extracellular substrate for mineral nucleation and maintenance; (2) an appropriate mineral component for nucleation; and (3) a crystal growth rate which matches tissue growth, a crystal growth limiter. It is increasingly evident that the osteoblast is the source of the nucleation substrate and probably determines its extracellular arrangement as well. Although bone contains predominantly type I collagen, a product of the osteoblast, other type I collagen-enriched tissues do not normally mineralize. Consequently, non-collagen proteins and their associated macromolecules, also of osteoblast origin, are visualized as participating in the nucleation process. In this fashion, agents that influence osteoblast behavior could also influence mineralization.

Osteoblasts may also contribute to mineralization by eliminating inhibitors of nucleation, such as pyrophosphate (124,129,392), and providing adequate amounts of inorganic phosphate for the mineralization process. Osteoblasts are enriched in a variety of phosphohydrolases that can serve both functions, including ATPases, pyrophosphohydrolase and alkaline phosphatase (9). The association of alkaline phosphatase with mineralization is well recognized, but its precise role is unclear. Isolated bone cells have been shown to mineralize a type I collagen-containing extracellular matrix, but only in the presence of an organic phosphate substrate such as β glycerol phosphate, a finding which is consistent with the notion that alkaline phosphate cleaves organic phosphates to yield inorganic phosphate at mineralization sites (9,109,434). Osteoblasts are also sources of matrix vesicles, extracellular membrane-invested structures replete with phosphatases, other hydrolases and phospholipids which may be the initial sites of nucleation during bone formation (see 7 for review). Whether matrix vesicles participate in mineralization associated with lamellar bone formation and physiological remodeling remains unclear, but they have been noted in osteoblast-associated mineralizing systems *in vivo* and *in vitro*. Finally, extracellular macromolecules of osteoblast origin, such as osteocalcin, may modulate crystal growth so that it keeps pace with the growth of the tissue in which the mineralization is occurring.

An important unanswered question is whether osteoblasts transport Ca^{2+} to mineralizing sites (apart from elaborating calcifiable matrix vesicles). Osteoblasts, like all mammalian cells, have elaborate enzymic systems for maintaining cytosolic free Ca^{2+} at a low and therefore non-toxic concentration (9,10,390). It will be interesting to determine whether osteoblasts, like intestinal cells and renal tubular epithelia, have specialized systems for transcellular calcium movement.

Osteoblasts and the Activation of Bone Remodeling

Evidence now indicates that in addition to forming bone the osteoblast plays a crucial role in the activation of remodeling. A variety of humoral agents can provoke osteoclast-mediated bone resorption *in vivo,* in complex organ systems *in vitro,* and in simplified *in vitro* systems in which isolated osteoclasts and bone segments are cocultured. These humoral agents include PTH, $1\alpha,25-(OH)_2D_3$, other vitamin D preparations, prostaglandins, osteoclast-activating factor, and growth factors (e.g., interleukin I and platelet-derived, epidermal and transforming growth factors) *(vide infra).* It had been assumed that osteoclasts possess receptors for and respond directly to these agents with a burst of resorbing activity. Although this hypothesis has not been disproven, a large body of experimentally derived information has accumulated which suggests that it is incorrect.

Initial evidence against this hypothesis came from studies employing partially separated populations of osteoclast-like and osteoblast-like cells. The cyclic AMP response to PTH, believed to mediate its effect on resorption, was exhibited mainly by osteoblast-like cells (33,239,316,476). By contrast, it was the osteoclast-like cells which responded to calcitonin, a resorption inhibitor, with an increase in cyclic AMP (239,476). Subsequent experiments have yielded strong evidence that another cell, such as an osteoblast or an osteoblast-derived cell (bone-lining cells) and not the osteoclast, is the primary target for the major resorption stimulators (369). Key elements of this evidence are as follows:

1. Osteoblasts have been shown to have receptors for and/or exhibit a variety of metabolic responses to PTH, $1\alpha,25-(OH)_2D_3$, prostaglandins of the ''E'' series, and other resorption stimulators *(vide infra,* descriptions of specific hormones and factors).
2. Definitive evidence for such receptors *and* responses in osteoclasts is lacking.
3. Isolated osteoclast-like cells will not resorb cultured bone segments lined by an intact cell envelope (486).
4. Resorption-stimulating agents such as PTH and PGE_2 cause changes in osteoblast function, notably shape change and secretion

of collagenase and of plasminogen activator (15,160,167,274,307,308,339,379,380), that may serve to expose the underlying bone surface and to modify it for osteoclast attack. Monensin, a monovalent cation ionophore which inhibits PTH-mediated bone resorption, decreases collagenase production by osteoblasts and by resorbing bones *in vitro* (89).

5. The presence of osteoblasts is required for the hormonal enhancement of bone resorption by isolated osteoclasts *in vitro* and for the formation of osteoclasts from their progenitors (37,58,385).
6. Periosteal tissue has been found to release a peptide stimulator of bone resorption and collagenase release (168).

This accumulation of indirect though relevant evidence suggests strongly that resorption stimulators act via an intermediate cell, perhaps an osteoblast or lining cell, as originally postulated by Rodan and Martin (369). The ''second'' message for resorption may either be the exposed, prepared bone surface itself or a humoral factor of lining cell (osteoblast) origin, or both. According to this theory, hormonal activation of a remodeling sequence requires first the disruption of the lining cell layer, thus exposing the underlying bone surface, and second, the preparation of that surface for osteoclast attraction and attachment. Exposure is achieved by the hormonally induced contraction of individual lining cells. PTH and prostaglandins of the ''E'' series, known resorption stimulators, convert isolated, cultured osteoblast-like cells from a flattened to a stellate shape *in vitro,* and cause similar changes in endosteal lining cells *in vitro.* This effect occurs rapidly and at low hormone concentrations, appears to be cyclic AMP-mediated and is triggered by changes in the contractile apparatus of the cell.

Preparation of the bone surface may well involve the enzymatic removal of organic materials which hinder osteoclast binding to bone, and the exposure of mineral-associated osteoclastic attractants such as osteocalcin. Collagenase secretion by osteoblasts, also demonstrated in response to resorption-stimulating agents, is one mechanism for organic matrix removal. Collagenase is secreted as a zymogen, procollagenase, in association with a peptide collagenase inhibitor, the removal (inactivation) of which may be associated with zymogen activation (377,382,455). Osteoclast-like cells also elaborate plasminogen activator which could convert procollagenase to collagenase (160). It is also possible that procollagenase, in close association with its inhibitor, may be secreted by osteoblasts as part of the organic matrix of bone, awaiting subsequent activation during osteoclastic resorption.

The Osteocyte-Lining Cell Complex

Some active osteoblasts are incorporated into the matrix they synthesize, and are buried beneath the subsequently deposited matrix. They maintain contact with each other and with surface osteoblasts/bone lining cells by slender processes that traverse the canaliculi of bone. Menton et al. found with scanning electron microscopy that trapped osteoblasts begin to form osteocyte lacunae by depositing collagen fibrils which roof them over, and that the lucunar walls mineralize quickly (265). Several functions have been assigned to osteocytes, including perilacunar bone resorption (osteocytic osteolysis) and bone formation. Osteocytes are envisaged as functioning in concert with superficial bone-lining cells (inactive osteoblasts), with which they are contiguous, to partition bone fluid from extracellular fluid (260,295,301). There is evidence of contiguity between the squamous bone lining cells and underlying osteocytes, gap junctions having been described between these various cellular elements (105,191).

The bone lining cell–osteocyte complex could mediate a rapid flux system for Ca^{2+} (see 422 for review). Since influx is not thought to be controlled, it is efflux that would be the regulated step. Consequently, by a process which is PTH-stimulated and calcitonin-inhibited, these cells may rapidly conduct Ca^{2+} from intraskeletal lacunae and from bone surfaces to

the extracellular fluids. Morphological studies suggest that this system responds within several minutes of exposure to hormone (91, 259,301). It functions in concert with osteoclast-mediated bone resorption, which exhibits the same directional responsivity to PTH and calcitonin, but does so only after 15–30 min (178,272).

Although osteocytes may well aid in storing Ca^{2+} postprandially and in conducting mineral from deeper skeletal recesses via the bone fluid to the extracellular fluid compartment, persuasive evidence of osteocytic osteolysis has not been obtained under conditions of enhanced bone resorption. Yet another role for osteocytes must be considered. One interpretation of the results of studies of explanted human bone tissue in primary culture is that osteocytes emerge from their lacunae and become osteoblast-like in nature, acquiring the ability to synthesize highly specialized matrix proteins (365). Consequently, osteocytes may be involved in the repair of microfractures and, at least theoretically, in the repair of resorption-mediated defects as well. Finally, osteocytes and their processes may stabilize bone mineral by maintaining an appropriate local ionic milieu.

The Mast Cells

Appreciable evidence has accumulated which indicates that mast cells participate in the regulation of remodeling, especially bone resorption (see 263 for review). Mast cells are situated in bone, where they increase in number with advancing age and in states of high remodeling (127). Localized and generalized losses of bone tissue accompany mast cell decreases (mastocytosis and urticaria pigmentosa) (112,376). Heparin, a known mast cell product, appears to enhance bone collagenase activity and is known to promote bone resorption (143,378). Furthermore, protamine, a basic 4.3 Kd polypeptide antagonist of heparin, inhibits bone resorption *in vivo* and blocks the effect of heparin on bone collagenase and resorption (331,381). Recently, Glowacki has reported the presence of mast cells in the vicinity of bone particles undergoing resorption following implantation *in vivo* (141). Exogenous heparin augmented and protamine decreased the resorptive processes. From these observations, mast cells, via the release of heparin, would seem to be important regulators of bone resorption.

Monocytes and Macrophages

It is now apparent that cells of the monocyte-macrophage series may, in addition to their roles in host defense, modify tissue development, organization, remodeling and repair (see 293 for review). Attributes that make these cells attractive as "local" regulatory elements include their (a) remarkably broad biosynthetic potential (they are capable of manufacturing many diverse regulatory molecules); (b) responsivity to a multiplicity of external signals; (c) wide tissue distribution; (d) capacity to migrate via the circulation and through tissues; (e) phagocytic characteristics; and (f) functional adaptability and diversity. Macrophages, then, are ideally suited to act as transducers, coordinators, and interpreters of local and systemic regulatory signals.

In skeletal remodeling, macrophages may act as possible (yet to be excluded) osteoclast progenitors (or at least as contributors to osteoclast polykaryons) *(vide supra),* as elaborators of soluble or surface factors which may regulate (stimulate or inhibit) bone resorption and formation, and as phagocytic cells which produce proteolytic enzymes and thereby aid in scavenging the products of osteoclast-mediated bone resorption. The anatomical proximity of macrophages to remodeling loci, their enormous biological potential, and their now-recognized capacity to secrete products which affect bone cell metabolism, make them reasonable candidates as participants in skeletal remodeling.

According to currently held concepts, cells of the macrophage/monocyte line derive from marrow-located hematopoietic stem cells. The application of cloning methodology to the culture of various marrow elements has led to the detailing of the macrophage/monocyte-bone cell genesis along the following lines (see 312 for review). An undifferentiated hematopoietic stem cell, referred to as CFU-S (colony-forming unit–spleen) in recognition of its ability to form colonies *in vitro,* can specialize along four different lines: lymphoid, erythroid, megakaryocytic, and granulocytic/monocytic. Factors that modulate the growth and/or specialization of these cells have been identified through the use of *in vitro* systems. For example, multiple glycoproteins derived from a variety of cell types have been found to stimulate the growth of myeloid progenitors: the colony-stimulating factors, or CSFs (e.g., macrophage CSF, granulocyte/macrophage CSF, and granulocyte CSF) (82,267,406). It will be important to determine whether CSFs play a role in the development of osteoclasts. Among the macrophage products which may affect bone remodeling are prostaglandins (39,407, and *vide infra*), interleukin 1 (IL-1) and a bone cell growth stimulator distinct from IL-1 *(vide infra).* Macrophages can also produce 1α, $25-(OH)_2D_3$ from $25-(OH)D_3$; conceivably, macrophages could release this stimulator locally at remodeling sites (86,212,303).

IL-1 is a peptide hormone produced by activated macrophages which promotes the proliferation, differentiation, and activation of many cell types (see 103 for review). One of its main functions is to maintain the spontaneous growth of T-lymphocytes and enhance the growth of antigen-exposed mature T-cells, by provoking the T-cells to elaborate a mitogen terminal interleukin 2 (IL-2). Murine and human IL-1 species and their precursors have been isolated (through the use of cloned cDNA preparations). At least two distinct species of IL-1 have been identified (IL-1α and IL-1β) (40,251). IL-1 has a molecular weight of approximately 17,500 daltons and its precursor approximately 31,000 daltons (17,234). Macrophages not only secrete IL-1 but also contain surface-bound IL-1 thought to activate T-cells that bind to macrophages (225). Other cell types, including keratinocytes and B-lymphocytes, produce IL-1 (137,258). Recently, Hanazawa et al. reported the isolation of IL-1-like material from the incubation medium conditioned by the mouse osteoblastic cell line MC3T3-E$_1$ (161). Among the diverse effects in various tissues that have been attributed to IL-1 are pyrogenic activity, neutrophil chemotaxis, proteolysis in muscle, the production of acute phase proteins, the production of collagenase by fibroblasts and synovial cells, and fibroblast proliferation (103).

Interest in IL-1 as a regulator of bone cell activity stemmed from the observation that it stimulated cartilage breakdown as well as the production of collagenase and other enzymes by synovial cells and chondrocytes (146,279). Subsequently, IL-1 was found to be a potent stimulator of bone resorption *in vitro* at concentrations as low as 25 pM (147,169). Dewhirst et al. have discovered an amino terminal sequence homology between IL-1 and human osteoclast activating factor (OAF) obtained from peripheral blood mononuclear cells (99). IL-1 may also influence bone formation. Beresford et al. found that exposure of organcultured bones and human bone cells to IL-1 *in vitro* enhances DNA and collagen synthesis (25). Canalis also found a stimulatory effect of IL-1 on DNA, collagen and non-collagen protein synthesis in bone *in vitro,* and showed that high doses or prolonged treatment periods actually inhibited collagen synthesis (48).

An anabolic effect of IL-1 on bone cells would not be unexpected, since prior studies had disclosed that material with IL-1 activity could stimulate fibroblast proliferation as well (103). The recognition that, under certain circumstances, macrophages produce a fibroblast growth stimulator which is devoid of IL-1 activity prompted us to examine the possibility that macrophages synthesize a non-IL-1 stimulator of osteoblast activity. We found that cultured resident peritoneal macrophages release a potent growth stimulator for osteoblast-like cells which has no IL-1 activity (359). It will be of interest to determine whether preosteoclasts or osteoclasts exhibit similar properties and, in addition, whether there is a dedicated subset of the macrophage population that is specifically responsible for the local regulation of bone remodeling.

Lymphoid Cells

A substantial body of evidence indicates that cells of the lymphoid system influence the development and activity of bone cells (see 23 for review). Pertinent observations have been made in animals with congenital and acquired osteopetrosis. Milhaud and co-workers demonstrated the presence of thymus atrophy in the osteopetrotic rat, and reported that transplantation of normal thymus tissue, but not normal bone marrow, cured the osteopetrosis (269, 270). Dichloromethylene bisphosphonate (Cl$_2$MBP)-induced osteopetrosis (*vide infra* for discussion of bisphosphonates) is also associated with thymus atrophy (226,271). Thymic lymphocytes (T-lymphocytes) are known to produce a fusion factor for macrophages (polykaryon-promoting factor) which may be involved in osteoclast development as well (1,404). Activated T- and B-lymphocytes also have receptors for $1\alpha,25$–(OH)$_2$D$_3$ and may depend on this vitamin for maturation (26, 338,356). Thymocytes have demonstrated responsivity to PTH and calcitonin, and receptors for parathyroid hormone and calcitonin on these cells have been described (256,264, 324,471,480).

This circumstantial evidence for a relationship between T-lymphocytes and bone cell activity achieves particular relevance in light of the fact that lymphocytes produce lymphokines which can affect bone cell metabolism. It is well-established that T-cells elaborate one or more species of protein which stimulate(s) osteoclast activity directly. The first such factor to be identified was termed osteoclast activating factor (OAF) (181). OAF has been linked to the excessive bone loss associated with periodontal disease, multiple myeloma, lymphosarcoma, and other malignancies (285). Evidence favoring the T-cell rather than the B-cell as the site of OAF production has been summarized by Baron et al. (180; see 23 for review), though Chen et al. have reported OAF formation by activated B-lymphocytes (70).

The requirement for macrophage stimulation may reflect the elaboration by macrophages of interleukin 1 (IL-1), which stimulates T-lymphocytes to synthesize the autocrine mitogen interleukin 2 (IL-2), thereby eliciting T-lymphocyte proliferation *(vide supra)* (103). Alternatively, macrophage-derived prostaglandins may be responsible for promoting OAF production (180,483). The chemical nature of OAF remains uncertain; in reality, OAF refers to a biological activity which appears to reside in multiple molecules of lymphoid tissue origin. Following its original identification, Mundy et al. reported OAF activity to reside in two molecular forms, termed big OAF (12–25 Kd) and little OAF (1.3–3.5 Kd), respectively (287). Subsequently, Luben reported the purification of a 9 Kd OAF from human tonsils (238). There is evidence that OAF and IL-1 are identical (99). Other lymphokines, such as lymphotoxin, a now purified molecule derived from stimulated lymphocytes (148), and the partly homologous lymphokine tumor necrosis factor β (TNF β) may also participate in the regulation of bone cell function (323,418); another species of TNF, TNFα, is produced by macrophages.

By contrast to resorption-stimulating lymphokines, γIFN inhibits "basal" bone resorption and the enhancement of resorption caused by added stimulators (194,326). Interferons represent a class of glycoproteins produced by lymphocytes (and macrophages) following proliferative stimulation which have antiviral properties but which also appear to modify cellular differentiation and proliferation (366). Of the known interferons, γIFN is thought to play a special role in immune regulation, acting mainly to promote immune and inflammatory responses in lymphocytes and macrophages. Three possible mechanisms have been proposed for the resorption inhibitory effect of γIFN: inhibition of endogenous prostaglandin (PG) synthesis, a known consequence of γIFN action ("basal" resorption has been attributed to endogenous PG production); a direct calci-tonin-like effect; and inhibition of osteoclast recruitment. Favoring the latter thesis is the finding of Jilka that γIFN inhibited the resorption of organ cultured bones only when added before and during the activation period (194). γIFN is known to promote polykaryon formation (468), an action which might be expected to increase osteoclast production, but it also reduces CSF-induced monocytopoiesis [as well as the proliferation of other marrow hemopoietic precursors (247)], and the net effect may be to decrease osteoclast precursor availability. Since γIFN also promotes macrophage specialization (19,421), inhibition of resorption may well reflect the predominance of its antiproliferative effect. Although the effects of γIFN on bone have been demonstrated using purified soluble preparations, at least some of the nonskeletal effects of γIFN appear to require cell-cell contact. Consequently, γIFN may act by virtue of its association with cells in intimate contact with the multicellular units of remodeling.

LOCAL AND SYSTEMIC FACTORS THAT REGULATE BONE CELL FUNCTION

Growth Factors

It is difficult to visualize systemic humoral agents as regulators of the complex cellular events which occur at a remodeling locus. Rather, regulation at the local level more reasonably explains the sequential, coordinated migration, activation and deactivation of diverse bone cell types, the balance between resorption and formation, the geographical restriction of remodeling loci, and the appropriately timed development of bone cell progenitors. That systemically secreted humoral agents do affect remodeling is beyond question *(vide infra);* they function as operational links between the bone compartment and somatic homeostasis, sensitive as they are to systemic rather than local events. On the other hand, locally posited and synthesized factors working in conjunction with the systemic humoral milieu appear to initiate and perpetuate skeletal turnover by modifying bone cell proliferation, specialization and activity. The identification of locally produced substances that influence bone cell behavior supports this view. Many types of factors have received attention as possible local determinants of remodeling: the polypeptide growth factors, the prostaglandins, adenosine and the matrix-located chemotactic and stabilizing factors. In addition, mechanical and electrical phenomena within bones are doubtless of regulatory significance.

Polypeptide Growth Factors

Growth factors are defined as extracellular proteins which promote cell proliferation, though many have effects on cell differentiation as well (see references 188 and 189 for reviews). They are commonly classified according to the responses they elicit: transforming and nontransforming, competency and progression, and inducing and noninducing. Transforming growth factor (TGFs), but not nontransforming factors, have the special ability to initiate proliferative events in anchorage-dependent cells, in essence causing them to behave like transformed cells. Competency factors convert resting cells to a proliferative mode but cannot alone cause movement through an entire cell cycle; that is a property of progression factors. Inducing factors elicit a directional change in the expression of specialized cell activities—for example, expediting the modulation of mesenchymal cells into chondrocytes. These assignments of function are based principally on *in vitro* assay systems, and certainly are not absolute. One factor may exhibit different activities in different test systems.

The number of identified and well-characterized growth factors has expanded dramatically in the past 10 years. Of key import, from the standpoint of this discussion, are those factors which are produced and act locally in bone. Before the identification of so-called intrinsic growth factors, growth factors isolated from non-skeletal tissue were shown to have effects

on bone cells, and it is important to review these effects for two reasons: (1) there may be bone cell-derived analogs of the extrinsic growth factors; and (2) the extrinsic factors may be particularly important in embryonic bone development as well as in bone repair. Consequently, we will consider separately the nature and effects on bone metabolism of growth factors thus far obtained principally from non-skeletal sources (extrinsic factors) and those derived from bone (intrinsic). This distinction is arbitrary, however, since bone tissues seem to elaborate some factors which were previously regarded as exclusively extraskeletal in origin.

Nature and effects on bone metabolism of growth factors derived principally from nonskeletal sources.

These factors (see 44,46,284,398 for reviews) include: epidermal growth factor (EGF), the transforming growth factors (TGFα and β), fibroblast growth factor (FGF), platelet-derived growth factor (PrDGF), prostate-derived growth factor (PrDGF), and various somatomedins, as well as insulin (Table 1).

EGF, a 6-kilodalton (Kd) polypeptide originally isolated from mouse submaxillary gland and human urine (urogastrone) (87), increases bone resorption (348,426), enhances the proliferation of osteoblast-like cells, and decreases osteoblast specialization, reducing alkaline

TABLE 1. *Growth factors derived principally from nonskeletal sources acting on bone cells*

	Major effects[a]
Epidermal growth factor (EGF)	↑R, ↑P, ↓F
Transforming growth factor alpha (TGFα)	↑R, ↑P, ↓F
Transforming growth factor beta (TGFβ)[b]	↑R, ↑P
Fibroblast growth factor (FGF)	↑P
Platelet-derived growth factor (PDGF)	↑R, ↑P, ↑F
Prostate-derived growth factor (PrDGF)	↑P, ↑F
Somatomedins (Sm)[b]	↑P, ↑F
Insulin	↑P, ↑F

[a]R = resorption; P = bone cell proliferation; F = biochemical evidence of formation.
[b]May also be elaborated by bone cells.

phosphatase activity and type I collagen synthesis (54,297,396). EGF receptors have been identified in mouse calvaria and in osteosarcoma cells (394,395). At least in the mouse, if not in the rat, the resorptive effect of EGF may be indirect, mediated by the local release of resorption-stimulating PGs (426). In the MC3T3-F_1 clone of osteoblast-like cells, EGF continued to inhibit alkaline phosphatase activity and collagen synthesis despite the addition of indomethacin, an inhibitor of PG synthesis, to the test system (396).

It is thought that certain growth factors, such as EGF, trigger the phosphorylation of cell proteins, including the receptor itself, via a tyrosine-specific protein kinase. Bone cells have been reported to contain phosphotyrosine phosphatase, an enzyme believed to be involved in the regulation of cell division (340). The notion that bone cells possess the ability to hydrolyze free phosphotyrosine would be consonant with the presence of a tyrosine protein kinase regulatory system in bone cells. Interestingly, both parathyroid hormone (PTH) and $1\alpha,25-(OH)_2D_3$ stimulated phosphotyrosine phosphatase activity over a 3-day period; hormone effects were dose-dependent. Phosphotyrosine phosphatase shares many properties in common with alkaline phosphatase, and the two may be identical.

Although the significance of EGF in bone growth and remodeling is unknown, the EGF receptor may transmit the effect of TGFα, a possible mediator of hypercalcemia associated with certain mammalian neoplasms, e.g., humoral hypercalcemia of malignancy (HHM). TGFα is a 50 amino-acid polypeptide found in tumor cell culture and in normal embryonic tissue (363). It binds to and activates the tyrosine kinase of the EGF receptor (443). Human recombinant or synthetic rat TGFα mimics the skeletal effects of EGF (187,284,409,428). TGFα promotes bone resorption at concentrations lower than does PTH and elicits PG production in resorbing mouse bone *in vitro* (428). Evidence points to TGFα as one mediator of the excessive bone resorption in HHM (284). It will be interesting to discover whether TGFα

is also responsible for the suppressed bone formation seen in that syndrome.

TGFβ is a 24 Kd dimer elaborated by normal adult tissue as well as neoplastic tissue; it does not occupy the EGF receptor, but requires EGF or PDGF for activity (284,362). It stimulates PG formation and bone resorption (428), and has also been postulated to be a mediator of HHM (284). Of special interest is that this material exhibits dose-dependent mitogenic activity for bone cells, thus mimicking EGF. There is reason to believe that bone cells elaborate TGFβ (57). TGFβ appears to be similar to a mitogen derived from media conditioned by organ-cultured rodent bones (57).

PDGF is another mitogenic protein that enhances bone resorption, ostensibly via local prostaglandin release, and stimulates bone cell growth (425). In contrast to EGF (and FGF, *vide infra*), PDGF elicits enhanced protein synthesis in bone [collagen as well as noncollagen protein (43)]; there is reason to believe that PDGF may be a competency factor, permitting stimulation of DNA synthesis by progression factors such as the somatomedins (see 171 for review). Native PDGF is in reality several, approximately 30 Kd peptides consisting of two chains (A and B); its heterogeneity may reflect partial degradation during purification, chiefly from platelets. PDGF contains structural homologies with oncogene products. Its B chain is virtually identical to p 28 sis, the transforming protein of simian sarcoma virus (SSV), and identical also to a portion of the counterpart of p 28 sis, c-sis, found in sarcoma and glioma cell lines, and others as well. Thus, PDGF may be responsible for the autocrine promotion of tumor cell growth. It is also a candidate for an HHM mediator, acting in concert with other growth factors (284).

Fibroblast growth factor (FGF) is a polypeptide which has been isolated principally from brain tissue and pituitary gland, although FGF immunoreactivity has been demonstrated in other tissues (30,111). It is mitogenic for mesenchymal and neuro-ectodermal cells of various types, most notably endothelial cells, and promotes osteoblast proliferation (53). Both acidic and basic growth factors for endothelial cells have been identified, and the concept of acidic and basic FGFs has emerged. Their major activity *in vivo* may well be to promote endothelial cell proliferation. Recently, Thomas et al. have reported a partial sequence homology between bovine brain acidic FGF and human IL-1 (442); recall that IL-1 of macrophage origin is a bone resorption stimulator and may promote human bone cell differentiation.

The recognition that the skeletal metastases of prostate cancer are often intensely osteoblastic has prompted a search for a prostate-associated bone growth factor. Recently, the PL-3 human prostatic cancer cell line has been shown to produce a peptide stimulator of bone cell proliferation, alkaline phosphatase activity and collagen synthesis. Furthermore, an 1800 base mRNA for this factor has been isolated from PL-3 (399).

Somatomedins, or insulin-like growth factors, comprise a family of low molecular weight, insulin-like peptides (about 7–8 Kd) made by a variety of tissues (see 413 for review). IGF I (somatomedin C) is synthesized principally in the liver, by a growth hormone-dependent process, and represents the circulating second messenger of postembryonic bone growth hormone effects, principally those on cartilage. IGF II (somatomedin A) and its murine counterpart, multiplication stimulating activity (MSA), appear to function in embryonic growth and development.

It is characteristic of the somatomedins that they promote not only cell proliferation, but also expressions of differentiated function, such as collagen and proteoglycan synthesis. For example, IGF I has been shown to increase bone cell growth and activity, and IGF I, like insulin, which it resembles structurally, exerts a specific effect on osteoblast collagen synthesis (42,50,386). Stracke et al. have obtained evidence that bones can produce IGF1 (IGF1 then becomes an autocrine/paracrine growth factor) and do so in response to growth hormone (412). They have postulated that local production of IGF1 may mediate the skeletal effects of growth hormone.

Insulin, closely related to the somatomedins, also has effects on bone cell function (49). Kream *et al.* have analyzed in detail the impact of insulin on collagen synthesis in fetal rat bone (219). Results of those experiments disclose that low insulin concentrations directly stimulate synthesis of the protein by osteoblasts, and high concentrations promote the multiplication of collagen synthesizing cells. Moreover, insulin increases procollagen in mRNA levels in bone (217; also unpublished observations noted in 219).

The intrinsic growth factors of bone.

Proteins capable of stimulating bone cell proliferation and/or function have been identified as secretory products of bone cells themselves, as components of the extracellular organic matrix (presumably derived from bone cells), and as products of cells of the monocyte-macrophage series (see 57,398 for reviews) (Table 2). Some factors (e.g., TGFβ, IGF I) are produced by nonskeletal tissues;

TABLE 2. *Local factors regulating bone cells*

Cell of origin	Factor	Major effects[a]
Lymphocyte	OAF/IL-1[b]	↑R, ↑F
	lymphotoxin	↑R
	TNF β	↑R
	γIFN[c]	↓R,
Macrophage	IL-1	↑R, ↑F
	MDGF[d]	↑F
	PGE	↑R, ↑ + ↓ F[e]
Osteoblast (matrix)[f]	BDGF I	↑F
	BDGF II	↑F
	TGF β	↑R, ↑F
	HSGF	↑F
	BMP	M → C[g]
	PGE	↑R, ↑ + ↓ F[e]

[a]R = resorption; F = biochemical evidence of formation.
[b]Indicates possible OAF − IL-1 homology (24j).
[c]Also produced by macrophages.
[d]Macrophage-derived growth factor (26b).
[e]Refers to PGE as enhancing bone formation at lower concentration (and perhaps in periosteum) and inhibiting at high concentrations.
[f]Indicates factors elaborated by osteoblasts or extracted from bone matrix; they may be identical.
[g]Refers to mesenchymal cell → chondrocyte conversion.

others may be unique products of bone cells. These factors are to be differentiated functionally from endogenous inducers of endochondral bone development (*vide infra*), though the two types of factors may be similar. Growth factors of either variety, working singly or in combination, may be responsible for regulating formative events in modeling, remodeling, endochondral ossification, repair, and primary periosteal bone growth. Of particular interest are those which could link resorption and formation during the remodeling cycle ("coupling" factors). These include (a) factors extracted from organic matrix, perhaps of osteoblast origin, that may stimulate osteoblast growth following their resorption-associated release from the matrix, and (b) factors elaborated by specialized macrophages which reside in the vicinity of the remodeling locus (*vide supra*).

Best characterized of the endogenous growth factors are so-called bone-derived growth factors (BDGFs) and human skeletal growth factor (HSGF). Two BDGFs have been isolated from media conditioned by organ-cultured calvaria from rat fetuses *and* by isolated osteoblast-like cells *in vitro*: a mitogen (BDGF I, MW 20-30 Kd) and a second factor (BDGF II, 6-13 Kd), which mimics somatomedins in its capacity to promote specialized activities as well as growth in bone cell systems (51). In addition, bone tissue produces a TGFβ-like activity (57). BDGF II may be similar to the cartilage-derived growth factor (CDGF) which is active in bone and cartilage cell systems (204–206). Shen et al. have reported that isolated osteoblasts elaborate two mitogenic activities, only one of which is somatomedin-like (391). Interestingly, the pure mitogen (non-somatomedin) was elaborated *in vitro* during the proliferative phase of those cells in culture. By contrast, the somatomedin-like material, which promoted specialized functions, was released as the cells matured (391).

HSGF, extracted from human demineralized bone matrix, was originally reported to be an 83 Kd protein (113); preliminary reports of subsequent studies employing purification under dissociative conditions suggest that the active principle is considerably smaller (280), perhaps 9 Kd. This principle is thought to be analogous to putative coupling factor, a peptide released from resorbing bones *in vitro* which stimulates osteoblast growth (114,184).

Inducers of cartilage and bone development.

This group of agents, exemplified by bone morphogenetic protein (BMP) (see 165 and 355 for reviews), includes substances extracted from demineralized bone which induce hard tissue formation when implanted in skeletal muscle and subcutaneous tissue *in vivo*. Osteosarcoma tissue yields similar material (6,400). At least some of these substances have also been shown to act *in vitro,* where they promote the conversion of mesenchymal cells (419) and muscle cells (389) into chondrocytes. It is likely that the *de novo* emergence of functioning chondrocytes then triggers a cascade of events resembling the process of endochondral bone formation, ultimately yielding mature bone replete with hematopoietic marrow.

Although it has been known for decades that decalcified bone and dentin are osteoinductive (185,448), efforts to purify and characterize the active factor(s) have yielded progress slowly (384,450). Bone morphogenetic protein (BMP) of bovine or human origin is reported to have a molecular weight of 17–18 Kd (449–451). The presence of other proteins, particularly those involved in stabilizing the inductive factors *in situ* and providing an appropriate microsurface, may be required for the full expression of osteoinduction. The relatively insoluble matrix gla protein may be one of these facilitating factors (335).

Local Nonpeptide Factors in Bone Cell Regulation

Prostaglandins

Since Klein and Raisz's initial demonstration that PGs enhance bone resorption *in vitro* (211), a large body of data has accumulated which indicates that PGs may regulate the development, maturation and activity of bone-resorbing and bone-forming cells (see 346 for review).

PGs appear to mediate "basal active" bone resorption: that component of cellular resorption *in vitro* that occurs in the absence of added resorption stimulators (145,207,228).

In addition to their possible role in "basal active" resorption, PGs appear to facilitate or mediate the resorption-promoting effects of a variety of agents, including EGF and PDGF (Table 2), at least in mouse bone *in vitro*) (*vide supra*), but not including PTH or $1\alpha,25-(OH)_2D_3$. Coupled increases in PGE production and bone resorption also occur in response to a variety of non-humoral stimuli, including mechanical stimulation (403) and 2-chloroadenosine (230).

PGs are powerful stimulators of bone resorption when added to organ cultured bones (102,211,344,383,427). Particularly effective are PGE_2 and PGE_1, although 13,14 dihydro PGE_2, PGI_2 (prostacyclin), and 6-keto PGE_1 are also active *in vitro* (98,102). Prostaglandins are active at concentrations ranging from 10^{-5} to 10^{-9} M, and their effects develop more slowly and are less prolonged after pulse exposure than those of other resorption stimulators such as PTH and $1\alpha,25-(OH)_2 D_3$ (110).

PGs have been shown to replicate the actions of PTH and $1\alpha,25-(OH)_2 D_3$ in promoting osteoclast-mediated resorption (179). PGs also induce the appearance of osteoclast-like cells in a complex bone marrow culture system (186). This finding is in agreement with the observation of Nafussi and Baron that PGs increase the number of cortical and medullary osteoclasts in organ-cultured bones (294).

Whereas PGs stimulate resorption in bone segments, PGI_2, PGE_1 and PGE_2 inhibit the activity of isolated osteoclasts *in vitro*, and appear to do so by a cyclic AMP-mediated mechanism (4,61,63,65). Stimulatory effects on resorption, however, are indirect, probably mediated by osteoblast-like cells (60). Hence, any net impact of PGs on remodeling would reflect an imbalance between their direct and indirect effects on the various cellular participants. In this regard, both osteoblasts and osteoclast-like cells bind PGE_2, though the latter have a higher capacity (107).

PGs have been established as mediators of *in vitro* bone resorption, but have not been as clearly defined as physiological mediators of bone resorption *in vivo*. It is believed, however, that PGs cause the excessive bone resorption associated with inflammatory disorders and fractures (88,92,93,235,367), and may induce the hypercalcemia accompanying certain animal and human tumors (388,429,459). Although PGs are not commonly involved in the HHM syndrome, their release by tumors that are metastatic to bone may cause local bone dissolution (14,332).

There is also uncertainty about the effects of PGs on bone formation, at least in part because a suitable *in vitro* model has been lacking. Evidence has been obtained from *in vitro* studies that PGs may promote the differentiation of preosteoblasts into osteoblasts. Chyun and Raisz, for example, reported a transient stimulation by PGs of periosteal DNA synthesis in organ-cultured bone following enhanced collagen formation in the central areas of the cultured calvaria (81), supporting earlier studies demonstrating PG-mediated increases in collagen labeling in chick bone (29). Of particular interest is that PGs nullify the inhibitory effect of glucocorticoids on DNA and collagen synthesis (346), in keeping with the notion that glucocorticoids may act by suppressing endogenous PG synthesis (*vide supra*). At higher doses, PGE_2 inhibits collagen synthesis (345). The concept that PGs may exert a preferential effect on periosteal tissue is supported by the data of Nafussi and Baron, who showed increased periosteal osteoblast activity in PGE-treated bones *in vitro* (294). A differentiation-promoting effect has also been demonstrated in a clone of osteoblast-like cells derived from newborn mouse calvaria (MC3T3-E1); PGE_2 (as well as $1\alpha,25-(OH)_2D_3$) induced alkaline phosphatase activity by an actinomycin D and cycloheximide-inhibitable process (153,154).

These *in vitro* studies suggest that PGs might, in the long term, increase bone formation *in vivo*. Indeed, infusion of PGs in infants with cyanotic heart disease to maintain the patency of the ductus arteriosus caused enhancement of periosteal bone formation and hyperostosis (446). Administration of PGE to rats leads to increases in new-woven trabecular bone, metaphyseal hard tissue, and cortical endosteal bone formation (192,447).

There is little doubt that the osteoblast is a primary target cell for osteotropic PGs. Like PTH, PGs accumulate in osteoblasts and stimulate them to secrete collagenase and to initiate cyclic AMP production (13,90,107,354). They also promote the activity of cyclic AMP-dependent protein kinases (314). Interestingly, the effect of PGE_2 is limited to protein kinase isoenzyme 2, whereas the other PGs and PTH promote isoenzymes 1 and 2 about equally (233). Also like PTH, PGs acutely influence bone cell Ca^{2+} accumulation. Exogenous PGE_2 increased Ca^{2+} accumulation in osteoblastic cells *in vitro,* but only when endogenous PG production was inhibited, primarily because these cells generate large amounts of PGs *in vitro* (116). Exogenous PGE_2 was likewise stimulatory of Ca^{2+} accumulation in osteoclastic cells, which are not vigorous PG producers, and acted in the absence of cyclooxygenase inhibitors (116). Like PTH, PGs cause acute changes in the shape of osteoblast-like cells (15).

These considerations, taken together, point to PGs as important local regulators of bone cell behavior. Although their precise roles and modes of action remain unclear, it is more than speculative to suggest that endogenously produced PGs, released in response to hormonal, pharmacological, inflammatory, and mechanical perturbations, may increase bone remodeling. In these situations, one can envisage agonists eliciting PG production by osteoblasts, or bone lining cells, and the newly produced PGs acting in concert with the agonist. A second role for PGs may be to induce the differentiation of both osteoclast and osteoblast precur-

sors. A sufficiency of osteoclast precursors would ensure a supply of osteoclasts for bone resorption and an ample number of osteoblast precursors would facilitate the completion of a remodeling cycle. In addition, PGs may induce *de novo* periosteal bone formation which is not linked specifically to remodeling, i.e., endogenous PG release resulting from the application of mechanical stresses to periosteal surfaces may enhance periosteal bone accumulation.

Adenosine

Adenosine is a nucleoside that has been found to modify metabolic processes in a variety of nonskeletal cells. The initial observation that adenosine at micromolar concentrations increased adenylate cyclase activity and cyclic AMP levels in isolated bone cells suggested that it may also be a local regulator of bone cell function (317,318). These observations prompted largely unsuccessful efforts to demonstrate effects on bone resorption and formation, perhaps due to the rapid metabolism of the nucleoside in skeletal tissue. More recently, Lerner and Fredholm showed that the nonmetabolized analog of adenosine, 2-chloradenosine (2-CA), stimulates resorption in organ cultured bones (132,229,230). Subsequent studies indicate that the resorptive effect of 2-CA may arise by two mechanisms: direct and indirect, through the local production of PGs. Hence, adenosine, via cyclic AMP, may replicate the effects of PTH and PGs on osteoblasts, eliciting a series of events which culminate in activation. PGs and adenosine would act in concert to stimulate resorption (230). Since adenosine is a neurotransmitter, it will be interesting to know whether it is released locally, perhaps at gap junctional sites, in response to physical and electrical stimuli in bone tissue.

Fluoride

Fluoride is considered a local regulatory factor because it may act on bone cells by virtue of accumulating in bone tissue (see 360 for review). Exposure of mammals to high concentrations of fluoride causes profound changes in bone physiology. Fluoride ion substitutes for hydroxyl ions in the crystal lattice to form fluorohydroxyapatite, thereby increasing the crystallinity and reducing the solubility of bone crystals—in essence, mineral stabilization. The increases in trabecular mass of the axial skeleton associated with high-dose fluoride exposure undoubtedly reflect an alteration in bone remodeling. Three effects have been proposed: enhanced osteoblast activity stemming from the increased microelectric transducive capacity of fluorohydroxyapatite; direct stimulation of osteoblast activity; and inhibition of the resorptive process. Recently, Farley *et al.* have demonstrated that fluoride enhanced bone cell growth and specialization and promoted bone formation *in vitro,* and did so at concentrations similar to those found to be active *in vivo* (115). Although histomorphometric studies demonstrate that fluoride promotes osteoid production by osteoblasts in excess of osteoid mineralization, nevertheless fluoride is associated with an increase in the amount of mineralized bone, particularly in the presence of adequate amounts of calcium and phosphate.

Electrical Phenomena and Bone Cell Behavior

That local electrical potentials occur in bone tissue is now well established. Two kinds of signals have been described (see 35 for review): stress-generated (arising when bone is mechanically stressed) and resting or steady-state (bioelectric) potentials. Two mechanisms for stress-generated potentials may exist: *piezoelectricity,* extending from the deformation of crystalline material, and *streaming potentials,* caused by stress-initiated changes in fluid fluxes through pores.

A substantial body of evidence indicates that electricity can promote bone formation, not only in terms of fracture repair, but also epiphyseal bone growth. This recognition has prompted numerous studies to examine the effects of electricity in various forms on the function of skeletal cells, including matrix formation, calcification, and cell proliferation. Of particular interest are alterations in bone cell

growth, since the bulk of data point to a stimulatory effect (162,163,213,214,302). Electrical stimulation has been shown to have variable *in vitro* effects on cyclic AMP formation and Ca^{2+} accumulation in skeletal cell systems (see 35 for review). Electrical stimulation has also been shown to decrease the cyclic AMP response of bone cells to exogenous PTH (34,41,213,214). The cyclic AMP and proliferative responses of osteoblast-like cells are contingent upon the field strength and the extracellular Ca^{2+} concentration (27,28,215). Increased synthesis of PGE was found upon exposure of osteosarcoma cells to an inductively coupled signal (195), and electrical stimulation has been shown to promote actin polymerization in isolated bone cells (227). One might suggest that alterations in local electrical signals transduce mechanical effects on remodeling, perhaps culminating in prostaglandin release.

Phosphate, Pyrophosphate, and Bisphosphonates

Among the ions that might modify bone cell activity, phosphate-containing molecules are among the most studied. Increasing concentrations of inorganic phosphate inhibit bone resorption (347), and inorganic orthophosphate has been shown to stimulate matrix formation and mineralization *in vitro* (12). Inorganic pyrophosphates were recognized over 20 years ago as compounds that bind to hydroxyapatite (199) and inhibit skeletal mineralization (122,123,126), acting at least in part by inhibiting calcium phosphate crystallization and aggregation (125,164). Accordingly, tissue pyrophosphatases would regulate mineralization by controlling the local concentrations of pyrophosphate. It was the search for clinically useful analogs of pyrophosphate, resistant to pyrophosphatase attack, that led to the discovery of the bisphosphonates, in which carbon was substituted for the ester oxygen in the pyrophosphate moiety (see 121 for review). A detailed consideration of these nonphysiological compounds is beyond the scope of this review. It must be emphasized, however, that they have provided a useful tool for the investigation of bone cell kinetics. The bisphosphonates concentrate in the skeleton, inhibit bone resorption or bone formation (or both), at least in part via direct effects on bone cells and their precursors, in which they accumulate.

Systemic Hormones and Bone Cell Metabolism

The effects of hormones and other regulatory agents on bone cell metabolism have been studied *in vivo* and *in vitro,* using a variety of experimental approaches. Assignment of specific responses to individual cell types within the bone compartment has represented an appreciable and as yet partially unresolved methodological problem. Much of our information has derived from the use of isolated cell systems, particularly osteoblast-like cells released from well-differentiated skeletal tissues, osteoblast-like cell clones, and osteoblast-like cells obtained from animal osteogenic sarcomas. Accumulation of hormones in specific target cells has been identified *in vivo,* using radioautographic and immunological approaches. The following summary reflects a composite of data obtained from these multiple sources.

Parathyroid Hormone (PTH)

PTH has multiple effects on bone cell behavior (see 475 for review). Acutely, it stimulates bone resorption and inhibits bone formation (101,218,341). PTH may also increase bone formation, acting indirectly as a consequence of enhanced remodeling, and also as part of a direct stimulatory effect on osteoblasts (151,387,445). This stimulatory effect on osteoblasts develops more gradually and in response to lower concentrations of PTH than the inhibitory effects. It is currently held that the osteoblast (or bone lining cell-osteocyte complex) is the primary target cell for the effects of PTH on resorption as well as formation *(vide supra).* In this regard, histochemical and immunocytochemical studies have localized PTH to osteoblasts and preosteoblasts (as well as osteocytes) *in vivo* (22,353).

The first step in PTH action is the interaction between the hormone and specific receptors on the osteoblast surface. Studies of the binding of biologically active radioiodinated bovine PTH species to osteoblast-like cells have indicated dissociation constants (kDa) in the nanomolar to subnanomolar range (330,352,361). PTH is then thought to elicit the emergence of second (intracellular) messages which initiate a cascade of purposive biological responses. There is every reason to believe that both cyclic AMP and Ca^{2+} represent such "second messengers" for at least some of the actions of PTH. The earliest detectable responses of osteoblast-like cells to PTH are enhancement of adenylate cyclase activity and increases in cellular cyclic AMP levels and cellular Ca^{2+} accumulation (69,108,252,364). Cyclic AMP production is linked to activation of cyclic AMP-dependent protein kinase which in turn catalyzes the phosphorylative modification of various cell processes (314). Increases in cytosolic Ca^{2+}, via calmodulin, also regulate key cell functions. Ca^{2+} and cyclic AMP-regulating mechanisms may also interact; evidence indicates that Ca^{2+} potentiates the cyclic AMP response to PTH (321). Recognizing the participation of two second messengers in PTH action, Lowik et al. have proposed a model in which the cyclic AMP formation and Ca^{2+} accumulation are linked to separate PTH receptors, with activation of both receptors inducing the full biological response to the hormone (236). Osteoblastic cells also exhibit desensitization to PTH, a potentially important control mechanism, wherein prolonged exposure diminishes their cyclic AMP response (170, 320,474,477). Both homologous desensitization (PTH treatment blunting the response to PTH) (170) and heterologous desensitization (cross-desensitization by other adenylate cyclase stimulators such as PGE_2) have been described (174,320). Though the causes of desensitization are incompletely understood, reduced receptor availability is a likely contributor (361).

It is likely *(vide supra)* that PTH initiates

bone resorption via an interaction with osteoblasts or bone lining cells. Changes believed to be associated with enhancement of resorption include an acute shape change (conversion of osteoblasts from a flattened to a stellate shape) and elaboration of mammalian collagenase, and plasminogen activator (15,160,167,217, 274,307,308,339,379,380).

The fact that PTH can stimulate as well as inhibit bone formation may reflect predominant actions at different concentrations of the hormone. For example, in osteoblast-like cells isolated from chick calvaria, low concentrations of PTH enhance and high concentrations suppress alkaline phosphatase levels (155). Increases in alkaline phosphatase activity have also been observed at low concentrations of PTH in neonatal mouse calvaria cells (481), and in the cloned established osteoblast-like cell line MC3T3-E1 (291). Low concentrations of PTH have been reported to increase DNA synthesis and cell replication in mouse calvaria cells, while high concentrations were inhibitory in the latter system (457). PTH-mediated enhancement of ornithine decarboxylase (ODC) in bone cells lends further support to its direct anabolic action (32,237). ODC catalyzes the rate-limiting step in polyamine synthesis; polyamines appear to influence cell growth and specialization.

It is tempting to speculate that the direct stimulatory effects on osteoblasts by PTH at low concentrations may reflect a physiological process that insures a ready supply of osteoblasts for repair of resorption cavities in remodeling, in essence supplementing the activity of locally derived factors which might couple formation and resorption. Alternatively, this action of PTH may be significant in embryological bone formation but not in physiological remodeling. In fact, PTH is known to have anabolic effects on cartilage tissue.

Calcitonin

The major skeletal action of calcitonin (CT) is to inhibit osteoclast-mediated bone resorption (see 18 for review). Administration of CT to experimental animals rapidly causes osteo-

clasts to detach from bone surfaces and to lose their ruffled borders (240). Pseudopod retraction, cell rounding, reduced motility and cytoskeletal rearrangements typify the responses of isolated osteoclasts to CT (59,67). In organ cultured bones, CT inhibits not only basal resorption but also the augmented resorption caused by a variety of agents, including PTH, PGE, and $1\alpha,25-(OH)_2D_3$ (133,343). One of the several recently isolated CT gene-related peptides has been found to promote bone resorption as well, probably via the CT receptor (373). *In vitro* systems have permitted the delineation of (1) the time-course of CT action; (2) the dose-response relationships, (3) the relative efficacies of CT preparations from different sources; and (4) some information about CT action at the cellular level. Of interest has been the phenomenon of escape, the reappearance of stimulated resorption after its initial suppression by CT, usually within 24–48 hr, despite the continued presence of the hormone (469). This phenomenon must be distinguished from "down regulation" at the cellular level, that implies an adaptive alteration in a specific molecular component (or components) in the chain of events in hormone action. Escape from the action of CT *in vitro* may be due in part to "down regulation," reflecting a reduction in the number of CT receptors. Actual decreases in CT receptors were shown to accompany escape *in vitro,* but the number of residual receptors should have been sufficient to permit continued CT action (430). On the other hand, alterations in cell dynamics, with the emergence of a population of CT-insensitive resorbing cells may also be contributory. The blunting of escape by external irradiation (osteoclast precursors are radiosensitive) in both *in vivo* and *in vitro* systems supports this possibility (220,290).

There is every reason to believe that CT is a direct-acting inhibitor of osteoclast function. Chambers and Magnus reported that CT, at low concentrations, blocked cytoplasmic activity and caused cell process retraction in isolated osteoclasts (66,67) and inhibited their ability to absorb bone *in vitro* (68).

From these observations, it has been suggested that the osteoclast is a target cell for CT. The further observation that osteoclast-like but not osteoblast-like cells respond biochemically to CT, has in fact formed the basis for assigning isolated bone cells to specific functional classes. Bone cells isolated from rodent calvaria by sequential enzymic digestion or by mechanical separation of periosteal and subperiosteal tissues before enzymatic release of cells are classified as osteoblastic or osteoclastic according to their biochemical responses to PTH and CT, the osteoclastic cells responding principally to CT and the osteoblastic cells to PTH (33,316,476). (The osteoclast identity of the CT-responsive cells, however, has not been proven.) CT receptors and/or actions have been demonstrated in cells of the immune regulatory system, including lymphocytes, monocytes and macrophages. For example, T-lymphocytes have CT receptors, and CT blocks their cyclic AMP and proliferative responses to PTH and PGE (256,264,325,470). Both stimulatory and inhibitory effects have been demonstrated in macrophages. Most recently, Stock and Coderre showed that salmon CT at low concentrations inhibited cAMP accumulation and stimulated prostaglandin production prompted by latex particle exposure in human monocytes (410,411).

Cyclic AMP has been proposed as a second messenger for CT action in osteoclasts. The possible participation of alterations in intracellular Ca^{2+}, and consequently in Ca^{2+}-calmodulin relationships, has also received experimental support in nonskeletal systems (142). CT has been shown to decrease cell Ca^{2+} accumulation in a population of osteoclast-like cells *in vitro,* without effect on apparent osteoblasts (393).

Vitamin D

Vitamin D_3, via its biologically active metabolite, $1\alpha,25-(OH)_2D_3$, has profound structural and functional effects on the skeleton (see 94 and 172 for reviews). Although other metabolites, particularly 24R,25 $(OH)_2 D_3$, may also be influential (305), their physiological significance remains to be determined. In terms of current knowledge about $1\alpha,25-(OH)_2D_3$, the metabolite may be regarded as a mediator of osteoid mineralization and of bone resorption, the two most thoroughly analyzed of its skeletal effects. It is generally agreed that enhanced bone resorption represents a direct effect of the metabolite on bone. By contrast, the thesis that $1\alpha,25-(OH)_2D_3$ has a direct effect on bone formation remains unproven.

Raisz et al. demonstrated that low concentrations of $1\alpha,25-(OH)_2D_3$ stimulate resorption in organ-cultured bones (349). This resorption mimics that caused by PTH, reflecting an increase in the activity and number of osteoclasts (179). $1\alpha,25-(OH)_2D_3$, like PTH, appears to stimulate resorption indirectly, via a prior action on another type of skeletal cell, perhaps the osteoblast or bone lining cell. In this regard, labeled $1\alpha,25-(OH)_2D_3$ uptake *in vivo* has been demonstrated in osteoprogenitor cells and osteoblasts but not in osteoclasts (292). Like PTH, $1\alpha,25-(OH)_2D_3$ failed to modify bone resorption by isolated rabbit osteoclasts cultured on human bone segments, but was effective when osteoblast-like cells were incorporated into the culture system (62). Also contributing to the stimulatory effect of $1\alpha,25-(OH)_2D_3$ is the enhancement of osteoclast generation from bone marrow precursors (186).

A large body of evidence indicates that $1\alpha,25-(OH)_2D_3$ promotes the differentiation of many cell types, including cells of the monocyte-macrophage series and lymphocytes (5,21, 278,358,414,415). Human peripheral monocytes, activated T- and B-lymphocytes, and lymphoid cell lines (but not normal resting lymphocytes) and other cell types have high affinity receptors (see 329 and 416 for reviews) for $1\alpha,25-(OH)_2D_3$ (26,266,268,338). $1\alpha,25-(OH)_2D_3$ inhibition of lymphocyte growth may derive from reduced formation of the autocrine lymphocyte growth factor interleukin 2 (IL-2). $1\alpha,25-(OH)_2D_3$ and its analogs can induce differentiation of normal and leukemic stem cells. For example, $1\alpha,25-(OH)_2D_3$ causes the maturation of human promyelocytic leukemia cells (HL60) into mono- and multinucleated macrophage-like cells which can then bind to and resorb devitalized bone (21,262,423,424). This effect has been associated with a reversible decrease in the expression of the c-myc oncogene (357). $1\alpha,25-(OH)_2D_3$ also inhibits cell growth and induces macrophagic conversion of mouse leukemic cells (M1) and the human histiocytic lymphoma cell line U937 (5,278). In that cell line, vitamin D induces a dose-dependent decrease in proliferation and an increase in specialization-associated properties reminiscent of the macrophage. Furthermore, treated cells acquire the electron microscopic characteristics of macrophages. These results are consistent with the notion that $1\alpha,25-(OH)_2D_3$ stimulates bone resorption, at least in part, by promoting the specialization of osteoclast precursors in bone marrow.

In addition to precursor cell maturation, multinucleation (polykaryon formation) is required for the full expression of osteoclast function. $1\alpha,25-(OH)_2D_3$ not only enhances the fusion and activation of alveolar macrophages (1,2), but also stimulates the emergence of multinucleated cells with osteoclast characteristics in long-term cultures of feline bone marrow (186).

The foregoing information indicates that $1\alpha,25-(OH)_2D_3$ plays two basic roles in bone resorption; first, enhancing osteoclast development; and second, promoting the maturation of lymphoid cells, thus enhancing their capacity to elaborate bone resorption-stimulating lyphokines such as osteoclast-activating factor.

Difficulties encountered in studying bone formation *in vivo* and *in vitro* have complicated the assessment of possible direct effects of $1\alpha,25-(OH)_2D_3$. Yet high affinity (Kd–0.1 to 0.2 nM), 3.2–3.7 S receptors for $1\alpha,25-(OH)_2D_3$ have been identified in osteoblasts and in osteoblast-like malignant cells (80, 216,249,467) and the activity of these receptors correlates with biological responses to the metabolite (74,75,104,467). Low concentrations of $1\alpha,25-(OH)_2D_3$ exert multiple effects on bone cell metabolism in various osteoblast models; in general, the dose-response relationships of these effects parallel receptor binding kinetics. These effects include inhibition of bone cell proliferation (84,104,128), collagen synthesis (in association with decreases in procollagen mRNA content) (374,477), and citrate decarboxylation (477). $1\alpha,25-(OH)_2D_3$ has also been reported to increase or decrease the acute cyclic AMP response to parathyroid hormone and also to be without effect (173,232,242, 319,477), though most recent studies suggest that attenuation is the predominant effect, particularly at high concentrations (56,79). Although $1\alpha,25-(OH)_2 D_3$ reduces alkaline phosphatase activity in organ-cultured bones (44,351), it raises alkaline phosphatase activity in osteoblasts and in osteogenic sarcoma cells (134,224,244,250). Noteworthy is the fact that $1\alpha,25-(OH)_2D_3-26,23$-lactone, which increases alkaline phosphatase activity in an established cell line, has been shown to block the resorptive action of $1\alpha,25-(OH)_2D_3$, but not that of PTH *in vivo* (210). Furthermore, recent studies with human bone cells indicate that very low concentrations (5×10^{-12} M) $1\alpha,25-(OH)_2 D_3$ increase proliferation, whereas dose-dependent inhibitory effects were noted at 5×10^{-9} to 5×10^{-6} M (400). $1\alpha,25-(OH)_2 D_3$, among other bone resorption-stimulating hormones, also promotes the activity of plasminogen activator in UMR106-01 osteosarcoma cells and in osteoblast-rich calvarial cells (160). It is reasonable to suggest that $1\alpha,25-(OH)_2 D_3$ acts by modifying *de novo* protein synthesis in these target cells following its association with specific cytosolic receptors, translation of the receptor-hormone complex to the nucleus, and subsequent alteration in DNA-dependent mRNA production (94,172,329).

Two recent findings provide long-awaited evidence for a direct effect of $1\alpha,25-(OH)_2 D_3$ on bone mineralization: (1) stimulation of osteocalcin synthesis (16,24,203,231,334) and citrate secretion (337), effects which could collaborate to inhibit hydroxyapatite growth; and (2) alterations in phospholipid metabolism in UMR106 osteosarcoma cells—increased phosphatidyl serine (PS) and decreased phosphatidyl ethanolamine (PE) formation (257). PS may facilitate mineralization by binding calcium and phosphorus. New protein synthesis was required for this effect, as it is for many (if not all) of the other skeletal effects of $1\alpha,25-(OH)_2 D_3$.

In systems of osteoblast-like cells, receptors for vitamin D appear to be regulated, exhibiting species variations and, in some cell systems, endogenous rhythms. For example, although the affinity constant and the sedimentation coefficient for the $1\alpha,25-(OH)_2 D_3$ receptors is the same in osteoblasts derived from the mouse and the rat, the receptor content is lower in the rat cells and fails to exhibit the growth rate dependence found in the mouse cells (75). Recently, vitamin A acid (retinoic acid) has been noted to increase the number of specific $1\alpha,25-(OH)_2$ vitamin D receptors in osteoblast-like osteosarcoma cells, indicating an interaction between these two fat-soluble vitamins (327). The physiological significance of these effects is unclear. Since many have been demonstrated in embryonic tissues and cells, or in transformed or established cell lines, their principal relevance may be related to embryologic bone development.

Glucocorticoids

Glucocorticoids inhibit bone growth and fracture healing, and cause osteoporosis in several species, including humans (see 140 for review). It is classically taught that glucocorticoid-mediated osteoporosis results from a decrease in osteoblast number and/or activity coupled with an increase in the rate of bone resorption. The osteoblast effect is regarded as a direct one, stemming from inhibition of osteoblast precursor proliferation and perhaps inhibition of specific differentiated functions. The increase in resorption is thought to be indirect, stemming from secondary hyperparathyroidism associated with reduced intestinal absorption of calcium.

In vitro studies using organ-cultured bones and various isolated cell systems have disclosed that the effects of glucocorticoids are complex and diverse, and differ in various species and, within isolated cell systems, at various times in the progression of the cell culture. In so-called bone-forming systems, glucocorti-

coids cause a transient, short-term increase in type I collagen synthesis and alkaline phosphatase activity, followed by a long-term decrease, in association with decreases in labeled thymidine incorporation into DNA and in net DNA content (45). These results are most consistent with an early differentiation-promoting effect followed by a late predominantly inhibitory effect on osteoblasts and osteoblast precursors. Hahn, Westbrook and Halsted demonstrated that exposure of an intact bone preparation from neonatal rat calvaria to as little as 100 nM cortisol for 24 hr increased alkaline phosphatase, citrate decarboxylation, thymidine incorporation, and total DNA (152). More recently, Canalis has shown that the impact of glucocorticoids on an isolated, intact bone system reflects the integrated responses of several cell types within the tissue itself (47). By examining the effects of glucocorticoids on periosteal tissues and on central nonperiosteal bone, presumably osteoblast-enriched, Canalis obtained data which suggest that cortisol does not inhibit the function of mature osteoblasts directly. Its predominant long-term effect is to diminish periosteal cell replication. The stimulatory effect of cortisol on the incorporation of radioactively labeled proline into collagen required the presence of intact periosteal and nonperiosteal bones. By contrast, cortisol stimulated alkaline phosphatase activity in central nonperiosteal bone. In a chick periosteal explant model, dexamethasone was found to enhance alkaline phosphatase activity and the proliferation of progenitor cells, culminating in an increased number of functioning osteoblasts (435). From these data, it would appear that glucocorticoids at physiological concentration promote the acquisition and preservation of the differentiated state in osteoblasts, and at higher concentrations or for longer periods of treatment, reduce the replication of osteoblast precursors.

The effects of glucocorticoids have also been examined in isolated osteoblasts and in osteoblast-like osteosarcoma cells, which have been found to contain specific, high affinity glucocorticoid receptors (71,78,117,166). Interestingly, glucocorticoids (a) decrease the synthesis of collagen and non-collagen protein (315), and (b) promote RNA degradation (322). Chen, Cone and Feldman reported that dexamethasone decreased the proliferation of sparsely and densely cultured mouse osteoblast-like cells, and sparsely cultured rat osteoblast-like cells, but increased proliferation of densely cultured rat cells (73). Hence, the actions of glucocorticoids on osteoblast-like cells *in vitro* are related to the species and to the cell density at the time of culture. Glucocorticoids have also been demonstrated to increase alkaline phosphatase activity and decrease cell growth in ROS17/2.8 osteosarcoma cells, an effect which is antagonized by cyclic AMP elevating agents such as parathyroid hormone, isoproterenol and 8-bromo cyclic AMP (243). Cortisol increases bicarbonate ATPase and alkaline phosphatase in cultured rabbit endosteal osteoblast-like cells (10), and has divergent effects on the homotypic desensitization of the cyclic AMP response to PTH, PGE_2 and calcitonin (193).

Two additional cellular effects of glucocorticoids deserve mention. First, glucocorticoids have been found to magnify the cyclic AMP response of bone cells to PTH (76,78, 296,368). This effect may be the summation of multiple individual actions on various components of the cyclic AMP-generating system, ultimately reflecting a general effect on membrane structure or composition (56). Not surprisingly, therefore, glucocorticoids can potentiate some of the metabolic responses of bone cells to PTH which are believed to be cyclic AMP-mediated. For example, Hahn, Westbrook and Halsted demonstrated that cortisol enhanced the suppressive effect of PTH on alkaline phosphatase, collagen synthesis and citrate decarboxylation in neonatal rat calvaria (152). Enhanced sensitivity to PTH was envisaged as one mechanism for the development of glucocorticoid-mediated osteopenia. A second effect of glucocorticoids is to modulate the high affinity receptor for $1\alpha,25-(OH)_2 D_3$ in osteoblasts (74,75,248). In mouse osteoblasts, the effects of glucocorticoids on the $1\alpha,25-$ $(OH)_2 D_3$ receptor concentration depended upon the gross growth phase of the cell: a reduction appeared early in log phase, a transient increase late in log phase, and a decrease in receptor number after the cells had achieved confluence (74). By contrast with the mouse bone cell system, in rat osteoblast-like cells, glucocorticoids increased receptor number throughout the entire culture cycle (75).

Glucocorticoids in combination with vitamin D create diverse effects on bone cell systems. Glucocorticoids modify certain of the effects of $1\alpha,25-(OH)_2 D_3$ in bone cell systems; for example, glucocorticoids blunt the $1\alpha,25-(OH)_2 D_3$-mediated stimulation of osteocalcin synthesis in human osteoblasts while promoting the inhibitory effect of the vitamin on collagen synthesis and citrate decarboxylation (400,478). Furthermore, glucocorticoids prevented the increased plasminogen activator activity caused by $1\alpha,25-(OH)_2 D_3$ in UMR106-01 rat osteogenic sarcoma cells (they prevented the effects of PTH as well) (160).

Although glucocorticoids appear to enhance bone resorption *in vivo* by an indirect mechanism, inhibitory effects have been observed *in vitro* (350). Glucocorticoids decreased the generation of osteoclast-like cells and the activity of existing osteoclasts in cultures of cat bone marrow (417). By contrast, glucocorticoids promote the dissolution of devitalized bone particles by mononuclear phagocytes and mononuclear polykaryons (432). Recently, Bar-Shavit et al. have reported that glucocorticoids stimulated the attachment of rat thioglycollate-elicited peritoneal macrophages to bone surfaces, in association with enhanced exposure of plasma membrane-associated sugar residues which appear to be pivotal in macrophage binding (20).

Sex Steroids (Estrogens, Androgens, and Progestins)

Estrogens influence skeletal physiology *in vivo*; there is appreciable evidence to indicate that estrogen deficiency accelerates bone loss, and may contribute significantly to osteoporosis in women (see 196 for review). However, convincing evidence for direct effects of estrogens on bone metabolism is lacking (52,55,408) and efforts to demonstrate specific bone receptors for estrogen in subhuman species have not been rewarding (77,458). Recently, Vaishnav et al. reported that estradiol 17β at low concentrations (10^{-10}–10^{-11} M) stimulated radioactive thymidine incorporation into DNA in the human bone cell system (456). Stanozolol, an anabolic steroid, also increased thymidine incorporation in the human bone cell systems, and expanded cell number and collagen synthesis as well (456). Such findings must certainly encourage and enliven efforts to identify sex steroid hormone receptors in human bone cell systems.

Sex steroids may also affect bone metabolism indirectly, via the immune regulatory system (3,176; see 149 for review). Thymic tissue concentrates and contains specific receptors for estrogens, androgens and progestins (85,281). Of interest is that, among human peripheral lymphocytes, estrogen receptors are restricted to those bearing the ''suppressor-cytotoxic'' phenotype (OKT8) (85). Receptors for and actions of estrogens have also been demonstrated in blast lymphoid cells (150). The bulk of studies indicate that estrogenic hormones markedly suppress many, if not all, of the major functions attributed to the cell-mediated immune system, e.g., tissue rejection and T-lymphocyte mitogen reactivity. Suppression of the elaboration of bone resorption-stimulating lymphokines may be one action of estrogenic hormones.

Thyroid Hormone

Thyroid hormone is known to stimulate trabecular bone remodeling, increasing both resorption and formation on trabecular surfaces. In adult dogs, thyroxin increases trabecular bone mass, perhaps by expediting the conversion from resorption to formation and prolonging the formative phase in remodeling loci (175). Both T4 and T3 enhance the resorption of organ-cultured long bone from rat fetus, by a process which is calcitonin- and cortisol-inhibitable but not blocked by indomethacin (288).

Vitamin A

Vitamin A is known to stimulate bone resorption *in vivo* and *in vitro*, by a mechanism which hinges on *de novo* protein and RNA synthesis (118,342). The fact that retinoic acid enhances $1\alpha,25$–$(OH)_2 D_3$ binding in osteosarcoma cells suggests that $1\alpha,25$–$(OH)_2 D_3$ might contribute to its skeletal effects. In addition, vitamin A and related compounds modify osteoblast activity. Dickson and Walls reported that retinol reversibly inhibits collagen synthesis without affecting the formation of non-collagen protein in isolated chick and mouse calvaria (100).

OVERVIEW

Bone remodeling is a coordinated sequence of cellular events that is closely regulated by systemically and locally elaborated agents. Cellular participants include osteoclasts and osteoblasts (and their precursors), osteocytes and bone lining cells (resting osteoblasts), cells of the monocyte/macrophage series, lymphocytes and mast cells. Systemically elaborated chemical agents (e.g., PTH, $1\alpha,25$–$(OH)_2 D_3$) may activate the remodeling cycle, but there must be a mechanism for targeting those systemic messages to specific sites or sets of sites, a local state of readiness or receptivity. Mechanical and electrical forces may increase the statistical likelihood that resistance to activation will be overcome at a given locus. Osteocytes may transmit mechanical or electrical messages from areas deep within bone to surface lining cells with which they are connected by gap junctions. Adenosine could be a transmitter of those messages.

According to prevailing evidence, the bone lining cell transduces activation impulses to the potential resorption apparatus by site preparation and perhaps by hormonal stimulation. Prostaglandins (e.g., PGE_2) released by lining cells themselves during initiation can in turn aid in site preparation and in osteoclast recruitment. Systemic (as well as local) regulators may also facilitate the maturation of osteoclasts and their emergence from the hemopoietic precursor pool.

Osteoblasts are then recruited and activated, perhaps in response to locally generated (released) peptides and prostanoids. Autocrine and paracrine growth factors of osteoblast origin ensure a sufficient supply of osteoblast precursors for bone formation. We know virtually nothing about the signals that terminate osteoclast and osteoblast activity, though disorders of termination appear to exist (e.g., Paget's disease of bone).

And what of the immunoregulatory cells in the remodeling scenario? Macrophages and lymphoid cells elaborate many substances (monokines, lymphokines) that influence bone cell behavior; some have been identified, and more are likely to be described. Macrophages themselves have the machinery to regulate remodeling events, and also to modify bone surfaces and digest components of the organic matrix. Various immunoregulatory cells can be visualized as participating in embryological bone development and in posttraumatic and postinflammatory repair. A role for such cells in physiological remodeling remains to be established.

Areas of future investigation include the following:

1. Local regulatory factors and their relationship to systemic controls.
2. *In vitro* and *in vivo* systems for studying human bone cell physiology and biochemistry.
3. The lineage of bone cells, and the relationship between remodeling and the immune regulatory and hematopoietic systems.
4. The processes of initiation and activation of remodeling, and the process whereby remodeling is terminated.
5. Matrix components and their relationships to cellular events in remodeling.
6. Interactions between remodeling units; the skeletal intermediary organization.
7. The biochemistry of bone cell-factor (hormone) interactions and subsequent responses.
8. Assay systems for testing the actions of pharmacological agents that might affect remodeling in humans.

ACKNOWLEDGMENTS

The authors gratefully acknowledge the editorial assistance of Mr. James Havranek. This grant was supported by National Institutes of Health Grant 2R01 AM19855.

REFERENCES

1. Abe, E., Miyaura, C., Tanaka, H., Shina, Y., Kuribayashi, T., Suda, S., Nishii, Y., DeLuca, H.F., and Suda, T. (1983): $1\alpha,25$–Dihydroxyvitamin D_3 promotes fusion of mouse alveolar macrophages both by a direct mechanism and by a spleen cell-mediated indirect mechanism. *Proc. Natl. Acad. Sci. USA,* 80:5583–5587.
2. Abe. E., Shina, Y., Miyaura, C., Tanaka, H., Hayashi, T., Kanegasaki, S., Saito, M., Nishii, Y., DeLuca, H.F., and Suda, T. (1984): Activation and fusion induced by $1\alpha,25$-dihydroxyvitamin D_3 and their relation in alveolar macrophages. *Proc. Natl. Acad. Sci. USA,* 81:7112–7116.
3. Ahmed, S.A., Dauphinee, M.J., and Talal, N. (1985): Effects of short-term administration of sex hormones on normal and autoimmune mice. *J. Immunol.,* 134:204–210.
4. Ali, N.N., and Chambers, T.J. (1983): The effect of prostaglandin I_2 and 6a-Carba-PGI_2 on the motility of isolated osteoclasts. *Prostaglandins,* 25:603–608.
5. Amento, E.P., Bhalla, A.K., Kurnick, J.T., Kradin, R.L., Clemens, T.L., Holick, S.A., Holick, M.F., and Krane, S.M. (1984): $1\alpha,25$-Dihydroxyvitamin D_3 induces maturation of the human monocyte cell line U937, and, in association with a factor from human T lymphocytes, augments production of the monokine, mononuclear cell factor. *J. Clin. Invest.,* 73:731–739.
6. Amitani, K., Nakata, Y., and Stevens, J. (1974): Bone induction by lyophilized osteosarcoma in mice. *Calcif. Tissue Res.,* 16:305–313.
7. Anderson, H.C. (1985): Matrix calcification: review and update. In: *Bone and Mineral Research/3,* edited by W.A. Peck, pp. 109–149. Elsevier, Amsterdam.
8. Anderson, R.E., Jee, W.S., and Woodbury, D.M. (1985): Stimulation of carbonic anhydrase in osteoclasts by parathyroid hormone. *Calcif. Tissue Int.,* 37:646–650.
9. Anderson, R.E., Kemp, J.W., Jee, W.S., and Woodbury, D.M. (1984): Ion transporting ATPases and matrix mineralization in cultured osteoblastlike cells. *In Vitro,* 20:837–846.

10. Anderson, R.E., Kemp, J.W., Jee, W.S.S., and Woodbury, D.M. (1984): Effects of cortisol and fluoride on ion-transporting ATPase activities in cultured osteoblastlike cells. *In Vitro,* 20:847–855.

11. Anderson, R.E., Shraer, H., and Gay, C.V. (1982): Ultrastructural immunocytochemical localzation of carbonic anhydrase in normal and calcitonin-treated chick osteoclasts. *Anat. Rec.,* 204:9–20.

12. Asher, M.A., Sledge, C.B., and Glimcher, M.J. (1974): The effect of inorganic orthophosphate on the ratio of collagen formation and degradation in bone and cartilage in tissue culture. *J. Clin. Endocrinol. Metab.,* 38:376–389.

13. Atkins, D., and Martin, T.J. (1977): Rat osteogenic sarcoma cells: effects of some prostaglandins, their metabolites and analogues on cyclic AMP production. *Prostaglandins,* 13:861–871.

14. Atkins, D., Ibbotson, K.J., Hillier, K., Hunt, N.H., Hammonds, J.C., and Martin, T.J. (1977): Secretion of prostaglandins as bone-resorbing agents by renal cortical carcinoma in culture. *Br. J. Cancer,* 36:601–607.

15. Aubin, J.E., Alders, E., and Heersche, J.N.M. (1983): A primary role for microfilaments, but not microtubules, in hormone induced cytoplasmic retraction. *Exp. Cell. Res.,* 143:439–450.

16. Auf-mkolk, B., Hauschka, P.V., and Schwartz, E.R. (1985): Characterization of human bone cells in culture. *Calc. Tissue Int.,* 37:229–235.

17. Auron, P.E., Webb, A.C., Rosenwasser, L.J., Mucci, S.F., Rich, A., Wolff, S.M., and Dinarello, C.A. (1984): Nucleotide sequence of human monocyte interleukin 1 precursor cDNA. *Proc. Natl. Acad. Sci. USA,* 81:7907–7911.

18. Austin, L.A., and Heath, H., III (1981): Calcitonin: physiology and pathophysiology. *N. Engl. J. Med.,* 304:269–278.

19. Ball, E.D., Guyre, P.M., Shen, L., Glynn, J.M., Maliszewski, C.R., Baker, P.E., and Fanger, M.W. (1984): Gamma interferon induces monocytoid differentiation in the HL-60 cell line. *J. Clin. Invest.,* 73:1072–1077.

20. Bar-Shavit, B., Kahn, A.J., Pegg, L.E., Stone, K.R., and Teitelbaum, S.L. (1984): Glucocorticoids modulate macrophage surface oligosaccharides and their bone binding activity. *J. Clin. Invest.,* 73:1277–1283.

21. Bar-Shavit, Z., Teitelbaum, S.L., Reitsma, P., Hall, A., Pegg, L.E., Trail, J., and Kahn, A.J. (1983): Induction of monocytic differentiation and bone resorption by 1,25-dihydroxyvitamin D_3. *Proc. Natl Acad. Sci. USA,* 80:5907–5911.

22. Barling, P.M., and Bibby, N.J. (1985): Study of the localization of [^{3}H] bovine parathyroid hormone in bone by light microscope autoradiography. *Calcif. Tissue Int.,* 37:441–46.

23. Baron, R., Vignery, A., and Horowitz, M. (1984): Lymphocytes, macrophages, and the regulation of bone remodeling. In: *Bone and Mineral Research, Annual 2,* edited by W.A. Peck, pp. 175–243. Elsevier, Amsterdam.

24. Beresford, J.N., Gallagher, J.A., Poser, J.W., and Russell, R.G.G. (1984): Production of osteocalcin by human bone cells in vitro. Effects of $1,25(OH)_2D_3$, $24,25(OH)_2D_3$, parathyroid hormone, and glucocorticoids. *Metab. Bone Dis. Relat. Res.,* 5:229–234.

25. Beresford, J.N., Gallagher, J.A., Gowen, M., Couch, M., Poser, J., Wood, D.D., and Russell, R.G.G. (1984): The effects of monocyte-conditioned medium and interleukin 1 on the synthesis of collagenous and non-collagenous proteins by mouse bone and human bone cells in vitro. *Bicheim. Biophys. Acta,* 801:58–65.

26. Bhalla, A.K., Amento, E.P., Clemens, T.L., Holick, M.F., and Krane, S.M. (1983): Specific high-affinity receptors for 1,25–dihydroxyvitamin D_3 in human peripheral blood mononuclear cells: presence in monocytes and induction in T lymphocytes following activation. *J. Clin. Endocrinol. Metab.,* 57:1308–1310.

27. Binderman, I., Somjen, D., Shimshoni, Z., Berger, E., Fischler, H., and Korenstein, R. (1984): Role of calcium in electric field stimulation of bone cells in culture [abstract]. *Transactions of the Bioelectrical Repair and Growth Society,* 4:33.

28. Binderman, I., Somjen, D., Shimshoni, Z., Levy, J., Fischler, H., and Korenstein, R. (1985): Stimulation of skeletal-derived cultures by different electric field intensities is cell specific. *Biochim. Biophys. Acta,* 844:273–279.

29. Blumenkrantz, N., and Sondergaard, J. (1972): Effect of prostaglandins E_1 and F_1 on biosynthesis of collagen. *Nature [New Biol.],* 239:246.

30. Böhlen, P., Esch, F., Baird, A., Jones, K.L., and Gospodarowicz, D. (1985): Human brain fibroblast growth factor; isolation and partial chemical characterization. *FEBS Lett.,* 185:177–181.

31. Bonucci, E. (1981): New knowledge on the origin, function and fate of osteoclasts. *Clin. Orthop.,* 158:252–269.

32. Boonekamp, P.M. (1985): The effect of calcium and $3',5'$ cAMP on the induction of ornithine decarboxylase activity in bone and bone cells. *Bone,* 6:37–42.

33. Braidman, I.P., Anderson, D.C., Jones, C.J.P., and Weiss, J.B. (1983): Separation of two bone cell populations from fetal rat calvaria and a study of their responses to parathyroid hormone and calcitonin. *J. Endocrinol.,* 99:387–399.

34. Brighton, C., and McCluskey, W. (1983): The early response of bone cells in culture to a capacitively coupled electric field (abstr.). *Transactions of the Bioelectrical Repair and Growth Society,* 3:10.

35. Brighton, C.T., and McCluskey, W.P. (1986): Cellular response and mechanisms of action of electrically induced osteogenesis. In: *Bone and Mineral Research/4,* edited by W.A. Peck, pp. 213–254. Elsevier, Amsterdam.

36. Burger, E.H., Van der Meer, J.W.M., Van de Gevel, J.S., Gribnau, J.C., Wil Thesingh, C., and Van Furth, R. (1982): In vitro formation of osteoclasts from long-term cultures of bone marrow mononuclear phagocytes. *J. Exp. Med.,* 156:1604–1614.

37. Burger, E.H., Van der Meer, J.W.M., and Nij-

weide, P.J. (1984): Osteoclast formation from mononuclear phagocytes: role of bone-forming cells. *J. Cell Biol.*, 99:1901–1905.

38. Burmester, G.R., Winchester, R.J., Dimitriu-Bona, A., Klein, M., Steiner, G., and Sissons, H.A. (1983): Delineation of four cell types comprising the giant cell tumor of bone; expression of Ia and monocyte-macrophage lineage antigens. *J. Clin. Ivest.*, 71:1633–1648.

39. Cahill, J., and Hopper, K.E. (1982): Immunoregulation by macrophages: differential secretion of PGE and IL1 during infection with salmonella enteritidis. *Cell. Immunol.*, 67:229–240.

40. Cameron, P., Limjvco, G., Rodkey, J., Bennett, L., and Schmidt, J.A. (1985): Amino acid sequence analysis of human interleukin 1 (IL-1). Evidence for biochemically distinct forms of IL-1. *J. Exp. Med.*, 162:790–801.

41. Cameron, R., and Brighton, C. (1985): Effects of a capacitively coupled electrical signal on cAMP concentration and on PTH stimulation of cAMP concentration in bone cell monolayers (abstr.). *Transact. Orthop. Res. Soc.*, 31:109.

42. Canalis, E. (1980): Effect of insulinlike growth factor I on DNA and protein synthesis in cultured rat calvaria. *J. Clin. Invest.*, 66:709–719.

42. Canalis, E. (1981): Effect of platelet-derived growth factor on cultured fetal rat calvaria. *Metabolism*, 30:970–975.

44. Canalis, E. (1983): Effect of hormones and growth factors on alkaline phosphatase activity and collagen synthesis in cultured rat calvariae. *Metabolism*, 32:14–20.

45. Canalis E. (1983): Effect of glucocorticoids on type I collagen synthesis, alkaline phosphatase activity, and deoxyribonucleic acid content in cultured rat calvariae. *Endocrinology*, 112:931–939.

46. Canalis E. (1983): The hormonal and local regulation of bone formation. *Endocr. Rev.*, 4:62–77.

47. Canalis, E. (1984): Effect of cortisol on periosteal and nonperiostal collagen and DNA synthesis in cultured rat calvariae. *Calcif. Tissue Int.*, 36:158–166.

48. Canalis, E. (1986): Interleukin-1 has independent effects on deoxyribonucleic acid and collagen synthesis in cultures of rat calvariae. *Endocrinology*, 118:74–81.

49. Canalis, E.M., Dietrich, J.W., Maina, D.M., and Raisz, L.G. (1977): Hormonal control of bone collagen synthesis *in vitro*: effects of insulin and glucagon. *Endocrinology*, 100:668–674.

50. Canalis, E.M., Hintz, R.L., Dietrich, J.W., Maina, D.M., and Raisz, L.G. (1971): Effect of somatomedin and growth hormone on bone collagen synthesis in vitro. *Metabolism*, 26:1079–1087.

51. Canalis, E., Peck, W.A., and Raisz, L.G. (1980): Stimulation of DNA and collagen synthesis by autologous growth factor in cultured fetal rat calvaria. *Science*, 210:1021–1023.

52. Canalis, E. and Raisz, L.G. (1978): Effect of sex steroids on bone collagen synthesis *in vitro*. *Calcif. Tissue Res.*, 25:105–110.

53. Canalis, E. and Raisz, L.G. (1980): Effect of fibroblast growth factor on cultured fetal rat calvaria. *Metabolism*, 29:108–114.

54. Canalis, E. and Raisz, L.G. (1979): Effect of epidermal growth factor on bone formation in vitro. *Endocrinology*, 104:862–869.

55. Caputo, C.B., Meadows, D., and Raisz, L.G. (1976): Failure of estrogens and androgens to inhibit bone resorption in tissue culture. *Endocrinology*, 98:1065–1068.

56. Catherwood, B.D. (1985): 1,25-Dihydroxycholecalciferol and glucocorticosteroid regulation of adenylate cyclase in an osteoblast-like cell line. *J. Biol. Chem.*, 260:736–743.

57. Centrella, M. and Canalis, E. (1985): Transforming and nontransforming growth factors are present in medium conditioned by fetal rat calvariae. *Proc. Natl. Acad. Sci. USA*, 82:7335–7339.

58. Chambers, T.J. (1982): Osteoblasts release osteoclasts from calcitonin-induced quiescence. *J. Cell Sci.* 57:247–260.

59. Chambers, T.J., Athanasou, N.A., and Fuller, K. (1984): Effect of parathyroid hormone and calcitonin on the cytoplasmic spreading of isolated osteoclasts. *J. Endocr.*, 102:281–286.

60. Chambers, T.J., Bristow, K., and Athanasou, N.A. (in press): Prostaglandins act as direct inhibitors and indirect stimulators of osteoclast motility. *Br. J. Exp. Pathol.*

61. Chambers, T.J., and Dunn, C.J. (1982): The effect of parathyroid hormone, 1,25-dihydroxycholecalciferol and prostaglandins on the cytoplasmic activity of isolated osteoclasts. *J. Pathol.*, 137:193–203.

62. Chambers, T.J., and Fuller, K. (1985): Bone cells predispose bone surfaces to resorption by exposure of mineral to osteoclastic contact. *J. Cell Sci.*, 76:155–165.

63. Chambers, T.J., Fuller, K., and Athanasou, N.A. (1984): The effect of prostaglandins I_2, E_1, E_2 and dibutyryl cyclic AMP on the cytoplasmic spreading of rat osteoclasts. *Br. J. Exp. Pathol.*, 65:557–566.

64. Chambers, T.J., and Horton, M.A. (1984): Failure of cells of the mononuclear phagocyte series to resorb bone. *Calcif. Tissue Int.*, 36:556–558.

65. Chambers, T.J., McSheehy, P.M.J., Thomson, B.M., and Fuller, K. (1985): The effect of calcium-regulating hormones and prostaglandins on bone resorption by osteoclasts disaggregated from neonatal rabbit bones. *Endocrinology*, 116:234–239.

66. Chambers, T.J., and Magnus, C.J (1982): Calcitonin alters behavior of isolated osteoclasts. *J. Pathol.*, 136:27–39.

67. Chambers, T.J., and Moore, A. (1983): The sensitivity of isolated osteoclasts to morphological transformation by calcitonin. *J. Clin. Endocrinol. Metab.*, 57:819–824.

68. Chambers, T.J., Revell, P.A., Fuller, K., and Athanasou, N.A. (1984): Resorption of bone by isolated rabbit osteoclasts. *J. Cell Sci.*, 66:383–399.

69. Chase, L.R., and Aurbach, G.D. (1970): The effect of parathyroid hormone on the concentration of adenosine 3′5′-monophosphate in skeletal tissue in vitro. *J. Biol. Chem.*, 245:1520–1526.

70. Chen, P., Trummel, C., Horton, J., Baker, J.J., and Oppenheim, J.J. (1976): Production of osteoclast-activiating factor by normal human periph-

eral blood rosetting and nonrosetting lymphocytes. *Eur. J. Immunol.*, 6:732–736.

71. Chen, T.L., Aronow, L., and Feldman, D. (1977): Glucocorticoid receptors and inhibition of bone cell growth in primary culture. *Endocrinology*, 100:619–628.

72. Chen, T.L., Cone, C.M., and Feldman, D. (1983): Effects of $1\alpha,25$-dihydroxyvitamin D_3 and glucocorticoids on the growth of rat and mouse osteoblast-like bone cells. *Calcif. Tissue Int.*, 35:806–811.

73. Chen, T.L., Cone, C.M., and Feldman, D. (1983): Glucocorticoid modulation of cell proliferation in cultured osteoblast-like bone cells: Differences between rat and mouse. *Endocrinology*, 112:1739–1745.

74. Chen, T.L., Cone, C.M., Morey-Holton, E., and Feldman, D. (1982): Glucocorticoid regulation of $1,25(OH)_2$-Vitamin D_3 receptors in cultured mouse bone cells. *J. Biol. Chem.*, 257:13564–13569.

75. Chen, T.L., Cone, C.M., Morey-Holton, E., and Feldman, D. (1983): $1,25$-dihydroxyvitamin D_3 receptors in cultured rat osteoblast-like cells; glucocorticoid treatment increases receptor content. *J. Biol. Chem.*, 258:4350–4355.

76. Chen, T.L., and Feldman, D. (1978): Glucocorticoid potentiation of the adenosine $3',5'$-monophosphate response to parathyroid hormone in cultured rat bone cells. *Endocrinology*, 102:589–596.

77. Chen, T.L., and Feldman, D. (1978): Distinction between alpha-fetoprotein and intracellular estrogen receptors: evidence against the presence of estradiol receptors in rat bone. *Endocrinology*, 102:236–244.

78. Chen, T.L., and Feldman, D. (1979): Glucocorticoid receptors and actions in subpopulations of cultured rat bone cells; mechanism of dexamethasone potentiation of parathyroid hormone-stimulated cyclic AMP production. *J. Clin. Invest.*, 63:750–758.

79. Chen, T.L., and Feldman, D. (1984): Modulation of PTH-stimulated cyclic AMP in cultured rodent bone cells; the effects of $1,25(OH)_2$ vitamin D_3 and its interaction with glucocorticoids. *Calcif. Tissue Int.*, 36:580–585.

80. Chen, T.L., Hirst, M.A., and Feldman, D. (1979): A receptor-like binding macromolecule for 1α-dihydroxycholecalciferol in cultured mouse bone cells. *J. Biol. Chem.*, 254:7491–7494.

81. Chyun, Y.S., and Raisz, L.G. (1984): Stimulation of bone formation by prostaglandin E_2. *Prostaglandins*, 27:97–103.

82. Clark-Lewis, I., Kent, S.B.H., and Schrader, J.W. (1984): Purification to apparent homogeniety of a factor stimulating the growth of multiple lineages of hemopoietic cells. *J. Biol. Chem.*, 259:7488–7492.

83. Coccia, P.F. (1984): Cells that resorb bone. *N. Engl. J. Med.*, 310:456–458.

84. Coccia, P.F., Krivit, W., Cervenka, J., Clawson, C., Kersey, J.H., Kim, T.H., Nesbit, M.E., Ramsay, N.K.C., Warkentin, P.I., Teitelbaum, S.L., Kahn, A.J., and Brown, D.M. (1980): Successful bone marrow transplantation for infantile malignant osteopetrosis. *N. Engl. J. Med.*, 302:701–708.

85. Cohen, J.H.M., Daniel, L., Cordier, G., Saez, S., and Revillard, J.-P. (1983): Sex steroid receptors in peripheral T cells: Absence of androgen receptors and restriction of estrogen receptors to OKT8-positive cells. *J. Immunol.*, 131:2767–2771.

86. Cohen, M.S., and Gray, T.K. (1984): Phagocytic cells metabolize 25-hydroxyvitamin D_3 in vitro. *Proc. Natl. Acad. Sci. USA*, 81:931–934.

87. Cohen, S. (1983): The epidermal growth factor. *Cancer*, 51:1787–1791.

88. Corbett, M., Dekel, S., Puddle, B., Dickson, R.A., and Francis, M.J.O. (1979): The production of prostaglandins in response to experimentally induced osteomyelitis in rabbits. *Prostagland. Med.*, 2:403–412.

89. Cowen, K.S., Sakamoto, M., and Sakamoto, S. (1985): Monensin inhibits collagenase production in osteoblastic cell cultures and also inhibits both collagenase release and bone resorption in mouse calvaria cultures. *Biochem. Int.*, 11:273–280.

90. Crawford, A., Atkins, D., and Martin, T.J. (1978): Rat osteogenic sarcoma cells: comparison of the effects of prostaglandins E_1, E_2, I_2 (prostacyclin), 6-keto F_1 and thromboxane B_2 on cyclic AMP production and adenylate cyclase activity. *Biochem. Biophys. Res. Commun.*, 82:1195–1201.

91. Davis, W.L., Matthews, J.L., Martin, J.H., Kennedy, J.W., and Talmage, R.V. (1974): The endosteum as a functional membrane. In: *Calcium-Regulating Hormones*, International Congress Series 346, edited by R. Talmage, M. Owens, and J. Parsons, pp. 275–283. Excerpta Medica, Amsterdam.

92. Dekel, S., and Francis, M.J.O. (1981): The treatment of osteomyelitis of the tibia with sodium salicylate. *J. Bone Joint Surg.*, 63B:178–184.

93. Dekel, S., Lenthall, G., and Francis, M.J.O. (1981): Release of prostaglandins from bone and muscle after tibial fracture. An experimental study in rabbits. *J. Bone Joint Surg.*, 63:185–189.

94. DeLuca, H.F. (1982): Metabolism and mechanism of action of vitamin D- 1982. In: *Bone and Mineral Research, Annual 1*, edited by W.A. Peck, pp. 7–73. Excerpta Medica, Amsterdam.

95. Delaissé, J.-M., Eeckhout, Y., and Vaes, G. (1980): Inhibition of bone resorption in culture by inhibitors of thiol proteinases. *Science*, 192:1340–1343.

96. Delaissé, J.-M., Eeckhout, Y., and Vaes, G. (1984): In vivo and in vitro evidence for the involvement of cysteine proteinases in bone resorption. *Biochem. Biophys. Res. Commun.*, 125:441–447.

97. Denholm, L.J., Termine, J.D., Gehron Robey, P., Fisher, L.W., Drum, M.A., Shimokawa, H., Hawkins, G.R., Cruz, J.B., Thompson, K.G., and Boyce, R.A. (1985): Bone-specific protein defects in osteogenesis imperfecta. In: *Current Advances in Skeletogenesis*, edited by A. Ornoy, A. Harell, and J. Sela, pp. 291–296. Elsevier, Amsterdam.

98. Dewhirst, F.E. (1984): 6-Keto-prostaglandin E_1-stimulated bone resorption in organ culture. *Calcif. Tissue Int.*, 36:380–383.

99. Dewhirst, F.E., Stashenko, P.P., Mole, J.E., and Tsurumachi, T. (1985): Purification and partial sequence of human osteoclast-activating factor: identity with interleukin 1. *J. Immunol.*, 135:2562–

2568.

100. Dickson, I., and Walls, J. (1985): Vitamin A and bone formation. Effect of an excess of retinol on bone collagen synthesis in vitro. *Biochem. J.,* 226:789–795.

101. Dietrich, J.W., Canalis, E.M., Maina, D.M., and Raisz, L.G. (1976): Hormonal control of bone collagen synthesis in vitro: effects of parathyroid hormone and calcitonin. *Endocrinology,* 98:943–949.

102. Dietrich, J.W., Goodson, J.M., and Raisz, L.G. (1975): Stimulation of bone resorption by various prostaglandins in organ culture. *Prostaglandins,* 10:231–240.

103. Dinarello, L.A. (1984): Interleukin I. *Rev. Infect. Dis.,* 6:51–95.

104. Dokoh, S., Donaldson, C.A., and Haussier, M.R. (1984): Influence of 1,25-dihydroxyvitamin D_3 on cultured osteogenic sarcoma cells: correlation with the 1,25-dihydroxyvitamin D_3 receptor. *Cancer Res.,* 44:2103–2109.

105. Doty, S.B. (1981): Morphological evidence of gap junctions between bone cells. *Calcif. Tissue Int.,* 33:509–512.

106. Doty, S.B., and Schofield, B.H. (1976): Enzyme histochemistry of bone and cartilage cells. *Prog. Histochem. Cytochem.,* 8:1–38.

107. Dziak, R.M., Hurd, D., Miyasaki, K., Brown, M., Weinfeld, H., and Hausmann, E. (1982): Prostaglandin E_2 binding and cyclic AMP production in isolated bone cells. *Calcif. Tissue Int.,* 35:243–249.

108. Dziak, R., and Stern, P.H. (1975): Calcium transport in isolated bone cells. III. Effects of parathyroid hormone and cyclic 3′,5′-AMP. *Endocrinology,* 97:1281–1287.

109. Ecarot-Charrier, B., Glorieux, F.H., van der Rest, M., and Pereira, G. (1983): Osteoblasts isolated from mouse calvaria initiate matrix mineralization in culture. *J. Cell Biol.,* 96:639–643.

110. Eilon, G., and Raisz, L.G. (1978): Comparison of the effects of stimulators and inhibitors of resorption on the release of lysosomal enzymes and radioactive calcium from fetal bone in organ culture. *Endocrinology,* 103:1969–1975.

111. Esch, F., Baird, A., Ling, N., Ueno, N., Hill, F., Denoroy, L., Klepper, R., Gospodarowicz, D., Böhlen, P., and Guillemin, R. (1985): Primary structure of bovine pituitary basic fibroblast growth factor (FGF) and comparison with the amino-terminal sequence of bovine brain acidic FGF. *Proc. Natl. Acad. Sci (USA),* 82:6507–6511.

112. Fallon, M.D., Whyte, M.P., and Teitelbaum, S.L. (1981): Systemic mastocytosis associated with generalized osteopenia; histopathological characterization of the skeletal lesion using undecalcified bone from two patients. *Hum. Pathol.,* 12:813–820.

113. Farley, J.R., and Baylink, D.J. (1982): Purification of a skeletal growth factor from human bone. *Biochemistry,* 21:3502–3507.

114. Farley, J.R., and Baylink, D.J. (1981): A putative coupling factor from human bone: effects on bone cells in vitro [abstract]. *Calcif. Tissue Int.,* 33:292.

115. Farley, J.R., Wergedal, J.E., and Baylink, D.J. (1983): Fluoride directly stimulates proliferation and alkaline phosphatase activity of bone-forming cells. *Science,* 222:330–332.

116. Farr, D., Pochal, W., Brown, M., Shapiro, E., Weinfeld, N., and Dziak, R. (1984): Effects of prostaglandins on rat calvarial bone cell calcium. *Arch. Oral Biol.,* 29:885–891.

117. Feldman, D., Dziak, R., Koehler, R., and Stern, P. (1975): Cytoplasmic glucocorticoid binding proteins in bone cells. *Endocrinology,* 96:29–36.

118. Fell, H.B., and Mellanby, E. (1952): The effect of hypervitaminosis A on embryonic limb-bones cultivated *in vitro. J. Physiol.,* 116:320–349.

119. Fisher, L.W., Termine, J.D., Dejter, S.W., Whitson, S.W., Yanagishita, M., Kimura, J.H., Hascall, V.C., Kleinman, H.K., Hassell, J.R., and Nilsson, B. (1983): Proteoglycans of developing bone. *J. Biol. Chem.,* 258:6588–6594.

120. Fisher, L.W., Whitson, S.W., Avioli, L.V., and Termine, J.D. (1983): Matrix sialoprotein of developing bone. *J. Biol. Chem.,* 258:12723–12727.

121. Fleisch, H. (1982): Bisphosphonates: mechanisms of action and clinical applications. In: *Bone and Mineral Research, Annual 1,* edited by W.A. Peck, pp. 319–357. Elsevier, Amsterdam.

122. Fleisch, H., and Bisaz, S. (1962): Mechanism of calcification: inhibitory role of pyrophosphate. *Nature,* 195:911.

123. Fleisch, H., and Neuman, W.F. (1961): Mechanisms of calcification: role of collagen, polyphosphates, and phosphatase. *Am. J. Physiol.,* 200:1296–1300.

124. Fleisch, H., Russell, R.G.G., and Francis, M.D. (1969): Diphosphonates inhibit hydroxyapatite dissolution in vitro and bone resorption in tissue culture and in vivo. *Science,* 165:1262–1264.

125. Fleisch, H., Russell, R.G.G., Bisaz, S., Termine, J.D., and Posner, A.S. (1968): Influence of pyrophosphate on the transformation of amorphous to crystalline calcium phosphate. *Calcif. Tissue Res.,* 2:49–59.

126. Fleisch, H., Straumann, F., Schenk, R., Bisaz, S., and Allgöwer, M. (1966): Effect of condensed phosphates on calcification of chick embryo femurs in tissue culture. *Am. J. Physiol.,* 211:821–825.

127. Frame, B. and Nixon, R.K. (1968): Bone-marrow mast cells in osteoporosis of aging. *N. Engl. J. Med.,* 279:626–630.

128. Franceschi, R.T., James, W.M., and Zerlauth, G. (1985): 1α,25-dihydroxyvitamin D_3 specific regulation of growth, morphology, and fibronectin in a human osteosarcoma cell line. *J. Cell. Physiol.,* 123:401–409.

129. Francis, M.D. (1969): The inhibition of calcium hydroxyapatite crystal growth by polyphosphonates and polyphosphates. *Calcif. Tissue Res.,* 3:151–162.

130. Franzen, A., and Heinegard, D. (1984): Extraction and purification of proteoglycans from mature bovine bone. *Biochem. J.,* 224:47–58.

131. Franzen, A., and Heinegard, D. (1984): Characterization of proteoglycans from the calcified matrix of bovine bone. *Biochem. J.,* 224:59–66.

132. Fredholm, B.B., and Lerner, U. (1984): Adenine nucleotide levels and adenosine metabolism in cultured calvarial bone. *Acta Physiol. Scand.,* 120:551–555.

133. Friedman, J., and Raisz, L.G. (1965): Thyrocalcitonin: inhibitor of bone resorption in tissue culture. *Science*, 150:1465–1467.

134. Fritsch, J., Grosse, B., Lieberherr, M., and Balsan, S. (1985): 1,25-Dihydroxyvitamin D_3 is required for growth-independent expression of alkaline phosphatase in cultured rat osteoblasts. *Calcif. Tissue Int.*, 37:639–645.

135. Frost, H.M. (1964): *Bone Biodynamics*. Little, Brown, Boston.

136. Frost, H.M. (1966): *The Bone Dynamics in Osteoporosis and Osteomalacia*. Charles C. Thomas, Springfield, Illinois.

137. Gahring, L.C., Buckley, A., and Daynes, R.A. (1985): Presence of epidermal-derived thymocyte activating factor-interleukin 1 in normal human stratum corneum. *J. Clin. Invest.*, 76:1585–1591.

138. Gay, C.V., Ito, M.B., and Schraer, H. (1983): Carbonic anhydrase activity in isolated osteoclasts. *Metab. Bone Dis. Relat. Res.*, 5:33–39.

139. Gebhardt, M.C., Lippiello, L., Bringhurst, F.R., and Mankin, H.J. (1985): Prostaglandin E_2 synthesis by human primary and metastatic bone tumors in culture. *Clin. Orthop.*, 196:300–305.

140. Gennari, C. (1985): Glucocorticoids and bone. In: *Bone and Mineral Research/3*, pp. 213–231, edited by W.A. Peck. Elsevier, Amsterdam.

141. Glowacki, J. (1983): The effects of heparin and protamine on resorption of bone particles. *Life Sci.*, 33:1019–1024.

142. Gnessi, L., Camilloni, G., Fabbri, A., Politi, V., DeLuca, G., DiStazio, G., Moretti, C., and Fraioli, F. (1984): In vitro interaction between calcitonin and calmodulin. *Biochem. Biophys. Res. Commun.*, 118:648–654.

143. Goldhaber, P. (1965): Heparin enhancement of factors stimulating bone resorption in tissue culture. *Science*, 147:407–408.

144. Goldstein, D.J., Rogers, C.E., and Harris, H. (1980): Expression of alkaline phosphatase loci in mammalian tissues. *Proc. Natl. Acad. Sci. (USA)*, 77:2857–2860.

145. Goodson, J.M., Offenbacher, S., Dewhirst. F.E., and Bloomfield, R.B. (1980): Inhibition of fetal bone growth and augmentation of PGE_2 resorptive response by indomethacin. *Adv. Prostaglandin Thromboxane Res.*, 7:901–904.

146. Gowen, M., Wood, D.D., Ihrie, E.J., Meats, J.E., and Russell, R.G.G. (1984): Stimulation by human interleukin 1 of cartilage breakdown and production of collagenase and proteoglycanase by human chondrocytes but not by human osteoblasts *in vitro. Biochem. Biophys. Acta*, 797:186–193.

147. Gowen, M., Wood, D.D., Ihrie, E.J., McGuire, M.K.B., and Russell, R.G.G. (1983): An interleukin 1 like factor stimulates bone resorption *in vitro. Nature*, 306:378–389.

148. Gray, P.W., Aggarwal, B.B., Benton, C.V., Bringman, T.S., Henzel, W.J., Jarrett, J.A., Leung, D.W., Moffat, B., Ng, P., Svedersky, L.P., Palladino, M.A., and Nedwin, G.E. (1984): Cloning and expression of cDNA for human lymphotoxin, a lymphokine with tumour necrosis activity. *Nature*, 312:721–724.

149. Grossman, C.J. (1984): Regulation of the immune system by sex steroids. *Endocr. Rev.*, 5:435–455.

150. Gulino, A., Screpanti, I., Torrisi, M.R., and Frati, L. (1985): Estrogen receptors and estrogen sensitivity of fetal thymocytes are restricted to blast lymphoid cells. *Endocrinology*, 117:47–54.

151. Gunness-Hey, M., and Hock, J.M. (1984): Increased trabecular bone mass in rats treated with human synthetic parathyroid hormone. *Metab. Bone Dis. Relat. Res.*, 5:117–182.

152. Hahn, T.J., Westbrook, S.L., and Halstead, L.R. (1984): Cortisol modulation of osteoblast metabolic activity in cultured neonatal rat bone. *Endocrinology*, 114:1864–1870.

153. Hakeda, Y., Nakatani, Y., Kurihara, N., Ikeda, E., Maeda, N., and Kumegawa, M. (1985): Prostaglandin E_2 stimulates collagen and non-collagen protein synthesis and prolyl hydroxylase activity in osteoblastic clone MC3T3-E1 cells. *Biochem. Biophys. Res. Commun.*, 126:340–345.

154. Hakeda, Y., Nakatani, Y., Hiramatsu, M., Kurihara, N., Tsunoi, M., Ikeda, E., and Kumegawa, M. (1985): Inductive effects of prostaglandins on alkaline phosphatase in osteoblastic cells, Clone MC3T3-E1. *J. Biochem.* 97:97–104.

155. Hall, A.K., and Dickson, I.R. (1985): The effects of parathyroid hormone on osteoblast-like cells from embryonic chick calvaria. *Acta Endocrinol.*, 108:217–223.

156. Hall, G.E., and Kenny, A.D. (1983): Parathyroid hormone increases carbonic anhydrase activity in cultured mouse calvaria [abstract]. *Calcif. Tissue Int.*, 35:682.

157. Hall, G.E., and Kenny, A.D. (1984): Carbonic anhydrase and 1,25-dihydroxycholecalciferol-induced bone resorption [abstract]. *Calcif. Tissue Int.*, 36:461.

158. Hall, G.E., and Kenny, A.D. (1985): Role of carbonic anhydrase in bone resorption induced by 1,25 dihydroxyvitamin D_3 *in vitro. Calcif. Tissue Int.*, 37:134–142.

159. Hall, G.E., and Kenny, A.D. (1985): Role of carbonic anhydrase in bone resorption induced by prostaglandin E_2 in vitro. *Pharmacology*, 30:339–347.

160. Hamilton, J.A., Lingelbach, S., Partridge, N.C., and Martin, T.J. (1985): Regulation of plasminogen activator production by bone-resorbing hormones in normal and malignant osteoblasts. *Endocrinology*, 116:2186–2191.

161. Hanazawa, S., Ohmori, Y., Amano, S., Miyoshi, T., Kumegawa, M., and Kitano, S. (1985): Spontaneous production of interleukin-1-like cytokine from a mouse osteoblastic cell line (MC3T3-G1). *Biochem. Biophys. Res. Commun.*, 131:774–779.

162. Hanks, C.T., Geister, D.E., Kim, J.S., Knizner, A.E., Ash, M.M., and Avery, J.K. (1981): DNA synthesis in fetal rat calvarium cells stimulated by microprocessor generated signal (abstr.). *Transactions of the Bioelectrical Repair and Growth Society*, 1:3.

163. Hanley, K., Norton, L., and Rodan, G. (1982): The effects of pulsed electromagnetic fields upon periosteal and osteoblast-like cells grown in culture (abstr.). *Transactions of the Bioelectrical Repair and Growth Society*, 2:46.

164. Hansen, N.M., Jr., Felix, R., Bisaz, S., and Fleisch, H. (1976): Aggregation of hydroxyapatite crystals. *Biochim. Biophys. Acta,* 451:549–559.

165. Harakas, N.K. (1984): Demineralized bone-matrix-induced osteogenesis. *Clin. Orthop.,* 188:239–251.

166. Haussler, M.R., Manolagas, S.C., and Deftos, L.J. (1980): Glucocorticoid receptor in clonal osteosarcoma cell lines: a novel system for investigating bone active hormones. *Biochem. Biophys. Res. Commun.,* 94:373–380.

167. Heath, J.K., Atkinson, S.J., Meikle, M.C., and Reynolds, J.J. (1984): Mouse osteoblasts synthesize collagenase in response to bone resorbing agents. *Biochim. Biophys. Acta,* 802:151–154.

168. Heath, J.K., Meikle, M.C., Atkinson, S.J., and Reynolds, J.J. (1984): A factor synthesized by rabbit periosteal fibroblasts stimulates bone resorption and collagenase production by connective tissue cells. *Biochim. Biophys. Acta,* 800:301–305.

169. Heath, J.K., Saklatvala, J., Meikle, M.C., Atkinson, S.J., and Reynolds, J.J. (1985): Pig interleukin 1 (catabolin) is a potent stimulator of bone resorption in vitro. *Calcif. Tissue Int.,* 37:95–97.

170. Heersche, J.N.M., Heyboer, M.P.M., and Ng, B. (1978): Hormone-specific suppression of adenosine 3′,5′-monophosphate responses in bone *in vitro* during prolonged incubation with parathyroid hormone, prostaglandin E, and calcitonin. *Endocrinology,* 103:333–340.

171. Heldin, C.-H., Wasteson, A., and Westermark, B. (1985): Platelet-derived growth factor. *Mol. Cell. Endocrinol.,* 39:169–187.

172. Henry, H.L., and Norman, A.W. (1984): Vitamin D: Metabolism and biological actions. *Ann. Rev. Nutr.,* 4:493–520.

173. Herrman-Erlee, M.P.M., and Gaillard, P.J. (1978): The effects of 1,25-dihydroxycholecalciferol on embryonic bone in vitro: a biochemical and histological study. *Calcif. Tissue Res.,* 25:111–118.

174. Hermann-Erlee, M.P.M., van der Meer, J.M., and Hekkelman, J.W. (1980): In vitro studies of the adenosine 3′,5′-monophosphate (cAMP) response of embryonic rat calvaria to bovine parathyroid hormone-(1-84) [bPTH-(1-84)], bPTH-(1-34), and bPTH-(3-34) and the loss of cAMP responsiveness after prolonged incubation. *Endocrinology,* 106:2013–2018.

175. High, W.B., Capen, C.C., and Black, H.E. (1981): The effects of 1,25-dihydroxycholecalciferol, parathyroid hormone, and thyroxine on trabecular bone remodeling in adult dogs: A histomorphometric study. *Am. J. Pathol.,* 105:279–287.

176. Holdstock, G., Chastenay, B.F., and Krawitt, E.L. (1982): Effects of testosterone, oestradiol and progesterone on immune regulation. *Clin. Exp. Immunol.,* 47:449–456.

177. Holtrop, M.E. (1975): The ultrastructure of bone. *Ann. Clin. Lab. Sci.,* 5:264–271.

178. Holtrop, M.E., King, G.J., Cox, K.A., and Reit, B. (1979): Time-related changes in the ultrastructure of osteoclasts after injection of parathyroid hormone in young rats. *Calcif. Tissue Int.,* 27:129–135.

179. Holtrop, M.E., and Raisz, L.G. (1979): Comparison of the effects of 1,25-dihydroxycholecalciferol, prostaglandin E_2, and osteoclast-activating factor with parathyroid hormone on the ultrastructure of osteoclasts in cultured long bones of fetal rats. *Calcif. Tissue Int.,* 29:201–205.

180. Horowitz, M., Vignery, A., Gershon, R.K., and Baron, R. (1984): Thymus-derived lymphocytes and their interactions with macrophages are required for the production of osteoclast-activating factor in the mouse. *Proc. Natl. Acad. Sci. (USA),* 821:2181–2185.

181. Horton, J.E., Raisz, L.G., Simmons, H.A., Oppenheim, J.J., and Mergenhagen, S.E. (1972): Bone resorbing activity in supernatant fluid from cultured human peripheral blood leukocytes. *Science,* 177:793–795.

182. Horton, M.A., Rimmer, E.F., and Lewis, D. (1984): Cell surface characterization of the human osteoclast: phenotypic relationship to other bone marrow-derived cell types. *J. Pathol.,* 144:281–294.

183. Horton, M.A., Rimmer, E.F., Moore, A., and Chambers, T.J. (1985): On the origin of the osteoclast: the cell surface phenotype of rodent osteoclasts. *Calcif. Tissue Int.,* 37:46–50.

184. Howard, G.A., Bottemiller, B.L., Turner, R.T., Rader, J.I., and Baylink, D.J. (1981): Parathyroid hormone stimulates bone formation and resorption in organ culture: evidence for a coupling mechanism. *Proc. Natl. Acad. Sci. (USA),* 78:3204–3208.

185. Huggins, C., Wiseman, S., and Reddi, A.H. (1970): Transformation of fibroblasts by allogeneic and xenogeneic transplants of demineralized tooth and bone. *J. Exp. Med.,* 132:1250–1258.

186. Ibbotson, K.J., Roodman, G.D., McManus, L.M., and Mundy, G.R. (1984): Identification and characterization of osteoclast-like cells and their progenitors in cultures of feline marrow mononuclear cells. *J. Cell Biol.,* 99:471–480.

187. Ibbotson, K.J., Twardzik, D.R., D'Souza, S.M., Hargreaves, W.R., Todaro, G.J., and Mundy, G.R. (1985): Stimulation of bone resorption in vitro by synthetic transforming growth factor-alpha. *Science,* 228:1007–1009.

188. James, R. (1984): Polypeptide growth factors. *Annu. Rev. Biochem.,* 53:259–292.

189. James, R., and Bradshaw, R.A. (1984): Polypeptide growth factors. *Annu. Rev. Biochem.,* 53:259–292.

190. Jaworski, Z.F.G. (1984): Coupling of bone formation to bone resorption: a broader view. *Calcif. Tissue Int.,* 36:531–535.

191. Jeansonne, B.G., Feagin, F.F., McMinn, R.W., Shoemaker, R.L., and Rehm, W.S. (1979): Cell-to-cell communication of osteoblasts. *J. Dent. Res.,* 58:1415–1423.

192. Jee, W.S.S., Ueno, K., Deng, Y.P., and Woodbury, D.M. (1985): The effects of prostaglandin E_2 in growing rats: increased metaphyseal hard tissue and cortico-endosteal bone formation. *Calcif. Tissue Int.,* 37:148–157.

193. Jez, D.H., and Heersche, J.N.M. (1983): The recovery of hormone responsiveness in desensitized neonatal rat calvariae. *Endocrinology,* 112:1036–

1041.

194. Jilka, R.L., and Hamilton, J.W. (1984): Inhibition of parathormone-stimulated bone resorption by type I interferon. *Biochem. Biophys. Res. Commun.,* 120:553–558.

195. Johnson, D., and Rodan, G. (1982): The effect of pulsating electromagnetic fields on prostaglandin synthesis in osteoblast-like cells [abstract]. *Transactions of the Bioelectrical Repair and Growth Society,* 2:7.

196. Johnston, C.C., Jr. (1985): Studies on prevention of age-related bone loss. *Bone and Mineral Research/3,* edited by W.A. Peck, pp. 233–257. Elsevier, Amsterdam.

197. Jones, S.J., Boyde, A., and Pawley, J.B. (1975): Osteoblasts and collagen orientation. *Cell Tissue Res.,* 159:73–80.

198. Jones, S.J., Hogg, N.M., Shapiro, I.M., Slusarenko, M., and Boyde, A. (1981): Cells with Fc receptors in the cell layer next to osteoblasts and osteoclasts on bone. *Metab. Bone Dis. Relat. Res.,* 2:357–362.

199. Jung, A., Bisaz, S., and Fleisch, H. (1973): The binding of pyrophosphate and two diphosphonates on hydroxyapatite crystals. *Calcif. Tissue Res.,* 11:269–280.

200. Kahn, A.J., Fallon, M.D., and Teitelbaum, S.L. (1984): Structure-function relationships in bone: an examination of events at the cellular level. In: *Bone and Mineral Research, Annual 2,* edited by W.A. Peck, pp. 125–174. Elsevier, Amsterdam.

201. Kahn, A.J., Stewart, C.C., and Teitelbaum, S.L. (1978): Contact-mediated bone resorption by human monocytes, *in vitro. Science,* 199:988–990.

202. Kallio, D.M., Garant, P.R., and Minkin, C. (1971): Evidence of coated membranes in the ruffled border of the osteoclast. *J. Ultrastruct. Res.,* 37:169–177.

203. Kaplan, G.C., Eilon, G., Poser, J.W., and Jacobs, J.W. (1985): Constitutive biosynthesis of bone Gla protein in a human osteosarcoma cell line. *Endocrinology,* 117:1235–1238.

204. Kato, Y., Nomura, Y., Tsuji, M., Kinoshita, M., Ohmae, H., and Suzuki, F. (1981): Somatomedin-like peptide(s) isolated from fetal bovine cartilage (cartilage-derived factor): isolation and some properties. *Proc. Natl. Acad. Sci. (USA),* 78:6831–6835.

205. Kato, Y., Watanabe, R., Hiraki, Y., Suzuki, F., Canalis, E., Raisz, L.G., Nishikawa, K., and Adachi, K. (1982): Selected stimulation of sulfated glycosaminoglycan synthesis by multiplication-stimulating activity, cartilage-derived factors and bone-derived growth factor. *Biochim. Biophys. Acta,* 716:232–239.

206. Kato, Y., Watanabe, R., Nomura, Y., Tsuji, M., Suzuki, F., Raisz, L.G., and Canalis, E. (1982): Effect of bone-derived growth factor on DNA, RNA and proteoglycan synthesis in cultures of rabbit costal chondrocytes. *Metabolism,* 31:812–815.

207. Katz, J.M., Skinner, S.J.M., Wilson, T., and Gray, D.H. (1983): The in vitro effect of indomethacin on basal bone resorption, on prostaglandin production and on the response to added prostaglandins. *Prostaglandins,* 26:545–555.

208. Kenny, A.D. (1985): Role of carbonic anhydrase in bone: Partial inhibition of disuse atrophy of bone by parenteral acetazolamide. *Calcif. Tissue Int.,* 37:126–133.

209. King, G.J., and Holtrop, M.E. (1975): Actin-like filaments in bone cells of cultured mouse calvaria as demonstrated by binding to heavy meromyosin. *J. Cell Biol.,* 66:445–51.

210. Kiyoki, M., Kurihara, N., Ishizuka, S., Ishii, S., Hakeda, Y., Kumegawa, M., and Norman, A.W. (1985): The unique action for bone metabolism of $1\alpha,25\text{-}(OH)_2D_3\text{-}26,23\text{-lactone}$. *Biochem. Biophys. Res. Commun.,* 127:693–698.

211. Klein, D.C., and Raisz, L.G. (1970): Prostaglandin stimulation of bone resorption in tissue culture. *Endocrinology,* 86:1436–1440.

212. Koeffler, H.P., Reichel, H., Bishop, J.E., and Norman, A.W. (1985): γ-Interferon stimulates production of 1,25-dihydroxyvitamin D_3 by normal human macrophages. *Biochem. Biophys. Res. Commun.,* 127:596–603.

213. Korenstein, P., Somjen, D., Danon, A., Fischler, H., and Binderman, I. (1981): Pulsed capacitive electric induction of cyclic-AMP changes, calcium^{45} uptake and DNA synthesis in bone cells [abstract]. *Transactions of the Bioelectrical Repair and Growth Society,* 1:34.

214. Korenstein, R., Somjen, D., Fischler, H., and Binderman, I. (1984): Capacitative pulsed electric stimulation of bone cells. Induction of cyclic-AMP changes and DNA synthesis. *Biochim. Biophys. Acta,* 803:302–307.

215. Korenstein, R., Somjen, D., Fischler, H., and Binderman, I. (1982): Primary induced cellular changes and cell specificity in pulsed capacitive stimulation of bone cells *in vitro. Transactions of the Bioelectrical Repair and Growth Society,* 2:5.

216. Kream, B.E., Jose, M., Yamada, S., and DeLuca, H.F. (1977): A specific high-affinity binding macromolecule for 1,25-dihydroxy vitamin D_3 in fetal bone. Science, 197:1086–1088.

217. Kream, B.E., Rowe, D.W., Gworek, S.C., and Raisz, L.G. (1979): Insulin and parathyroid hormone after collagen synthesis and procollagenase messenger RNA levels in fetal rat bone in vitro [abstract]. *Calcif. Tissue Int.,* 28:148.

218. Kream, B.E., Rowe, D.W., Gworek, S.C., and Raisz, L.G. (1980): Parathyroid hormone alters collagen synthesis and procollagen mRNA levels in fetal rat calvaria. *Proc. Natl. Acad. Sci. (USA),* 77:5654–5658.

219. Kream, B.E., Smith, M.D., Canalis, E., and Raisz, L.G. (1985): Characterization of the effect of insulin on collagen synthesis in fetal rat bone. *Endrocrinology,* 116:296–302.

220. Krieger, N.S., Feldman, R.S., and Tashjian, A.H., Jr. (1982): Parathyroid hormone and calcitonin interactions in bone: irradiation-induced inhibition of escape in vitro. *Calcif. Tissue Int.,* 34:197–203.

221. Krieger, N.S., and Tashjian, A.H., Jr. (1980): Parathyroid hormone stimulates bone resorption via a Na-Ca exchange mechanism. *Nature,* 287:843–845.

222. Krieger, N.S., and Tashjian, A.H., Jr. (1982): In-

hibition of parathyroid hormone-stimulated bone resorption by monovalent cation ionophores. *Calcif. Tissue Int.*, 34:239–244.

223. Krieger, N.S., and Tashjian, A.H., Jr. (1983): Inhibition of stimulated bone resorption by vanadate. *Endocrinology*, 113:324–328.

224. Kumegawa, M., Ikeda, E., Tanaka, S., Haneji, T., Yora, T., Sakagishi, Y., Minami, N., and Hiramatsu, M. (1984): The effects of prostaglandin E$_2$, parathyroid hormone, 1,25 dihydroxycholecalciferol, and cyclic nucleotide analogs on alkaline phosphatase activity in osteoblastic cells. *Calcif. Tissue Int.*, 36:72–76.

225. Kurt-Jones, E.A., Beller, D.I., Mizel, S.B., and Unanue, E.R. (1985): Identification of a membrane-associated interleukin 1 in macrophages. *Proc. Natl. Acad. Sci. (USA)*, 82:1204–1208.

226. Labat, M.L., Tzehoval, E., Moricard, Y., Feldman, M., and Milhaud, G. (1983): Lack of a T-cell dependent subpopulation of macrophages in (dichloromethylene) diphosphonate-treated mice. *Biomed. Pharmacother.*, 37:270–276.

227. Laub, F. and Korenstein, R. (1984): Actin polymerization induced by pulsed electric stimulation of bone cells *in vitro*. *Biochim. Biophys. Acta*, 803:308–313.

228. Lerner, U. (1982): Indomethacin inhibits bone resorption *in vitro* without affecting bone collagen synthesis. *Agents Actions*, 12:466–470.

229. Lerner, U. and Fredholm, B.B. (1982): 2-Chloroadenosine increases calcium mobilization from mouse calvaria in vitro. *Acta Endocrinol.*, 100:313–320.

230. Lerner, U. and Fredholm, B.B. (1985): Prostaglandin E$_2$ and 2-Chloroadenosine act in concert to stimulate bone resorption in culture murine calvarial bones. *Biochem. Pharmacol.*, 34:937–940.

231. Lian, J.B., Coutts, M., and Canalis, E. (1985): Studies of hormonal regulation of osteocalcin synthesis in cultured fetal rat calvariae. *J. Biol. Chem.*, 260:8706–8710.

232. Lieberherr, M., Garabedian, M., Guillozo, H., Thil, C.L., and Balsan, S. (1980): In vitro effects of vitamin D$_3$ metabolites in rat calvaria cAMP content. *Calcif. Tissue Int.*, 30:209–216.

233. Livesey, S.A., Kemp, B.E., Re, C.A., Partridge, N.C., and Martin, T.J. (1983): Selective hormonal activation of cyclic AMP-dependent protein kinase isoenzymes in normal and malignant osteoblasts. *J. Biol. Chem.*, 257:14983–14987.

234. Lomedico, P.T., Gubler, U., Hellmann, C.P., Dukovich, M., Giri, J.G., Pan, Y.-C.E., Collier, K., Semionow, R., Chua, A.O., and Mizel, S.B. (1984): Cloning and expression of murine interleukin-1 cDNA in *Escherichia coli*. *Nature*. 312:458–462.

235. Loning, T., Albers, H.-K., Lisboa, B.P., Burkhardt, A., and Caselitz, J. (1980): Prostaglandin E and the local immune response in chronic periodontal disease. Immunohistochemical and radioimmunological observations. *J. Periodont. Res.*, 15:525–535.

236. Löwik, C.W.G.M., van Leeuwen, J.P.T.M., van der Meer, J.M., van Zeeland, J.K., Schevan, B.A.A., and Hermann-Erlee, M.P.M. (1985): A

237. Löwik, C.W.G.M., van Zeeland, J.K., and Herrmann-Erlee, M.P.M. (1986): An *in situ* assay system to measure ornithine decarboxylase activity in primary cultures of chicken osteoblasts. Effect of bone-seeking hormones. *Calcif. Tissue Int.*, 38:21–26.

two-receptor model for the action of parathyroid hormone on osteoblasts: a role for intracellular free calcium and cAMP. *Cell Calcium*, 6:311–326.

238. Luben, R.A. (1978): Purification of a lymphokine: osteoclast activating factor from human tonsil lymphocytes. *Biochem. Biophys. Res. Commun.*, 84:15–22.

239. Luben, R.A., Wong, G.L., and Cohn, D.V. (1976): Biochemical characterization with parathyroid and calcitonin of isolated bone cells: provisional identification of osteoclasts and osteoblasts. *Endocrinology*, 99:526–534.

240. Lucht, U. (1973): Effects of calcitonin on osteoclasts in vivo: an ultrastructural and histochemical study. *Z. Zellforsch.*, 145:75–87.

241. Lucht, U. (1976): Osteoclasts and their relationship to bone as studied by electron microscopy. *Z. Zellforsch M. Krosk. Anat.*, 135:211.

242. Mahgoub, A., and Sheppard, H. (1975): Early effect of 25-hydroxy-cholecalciferol (25-OH-D$_3$) and 1,25-dihydroxycholecalciferol (1,25-(OH)$_2$-D$_3$) on the ability of parathyroid hormone (PTH) to elevate cyclic AMP of intact bone cells. *Biochem. Biophys. Res. Commun.*, 62:901–907.

243. Majeska, R.J., Nair, B.C., and Rodan, G.A. (1985): Glucocorticoid regulation of alkaline phosphatase in the osteoblastic osteosarcoma cell line ROS 17/2.8. *Endocrinology*, 116:170–179.

244. Majeska, R.J., and Rodan, G.A. (1982): The effect of 1,25-(OH)$_2$-D$_3$ on alkaline phosphatase activity in osteoblastic by osteosarcoma cell lines. *J. Biol. Chem.*, 257:3362–3365.

245. Malkani, K., Luxembourger, M.M., and Rebel, A. (1973): Cytoplasmic modifications at the contact zone of osteoclasts and calcified tissue in the diaphyseal growing plate of foetal guinea pig tibia. *Calcif. Tissue Res.*, 11:258–264.

246. Malone, J.D., Teitelbaum, S.L., Griffin, G.L., Senior, R.M., and Kahn, A.J. (1982): Recruitment of osteoclast precursors by purified bone matrix constituents. *J. Cell Biol.*, 92:227–230.

247. Mamus, S.W., Beck-Schroeder, S., and Zanjani, E.D. (1985): Suppression of normal human erythropoiesis by gamma interferon in vitro; role of monocytes and T lymphocytes. *J. Clin. Invest.*, 75:1496–1503.

248. Manolagas, S.C., Abare, J., and Deftos, L.J. (1984): Glucocorticoids increase the 1,25(OH)$_2$D$_3$ receptor concentration in rat osteogenic sarcoma cells. *Calcif. Tissue Int.*, 36:153–157.

249. Manolagas, S.C., Haussler, M.R., and Deftos, L.J. (1981): 1,25-Dihydroxyvitamin D$_3$ receptor-like macromolecule in rat osteogenic sarcoma cell lines. *J. Biol. Chem.*, 255:4414–4417.

250. Manolagas, S.C., Spiess, Y.H., Burton, D.W., and Deftos, L.J. (1983): Mechanism of action of 1,25-dihydroxyvitamin D$_3$-induced stimulation of alkaline phosphatase in cultured osteoblast-like cells. *Mol. Cell. Endocrinol.*, 33:27–36.

251. March, C.J., Mosley, B., Larsen, A., Cerretti, D.P., Braedt, G., Price, V., Gillis, S., Henney, C.S., Kronheim, S.R., Grabstein, K., Conlon, P.J., Hopp, T.P., and Cosman, D. (1985): Cloning, sequence and expression of two distinct human interleukin-1 complementary DNAs. *Nature,* 315:641–649.

252. Marcus, R., and Orner, F.B. (1980): Parathyroid hormone as a calcium ionophore: test of specificity. *Calcif. Tissue Int.,* 32:207–211.

253. Marks, C.R., Seifert, M.F., and Marks, S.C., III (1984): Osteoclast populations in congenital osteopetrosis: additional evidence of heterogeneity. *Metab. Bone Dis. Relat. Res.,* 5:259–264.

254. Marks, S.C., Jr. (1983): The origin of osteoclasts: evidence, clinical implications and investigative challenges of an extra-skeletal source. *J. Pathol.,* 12:226–256.

255. Marks, S.C., Jr. (1984): Congenital osteopetrotic mutations as probes of the origin, structure and function of osteoclasts. *Clin. Orthop.,* 189:239–263.

256. Marx, S.J., Aurbach, G.D., Gavin, J.R., and Buell, D.W. (1974): Calcitonin receptors on cultured human lymphocytes. *J. Biol. Chem.,* 249:6812–6816.

257. Matsumoto, T., Kawanobe, Y., Morita, K., and Ogata, E. (1985): Effect of 1,25-dihydroxyvitamin D_3 on phospholipid metabolism in a clonal osteoblast-like rat osteogenic sarcoma cell line. *J. Biol. Chem.,* 260:13704–13709.

258. Matsushima, K., Kuang, Y.O., Tosato, G., Hopkins, S.J., and Oppenheim, J.J. (1985): B-cell derived interleukin 1 (IL-1)-like factor. I. Relationship of production of IL-1-like factor to accessory cell function of Epstein-Barr virus-transformed human B-lymphoblast lines. *Cell. Immunol.,* 94:406–417.

259. Matthews, J.L., and Talmage, R.V. (1981): Influences of parathyroid hormone on bone cell ultrastructure. *Clin. Orthop.,* 156:27–38.

260. Matthews, J.L., Talmage, R.V., and Doppelt, S.H. (1980): Rapid response of the osteocyte-lining cell complex to calcitonin. *Metab. Bone Dis. Relat. Res.,* 2:113–122.

261. McArthur, W., Yaari, A.M., and Shapiro, I.M. (1980): Bone solubilization by mononuclear cells. *Lab. Invest.,* 42:450–456.

262. McCarthy, D.M., San Miguel, J.F., Freake, H.C., Green, P.M., Zola, H., Catovsky, D., and Goldman, J.M. (1983): 1,25-Dihydroxyvitamin D_3 inhibits proliferation of human promyelocytic leukemia (HL60) cells and induces monocyte-macrophage differentiation in HL60 and normal human bone marrow cells. *Leuk. Res.,* 7:51–55.

263. McKenna, M.J., and Frame, B. (1985): The mast cell and bone. *Clin. Orthop.,* 200:226–233.

264. McManus, J.P., and Whitfield, J.F. (1970): Inhibition by thyrocalcitonin of the mitogenic actions of parathyroid hormone and cyclic adenosine 3',5'-monophosphate on rat thymocytes. *Endocrinology,* 86:934–939.

265. Menton, D.N., Simmons, D.J., Chang, S.L., and Orr, B.Y. (1984): From bone lining cell to osteocyte—an SEM study. *Anat. Rec.,* 209:29–39.

266. Merke, J., Senst, S., and Ritz, E. (1984): Demonstration and characterization of 1,25-dihydroxyvitamin D_3 receptors in human mononuclear blood cells. *Biochem. Biophys. Res. Commun.,* 120:199–205.

267. Metcalf, D. (1985): The granulocyte-macrophage colony-stimulating factors. *Science,* 229:16–22.

268. Mezzetti, G., Bagnara, G., Monti, M.G., Bonsi, L., Brunelli, M.A., and Barbiroli, B. (1984): 1α,25-Dihydroxycholecalciferol and human histiocytic lymphoma cell line (U-937): the presence of receptor and inhibition of proliferation. *Life Sci.,* 34:2185–2191.

269. Milhaud, G., and Labat, M.L. (1978): Thymus and osteopetrosis. *Clin. Orthop.,* 135:260–271.

270. Milhaud, G., Labat, M.L., Parant, M., Damais, C., and Chedid, L. (1977): Immunological defect and its correction in the osteopetrotic mutant rat. *Proc. Natl. Acad. Sci. (USA),* 74:339–342.

271. Milhaud, G., Labat, M.L., and Moricard, Y. (1983): (Dichloromethylene diphosphonate) induced impairment of T-lymphocyte function. *Proc. Natl. Acad. Sci. (USA),* 80:4469–4473.

272. Miller, S.C. (1978): Rapid activation of the medullary bone osteoclast cell surface by parathyroid hormone. *J. Cell Biol.,* 76:615–618.

273. Miller, S.C. (1985): The rapid appearance of acid phosphatase activity at the developing ruffled border of parathyroid hormone activated medullary bone osteoclasts. *Calcif. Tissue Int.,* 37:526–529.

274. Miller, S.S., Wolf, A.M., and Arnaud, C.D. (1976): Bone cells in culture: morphologic transformation by hormones. *Science,* 192:1340–1342.

275. Minkin, C. (1982): Bone acid phosphatase: tartrate-resistant acid phosphatase as a marker of osteoclast function. *Calcif. Tissue Int.,* 34:285–290.

276. Minkin C., and Jennings, J.M. (1972): Carbonic anhydrase and bone remodeling: sulfonamide inhibition of bone resorption in organ culture. *Science,* 176:1031–1033.

277. Minkin, C., Posek, R., and Newbrey, J. (1981): Mononuclear phagocytes and bone resorption: identification and preliminary characterization of a bone-derived macrophage chemotactic factor. *Metab. Bone Dis. Relat. Res.,* 2:363–369.

278. Miyaura, C., Abe, E., and Suda, T. (1984): Extracellular calcium is involved in the mechanism of differentiation of mouse myeloid leukemia cells (M1) induced by 1α,25-dihydroxyvitamin D_3. *Endocrinology,* 115:1891–1896.

279. Mizel, S.B., Dayer, J.-M., Krane, S.M., and Mergenhagen, S.E. (1981): Stimulation of rheumatoid synovial cell collagenase and prostaglandin production by partially purified lymphocyte-activating factor (interleukin 1). *Proc. Natl. Acad. Sci. (USA),* 78:2474–2477.

280. Mohan, S., Jennings, J., Linkhart, T., Taylor, A., and Baylink, D. (1985): Purification and characterization of a small molecular weight human skeletal growth factor (hSGF) (abstr.). In: *Program and Abstracts, Seventh Annual Scientific Meeting of the American Society for Bone and Mineral Research,* Abstract 9.

281. Morgan, D.D., and Grossman, C.J. (1984): Analysis and properties of the cytosolic estrogen receptor

from rat thymus. *Endocr. Res.*, 10:193–207.

282. Mundy, G.R., Altman, A.J., Gondek, M.D., and Bandelin, J.G. (1977): Direct resorption of bone human monocytes. *Science,* 196:1109–1111.

283. Mundy, G.R., DeMartino, S., and Rowe, D.W. (1981): Collagen and collagen-derived fragments are chemotactic for tumor cells. *J. Clin. Invest.*, 68:1102–1105.

284. Mundy, G.R., Ibbotson, K.J., and D'Souza, S.M. (1985): Tumor products and the hypercalcemia of malignancy. *J. Clin. Invest.*, 76:391–394.

285. Mundy, G.R., Luben, R.A., Raisz, L.G., Oppenheim, J.J., and Buell, D.N. (1974): Bone-resorbing activity in supernatants from lymphoid cell lines. *N. Engl. J. Med.*, 290:867–871.

286. Mundy, G.R., and Poser, J.W. (1983): Chemotactic activity of γ-carboxyglutamic acid containing protein in bone. *Calcif. Tissue Int.*, 35:164–168.

287. Mundy, G.R., Raisz, L.G., Shapiro, J.L., Bandelin, J.G., and Turcotte, R.J. (1977): Big and little forms of osteoclast activating factor. *J. Clin. Invest.*, 60:122–128.

288. Mundy, G.R., Shapiro, J.L., Bandelin, J.G., Canalis, E.M., and Raisz, L.G. (1976): Direct stimulation of bone resorption by thyroid hormones. *J. Clin. Invest.*, 58:529–534.

289. Nagayama, M., Sakamoto, S., and Sakamoto, M. (1984): Mouse bone collagenase inhibitor: Purification and partial characterization of the inhibitor from mouse calvaria cultures. *Arch. Biochem. Biophys.*, 228:653–658.

290. Nakamura, T., Toyofuku, F., and Kanda, S. (1985): Whole-body irradiation inhibits the escape phenomenon of osteoclasts in bones of calcitonin-treated rats. *Calcif. Tissue Int.*, 37:42–45.

291. Nakatani, Y., Tsunoi, M., Hakeda, Y., Kurihara, N., Fujita, K., and Kumegawa, M. (1984): Effects of parathyroid hormone on cAMP production and alkaline phosphatase activity in osteoblastic clone MC3T3-E1 cells. *Biochem. Biophys. Res. Commun.*, 123:894–899.

292. Narbaitz, R., Stumpf, W.E., Sar, M., Huang, S., and DeLuca, H.F. (1983): Autoradiographic localization of target cells for 1α,25-dihydroxyvitamin D₃ in bones from fetal rats. *Calcif. Tissue Int.*, 35:177–182.

293. Nathan, C.F., Murray, H.W., and Cohn, Z.A. (1980): The macrophage as an effector cell. *N. Engl. J. Med.*, 303:622–626.

294. Nefussi, J.-R., and Baron, R. (1985): PGE₂ stimulates both resorption and formation of bone *in vitro:* Differential responses of the periosteum and the endosteum in fetal rat long bone cultures. *Anat. Rec.*, 211:9–16.

295. Neuman, W.F. (1972): The bone:blood equilibrium: a possible system for its study in vitro. In: *Calcium, Parathyroid Hormone and the Calcitonins,* International Congress Series 243, edited by R. Talmage and P. Munson, pp. 389–398. Excerpta Medica, Amsterdam.

296. Ng, B., Hekkelman, J.W., and Heersche, J.N.M. (1979): The effect of cortisol on the adenosine 3′,5′-monophosphate response to parathyroid hormone of bone *in vitro. Endocrinology,* 104:1130–1135.

297. Ng, K.W., Partridge, N.C., Niall, M., and Martin, T.J. (1983): Stimulation of DNA synthesis by epidermal growth factor in osteoblast-like cells. *Calcif. Tissue Int.*, 35:624–628.

298. Nishimoto, S.K., and Price, P.A. (1979): Proof that the γ-carboxyglutamic acid-containing bone protein is synthesized in calf bone; comparative synthesis rate and effect of coumarin on synthesis. *J. Biol. Chem.*, 254:437–441.

299. Nishimoto, S.K., and Price, P.A. (1980): Secretion of the vitamin K-dependent protein of bone by rat osteosarcoma cells. Evidence for an intracellular precursor. *J. Biol. Chem.*, 255:6579–6583.

300. Nolan, R.D., Partridge, N.C., Godfrey, H.M., and Martin, T.J. (1983): Cyclo-oxygenase products of arachidonic acid metabolism in rat osteoblasts in culture. *Calcif. Tissue Int.*, 35:294–297.

301. Norimatsu, M., Vanderwiel, C.J., and Talmage, R.V. (1979): Morphological support of a role for cells lining bone surfaces in maintenance of plasma calcium concentration. *Clin. Orthop.*, 138:254–262.

302. Norton, L.A., Shleyer, A., and Rodan, G. (1980): Electromagnetic field effects on DNA synthesis in bone cells (abstr.). *J. Electrochem. Soc.*, 127:129c.

303. Okabe, T., Ishizuka, S., Fujisawa, M., Watanabe, J., and Takaku, F. (1985): Human myeloid leukemia cells metabolize 25-hydroxyvitamin D₃ in vitro. *Biochem. Biophys. Res. Commun.*, 127:635–641.

304. Olsen, B.R. (1981): Collagen biosynthesis. In: *Cell Biology of Extracellular Matrix,* edited by E.D. Hay, pp. 139–177. Plenum Press, New York.

305. Ornoy, A., Goodwin, D., Hoft, D., Edelstein, S. (1978): 24,25-dihydroxyvitamin D is a metabolite of vitamin D essential for bone formation. *Nature,* 276:517–519.

306. Osdoby, P., Martini, M.C., and Caplan, A.I. (1982): Isolated osteoclasts and their presumed progenitor cells, the monocyte, in culture. *J. Exp. Zool.*, 224:331–344.

307. Otsuka, K., Sodek, J., and Limeback, H.F. (1984): Collagenase synthesis by osteoblast-like cells. *Calcif. Tissue Int.*, 36:722–724.

308. Otsuka, K., Sodek, J., and Limeback, H.F. (1984): Synthesis of collagenase and collagenase inhibitors by osteoblast-like cells in culture. *Eur. J. Biochem.*, 145:123–129.

309. Otsuka, K., Yao, K.-L., Wasi, S., Tuna, P.S., Aubin, J.E., Sodek, J., and Termine, J.D. (1984): Biosynthesis of osteonectin by fetal porcine calvarial cells in vitro. *J. Biol. Chem.*, 259:9805–9812.

310. Oursler, M.J., Bell, L.V., Clevinger, B., and Osdoby, P. (1985): Identification of osteoclast-specific monoclonal antibodies. *J. Cell Biol.*, 100:1592–1600.

311. Owen, M. (1978): Histogenesis of bone cells. *Calcif. Tissue Res.*, 25:205–207.

312. Owen, M. (1985): Lineage of osteogenic cells and their relationship to the stromal system. In: *Bone and Mineral Research/3,* edited by W.A. Peck, pp. 1–25. Elsevier, Amsterdam.

313. Parfitt, A.M. (1984): The cellular basis of bone remodeling: the quantum concept reexamined in light of recent advances in the cell biology of bone. *Calcif. Tissue Int.*, 36:S37–S45.

314. Partridge, N.C., Kemp, B.E., Veroni, M.C., and

Martin, T.J. (1981): Activation of adenosine 3',5'-monophosphate-dependent protein kinase in normal and malignant bone cells by parathyroid hormone, prostaglandin E_2 and prostacyclin. *Endocrinology,* 108:220–225.

315. Peck, W.A., Brandt, J., and Miller, I. (1967): Hydrocortisone-induced inhibition of protein synthesis and uridine incorporation in isolated bone cells. *Proc. Natl. Acad. Sci. (USA),* 57:1599–1606.

316. Peck, W.A., Burks, J.A., Wilkins, J., Rodan, S.B., and Rodan, G.A. (1977): Evidence for preferential effects of parathyroid hormone, calcitonin and adenosine on bone and periosteum. *Endocrinology,* 100:1357–1364.

317. Peck, W.A., Carpenter, J., and Messinger, K. (1974): Cyclic 3',5'-adenosine monophosphate in isolated bone cells. II. Responses to adenosine and parathyroid hormone. *Endocrinology,* 94:148–154.

318. Peck, W.A., Carpenter, J.G., and Schuster, R.J. (1976): Adenosine-mediated stimulation of bone cell adenylate cyclase activity. *Endocrinology,* 99:901–909.

319. Peck, W.A., and Dowling, I (1976): Failure of 1,25-dihydroxycholecalciferol [1,25-$(OH)_2D_3$] to modify cyclic AMP levels in parathyroid hormone-treated and untreated bone cells. *Endocrine Res. Commun.,* 3:157–166.

320. Peck. W.A., and Kohler, G. (1980) Hormonal and non-hormonal desensitization in isolated bone cells. *Calcif. Tissue Int.,* 32:95–103.

321. Peck, W.A., Kohler, G., and Barr, S. (1981): Calcium-mediated enhancement of the cyclic AMP response in cultured bone cells. *Calcif. Tissue Int.,* 33:409–416.

322. Peck, W.A., Messinger, K., Brandt, J., and Carpenter, J. (1969): Impaired accumulation of ribonucleic acid precursors and depletion of ribonucleic acid in glucocorticoid-treated bone cells. *J. Biol. Chem.,* 244:4174–4184.

323. Pennica, D., Nedwin, G.E., Hayflick, J.S., Seeburg, P.H., Derynck, R., Palladino, M.A., Kohr, W.J., Aggarwal, B.B., and Goeddel, D.V. (1984): Human tumour necrosis factor: precursor structure, expression and homology to lymphotoxin. *Nature,* 312:724–729.

324. Perris, A.D., Whitfield, J.F., and Rixon, R.H. (1967): Stimulation of mitosis in bone marrow and thymus of normal and irradiated rats by divalent cations and parathyroid extract. *Radiat. Res.,* 32:550–563.

325. Perry, H.M., Chappel, J.C., Bellorin-Font, E., Martin, K.J., and Teitelbaum, S.L. (1982): Parathyroid hormone receptors on human circulating mononuclear leukocytes (abstr.). *Calcif. Tissue Int.,* 34:S13.

326. Peterlik, M., Hoffmann, O., Swetly, P., Klaushofer, K., and Koller, K. (1985): Recombinant γ-interferon inhibits prostaglandin-mediated and parathyroid hormone-induced bone resorption in cultured neonatal mouse calvaria. *FEBS Lett.,* 185:287–290.

327. Petkovich, P.M., Heersche, J.N.M., Tinker, D.O., and Jones, G. (1984): Retinoic acid stimultes 1,25-dihydroxyvitamin D_3 binding in rat osteosarcoma cells. *J. Biol. Chem.,* 259:8274–8280.

328. Pierce, W.M., Jr., Lineberry, M.D., and Waite, L.C. (1982): Effect of sulfonamides on the hypercalcemic response to vitamin D. *Horm. Metab. Res.,* 14:670–673.

329. Pike, J.W. (1985): Intracellular receptors mediate the biologic action of 1,25-dihydroxyvitamin D_3. *Nutr. Rev.,* 43:161–168.

330. Pliam, N.B., Nyiredy, K.A., and Arnaud, C.D. (1982): Parathyroid hormone receptors in avian bone cells. *Proc. Natl. Acad. Sci. (USA),* 79:2061–2063.

331. Potts, M., Doppelt, S., Taylor, S., Folkman, J., Neer, R., and Potts, J.T., Jr. (1984): Protamine: a powerful *in vivo* inhibitor of bone resorption. *Calcif. Tissue Int.,* 36:189–193.

332. Powles, T.J., Dowsett, M., Easty, D.M., Easty, G.C., and Neville, A.M. (1976): Breast-cancer osteolysis, bone metastases and anti-osteolytic effect of aspirin. *Lancet,* 1:608–610.

333. Price, P. (1982): Osteocalcin. In: *Bone and Mineral Research,* Volume 1, edited by W.A. Peck, pp. 157–190. Excerpta Medica, Amsterdam.

334. Price, P.A., and Baukol, S.A. (1980): 1,25-dihydroxyvitamin D_3 increases the synthesis of the vitamin K-dependent bone protein by osteosarcoma cells. *J. Biol. Chem.,* 255:11660–11663.

335. Price, P.A., Urist, M.R., and Otawara, Y. (1983): Matrix Gla protein, a new γ-carboxyglutamic acid-containing protein which is associated with the organic matrix of bone. *Biochem. Biophys. Res. Commun.,* 117:765–771.

336. Price, P.A., Williamson, M.K., Haba, T., Dell, R.B., and Jee, W.S.S. (1982): Excessive mineralization with growth plate closure in rats on chronic warfarin treatment. *Proc. Natl. Acad. Sci. (USA),* 79:7734–7739.

337. Price, P.A., Williamson, M.K., and Sloper, S.A. (1984): 1,25-dihydroxyvitamin D_3 increases citrate secretion from osteosarcoma cells. *J. Biol. Chem.,* 259:2537–2540.

338. Provvedini, D.M., Tsoukas, C.D., Deftos, L.J., and Manolagas, S.C. (1983): 1,25-Dihydroxyvitamin D_3 receptors in human leukocytes. *Science,* 221:1181–1183.

339. Puzas, J.E., and Brand, J.S. (1976): Collagenolytic activity from isolated bone cells. *Biochim. Biophys. Acta,* 429:914–974.

340. Puzas, J.H., and Brand, J.S. (1985): Bone cell phosphotyrosine phosphatase: characterization and regulation by calcitropic hormones. *Endocrinology,* 116:2463–2468.

341. Raisz, L.G. (1963): Stimulation of bone resorption by parathyroid hormone in tissue culture. *Nature,* 197:1015–1016.

342. Raisz, L.G. (1965): Inhibition by actinomycin D of bone resorption induced by parathyroid hormone or vitamin A. *Proc. Soc. Exp. Biol. Med.,* 119:614–617.

343. Raisz, L.G. (1976): Mechanisms of bone resorption. In: *Handbook of Physiology,* Section 7, Vol. VII, edited by G.D. Aurbach, pp. 117–136. American Physiological Society, Washington, D.C.

344. Raisz, L.G., Dietrich, J.W., Simmons, H.A., Seyberth, H.W., Hubbard, W., and Oates, J.A. (1977): Effect of prostaglandin endoperoxides and metabolites on bone resorption in vitro. *Nature,* 267:532–534.

345. Raisz, L.G., and Koolemans-Beynen, A.R. (1974): Inhibition of bone collagen synthesis by prostaglandin E_2 in organ culture. *Prostaglandins*, 8:377–385.

346. Raisz, L.G., and Martin, T.J. (1984): Prostaglandins in bone and mineral metabolism. In: *Bone and Mineral Research, Annual 2*, edited by W.A. Peck, pp. 286–310. Elsevier, Amsterdam.

347. Raisz, L.G., and Niemann, I. (1969): Effect of phosphate, calcium and magnesium on bone resorption and hormonal responses in tissue culture. *Endocrinology*, 85:446–452.

348. Raisz, L.G., Simmons, H.A., Sandberg, A.L., and Canalis, E. (1980): Direct stimulation of bone resorption by epidermal growth factor. *Endocrinology*, 107:270–273.

349. Raisz, L.G., Trummel, C.L., Holick, H.F., and DeLuca, H.F. (1972): 1,25-Dihydroxycholecalciferol: a potent stimulator of bone resorption in tissue culture. *Science*, 175:768–769.

350. Raisz, L.G., Trummel, C.L., Wener, J.A., and Simmons, H. (1972): Effects of glucocorticoids on bone resorption in tissue culture. *Endocrinology*, 90:961–967.

351. Ramp, W.K., and Baker, R.L. (1985): 1,25-Dihydroxyvitamin D_3 decreases alkaline phosphatase activity in cultures of embryonic chick tibiae (42029). *Proc. Soc. Exp. Biol. Med.*, 178:437–442.

352. Rao, L.G., and Murray, T.M. (1985): Binding of intact parathyroid hormone to rat osteosarcoma cells: major contribution of binding sites for the carboxyl-terminal region of the hormone. *Endocrinology*, 117:1632–1638.

353. Rao, L.G., Murray, T.M., and Heersche, J.N.M. (1983): Immunohistochemical demonstration of parathyroid hormone binding to specific cell types in fixed rat bone tissue. *Endocrinology*, 113:805–810.

354. Rao, L.G., Ng, B., Brunette, D.M., and Heersche, J.N.M. (1977): Parathyroid hormone and prostaglandin E_2-response in a selected population of bone cells after repeated subculture and storage at −80° C. *Endocrinology*, 100:1233–1241.

355. Reddi, A.H. (1985): Regulation of bone differentiation by local and systemic factors. In: *Bone and Mineral Research/3*, edited by W.A. Peck, pp. 27–48. Elsevier, Amsterdam.

356. Reinhardt, T.A., Horst, R.L., Littledike, E.T., and Beltz, D.C. (1982): 1,25-Dihydroxyvitamin D_3 receptor in bovine thymus gland. *Biochem. Biophys. Res. Commun.*, 106:1012–1018.

357. Reitsma, P.H., Rothberg, P.G., Astrin, S.M., Trial, J., Bar-Shavit, Z., Hall, A., Teitelbaum, S.L., and Kahn, A.J. (1983): Regulation of *myc* gene expression in HL-60 leukaemia cells by a vitamin D metabolite. *Nature*, 306:492–494.

358. Ribgy, W.F.C., Shen, L., Ball, E.D., and Fanger,, M.W. (1985): 1,25-Dihydroxyvitamin D_3 induces a myelomonocytic phenotype with enhanced effector cell function in the HL-60 promyelocytic leukemia cell line. *Mol. Immunol.*, 22:567–572.

359. Rifas, L., Shen, V., Mitchell, K., and Peck, W.A. (1984): Macrophage-derived growth factor for os-teoblast-like cells and chondrocytes. *Proc. Natl. Acadm Sci. (USA)*, 81:4558–4562.

360. Riggs, B.L. (1984): Treatment of osteoporosis with sodium fluoride: an appraisal. In: *Bone and Mineral Research, Annual 2*, edited by W.A. Peck, pp. 366–393. Elsevier, Amsterdam.

361. Rizzoli, R.E., Somerman, M., Murray, T.M., and Aurbach, G.D. (1983): Binding of radioiodinated parathyroid hormone to cloned bone cells. *Endocrinology*, 113:1832–1838.

362. Roberts, A.B., Frolik, C.A., Anzano, M.A., Assoian, R.K., and Sporn, M.B. (1984): Purification of type β transforming growth factors from nonneoplastic tissues. In: *Methods for Preparation of Media Supplements, and Substrata for serum-free Animal Cell Culture*, pp. 181–194. Alan R. Liss, New York.

363. Roberts, A.B., Frolik, C.A., Anzano, M.A., and Sporn, M.B. (1983): Transforming growth factor from neoplastic and nonneoplastic tissues. *Fed. Proc.*, 42:2621–2625.

364. Robertson, W.G., Peacock, M., Atkins, D., and Webster, L.A. (1972): The effect of parathyroid hormone on the uptake and release of calcium by bone in tissue culture. *Clin. Sci.*, 43:715–718.

365. Robey, P.G., and Termine, J.D. Human bone cells *in vitro*. *Calcif. Tissue Int.*, 37:453–460.

366. Robinson, B.W.S., McLemore, T.L., and Crystal, R.G. (1985): Gamma interferon is spontaneously released by alveolar macrophages and lung T lymphocytes in patients with pulmonary sarcoidosis. *J. Clin. Invest.*, 75:1488–1495.

367. Robinson, D.R., Tashjian, A.H., Jr., and Levine, L. (1975): Prostaglandin stimulated bone resorption by rheumatoid synovia. Possible mechanisms for bone destruction in rheumatoid arthritis. *J. Clin. Invest.*, 56:1181–1188.

368. Rodan, S.B., Fischer, M.K., Egan, J.J., Epstein, P.M., and Rodan, G.A. (1984): The effect of dexamethasone on parathyroid hormone stimulation of adenylate cyclase in ROS 17/2.8 cells. *Endocrinology*, 115:951–958.

369. Rodan, G.A., and Martin, T.J. (1981): Role of osteoclasts in hormonal control of bone resorption—a hypothesis. *Calcif. Tissue Int.*, 33:349–351.

370. Rodan, G.A., and Rodan, S.B. (1984): Expression of the osteoblastic phenotype. In: *Bone and Mineral Research, Annual 2*, edited by W.A. Peck, pp. 244–285. Elsevier, Amsterdam.

371. Rodan, S.B., Rodan, G.A., Simmons, H.A., Walenga, R.W., Feinstein, M.B., and Raisz, L.G. (1981): Bone resorptive factor produced by osteosarcoma cells with osteoblastic features is PGE_2. *Biochem. Biophys. Res. Commun.*, 102:1358–1365.

372. Romberg, R.W., Werness, P.G., Lollar, P., Riggs, B.L., and Mann, K.G. (1985): Isolation and characterization of native adult osteonectin. *J. Biol. Chem.*, 260:2728–2736.

373. Roos, B.A., Fischer, J.A., Pignat, W., Alander, C.B., and Raisz, L.G. (1986): Evaluation of the *in vivo* and *in vitro* column-regulating actions of noncalcitonin peptides produced via calcitonin gene expression. *Endocrinology*, 118:46–51.

374. Rowe, D.W., and Kream, B.E. (1982): Regulation of collagen synthesis in fetal rat calvaria by 1,25 dihydroxyvitamin D₃. *J. Biol. Chem.*, 257:8009–8015.

375. Ryder, M.I., Jenkins, S.D., and Horton, J.E. (1981): The adherence to bone by cytoplasmic elements of osteoclast. *J. Dent. Res.*, 60:1349–1355.

376. Sagher, F., and Even-Paz, Z. (1967): *Mastocytosis and the Mast Cell*. Year Book Medical Publishers, Chicago.

377. Sakamoto, S., Goldhaber, P., and Glimcher, M.J. (1972): The further purification and characterization of mouse bone collagenase. *Calcif. Tissue Res.*, 10:142–151.

378. Sakamoto, S., and Sakamoto, M. (1981): *Chemistry and Biology of Heparin*, pp. 133–142, edited by R.L. Lundblad, W.V. Brown, K.G. Mann, and H.R. Roberts. Elsevier, Amsterdam.

379. Sakamoto, S., and Sakamoto, M. (1984): Osteoblast collagenase: collagenase synthesis by clonally derived mouse osteogenic (MC3T3-E1) cells. *Biochem. Int.*, 9:51–58.

380. Sakamoto, S., and Sakamoto, M. (1985): Biochemical and immunohistochemical studies on collagenase in resorbing bone in tissue culture. *J. Periodont. Res.*, 17:523–526.

381. Sakamoto, S., Sakamoto, M., Goldhaber, P., and Glimcher, M.J. (1975): Studies on the interaction between heparin and mouse bone collagenase. *Biochim. Biophys. Acta* 385:41–50.

382. Sakamoto, S., Sakamoto, M., Goldhaber, P., and Glimcher, M.J. (1978): Mouse bone collagenase: purification of the enzyme by heparin-Sepharose 4B affinity chromatography and preparation of specific antibody to the enzyme. *Arch. Biochem. Biophys.*, 188:438–449.

383. Sakamoto, S., Sakamoto, M., Goldhaber, P., and Glimcher, M.J. (1979): Collagenase activity and morphological and chemical bone resorption induced by prostaglandin E₂ in tissue culture. *Proc. Soc. Exp. Biol. Med.*, 161:99–103.

384. Sampath, T.K., and Reddi, A.H. (1981): Dissociative extraction and reconstitution of extracellular matrix components involved in local bone differentiation. *Proc. Natl. Acad. Sci. (USA)*, 78:7599–7603.

385. Scheven, B.A.A., Burger, E.H., Kawilarang-de Haas, E.W.M., Wassenaar, A.M., and Nijweide, P.J. (1985): Effects of ionizing irradiation on formation and resorbing activity of osteoclasts in vitro. *Lab. Invest.*, 53:72–79.

386. Schmid, C., Steiner, T., and Froesch, E.R. (1983): Insulin-like growth factors stimulate synthesis of nucleic acids and glycogen in cultured calvaria cells. *Calcif. Tissue Int.*, 35:578–585.

387. Selye, H. (1932): On the stimulation of new bone formation with parathyroid extract and irradiated ergosterol. *Endocrinology*, 16:547–558.

388. Seyberth, H.W., Segre, G.V., Morgan, J.L., Sweetman, B.J., Potts, J.T., Jr., and Oates, J.A. (1975): Prostaglandins as mediators of hypercalcemia associated with certain types of cancer. *N. Engl. J. Med.*, 293:1278–1283.

389. Seyedin, S.M., Thomas, T.C., Thompson, A.Y., Rosen, D.M., and Piez, K.A. (1985): Purification and characterization of two cartilage-inducing factors from bovine demineralized bone. *Proc. Natl. Acad. Sci. (USA)*, 82:2267–2271.

390. Shen, V., Kohler, G., and Peck, W.A. (1983): A high affinity, calmodulin-responsive (Ca²⁺ + Mg²⁺)-ATPase in isolated bone cells. *Biochim. Biophys. Acta*, 727:230–238.

391. Shen, V., Rifas, L., Kohler, G., and Peck, W.A. (1985): Fetal rat chondrocytes sequentially elaborate separate growth- and differentiation-promoting peptides during their development in vitro. *Endocrinology*, 116:920–925.

392. Shinoda, H., Adamek, G., Felix, R., Fleisch, H., Schenk, R., and Hagan, P. (1983): Structure-activity relationships of various bisphosphonates. *Calcif. Tissue Int.*, 35:87–89.

393. Shlossman, M., Brown, M., Shapiro, E., and Dziak, R. (1982): Calcitonin effects on isolated bone cells. *Calcif. Tissue Int.*, 34:190–196.

394. Shupnik, M.A., Ip, N.Y., and Tashjian, A.H., Jr. (1980): Characterization and regulation of receptors for epidermal growth factor in mouse calvaria. *Endocrinology*, 107:1738–1746.

395. Shupnik, M.A., and Tashjian, A.H., Jr. (1981): Functional receptors for epidermal growth factor on human osteosarcoma cells. *J. Cell. Physiol.*, 109:403–410.

396. Shupnik, M.A., and Tashjian, A.H., Jr. (1982): Epidermal growth factor and phorbol ester actions on human osteosarcoma cells; characterization of responsive and nonresponsive cell lines. *J. Biol. Chem.*, 257:12161–12164.

397. Shuttleworth, A., and Veis, A. (1972): The isolation of anionic phosphoproteins from bovine cortical bone via the periodate solubilization of bone collagen. *Biochim. Biophys. Acta*, 257:414–420.

398. Simpson, E. (1984): Growth factors which affect bone. *Trends Biomed. Sci.*, 9:527–530.

399. Simpson, E., Harrod, J., Eilon, G., Jacobs, J.W., and Mundy, G.R. (1985): Identification of a messenger ribonucleic acid fraction in human prostatic cancer cells coding for a novel osteoblast-stimulating factor. *Endocrinology*, 117:1615–1620.

400. Skjodt, H., Gallagher, J.A., Beresford, J.N., Couch, M., Poser, J.W., and Russell, R.G.G. (1985): Vitamin D metabolites regulate osteocalcin synthesis and proliferation of human bone cells in vitro. *J. Endocrinol.*, 105:391–396.

401. Slaughter, C.A., Coseo, M.C., and Harris, H. (1981): Detection of enzyme polymorphism by using monoclonal antibodies. *Proc. Natl. Acad. Sci. (USA)*, 78:1124–1128.

402. Sly, W.B., Hewett-Emmett, D., Whyte, M.P., Yu, S.L., and Tashjian, R.E. (1983): Carbonic anhydrase II deficiency identified as the primary defect in the autosomal recessive syndrome of osteopetrosis with renal tubular acidosis and cerebral calcification. *Proc. Natl. Acad. Sci. (USA)*, 80:2752–2756.

403. Somjen, D., Binderman, I., Berger, E., and Harell, A. (1980): Bone remodeling induced by physical stress is prostaglandin E₂ mediated. *Biochim. Biophys. Acta*, 627:91–100.

404. Sone, S., Bucana, C., Hoyer, L., and Fidler, I. (1981): Kinetics and ultrastructural studies of the induction of rat alveolar macrophage fusion by mediators released from mitogen-stimulated lymphocytes. *Am. J. Pathol.,* 103:234–246.

405. Spector, A.R., and Glimcher, M.J. (1972): The extraction and characterization of soluble anionic phosphoproteins from bone. *Biochim. Biophys. Acta.,* 263:593–603.

406. Stanley, E.R., Guilbert, L.J., Tushinski, R.J., and Bartelmez, S.H. (1983): CSF-1—a mononuclear phagocyte lineage-specific hemopoietic growth factor. *J. Cell. Biochem.,* 21:151–159.

407. Stenson, W.F., and Parker, C.W. (1980): Prostaglandins, macrophages and immunity. *J. Immunol.,* 125:1–5.

408. Stern, P.H. (1969): Inhibition by steroids of parathyroid hormone induced Ca^{45} release from embryonic rat bone *in vitro. J. Pharmacol. Exp. Ther.,* 168:211–217.

409. Stern, P.H., Krieger, N.S., Nissenson, R.A., Williams, R.D., Winkler, M.E., Derynck, R., and Strewler, G.J. (1985): Human transforming growth factor-alpha stimulates bone resorption in vitro. *J. Clin Invest.,* 76:2016–2019.

410. Stock, J.L., and Coderre, J.A. (1982): Calcitonin and parathyroid hormone inhibit accumulation of cyclic AMP in stimulated human mononuclear cells. *Biochem. Biophys. Res. Commun.,* 109:935–942.

411. Stock, J.L., and Coderre, J.A. (1984): Calcitonin enhances production of prostaglandins by stimulated human monocytes. *Prostaglandins,* 27:771–779.

412. Stracke, H., Shulz, A., Moeller, D., Rossol, S., and Schatz, H. (1984): Effect of growth hormone on osteoblasts and demonstration of somatomedin-C/IGF-1 in bone organ culture. *Acta Endocrinol.,* 107:16–24.

413. Straus, D.S. (1984): Growth-stimulatory actions of insulin in vitro and in vivo. *Endocr Rev.,* 5:356–369.

414. Studzinski, G.P., Bhandal, A.K., and Brelvi, Z.S. (1985): A system for monocytic differentiation of leukemic cells HL 60 by a short exposure to 1,25-dihydroxycholecalciferol (42098). *Proc. Soc. Exp. Biol. Med.,* 179:288–295.

415. Studzinski, G.P., Bhandal, A.K., and Brelvi, Z.S. (1985): Cell cyclic sensitivity of HL-60 cells to the differentiation-inducing effects of 1-α,25-Dihydroxy vitamin D₃. *Cancer Res.,* 45:3898–3905.

416. Suda, T., Miyaura, C., Abe, E., and Kuroki, T. (1987): Modulation of cell differentiation, immune responses and tumor promotion by vitamin D compounds. In: *Bone and Mineral Research/4,* edited by W.A. Peck, pp. 1–48. Elsevier, Amsterdam.

417. Suda, T., Testa, N.G., Allen, T.D., Onions, D., and Jarrett, O. (1983): Effect of hydrocortisone on osteoclasts generated in cat bone marrow cultures. *Calcif. Tissue Int.,* 35:82–86.

418. Sugarman, B.J., Aggarwal, B.B., Hass, P.E., Figari, I.S., Palladino, M.A., Jr., and Shepard, H.M. (1985): Recombinant human tumor necrosis factor-α; Effects on proliferation of normal and transformed cells in vitro. *Science,* 230:943–945.

419. Syftestad, G.T., Triffit, J.T., Urist, M.R., and Caplan, A.I. (1984): An osteo-inductive bone matrix extract stimulates the *in vitro* conversion of mesenchyme into chondrocytes. *Calcif. Tissue Int.,* 36:625–627.

420. Takaoka, K., Yoshikawa, H., Shimizu, N., Ono, K., Amitani, K., and Nakata, Y. (1982): Partial purification of bone-inducing substances from a murine osteosarcoma. *Clin. Orthop.,* 164:265–270.

421. Takei, M., Takeda, K., and Konno, K. (1984): The role of interferon-γ in induction of differentiation of human myeloid leukemia cell lines, ML-1, and HL-60. *Biochem. Biophys. Res. Commun.,* 124:100–105.

422. Talmage, R.V., Cooper, C.W., and Toverud, S.U. (1982): The physiological significance of calcitonin. *Bone and Mineral Research, Annual 1,* edited by W.A. Peck, pp. 74–143. Excerpta Medica, Amsterdam.

423. Tanaka, H., Abe, E., Miyaura, C., Kuribayashi, T., Konno, K., Nishii, Y., and Suda, T. (1982): 1α,25-Dihydroxycholecalciferol and human myeloid leukemia cell line (HL-60): The presence of receptors and induction of differentiation. *Biochem. J.,* 204:713–719.

424. Tanaka, H., Abe, E., Miyaura, C., Shiina, Y., and Suda, T. (1983): 1α,25-Dihydroxyvitamin D₃ induces differentiation of human promyelocytic leukemia cells (HL-60) into monocyte-macrophages, but not into granulocytes. *Biochem. Biophys. Res. Commun.,* 117:86–92.

425. Tashjian, A.H., Jr., Hohmann, E.L., Antoniades, H.N., and Levine, L. (1982): Platelet-derived growth factor stimulates bone resorption via a prostaglandin-mediated mechanism. *Endocrinology,* 111:118–124.

426. Tashjian, A.H., Jr., and Levine, L. (1978): Epidermal growth factor stimulates prostaglandin production and bone resorption in cultured mouse calvaria. *Biochem. Biophys. Res. Commun.,* 107:1738–1746.

427. Tashjian, A.H., Jr., Tice, J.E., and Sides, K. (1977): Biological activities of prostaglandin analogues and metabolites on bone in organ culture. *Nature,* 266:645–646.

428. Tashjian, A.H., Jr., Voelkel, E.F., Lazzaro, M., Singer, F.R., Roberts, A.B., Derynck, R., Winkler, M.E., and Levine, L. (1985): α and β human transforming growth factors stimulate prostaglandin production and bone resorption in cultured mouse calvaria. *Proc. Natl. Acad. Sci. (USA),* 82:4535–4538.

429. Tashjian, A.H., Jr., Voelkel, E.F., Levine, L., and Goldhaber, P. (1972): Evidence that the bone resorption stimulating factor produced by mouse fibrosarcoma cells is prostaglandin E₂. A new model for the hypercalcemia of cancer. *J. Exp. Med.,* 135:1329–1343.

430. Tashjian, A.H., Jr., Wright, D.R., Ivey, J.L., and Port, A. (1978): Calcitonin binding sites in bone: relationship to biological response and "escape." *Rec. Prog. Horm. Res.,* 34:285–331.

431. Teitelbaum, S.L., and Kahn, A.J. (1980): Mononuclear phagocytes, osteoclasts and bone resorption. *Mineral Electrolyte Metab.,* 3:2–9.

432. Teitelbaum, S.L., Malone, J.D., and Kahn, A.J. (1981): Glucocorticoid enhancement of bone resorption by rat peritoneal macrophages *in vitro*. *Endocrinology*, 108:795–799.

433. Teitelbaum, S.L., Stewart, C.C., and Kahn, A.J. (1979): Rodent peritoneal macrophages as bone resorbing cells. *Calcif. Tissue Int.*, 27:255–261.

434. Tenenbaum, H.C., and Heersche, J.N.M. (1982): Differentiation of osteoblasts and formation of mineralized bone in vitro. *Calcif. Tissue Int.*, 34:76–79.

435. Tenenbaum, H.C., and Heersche, J.N.M. (1985): Dexamethasone stimulates osteogenesis in chick periosteum in vitro. *Endocrinology*, 117:2211–2217.

436. Termine, J.D. (1987): Bone proteins and mineralization. In: *Rheumatology, Volume 10: Connective Tissue in Normal and Pathological States*, edited by K. Kuhn and T. Krieg. Karger Press, Basel.

437. Termine, J.D., Belcourt, A.B., Conn, K.M., and Kleinmann, H.K. (1981): Mineral and collagen binding proteins of fetal calf bone. *J. Biol. Chem.*, 256:10403–10408.

438. Termine, J.D., Gehron Robey, P., Fisher, L.W., Shimokawa, H., Drum, M.A., Conn, K.M., Hawkins, G.R., Cruz, J.B., and Thompson, K.G. (1984): Osteonectin, bone proteoglycan and phosphophoryn defects in a form of bovine osteogenesis imperfecta. *Proc. Natl. Acad. Sci. (USA)*, 81:2213–2217.

439. Termine, J.D., Kleinmann, H.K., Whitson, S.W., Conn, K.M., McGarvey, M.L., and Martin, G.R. (1981): Osteonectin, a bone specific protein linking mineral to collagen. *Cell*, 26:99–105.

440. Testa, N.G., Allen, T.D., Lajtha, L.G., Onim, D., and Jarrett, O. (1981): Generation of osteoclasts *in vitro*. *J. Cell. Sci.*, 47:127–137.

441. Thesingh, C.W., and Scherft, J.P. (1985): Fusion disability of embryonic osteoclast precursor cells and macrophages in the microphthalmic osteopetrotic mouse. *Bone*, 6:43–52.

442. Thomas, K.A., Rios-Candelore, M., Gimenez-Gallego, G., DiSalvo, J., Bennett, C., Rodkey, J., and Fitzpatrick, S. (1985): Pure brain-derived acidic fibroblast growth factor is a potent angiogenic vascular endothelial cell mitogen with sequence homology to interleukin 1. *Proc. Natl. Acad. Sci. (USA)*, 82:6409–6413.

443. Todaro, G.J., Fryling, C., and DeLarco, J.E. (1980): Transforming growth factors produced by certain tumor cells: polypeptides that interact with epidermal growth factor receptors. *Proc. Natl. Acad. Sci. (USA)*, 77:5258–5262.

444. Tran Van, P., Vignery, A., and Baron, R. (1982): An electron-microscopic study of the bone-remodeling sequence in the rat. *Cell Tissue Res.*, 225:283–292.

445. Turnbull, R.S., Heersche, J.N.M., Tam, C.S., and Howley, T.P. (1983): Parathyroid hormone stimulates dentin and bone apposition in the thyroparathyroidectomized rat in a dose-dependent fashion. *Calcif. Tissue Int.*, 35:586–590.

446. Ueda, K., Saito, A., Nakamo, H., Aoshima, M., Yokota, M., Muraoka, R., and Iwaya, T. (1980): Cortical hyperostosis following long-term administration of prostaglandin E_1 in infants with cyanotic congenital heart disease. *J. Pediatr.*, 97:834–836.

447. Ueno, K., Haba, T., Woodbury, D., Price, P., Anderson, R., and Jee, W.S.S. (1985): The effects of prostaglandin E_2 in rapidly growing rats: depressed longitudinal and radial growth and increased metaphyseal hard tissue mass. *Bone*, 6:79–86.

448. Urist, M.R. (1983): Bone formation by auto-induction. *Science*, 220:680–685.

449. Urist, M.R., Huo, Y.K., Brownell, A.G., Hohl, W.M., Buyske, J., Lietze, A., Tempst, P., Hunkapiller, M., and DeLange, R.J. (1984): Purification of bovine bone morphogenetic protein by hydroxyapatite chromatography. *Proc. Natl. Acad. Sci. (USA)*, 81:371–375.

450. Urist, M.R., Lietze, A., Mizutani, H., Takagi, K., Triffitt, J.T., Amstutz, J., DeLange, R., Termine, J., and Finerman, G.A.M. (1982): A bovine low molecular weight bone morphogenetic protein (BMP) fraction. *Clin. Orthop.*, 162:219–231.

451. Urist, M.R., Sato, K., Brownell, A.G., Malinin, T.I., Lietze, A., Huo, Y.-K., Prolo, D.J., Oklund, S., Finerman, G.A.M., and DeLange, R.J. (1983): Human bone morphogenetic protein (hBMP). *Proc. Soc. Exp. Biol. Med.*, 173:194–199.

452. Vaananen, H.K., and Parvinen, E.K. (1983): High activity isoenzyme of carbonic anhydrase in rat calvaria osteoclasts. Immunohistochemical study. *Histochemistry*, 78:481–485.

453. Vaes, G. (1965): Excretion of acid and lysosomal hydrolytic enzymes during bone resorption induced in tissue culture by parathyroid extract. *Exp. Cell. Res.*, 39:470–474.

454. Vaes, G. (1968): On the mechanism of bone resorption. The action of parathyroid hormone on the excretion and synthesis of lysosomal enzymes and on the extracellular release of acid by bone cells. *J. Cell. Biol.*, 39:676–697.

455. Vaes, G. (1972): The release of collagenase as an inactive proenzyme by bone explants in culture. *Biochem. J.*, 126:275–289.

456. Vaishnav, R., Gallagher, J.A., Beresford, J.N., Poser, J., and Russell, R.G.G. (1984): Direct effects of stanozolol and estrogens on human bone cell culture. In: *Osteoporosis I*, edited by C. Christiansen, C.D. Arnaud, A.M. Parfitt, W.A. Peck, and B.L. Riggs, pp. 485–487. Aalborg Stiftsbogtrykkeri, Copenhagen.

457. van der Plas, A., Feyen, J.H.M., and Nijweide, P.J. (1985): Direct effect of parathyroid hormone on the proliferation of osteoblast-like cells; a possible involvement of cyclic AMP. *Biochem. Biophys. Res. Commun.*, 129:918–925.

458. van Paassen, H.C., Poortman, J., Borgart-Creutzburg, I.H.C., Thijssen, J.H.H., and Duursma, S.A. (1978): Oestrogen binding proteins in bone cell cytosol. *Calcif. Tissue Res.*, 25:249–254.

459. Voelkel, E.F., Tashjian, A.H., Jr., Franklin, R., Wasserman, E., and Levine, L. (1975): Hypercalcemia and tumour-prostaglandins: the VX2 carcinoma model in the rabbit. *Metabolism*, 24:973–986.

460. Von Der Mark, K., Von Der Mark, H., and Gay, S. (1976): Study of differential collagen synthesis during development of the chick embryo by immu-

nofluorescence. II. Localization of type I and type II collagen during long bone development. *Dev. Biol.*, 53:153–170.

461. Waite, L.C. (1972): Carbonic anhydrase inhibitors, parathyroid hormone and calcium metabolism. *Endocrinology*, 91:1160–1165.

462. Waite, L.C., and Kenny, A.D. (1969): Acetazolamide inhibition of the hypercalcemic response to parathyroid hormone. *Pharmacologist*, 11:252.

463. Waite, L.C., Volkert, W.A., and Kenny, A.D. (1970): Inhibition of bone resorption by acetazolamide in the rat. *Endocrinology*, 87:1129–1139.

464. Walker, D.G. (1975): Bone resorption restored in osteopetrotic mice by transplants and normal bone marrow and spleen cells. *Science*, 190:784–785.

465. Walker, D.G. (1975): Control of bone resorption by hematopoietic tissue; the induction and reversal of congenital osteopetrosis in mice through use of bone marrow and splenic transplants. *J. Exp. Med.*, 142:651–663.

466. Walker, D.G. (1975): Spleen cells transmit osteopetrosis in mice. *Science*, 190:785–787.

467. Walters, M.R., Rosen, D.M., Norman, A.W., and Luben, R.A. (1982): 1,25-Dihydroxyvitamin D receptors in an established bone cell line; correlation with biochemical responses. *J. Biol. Chem.*, 257:7481–7484.

468. Weinberg, J.B., Hobbs, M.M., and Misukonis, M.A. (1984): Recombinant human γ-interferon induces human monocyte polykaryon formation. *Proc. Natl. Acad. Sci. (USA)*, 81:4554–4557.

469. Wener, J.A., Gerton, S.J., and Raisz, L.G. (1972): Escape from inhibition of resorption in cultures of fetal bone treated with calcitonin and parathyroid hormone. *Endocrinology*, 90:752–759.

470. Whitfield, J.F., McManus, J.P., Franks, D.J., Braceland, B.M., and Gillan, D.J. (1972): Calcium mediated effects of calcitonin on cAMP formation and lymphoblast proliferation in thymocyte populations. *J. Cell. Physiol.*, 80:315–328.

471. Whitfield, J.F., McManus, J.P., and Rixon, R.H. (1970): The possible mediation by cyclic AMP of parathyroid hormone-induced stimulation of mitotic activity and deoxyribonucleic acid synthesis in rat thymic lymphocytes. *J. Cell. Physiol.*, 75:213–224.

472. Whitson, S.W., Harrison, W., Dunlap, M.K., Bowers, D.E., Fisher, L.W., Gehron Robey, P., and Termine, J.D. (1984): Fetal bovine bone cells synthesize bone-specific matrix proteins. *J. Cell Biol.*, 99:607–614.

473. Wiestner, M., Fischer, S., Dessau, W., and Muller, P.K. (1981): Collagen types synthesized by isolated calvarium cells. *Exp. Cell Res.*, 133:115–125.

474. Wong, G.L. (1979): Induction of metabolic changes and down regulation of bovine parathyroid hormone-responsive adenylate cyclases are dissociable in isolated osteoclasts and osteoblastic bone cells. *J. Biol. Chem.*, 254:34–37.

475. Wong, G.L. (1987): Skeletal effects of parathyroid hormone. In: *Bone and Mineral Research/4*, edited by W.A. Peck, pp. 103–130. Elsevier, Amsterdam.

476. Wong, G., and Cohn, D.V. (1974): Separation of parathyroid hormone and calcitonin-sensitive cells from non-responsive bone cells. *Nature*, 272:713–715.

477. Wong, G.L., Luben, R.A., and Cohn, D.V. (1977): 1,25-Dihydroxycholecalciferol and parathormone: effects on isolated osteoclast-like and osteoblast-like cells. *Science*, 197:663–665.

478. Wong, G.L., Lukert, B.P., and Adams, J.S. (1980): Glucocorticoids increase osteoblast-like bone cell response to 1,25(OH)$_2$D$_3$. *Nature*, 285:254–257.

479. Wright, G.M., and Leblond, C.P. (1981): Immunohistochemical localization of procollagens. III. Type I procollagen antigenicity in osteoblasts and prebone (osteoid). *J. Histochem. Cytochem.*, 29:791–804.

480. Yamamoto, L., Potts, J.T., and Segre, G.V. (1983): Circulating bovine lymphocytes contain receptors for parathyroid hormone. *J. Clin. Invest.*, 71:404–407.

481. Yee, J.A. (1985): Stimulation of alkaline phosphatase activity in cultured neonatal mouse calvarial bone cells by parathyroid hormone. *Calcif. Tissue Int.*, 37:530–538.

482. Yeh, C.-K., and Rodan, G.A. (1984): Tensile forces enhance prostaglandin E synthesis in osteoblastic cells grown on collagen ribbons. *Calcif. Tissue Int.*, 36:S67–S71.

483. Yoneda, T., and Mundy, G.R. (1979): Monocytes regulate osteoclast-activating factor production by releasing prostaglandins. *J. Exp. Med.*, 150:338–350.

484. Zambonin Zallone, A., and Teti, A. (1985): Autoradiographic demonstration of *in vitro* fusion of blood monocytes with osteoclasts. *Basic Appl. Histochem.*, 29:45–48.

485. Zambonin Zallone, A., Teti, A., and Primavera, M.V. (1984): Monocytes from circulating blood fuse *in vitro* with purified osteoclasts in primary culture. *J. Cell Sci.*, 66:335–342.

486. Zambonin Zallone, A., Teti, A., and Primavera, M.V. (1984): Resorption of vital or devitalized bone by isolated osteoclasts in vitro: the role of lining cells. *Cell Tissue Res.*, 235:561–564.

487. Zambonin Zallone, A., Teti, A., Primavera, M.V., Naldini, L., and Marchisio, P.C. (1983): Osteoclasts and monocytes have similar cytoskeletal structures and adhesion property *in vitro*. *J. Anat.*, 137:57–70.

Osteoporosis: Etiology, Diagnosis, and Management, edited by B. Lawrence Riggs and L. Joseph Melton, III. Raven Press, New York © 1988.

2

Bone Remodeling: Relationship to the Amount and Structure of Bone, and the Pathogenesis and Prevention of Fractures

A. M. Parfitt

Bone and Mineral Research Laboratory, Department of Medicine, Henry Ford Hospital, Detroit, Michigan 48202

The term "bone remodeling" is ambiguous. In many nonclinical contexts it commonly refers to all processes of subtraction from or addition to a bone surface regardless of location, timing, magnitude, purpose or mechanism. But in the more restricted sense now customary in clinical contexts, and used in this chapter, it identifies the bone replacement mechanism in the adult skeleton of man and some other large animals, which is the cellular and morphologic substratum of bone turnover (55,120). Remodeling has the function of maintaining the biomechanical competence of the skeleton by preventing the accumulation of fatigue damage (99) and maintaining an adequate supply of young bone of relatively low mineral density to subserve mineral homeostasis (123). Remodeling occurs by the continuous removal and replacement of whole volumes of bone tissue, a process carried out by the osteoclasts and osteoblasts on bone surfaces which, together with their precursor cells, make up the remodeling system. Osteoclasts and osteoblasts are fully differentiated cells of finite life span that require continuous renewal from separate stem cell populations (see Chapter 1 *this volume*). The cellular events of bone remodeling differ in important ways from those of development, growth, repair and the osseous response to pathologic processes such as neoplasia and infection, and information relevant only to these topics rather than to normal adult remodeling will be considered only by way of contrast.

Bone remodeling is important in several ways to the understanding of osteoporosis. It mediates the effects, whether beneficial or harmful, of all agents—endocrine, nutritional, or mechanical—that act on the skeleton. The speed and extent of replacement regulate the rates of bone gain or loss at specific locations and times, of which the cumulative effects determine the three-dimensional distribution and amount of bone throughout the body. The rate of turnover determines the age of bone tissue and various physical and chemical properties of bone that depend on its age and may affect its function. Finally, the organization of the remodeling system (55) profoundly influences the response to therapeutic intervention and may determine its ultimate success or failure.

But before the remodeling system can be explained, a brief description is needed of what is being remodeled.

FUNCTION AND STRUCTURE OF BONE AND THE EFFECTS OF AGE

Bone is a specialized connective tissue in which a matrix consisting of collagen fibers, a large variety of other proteins and ground substance is impregnated with a solid mineral (see Chapter 3, *this volume*). Bone is the main constituent of the bones, which are the individual organs of the skeletal system. The amount of matrix determines the volume of bone and the extent of mineral deposition determines its density.[1] This relationship is important because most noninvasive methods of determining the amount of bone, referred to in this context as bone mass, in fact measure the amount of either total mineral or calcium. Old bone is more highly mineralized and therefore more dense than young bone, but the degree of mineralization and the proportion of unmineralized matrix or osteoid averaged over the whole skeleton do not often vary by more than 5% except in osteomalacia. Consequently, bone substance density changes much less with age than bone matrix volume, which is the main determinant of apparent bone density. Apparent density falls with age, giving rise to the seeming paradox that with increasing age the density of the bones declines but the density of bone shows little change.

The skeletal system has both biomechanical and metabolic funcitons. The hardness and rigidity of bone enable the skeleton to maintain the shape of the body, to protect the soft tissues, to provide a framework for the bone marrow, and to transmit the force of muscular contraction from one part of the body to another.

---

[1]For clarity, three uses of the term bone density (mass /unit volume) should be distinguished. The reference volume is bone matrix for bone substance density, or true bone density, bone tissue (including marrow and other soft tissues) for bone tissue density, and bone as an organ for apparent or whole bone density, as would be obtained by applying Archimedes' principle to an entire bone.

The mineral content of bone contributes to the regulation of extracellular fluid (ECF) composition, particularly the ionized calcium concentration. The solid phase of bone mineral is in contact with the bone ECF, which is separated from the systemic ECF by the flat cells which line all bone surfaces that are not currently active in remodeling. Distributed throughout the bone are osteocytes lying within lentil shaped lacunae, joined to each other and to the cells on the surface by filamentous prolongations of the cells that run within canaliculae. The bone ECF extends throughout the lacunar-canalicular system, and as on the surface, lies between the solid bone and the cells. Apart from the losses or gains of bone tissue in bulk, all transfers of ions between bone mineral and systemic ECF take place between or through the surface cells and osteocytes, which collectively make up the homeostatic system.

Cortical Bone and Trabecular Bone

It is convenient to distinguish two types of bone structure in the adult skeleton-cortical bone tissue (or compacta) and trabecular bone tissue (or spongiosa) (68,79,179). The porosity, or soft tissue content, is usually less than 10% by volume in cortical bone and more than 75% by volume in trabecular bone but, particularly in the aging skeleton, all degrees of porosity may be found. The ratio of surface to volume of bone is about four times higher in trabecular than in cortical bone, but because of the difference in porosity, the ratio of surface to volume of tissue is more nearly the same. Cortical bone provides about three quarters of total skeletal mass but only about one-third of the total surface (129). It forms the outer wall of all bones, but the bulk of cortical bone is in the shafts of the long bones of the appendicular skeleton. Trabecular bone provides the remaining one quarter of total skeletal mass and about two-thirds of the total surface. It consists of a complex three-dimensional network of curved plates and rods (trabeculae) 100 to 150 μm in thickness that are continuous with the inner side of the cortex and form interconnecting spaces of 500 to 1000 μm diameter that contain either hematopoietic or fatty marrow. Trabecular bone is found mainly in the bones of the axial skeleton and in the ends of the long bones.

Cortical and trabecular bone differ not only in porosity and surface: volume ratio, but in proximity to the bone marrow, blood supply, rapidity of turnover, timing and magnitude of loss with age, and influence on fracture risk. But treating each type of bone as a single compartment, although more accurate than failing to make this distinction, is still a considerable oversimplification. The transition between them is gradual rather than abrupt, especially in the elderly, with an intervening zone that is intermediate in both structural and functional characteristics (81). Furthermore, bone in different locations is subjected to very different biomechanical stresses, and cortical bone turnover is much higher in the axial than in the appendicular skeleton. In the spine, a rectangular lattice consisting of vertical and horizontal rods and perforated plates is the predominant structure beneath the endplates and a honeycomb of cylindrical spaces formed by mainly vertical plates is the predominant structure in the center (2,8). There are many other different structural types of trabecular bone (158,170) and at least three functional types with different rates of turnover, depending on proximity to a synovial joint, to hematopoietic marrow or to fatty marrow (144).

Bone Surfaces

All bone remodeling originates on a bone surface, and each bone has four surfaces: periosteal, intracortical (including both Haversian and Volkmann canals), endocortical and trabecular, the latter three being in continuity. A surface which is closed and unbounded and divides space into an inside and an outside may be referred to as an envelope (129). The periosteal envelope encloses all of the hard and soft tissues of a single bone, and the endosteal envelope, with its three subdivisions (trabecular, endocortical and intracortical) encloses all of the soft tissues within the bone with the ex-

ception of the osteocytes and their processes. Bone is therefore inside the periosteal envelope and outside the endosteal envelope, which demarcates bone from bone marrow. The behavior of bone cells and their responses to mechanical, chemical and hormonal stimuli differ significantly between the periosteal and endosteal envelopes. This is obvious during growth, but even in the adult skeleton there may simultaneously be a net gain of bone adjacent to the periosteum, and a net loss of bone adjacent to the endosteum. The distribution of remodeling activity and bone gain or loss between the three subdivisions of the endosteal envelope is also different at different ages, in different bones, and in different disease states.

Lamellar Bone and Woven Bone

The structural difference between cortical and trabecular bone is visible with the naked eye, but lamellar and woven bone are distinguished by the microscopic orientation of collagen fiber bundles (61,79,149). Normally all bone in the adult human skeleton, both cortical and trabecular, is laminated like multilayer plywood, consisting of layers about 3 μm thick within which there is a moderately uniform orientation of collagen fibers that remain parallel to one another at least over distances shorter than 50 μm. Adjacent lamellae are distinguishable by alternation in the principal fiber direction, although this transition appears more abrupt by light microscopy than by scanning electron microscopy (17). One pair of adjacent lamellae gives rise to one pair of light and dark lines of birefringence when examined by polarized light. The osteocyte lacunae lie between adjacent lamellae but are staggered so that canaliculae that run perpendicular to the lamellae usually connect osteocytes that are 2 to 3 lamellae apart. In cortical bone the lamellae are concentric, but in trabecular bone they are usually more flattened and have a more variable radius of curvature.

The most characteristic feature of woven bone (also referred to as fetal bone or fibrous bone) is that the collagen fibers run in all directions like a carpet underfelt, in contrast to the regular orientation of collagen fibers in lamellar bone (55,68). Woven bone may resemble either compacta or spongiosa in its three-dimensional structure, but is usually intermediate between cortical and trabecular bone in its porosity and in the size of its soft tissue spaces (61). The structural elements are randomly arranged without relation to lines of stress and are irregular and variable in thickness. Osteocytes are more frequent and are scattered at random with no relation to vascular channels and their lacunae are irregular in surface, larger and more variable in size and shape than in lamellar bone. Although typical examples of lamellar and woven bone are easy to distinguish, to classify bone only into these two types is an oversimplification since all degrees of randomness of collagen fiber orientation can be observed. Woven bone is invariably the first type of bone formed where no bone previously existed, and it is usually a temporary material whose normal fate is to be resorbed and replaced by lamellar bone.

Lamellar bone is made only in apposition to an existing surface; each osteoblast is coordinated with its neighbors, and together they make a continuous layer of bone laid down only on one side of the cell. How osteoblasts control and systematically vary the orientation of collagen fibers to produce the lamellar structure of mature bone is unknown, although the alignment of the most superficial fibers closely matches the shape and alignment of the osteoblasts (76). By contrast, woven bone is formed directly in condensations of fibrous tissue without the necessity for an adjacent free bone surface, by the rapid, uncoordinated and nonpolarized action of individual osteoblasts. Each forms an island of new matrix, and adjacent islands coalesce into nodules. Mineralization occurs rapidly and simultaneously in each nodule and without relation to collagen fibers or blood vessels, the process resembling somewhat the mineralizaiton of cartilage rather than of mature lamellar bone (17,79).

The differences between lamellar and woven bone are relevant to osteoporosis for several reasons. First, only woven bone can be formed in cell culture, which places certain constraints on the applicability of cell culture experiments to the pathogenesis and treatment of osteoporosis. Second, woven bone formation is less susceptible to endocrine and other regulation than is lamellar bone formation (55), which is why fracture healing may be quite normal even in osteoporotic patients with subnormal rates of bone formation and impaired osteoblast function. Third, the first bone formed in response to sodium fluoride administration, although deposited in apposition to an existing bone surface, has several of the features of woven bone (14), and is not as strong as an equivalent volume of lamellar bone. Finally, the controlled production of woven bone in specific locations may turn out to be an important strategy for the restoration of normal bone structure in severe osteoporosis.

Bone Structural Units

Histologists have long recognized that the skeleton is constructed of many small elements of bone made at different times (68,79,129); these will be referred to as bone structural units (BSU). As bricks are held together by mortar, so the BSU are held together by a highly mineralized but collagen poor connective tissue, which is visible in two-dimensional histologic sections as a cement line, but in three-dimensional reality is a cement plane or surface (Fig. 1). The strength of bone is increased by this method of construction, but slippage at the cement plane can be produced by prolonged mechanical stress (90). Almost all cement lines are reversal lines, which mark the furthest extent of a previous episode of bone resorption, and are recognized by their irregular scalloped appearance, acid phosphatase staining, discontinuity of canaliculae and abrupt change in lamellar orientation (129,149). A few cement lines are arrest lines, formed during a period of temporary interruption of bone formation, and recognized by their smooth surface, lack of acid phosphatase staining, and continuity of canaliculae and lamellar orientation. Arrest

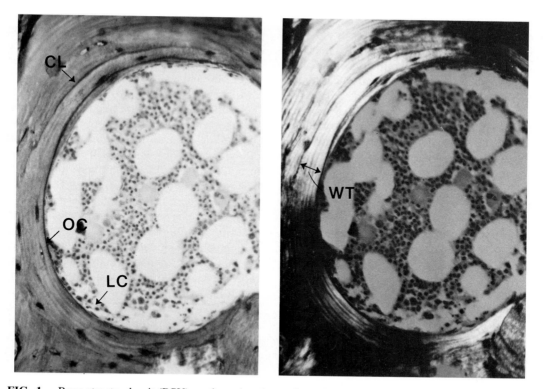

FIG. 1. Bone structural unit (BSU) on the trabecular surface. On the left normal illumination shows positive identification of cement line (CL). On the right polarized light shows corresponding pattern of lamellation. The distance between the cement line and the bone surface at any point is the wall thickness (WT); this distance averaged over the entire quiescent surface is mean wall thickness (MWT). LC = lining cell; OC = osteocyte. (Gallocyanine stain; original magnification × 160).

lines indicate that the BSU was completed in two or more separate periods rather than continuously, and increase in number with age (68).

The characteristic BSU of adult cortical bone is the secondary osteon or Haversian system, a cylinder about 200 to 250 μm in diameter roughly parallel to the long axis of the bone, with a central canal about 40 to 50 μm in diameter; the canals are connected to each other by transverse Volkmann's canals and periodically either divide or reunite to form a branching network. Within the canal run blood vessels, lymphatics, nerves and loose connective tissue which are all continuous with those of the bone marrow and the periosteum. The total length of a single canal from periosteum to endosteum is about 10,000 μm or 1 cm, but

the mean distance between branch points is approximately 2.5 mm (129). Osteons form approximately two-thirds of cortical bone volume, a proportion which falls with age, the remainder being made up of interstitial bone representing the remnants of previous generations of osteons, and the subperiosteal and subendosteal circumferential lamellae. The walls of the osteon, made up of 20 to 30 concentric lamellae, are about 70 to 100 μm thick.

In trabecular bone the BSU are flattened, as if an osteon had been slit open and unrolled, and lie roughly parallel to the plane of the trabecular plates; to emphasize the similarity in structure they are sometimes referred to as trabecular osteons. In two-dimensional sections the BSU which form the trabecular surface are shaped like thin crescents about 600 μm long and about 60 μm in depth at the center, tapering at each end. But in three-dimensional reality they are much larger and their shape is much more complex, with prolongations in different directions that interlock with adjacent BSU; as a result units that appear separate in a two-dimensional section could often have been made by the same team of osteoblasts in the same resorption cavity (88). It is useful to distinguish between surface BSU that resulted from remodeling in the previous 5 years or so and the intervening interstitial bone that may be much older. Surface BSU follow the shape of the trabecular surface, most of which is concave towards the marrow spaces, although the central area of large plates may be almost flat, and the rods and the edges of the plates are convex.

Age-related Changes in Amount of Bone

Changes in bone mass during the human life span fall into three periods. From conception until epiphyseal closure there is a progressive increase in bone volume, both trabecular from endochondral ossification, and cortical from net periosteal apposition supplemented at different times and places by net endosteal apposition. After cessation of growth there is a period of consolidation during which cortical porosity, still high in late adolescence, continues to fall and bone tissue density increases as bone turnover falls to a nadir (37,55,84). The cortices also become thicker because of net apposition on endosteal as well as on periosteal surfaces (56). Data on trabecular bone during the period of cortical consolidation is inconsistent. No new trabeculae can be made once endochondral ossification ceases with epiphyseal closure, but in autopsy studies of lumbar vertebrae (7), and ilium (96) the thickness of trabeculae and the total amount of trabecular bone both increased to a peak in the third decade. Other investigators have found no increase in the amount of trabecular bone after epiphyseal closure (29,39).

Peak adult bone mass, representing the summated contributions of growth (90 to 95%) and consolidation (5 to 10%), is reached at about age 35 to 40 for cortical bone and probably earlier for trabecular bone. Peak adult bone mass is about 25 to 30% higher in males than in females and about 10% higher in blacks than in whites, but within each demographic subgroup there are large differences among individuals, with a coefficient of variation (CV; standard deviation as a percentage of the mean) of about 15% (57). As a result one woman in forty (2.5%) has a peak adult bone mass which is less than the average bone mass for women at age 65. These individual differences make a substantial contribution to individual differences in fracture risk, both between and within demographic subgroups (106). The differences are partly under genetic control but must also reflect a variety of hormonal, nutritional and socioeconomic factors.

A few years after peak adult bone mass is attained, sooner in women than in men, age-related bone loss begins, a universal phenomenon of human biology that occurs regardless of sex, race, occupation, habitual physical activity, dietary habits, economic development, geographic location or historical epoch (7,29,37,39,56,57,84,96,106,109). In this it differs from the age-related increase in blood pressure which, although ubiquitous in the developed countries, does not occur in many communities remote from Western civilization. Bone is lost from every site amenable to measurement, but only from the endosteal surfaces in contact with the bone marrow, since the periosteal surface continues to gain bone slowly throughout life (59). No serial measurements have been reported in blacks, so it is not known whether they differ from whites in rates of bone loss as well as in peak adult bone mass.

In males, average cortical bone loss is about 0.3% of peak adult bone mass per year and trabecular bone loss slightly faster. In females, the average loss is about 1% of peak adult bone mass per year for both cortical and trabecular bone, with acceleration for about 5 years after menopause and a slower rate at both earlier and later times (89,154). The sex difference is greater for the femoral shaft than for the rib or the spine (7). After about age 90, the rate of endosteal loss may fall below the rate of periosteal gain, so that cortical thickness, having declined progressively for 40 to 50 years, very slowly increases (67). The absolute reduction in thickness is about the same in the mid diaphysis of a large bone such as the femur as in a small bone such as the metacarpal, with net endosteal loss of about 50 μm/year in both (7,122), so that the relative loss is greater in the smaller bone. In both sexes those with most bone lose most quickly, and there are large individual differences in rate of loss, but conforming to a Gaussian distribution (67).

BONE REMODELING—THE QUANTUM CONCEPT

Bone remodeling occurs in anatomically discrete foci which are active for 4 to 8 months (12,55,79,120). Precursor cells proliferate into a team of new osteoclasts which erodes a cavity on a bone surface. The osteoclasts then disappear and there is a quiescent interval or reversal phase during which the irregular floor of the cavity is smoothed off and a layer of cement substance is deposited. A team of osteoblasts derived from a different precursor cell pool are then assembled with the task of replacing as exactly as possible the recently removed bone. The wide variety of age-related changes just described can all in some manner be accounted for by modifications of this stereotyped sequence of events.

During remodeling, changes in the amount of bone are quite slow and changes in the shape of the bones are barely perceptible. This is in contrast to modeling, the totality of mechanisms that increase the size of bones and adapt their shape to mechanical load during growth, by moving bone surfaces through tissue space relative to some defined bodily axis, a type of movement referred to as ''drift'' (55). There are many differences between remodeling and modeling (Table 1), but the most fundamental is that in contrast to the cyclical erosion and repair of microscopic cavities with

TABLE 1. *Some differences between remodeling and modeling*

	Remodeling	Modeling
Timing	Cyclical	Continuous
Location of R and F	Same surface	Different surfaces
Extent	20% of surface	100% of surface
Activation[a]	Needed	Not needed
Apposition rate	0.3 to 1.0 μm/d	2 to 20 μm/d
Balance	Net loss	Net gain
Coupling	Local	Systemic

R = resorption; F = formation
[a]In sense of transformation of quiescent to active surface. Modified from Parfitt, ref. 131, with permission.

long periods of quiescence between cycles that characterizes remodeling, in modeling either bone resorption or bone formation occur continuously on one surface for long periods of time without interruption. The specialized collection of cells which accomplish one quantum of bone turnover—erosion of one cavity and its refilling to form one new BSU—is referred to as a bone remodeling unit (BRU). The life cycle of a single representative BRU on a trabecular surface will now be examined in more detail in five successive stages of quiescence, activation, resorption, reversal, formation and back to quiescence (12,131; Fig. 2).

Quiescence

In contrast to young growing animals, in which most free bone surfaces are either forming or resorbing, in adult large animals, including man, about 80% of the trabecular and inner cortical bone surfaces and about 95% of the intracortical bone surface are inactive with respect to bone remodeling (129,131). The bone surface is covered by a layer of extremely thin (0.1 to 1 μm) flattened lining cells about 50 μm in diameter (103,112,131) that arise by terminal transformation of osteoblasts, as will be described later. Because of their osteoblast lineage they probably retain the same hormonal receptors and responsiveness, but in adult human bone they appear to have lost the ability

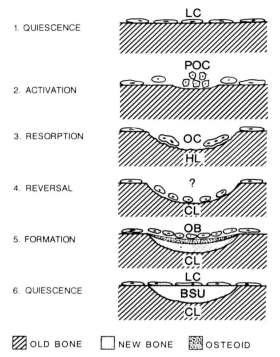

1. QUIESCENCE

2. ACTIVATION

3. RESORPTION

4. REVERSAL

5. FORMATION

6. QUIESCENCE

▨ OLD BONE   ☐ NEW BONE   ▧ OSTEOID

FIG. 2. The normal remodeling sequence in adult human trabecular bone. Schematic representation of successive events on the endosteal surface. LC = lining cell; POC = preosteoclast (mononuclear); OC = osteoclast (multinucleated); HL = Howship's lacuna; CL = cement line (reversal line); OB = osteoblast; BSU = bone structural unit. From Parfitt, ref. 131, with permission.

to synthesize collagen and should not be referred to as osteoblasts, resting or otherwise (12). Nevertheless they probably retain the ability to function as osteogenic precursor cells and to make osteoblast gene products other than collagen.

Between the lining cells and the bone is a thin (0.1 to 0.5 μm) layer of unmineralized connective tissue (113,164). The collagen fibers of this endosteal membrane are packed in smaller bundles and oriented more randomly than in the bone matrix, and are fewer in number with relatively more amorphous ground substance than in bone. The endosteal membrane, although it never mineralizes, is sometimes erroneously referred to as osteoid, a tissue that it may resemble under light

microscopy but from which it clearly differs both in ultrastructure (131) and in function, which is to protect the bone surface from attack by osteoclasts (23). On bone surfaces adjacent to fatty (yellow) marrow, the lining cells are separated by a similar connective tissue layer from the thin cytoplasm of the fat cells, and are frequently in close proximity to bone marrow capillaries (113). On bone surfaces adjacent to hematopoietic (red) marrow, the fat cell cytoplasm is replaced by the squamous cells of the marrow sac (79,131). The entire thickness of tissue separating the marrow from the bone, comprising two layers of cells and two layers of connective tissue, is only 1 to 2 μm.

Activation

The conversion of a small area of surface from quiescence to activity (with respect to remodeling) is referred to as activation. Initiating the cycle of remodeling requires first, the recruitment of osteoclasts; second, a means for them to gain access to the bone; and third, a mechanism for their attraction and attachment to the surface (12,131). In an adult skeleton of normal size; activation occurs somewhere about once every 10 sec (129). Apart from variations in whole body activation as a function of age, sex, race and metabolic state, there are systematic differences between different bones and between different surfaces in the same bone. Subject to these constraints, activation occurs partly at random and partly in response to focal structural or biomechanical requirements (129). The origin of osteoclasts, and their mechanisms of recruitment are discussed in Chapter 1 and in ref. 12 and 79. For intracortical remodeling, osteoclast precursor cells presumably travel in the circulation to the site of activation, which is either a Volkmann or a Haversian canal. Trabecular remodeling occurs preferentially in relation to hematopoietic rather than fatty marrow (175) and at least some of the precursor cells originate locally (12). In either case, the precursor cells must penetrate both the layer of marrow sac cells and the layer of lining cells, probably by inserting pseudopodia between the cells (12). After reaching the mineralized bone surface, the precursor cells undergo fusion into osteoclasts.

Why activation occurs at a particular location at a particular time is usually unknown. When it is induced experimentally by orthodontic tooth manipulation, the first observable change is the accumulation of cells positive for fluoride-inhibitible non-specific esterase adjacent to the site of impending resorption (11). Any theory of activation must account for the presence in osteoblasts, but not in osteoclasts, of receptors for many of the known stimuli of bone resorption (see Chapter 1, *this volume*), and must provide for specific local instruction of the osteoclasts. This has led to the concept that activation is initiated by focal events in the cellular and connective tissue investment of the bone surface, in which the lining cells of osteoblast lineage are assigned a crucial role. Recent experimental work has suggested a variety of ways in which the lining cells could be responsible for each of the three components necessary for activation (12,131), but the most important point is that the lining cells digest the endosteal membrane (23) and retract to expose the mineralized bone surface, which is chemotactic for osteoclast precursor cells (12,79,131).

Resorption

Once in contact with the bone, the newly formed team of osteoclasts begin to erode a cavity of characteristic shape and dimensions, referred to in trabecular bone as a Howship's lacuna and in cortical bone as a cutting cone (129). The osteoclast is motile, and can resorb bone over a domain which is 2 to 3 times larger than the area in contact with the cell at one time. The precise three-dimensional path of individual osteoclasts *in vivo* is unknown; a relationship to collagen bundle orientation is suggested by light microscopy (174) but not by scanning electron microscopy (76). In cortical bone the osteoclasts in the cutting cone travel about 20 to 40 μm/day roughly parallel to the

long axis of the bone and about 5 to 10 μm/day perpendicular to the main direction of advance (129). In trabecular bone, osteoclasts erode rapidly to a depth of about two-thirds of the final cavity, the remainder being eroded much more slowly by mononuclear cells (45). These could be potential precursor cells that have failed to fuse, resorbing monocytes, or disaggregated osteoclasts (12). When the cavity reaches a mean depth of about 50 μm from the surface in trabecular bone and about 100 μm from the center of the cone in cortical bone, which takes between one and three weeks, resorption at that location ceases, but how control is exerted on the size, shape and depth of a cavity is unknown (12,131).

In Haversian remodeling in the adult dog, labeled nuclei first appear in osteoclasts about 3 days after ^{3}H thymidine labeling (69); the mean life span of osteoclast nuclei was estimated at 12.5 days, with a corresponding turnover of 8%/day, so that a constant supply of new precursor cells is needed to replenish the nuclei at each resorptive site. Morphologic analysis of the time sequence of labeling suggested that these sustaining precursor cells are mostly derived from a locally proliferating population of cells near the bone surface rather than from circulating cells, although the origin of the proliferating cells could not be determined. Similar conclusions were reached concerning endosteal remodeling in the rat (12). The mean life span of the multinucleated cell is longer than of its nuclei, and both are longer than the time needed to complete excavation at one place because of the ability of the osteoclast to move across the bone surface. It is possible that some osteoclasts disaggregate into mononuclear resorbing cells (12), but other than this nothing is known of the fate either of the individual nucleus or of the whole cell.

Reversal

This is the time interval between completion of resorption and commencement of formation at a particular location, normally about one to two weeks in duration, when the events occur that underly the coupling of these processes (12,131). The timely appearance of a sufficient number of new osteoblasts at the base of the resorption cavity must involve both a stimulus to cell division and a mechanism for attracting the cells to a particular location on the surface. The histologic counterpart of the reversal period is a Howship's lacuna lacking osteoclasts, but containing mononuclear cells whose nature, origin, relationship to the cells that complete resorption, and role in coupling are unknown. Electron microscopy of the reversal phase in the rat periodontal ligament identified partially released osteocytes and mononuclear phagocytes. Some of the reversal cells partly smooth over the ragged surface left by the resorptive process and deposit a thin layer of cement substance, thus preparing the surface for bone formation (12). Other mononuclear cells observed during the reversal period are preosteoblasts, with pale cytoplasm and large nuclei indicating the G_1 phase of the cell cycle (145).

The coupling mechanism appears to be intrinsic to bone, locally regulated and automatic, in the sense that once activation has occurred, the cycle of remodeling proceeds inevitably to completion without the need for further intervention. A substance referred to as human skeletal growth factor has been isolated from human bone and shown to increase DNA synthesis in bone cells, stimulate osteoblast proliferation and induce bone formation (48), but this cannot be the only signal involved. In Haversian remodeling a substance released from matrix or cells during resorption would be present in highest concentration at the site where new osteoblasts are needed, but this does not apply to trabecular remodeling, where the local microcirculation is an open network rather than an isolated loop. Release of an osteoblast mitogen from resorbed bone may ensure that new osteoblasts arrive in the right number and at the right time, but other signals, such as chemotactic constituents of cement substance, are needed to ensure that they assemble in the right location and in the correct alignment, with uniform polarity as a continuous monolayer (12,131).

Formation

In contrast to bone resorption, bone formation occurs in two stages, matrix synthesis and mineralization, which are separated both in time and in space. Soon after deposition of the cement surface the team of new osteoblasts begins to deposit a layer of bone matrix, referred to as an osteoid seam. Apparently homogeneous by light microscopy, at the ultra-structural level osteoid contains several zones, the nascent collagen fibrils adjacent to the osteoblast showing increasing aggregation and alignment because of cross-linking before incorporation into mineralized bone (50,79). Because of the local geometry, osteoid seams in cortical bone appear as rings, but in trabecular bone as crescents tapering at each end. The new matrix begins to mineralize after about 5 to 10 days of maturation. As a result, matrix apposition and mineralization are systematically out of step as the osteoid seam first increases and then decreases in thickness. The rate of mineral apposition can be measured directly *in vivo* after double tetracycline labeling, as the mean distance between fluorescent bands divided by the time interval between the mid points of the periods of tetracycline administration (129). In experimental animals the rate of matrix apposition can be measured directly *in vivo* by autoradiography of bone after administration of a collagen precursor, such as labeled proline (97), but in human subjects only indirect measurement is possible, by relating osteoid seam width to the mineral apposition rate and to distance from the cement surface as an index of the passage of time (146).

The use of tetracycline labeling as a diagnostic tool is described in Chapter 9, but some additional details are important for the understanding of bone remodeling. Tetracycline chelates calcium, and when the blood level is raised it binds reversibly to every bone surface accessible to the circulation, but with preference for the most recently formed mineral which is of small crystal size and large surface area (see Chapter 3, *this volume*). During the time interval between the end of the second labeling period and the biopsy (preferably kept constant at four days), tetracycline is permanently fixed at sites of currently active mineralization because a layer of new mineral is deposited of sufficient thickness to prevent the escape of tetracycline when its blood level falls to zero, as occurs from all bone surfaces where there is no mineral deposition. The mineralization front, defined by tetracycline uptake or by toluidine blue staining (167), is located at, but is not synonymous with, the osteoid-mineralized bone interface (or zone of demarcation) which persists until the osteoid seam disappears, whether or not mineralization is occurring.

A double band of fluorescence establishes unequivocally that bone formation occurred during the relevant time period, but only a single label can be deposited if mineralization begins or ends between the periods of label administration, since most single labels are evidence of bone formation, especially if they are in continuity with double labels. The best estimate of the extent of bone surface currently undergoing mineralization is the mean length of the two labels, which is equivalent to the combined lengths of all double labels and half the single labels (29). If mineralization occurred continuously at a measureable rate throughout the life span of an osteoid seam, all osteoid would be labeled except that most recently formed which has not yet started to mineralize, and the proportion of labeled osteoid would normally be greater than 90%. But in practice, the currently mineralizing surface as just defined, averages only about 60 to 65% of the osteoid surface in normal premenopausal women and 50 to 55% in normal postmenopausal women. This discrepancy can be explained in two ways: First, there may be a temporary cessation of mineralization to form a so-called resting seam (55), for which there is suggestive evidence in normal dogs (64). Second, if mineral apposition is extremely slow, too few tetracycline molecules may be retained to exceed the threshold for visible fluorescence (129). Which mechanism is more important is unknown.

In considering the relationship between the

results of bone histomorphometry as usually performed and the sequential changes at an individual site of formation, it is important to distinguish between the *mean* values of various measured and derived quantities found in one individual and the *instantaneous* values that occur at different stages of osteoid seam development in that individual. Because much of the osteoid surface is unlabeled for one or other of the reasons mentioned earlier, the best estimate currently available for the mean rate of matrix apposition is the mineral appositional rate averaged over the entire osteoid surface according to the fraction of osteoid that is labeled, referred to as the osteoid appositional rate, otherwise known as effective appositional rate (143), or (in cortical bone) the radial closure rate (55,129). Although the instantaneous rates of matrix and mineral apposition are continually changing and out of phase, the mean rates averaged over the life span of the osteoid seam are identical, because in the absence of osteomalacia the volume of new mineralized bone is the same as the volume of new matrix. By relating the mean rate of matrix apposition to the mean wall thickness, which is the mean distance between the quiescent surface and the nearest reversal line (Fig. 1), the time taken to rebuild the average BSU at a single location can be estimated, and by extension the time taken to complete one entire cycle of remodeling, or the total remodeling period.

In both cortical and trabecular bone the instantaneous rate of matrix apposition is most rapid (2 to 3 μm/day) at the beginning, when the osteoblasts are strongly basophilic, columnar, and densely packed, and the osteoid seam reaches a maximum width of about 20 μm just before or shortly after the onset of mineralization 5 to 10 days later (44,129,146). The instantaneous rate of mineral apposition is initially 1 to 2 μm/day and exceeds the rate of matrix apposition until formation is completed. With time the osteoblasts and their nuclei become progressively flatter and broader and their cytoplasm less basophilic and less abundant. Corresponding to this morphologic change, there is a progressive reduction in the rates of both matrix and mineral apposition and in the thickness of the osteoid seam (44, 79,129,131,136). The apparent fall in osteoblast activity is due mainly to a reduction in cell surface density, but the morphologic changes (especially the reduction in cell volume) suggest that there is also a reduction in the rate of matrix output per cell. Eventually the osteoid seam disappears, and the cells remaining on the surface complete their morphologic and functional transformation to lining cells (129,131). Construction of the new BSU is now finished and the surface has returned to its original state of quiescence except that the bone is younger and will continue to increase its density until mineralization is complete. In both cortical and trabecular bone the duration of formation is about three months and the duration of the complete cycle about four months, but a further 3 to 6 months will be required for the bone to become fully mature.

According to this model, the durations of matrix synthesis and of mineralization overlap, but are neither coextensive nor necessarily identical. Three separate stages can be recognized (Fig. 3). In the first stage, matrix synthesis occurs alone without mineralization, in the second stage matrix synthesis and mineralization occur together, and in the third state mineralization occurs alone without matrix synthesis. During the first stage the osteoid seam rapidly increases in thickness from zero to a maximum value, and during the second and third stages it slowly gets progressively thinner until there remains only the endosteal membrane, which is the last tissue deposited by the osteoblast at the end of its life span. In an alternative model (44), the second and third stages are merged, matrix synthesis and mineralization terminating simultaneously. In either case, the third stage is probably when osteoblast activity may temporarily be interrupted

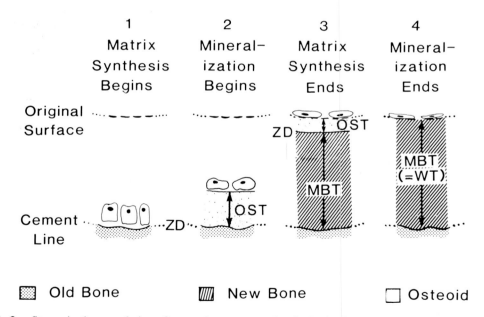

FIG. 3.   Stages in the completion of a new bone structural unit. In the first stage matrix synthesis occurs alone, in the second stage matrix synthesis and mineralization occur together, and in the third stage mineralization occurs alone. OST = osteoid seam thickness; MBT = mineralized bone thickness; WT = wall thickness of completed BSU; ZD = zone of demarcation—the junction between mineralized bone and osteoid. Note that the ZD moves progressively away from the cement line and that osteoblasts change progressively from cuboidal to flat. Modified from Parfitt, Osteomalacia and related disorders. In: *Metabolic Bone Disease,* 2nd ed., edited by L.V. Avioli and S.M. Krane. Grune and Stratton, Orlando (in press).

and when mineral apposition may sometimes be too slow for tetracycline fixation to occur.

Some investigators have proposed that several generations of osteoblasts are needed to complete each new BSU, but both morphologic and kinetic evidence make it much more likely that all the osteoblasts needed at each location are assembled on the cement surface before bone formation begins, and that at each point on the surface a single osteoblast makes all the bone matrix that is formed (73,125). Of the original cell population, some become osteocytes, some become lining cells and some disappear by an unknown mechanism (129). The concept of a single generation of osteoblasts has several implications. First, how completely the cavity is refilled probably depends more on the number of osteoblasts initially assembled than on their individual activity (125). Consequently, the many biomechanical and hormonal agents that regulate bone formation probably act more on osteoblast recruitment than on differentiated cell function (70). Second, the previously mentioned temporary interruptions in bone formation during the life span of one seam that become more frequent with increasing age, and especially in patients with osteoporosis (142), represent cyclic variation in activity of the same cells, rather than a pause for recruitment of new cells.

Remodeling and Turnover

Remodeling is the cellular basis of bone turnover, but the concepts are distinct. As already mentioned, turnover depends in part on the distribution of remodeling between different surfaces and different bones, the more even the distribution the greater the turnover for the same cellular activity. Less obviously, turnover is also influenced by the distribution of remodeling between regions of bone of different ages, which can occur in three ways (129). If each moiety of bone has the same probability of being remodeled regardless of its age, remodeling would be randomly distributed and the bone present at a particular time would dis-

appear exponentially; in the usual sedentary human condition, most remodeling is probably of this kind. A second possibility is selective remodeling, in which older and denser bone is preferentially removed (160), most likely in response to osteocyte senescence, local trauma or fatigue microdamage. Finally, there is redundant remodeling, in which younger bone is preferentially removed. Mean bone age (the weighted mean of all individual moieties of bone, some made very recently and some made many years ago) and its frequency distribution are affected differently by the three modes of remodeling (63). In an adult after skeletal maturity with normal rates of turnover and random remodeling, mean age would be about 20 years for cortical bone and about 4 years for trabecular bone. These values will be decreased by selective remodeling and increased by redundant remodeling.

The choice between random and redundant remodeling is partly dependent on the distance of different moieties of bone from the surface. For example, trabecular interstitial bone can be remodeled only if the resorption cavity is of greater than average depth; consequently, bone closer to the surface has a much higher chance of being replaced. In cortical bone, the distance from an existing surface is less important, because a cutting cone can travel far from its point of origin to create a new osteon with a new Haversian canal (160). But in another type of cortical remodeling focal reconstruction of an existing osteon occurs in a transverse or radial direction without longitudinal advance (100). The existence of this process has been conclusively demonstrated by serial sections (102) and it probably accounts for the presence within the same osteon of inner and outer regions (separated by a cement line) that are of different mineral density on microradiography. Such double-zone osteons represent about 10% of the total before age 30, increasing steadily to about 20% at age 80 (118). Although less well established, it is likely that a similar process occurs in trabecular bone. Whether focal reconstruction of this kind occurs in response to fatigue microdamage is unknown.

IMPLICATIONS OF QUANTAL REMODELING FOR THE UNDERSTANDING OF OSTEOPOROSIS

Quantal remodeling places certain constraints on the cellular mechanisms that underlie gains or losses of bone. First, after cessation of growth no mechanism exists for the *de novo* stimulation of lamellar bone formation without a preceding episode of bone resorption. Second, the rate of remodeling activation is the main determinant of whole body rates of resorption and formation and of the various biochemical and kinetic indices of bone turnover. Third, the focal bone balance in each remodeling unit, which is the difference between the total amount of bone resorbed by one team of osteoclasts and the total amount of bone formed by the succeeding team of osteoblasts, when summed for all units active on a surface in a defined time period, determines the direction of bone balance at that surface. Fourth, for a particular degree of focal remodeling imbalance as just defined, the magnitude of bone gain or loss at a surface is determined by the local rate of remodeling activation, and the summation of gain or loss at each surface in each bone determines the bone balance for the whole skeleton.

Quantal remodeling also imposes limitations on the accuracy with which serial measurements, whether of bone mass or indices of bone remodeling, can be extrapolated to determine future trends. The average duration of one complete cycle of remodeling—the remodeling period (or sigma in Frost's terminology)—constitutes a natural time unit for the skeleton because it is the minimum time required to establish a steady state response to any change in activation rate or in differentiated cell function. Observations made over a shorter time period will reflect mainly a variety of transient responses that are determined by the unchanging order in which remodeling events occur and the time intervals between them. As a particular and important instance of this generalization, each bone remodeling unit is associated with a reversible deficit of bone mineral that when integrated over the entire skeleton is of sufficient magnitude to influence measurements of bone mass and their interpretation. Consequently, there is a minimum duration of observation required to demonstrate the long-term response to therapeutic agents. This time period is determined by the biological characteristics of the remodeling system and cannot be shortened, no matter how much instrumental precision can be improved. Each of these points will now be examined in more detail.

No Lamellar Bone Formation in the Adult without Preceding Resorption

Because of its solidity, formation of new bone within the cortex can occur only where bone has been removed. This physical constraint does not apply to the periosteal or endosteal surface, and the evidence that here also bone formation is coupled spatially and temporally to bone resorption is less direct. Examination of the trabecular surface reveals only cavities in various stages of excavation and repair. Except for callus formation around an occasional microfracture (41,87), there are no localized excrescences such as would result from bone formation *de novo*. More compelling evidence is that (as in cortical bone) almost all cement lines have the scalloped configuration of reversal lines when examined in ground sections of unembedded bone (62). This important observation has recently been confirmed using an improved method for demonstrating cement lines in plastic embedded sections of trabecular bone (157). Consequently, the number, location and shape of the bone structural units are determined entirely by the number, location, and shape of the resorption cavities previously eroded by osteoclasts, and operating within this constraint, the osteoblasts control only the size of the newly formed structural units.

Some possible exceptions to this rule must be considered. Continued bone expansion after cessation of longitudinal growth, presumably by the subperiosteal apposition of new circumferential lamellae, has been demonstrated by sequential measurements in the metacarpal (122) and in the radius (67) and is probably a general phenomenon (59). But its extreme slowness, a net gain of 2.5 to 5.0 μm/year rather than 100 to 1000 μm/year as during growth, is much more in keeping with remodeling than with persistence of modeling, an interpretation that is strongly supported by histologic examination of ribs fortuitously labeled with tetracycline (43,122). Another candidate for direct transformation from a quiescent to a forming surface is the response to sodium fluoride administration (126), but it has recently been found that fluoride induced bone formation is preceded by a brief period of bone resorption, using the improved method of cement line demonstration previously mentioned (R.K. Schenk, personal communication). Yet another candidate is adaptation to mechanically induced strain (92), but there is no information on the initial cellular response.

If lining cells reverted directly to osteoblasts, some of the bone surface would temporarily lose its protective cellular covering. If this occurred without digestion of the endosteal membrane (23) it is conceivable that there could be recruitment of osteoblasts rather than osteoclasts, but the resultant new bone would be separated from the old bone by a thin layer of unmineralized tissue, which has never been observed. Direct transformation from quiescence to formation without intervening resorption is probably possible at the periosteum where there are usually two or more layers of potentially osteogenic cells. Apart from this, it seems likely that all apparent exceptions to the generalization that after cessation of growth lamellar bone formation does not occur without preceding resorption represent specialized forms of remodeling in which the balance within each cycle is shifted in favor of formation, to an extent that enables the new bone to spread beyond the confines of the resorption cavity and so to be no longer constrained by its shape.

Activation Determines Total Body Resorption and Formation

According to the quantum concept, the bone resorption rate (BRR) is the product of the number of new cavities eroded in a defined time period and the average volume of each cavity, and the bone formation rate (BFR) is the product of the number of new BSU completed in the same time period and the average volume of each new BSU. Each cavity and each new BSU is the result of one event of activation. Consequently, the number of new cavities and the number of new BSU are the same and are both equal to the rate of activation:

$$BRR = \text{activation rate} \times \text{mean cavity volume} \quad (1)$$

$$BFR = \text{activation rate} \times \text{mean BSU volume} \quad (2)$$

The average cavity and BSU volumes, although identical only for a short period after attainment of peak adult bone mass, do not usually differ by more than 10%, since the rate of bone loss averages about 1% of peak adult bone mass/year (57,109) and the whole body rate of turnover is about 10%/year, 4% in cortical bone and 25% in trabecular bone (129). These relationships hold whether resorption and formation are related to an area of bone surface, a volume of bone, a single whole bone, or the entire skeleton, and can be used to obtain internally consistent definitions of activation rate in terms of primary histologic measurements in both cortical and trabecular bone.

The essence of the argument is that differences between subjects are much greater for bone formation rate than for BSU volume, so that most of the individual variation in formation rate is the result of individual variation in rate of activation (91). It is difficult to measure BSU volume rigorously in three dimensions, but it is related to the two-dimensional measurement of mean wall thickness (MWT), which is the mean distance between the quiescent surface of a completed BSU and the nearest reversal line (Fig. 1). The CV for cortical bone formation rate in the rib is normally about 50%, but the CV for mean wall thickness is only about 7% (129). In the ilium, the CV for trabecular bone formation rate in normal premenopausal women is 55% whereas the CV for

MWT is 12%, with corresponding values for normal postmenopausal women of 50% and 11%. The CV for MWT is even smaller if the values are adjusted for the negative regression on age (4). Consequently, in both cortical and trabecular bone the resorption and formation rates are controlled by variation in the rate of activation rather than in the volumes of bone resorbed and formed by individual teams of osteoclasts and osteoblasts.

If bone turnover is increased or decreased it is often assumed that the individual cells, on which turnover depends, are working more quickly or more slowly, but this is to confuse the amount of work performed with the time taken to complete it. The relative constancy of mean wall thickness means that bone resorption and formation rates are largely independent of the rates of individual cell activity, which vary over a wide range (91). These conclusions are important for the interpretation of all kinetic and biochemical indices of bone turnover (139). Because they reflect the integrated remodeling activity of the entire skeleton, they are not affected by the sampling problems that are inescapable when bone remodeling is examined by histologic measurements on a bone biopsy. But from the preceding argument it is evident that all indices of whole body resorption or formation (see Chapter 9, *this volume*) are influenced mainly by changes in the whole body rate of remodeling activation and cannot be used to study the function of individual teams of osteoclasts and osteoblasts, still less the function of individual cells.

Events Within the Remodeling Unit Determine whether Bone is Gained or Lost

According to the quantum concept each bone remodeling unit adds or (more commonly) subtracts a small volume of bone, and it is the sum of all these small changes that constitutes bone balance at a particular surface, in each bone, and for the entire skeleton. If the average cavity is incompletely refilled with new bone this is both a necessary and a sufficient condition for bone to be lost at that surface (124,132). Consequently, the difference between resorption and formation necessary for the occurrence of bone gain or loss must be examined, not at the level of the whole body, but at the level of the individual remodeling unit. The cellular mechanisms responsible for focal remodeling imbalance will be examined in detail in a later section, but three general points will be made here.

First, there are systematic differences in the sign of focal balance between different surfaces. The average BRU adds a small volume of bone on the periosteal surface and subtracts a small volume of bone at the endosteal surface. There are also differences between the three subdivisions of the endosteal surface, imbalance being greatest on the endocortical, least on the intracortical, and intermediate on the trabecular surface (129). Especially noteworthy are the differences between the endocortical and trabecular surfaces, which are immediately adjacent to one another, have the same micro environment and have similar rates of activation, at least in the ilium. Second, during the brief plateau period after attainment of peak adult bone mass the average BRU neither adds nor subtracts bone, and with the onset of age-related loss the shift to net bone subtraction could result either from an increase in mean cavity depth with no change in the thickness of new bone deposited (osteoclast-dependent bone loss), or a decrease in thickness of new bone with no change in cavity depth (osteoblast-dependent bone loss), or from some combination of these changes (Fig. 4; 124). Third, once the BRU has run its course and the surface has reverted to quiescence, the remodeling transaction is completed, and any loss that resulted from the transaction is irrevocable and permanent. Replacement of the lost bone must await the next activation a few years later, and a favorable shift in balance in the BRU that will follow.

Activation Controls the Magnitude of Bone Gain or Loss

It is well-known that changes in the rate of bone turnover are associated with parallel

NORMAL – FOCAL
BONE BALANCE

OSTEOCLAST MEDIATED
BONE LOSS

OSTEOBLAST MEDIATED
BONE LOSS

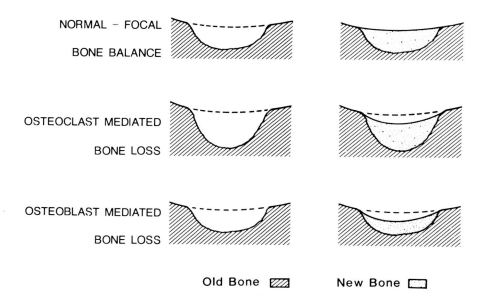

Old Bone 🔲   New Bone 🔲

FIG. 4. Possible mechanisms of focal remodeling imbalance. The upper panel shows a normal depth resorption cavity on the left, completely refilled with new bone on the right. The middle panel shows a resorption cavity of excessive depth that is incompletely refilled by a normal amount of new bone. The bottom panel shows a resorption cavity of normal depth that is incompletely refilled by a subnormal amount of new bone. Note that the extent of net bone loss resulting from a single cycle of remodeling, indicated by the difference between the new and old locations of the bone surface, can be the same, despite the difference in cellular mechanism. Modified from Parfitt, ref. 124, with permission.

changes in the rate of bone loss (26,159), a relationship that is a predictable consequence of quantal remodeling. Equations 1 and 2 in the previous section can be combined and rearranged to give:

(BRR-BFR) = Activation rate × (mean cavity volume–mean BSU volume)   (3)

As before, this relationship holds whether it refers to a single surface or to the entire skeleton or to any level in between. Consequently, for a given degree of remodeling imbalance, the rate of change in bone volume is proportional to the rate of remodeling activation. This holds for bone gain as well as for bone loss, and it explains why net periosteal apposition as well as net endosteal resorption are both faster in postmenopausal women than in men (58,122) and both faster in patients with primary hyperparathyroidism than in control subjects matched for age, sex and race (122,134). An increase in activation rate does not by itself cause bone loss (other than the temporary and reversible loss described on page 62), but amplifies the trend already established at a bone surface. Whether focal remodeling imbalance is the result of increased osteoclast number or efficiency or decreased osteoblast number or efficiency makes no difference to the relationship between the rate of activation and the rate of bone loss. It is for this reason that the defect in bone cell function responsible for bone loss cannot be inferred from any kinetic or biochemical indices of whole body bone turnover.

BRU Life Span is the Natural Time Unit of the Skeleton

If the skeleton is in a steady state, remodeling is asynchronous, with different cycles distributed randomly in time; some cycles have just begun, some are about to finish and most are somewhere in between. Bone lost at those locations where the BRU is in a resorptive stage is balanced by bone gained at other locations where the BRU is in a formative stage. If the steady state is disturbed, for example by an injury, or a large change in dietary calcium, or the onset of a disease, or the administration of a therapeutic agent, the initial response is usually a change in the rate of remodeling activation. This will be followed after a few weeks by a corresponding change in the rate of whole body bone resorption and a few months after that by a change in the same direction in whole body bone formation (55,120). Changes in the function of differentiated cells already present will also be followed by transient responses in a predictable sequence (129). The apparent effect of any perturbation will depend on the time of observation, and the long-term response can only be determined by waiting long enough for all remodeling transients to subside and a new steady state to be attained.

The waiting time required is related to but is longer than the remodeling period defined earlier. The time taken to complete a new BSU can be estimated from the relationship:

Formation period = mean wall thickness/osteoid apposition rate.

In a steady state fractions of space are equivalent to fractions of time, so that the resorption and reversal periods can be estimated from the relative surface extents of these activities in relation to the surface extent of formation, and the duration of the entire remodeling period derived. This is the time needed to rebuild from the cement line to the new surface *at a single location*. But the resorption front may continue to advance through the bone or across the surface after formation in one location has been completed (129). Consequently the life span of the entire BRU is longer, probably by at least a factor of 2, than the remodeling period as just defined. Since the immediate effects of the perturbation may not be fully developed for several weeks or months, the total time required to attain a new steady state after the onset of a perturbation is probably close to three times the remodeling period calculated on the basis of cross-sectional events at a single location on the bone surface.

This time is so long (close to a year) that mi-

nor perturbations of bone remodeling probably occur with sufficient frequency to ensure that no one's skeleton is ever strictly in a steady state. The resultant oscillations will in most cases be small, but will weaken the significance of changes observed in an individual subject over a short period of time, and make it more difficult to detect relationships in a group of subjects, such as between indices of resorption and formation. The oscillations will also complicate the interpretation of bone histomorphometry. Ideally, all equal intervals of time during the remodeling sequence should have an equal probability of being intercepted, but this is possible only if bone remodeling was in a steady state during the three weeks or so before the biopsy, adding the problem of sampling variation in time to the well-known problem of sampling variation in space (129).

Activation Controls the Remodeling-Dependent Reversible Mineral Deficit

Because of the time interval between resorption and formation, each BRU is associated with a temporary deficit of bone mineral, of which there are three components (121). First is the volume of bone that has been removed and will eventually be replaced, or remodeling space, which depends on the duration of the reversal phase. Because of the geometry of the cutting and closing cones the physical reality of the remodeling space is easy to appreciate in cortical bone (Fig. 5), but the resorption lacunae and osteoid seams on trabecular surfaces collectively exemplify the same concept (Fig. 6). The second component is the volume of new osteoid that will eventually be mineralized, which depends on the time between matrix apposition and mineralization, or the mean mineralization lag time; remodeling space and osteoid together can be regarded as potential bone. The third component arises from the low density of recently formed bone, and depends on the time required for completion of mineralization. Within a few days of the onset of mineralization bone density increases rapidly to about 1.4 g/cm^3 (primary mineralization) and

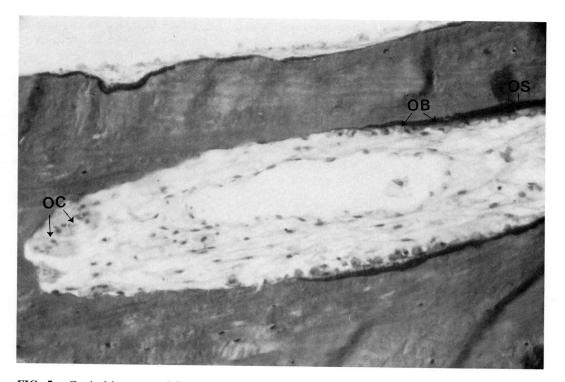

FIG. 5. Cortical bone remodeling unit in human iliac bone. Osteoclasts (OC) are eroding a longitudinal cavity from right to left, which is being refilled centripetally by osteoblasts (OB) lining an osteoid seam (OS). The cavity is currently filled with loose fibrous and vascular connective tissue most of which will eventually be replaced by osteonal bone, leaving only a Haversian canal.

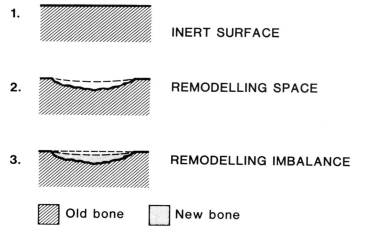

1.   INERT SURFACE

2.   REMODELLING SPACE

3.   REMODELLING IMBALANCE

Old bone   New bone

FIG. 6. Distinction between reversible and irreversible bone loss. Erosion of a resorption cavity on a previously inert trabecular bone surface creates a temporary deficit of bone referred to as remodeling space, most of which will be replaced. At the completion of bone formation, incomplete refilling of the cavity leaves a permanent bone deficit. Compare with Figure 2. From Parfitt, ref. 138, with permission.

then increases slowly to about 2.0 g/cm³ over the next 6 to 12 months (secondary mineralization). The sum of the three components is the total turnover related reversible mineral deficit (RMD); the deficit is reversible because replacement of each component is inevitable as the BRU completes its evolution and the new bone reaches maturity (121).

The sequential changes in bone and mineral balance produced by five stages in the life history of a single cortical BRU are shown dia-grammatically in Fig. 7, on the assumption that all of the bone removed is eventually replaced. For the first 20 days resorption occurs alone. For the next 80 days resorption continues at the same rate, and formation gradually increases until a complete osteon is formed. Resorption and formation then remain equal as the BRU continues to advance longitudinally. When, after an unknown time, the advance stops, resorption gradually diminishes over about 20 days, but formation continues at the

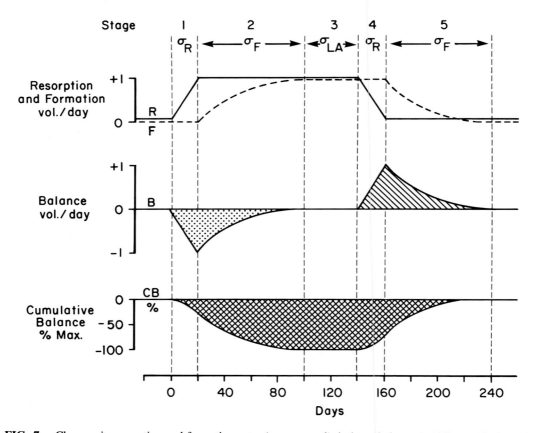

FIG. 7. Changes in resorption and formation rates *(upper panel)*, in bone balance *(middle panel)*, in arbitrary units of bone volume per day and in cumulative balance *(lower panel)* as percent of maximum deviation in balance, during five stages in the evolution of a single cortical remodeling unit. Curvilinear segments are due to more rapid bone formation or beginning of osteon closure. σ_R = duration of resorption in cross section (20 days), σ_F = duration of formation in cross section (80 days), and σ_{LA} = duration of longitudinal advance during which resorption and formation continue at the same rate; this duration is unknown but is arbitrarily taken as $0.5\sigma_F$. Note that entire life span of remodeling unit = $3\sigma_F$. From Parfitt and Kleerekoper. (1980): The divalent ion homeostatic system: Physiology and metabolism of calcium, phosphorus, magnesium and bone. In: *Clinical Disorders of Fluid and Electrolyte Metabolism,* 3rd ed., edited by M. Maxwell and C.R. Kleeman, pp. 269–398. McGraw Hill, New York, with permission.

same rate. Finally, after cessation of resorption, formation continues alone at a diminishing rate for a further 80 days until a new osteon is completed; for simplicity the continuation of secondary mineralization is not shown. These five stages are less clearly defined in trabecular BRU. The extent to which mineral homeostasis is disturbed by the BRU depends on the balance at any instant, but the extent to which bone mass is disturbed depends on the cumulative balance (Fig. 7); when the daily balance is maximally negative the cumulative negative balance is small, and when the cumulative balance is maximally negative the daily balance is zero.

From a large body of histomorphometric data, the combined volume of remodeling space and osteoid tissue in all the BRU in a skeleton with a normal rate of bone turnover is about 18cm^3 (121,129), corresponding to a deficit of about 11 g of calcium; the deficit includes phosphate, magnesium and other constituents of bone mineral, but is most conveniently specified in terms of calcium alone. The additional deficit associated with recently formed low density bone normally amounts to about 4 g calcium; the combined total RMD of 15 g, about 1.5% of total body calcium in a woman, is the amount by which total body calcium would increase if activation and remodeling were to fall to zero (121,123). Conversely, in response to an increase in the rate of remodeling activation, all three components of the RMD would increase in the same proportion. For example, if activation and turnover abruptly increased by four-fold, the RMD would increase to 60g and total body calcium would fall by about 4%.

The sequential changes in whole body bone and mineral balance that would result are shown diagrammatically in 7 stages in Fig. 8. For the first 80 days the balance gets progressively more negative. For the next 60 days the negative daily balance remains at the same level as the continued addition of new units offsets the progressive changes in existing units, but the cumulative balance continues to worsen. The negative daily balance then gradually diminishes over the next 80 days as the oldest systems enter their replacement phase, and the cumulative balance approaches a plateau. The daily balance then returns to zero, and a new steady state is achieved in which the cumulative bone and mineral deficit remains unchanged for as long as the increase in activation and turnover persists. When these return to the previous levels, the next three stages are mirror images of the first three (Figure 8). The relationship between daily and cumulative balance is similar for the aggregate of all units as for a single unit. The negative daily bone and mineral balance lasts for approximately 8 months, and the total calcium deficit of 45 g corresponds to an average daily loss of about 200 mg and a peak daily loss of about 300 mg, most of which will occur as increased urinary calcium excretion. Reverse changes of equal magnitude and equal duration occur when activation and turnover return to normal.

Expansion of remodeling space is radiographically more evident in cortical than in trabecular bone. The deficit in bone is relatively smaller in the cortex, but the increase in porosity is relatively much greater. Also, because of the difference in BRU geometry (Figs. 5 and 6), individual resorption cavities are much larger in the cortex and an increase in their number is visible on high quality radiographs as an increase in longitudinal striation (105, 172). Conversely, except in osteomalacia, an increase in cortical striation is a reliable index of an increase in remodeling activation and bone turnover. Such increases in radiographic as well as in biochemical indices of bone remodeling are evident soon after menopause (60,135). A reversible increase in cortical porosity is also found during the prepubertal growth spurt (84,135,172), during late pregnancy and lactation (123) and during the antler growth cycle in deer (123). In large animals, physiologic demands for calcium are met by drawing, not on trabecular bone, as is the popular belief, but on cortical bone, from which much more calcium can be removed with much less compromise to the structural integrity of the skeleton (123).

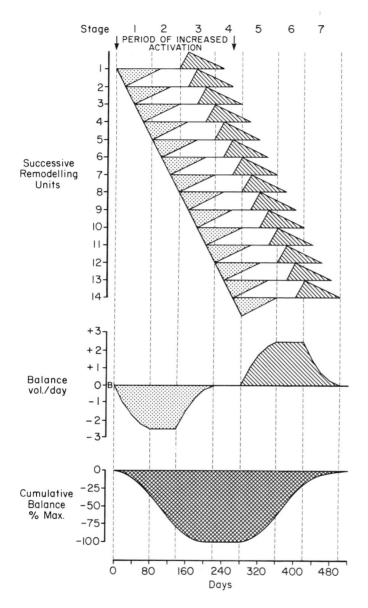

FIG. 8. Changes in bone balance caused by succession of new remodeling units initiated after an increase in activation at time zero *(upper panel)*. Each of units 1 to 14 is similar to the middle panel of Fig. 7, except that curvilinear segments are shown as linear for simplicity. No further new units are initiated after t = 250 days, when activation returns to the previous level. Summation of bone balances of individual units at different phases at the same time *(middle panel)* leads to seven stages in total response. For example, at 220 days the different stages of negative balance in units 8 to 11 offset exactly the different stages of positive balance in units 1 to 4, units 5 to 7 being in zero balance. The cumulative balance is shown in lower panel; scales as in Fig. 7. From Parfitt and Kleerekoper (1980): The divalent ion homeostatic system: Physiology and metabolism of calcium, phosphorus, magnesium and bone. In: *Clinical Disorders of Fluid and Electrolyte Metabolism,* 3rd ed., edited by M. Maxwell and C.R. Kleeman, pp. 269–398. McGraw Hill, New York, with permission.

MICROSTRUCTURAL CONSEQUENCES AND CELLULAR MECHANISMS OF BONE LOSS

Age-related bone loss at the macroscopic level was briefly described on page 50, but bone is a structural material that undergoes changes in internal architecture as well as in mass and external dimensions. An accurate description of the microanatomic changes is an essential basis for understanding the disorders of bone cell function that are responsible, and the possibilities for therapeutic intervention.

Cortical Bone Loss

This process is considered first because it is the major element in most descriptions of bone loss at the macroscopic level and because it is geometrically simpler than loss of trabecular bone. Removal of bone from the inner cortical surface is apparent from measurements on X-rays, but in some bones removal from within the cortex makes an additional contribution to the fall in total bone mineral mass. Detectable only by histologic examination or by measurement of bone tissue density, this permanent increase in cortical porosity must be distinguished from the temporary increase manifested radiographically as longitudinal striation that occurs in all states of high bone turnover, including menopausal estrogen deficiency. Age-related changes in porosity increase in severity from the periosteum to the endosteum. In the outer half of the cortex the total change is small (an increase of 1 to 2%) and is mostly accounted for by the rise in number of Haversian canals that inevitably follows the continued formation of new osteons (31,100), with a lesser contribution from increase in the size of some canals (7,77). In the inner half of the cortex the total change in porosity is much greater (an increase of 5 to 10%) and is due mainly to an increase in the size of the spaces rather than in their number.

The differences in type and extent of porosity between the outer and inner regions of the cortex are related to the mechanism of cortical thinning (132). Many of the large spaces originate from resorption cavities on the endocortical surface rather than from intracortical canals, so that the subendosteal spaces communicate with, and can be regarded as extensions of, the marrow cavity, which consequently expands in volume (7,9,81). Enlargement and coalescence of the cavities transforms the inner third or more of the original cortex into a tissue that resembles trabecular bone in porosity and surface:volume ratio but with structural elements that are thicker and more irregular in size and shape (Fig. 9). The discontinuity of radiographic image that results from a sufficient increase in inner cortical porosity underlies the measured reduction in cortical thickness with age. When this process occurs next to existing trabecular bone, as in the ilium, it forms the so-called transitional zone (81). Adding to the volume of trabecular bone tissue

in this manner partly offsets loss of some of the original bone in the marrow cavity, so that the absolute volume of trabecular bone may not change much even though its relative volume (analogous to concentration) falls.

Trabecular Bone Loss

Despite the complexity of structure of trabecular bone, until recently most histologic studies reported only the single measurement of the proportion of tissue occupied by bone, or trabecular bone volume. It is often stated by nonhistologists that trabecular bone loss occurs mainly because the structural elements become thinner, but the fall in amount is relatively much greater than the fall in thickness. If the predominant structural element is a plate, mean trabecular thickness can be estimated from the perimeter and area of bone in two-dimensional histologic sections (141). If the predominant structural element is a rod, the method underestimates the mean diameter (95), but the reasonable agreement between direct and indirect methods supports the plate model at least as a first approximation. Assuming the plates to be parallel, the density (number/mm) and separation of the trabeculae can be calculated, and the total amount of bone partitioned into independent components of trabecular thickness and trabecular density. Although this is a considerable oversimplification, it is an improvement on ignoring microstructure altogether. The calculated value for trabecular density is a reasonable index of the probability that a scanning line will intercept a structural element of bone, and the calculated separation is a reasonable index of the average diameter of the marrow cavities between the structural elements of bone. Consequently, a fall in plate density and an increase in plate separation both indicate that some structural elements have been completely removed, and that those remaining are less completely connected (85,141).

Using this simple model, loss of axial trabecular bone in women after menopause can be shown to occur predominantly by reduction in the ''number'' of trabeculae, rather than in

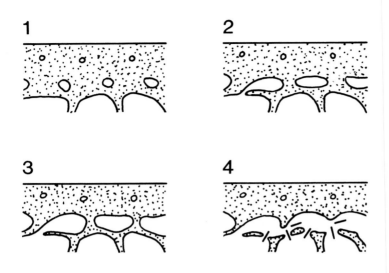

FIG. 9. Microscopic evolution of cortical bone loss. Successive stages in osteoclast-dependent thinning of cortical bone. 1. Normal adult cortex with larger Haversian canals closer to the inner cortical surface. 2. Enlargement of subendosteal spaces and communication with the marrow cavity. 3. Further enlargement and conversion of the inner third of the cortex to a structure that topologically resembles trabecular bone, with expansion of the marrow cavity. 4. Perforation and disconnection of the new trabecular structures. From Parfitt, ref. 132, with permission.

their thickness (85,141). More accurately, there is loss of the central regions of the plates, a process that begins with focal perforation (5), and continues by enlargement of the perforation to a window 100 to 400 μm wide (fenestration; 40). The border of the window is topologically a saddle surface, since the local curvature is concave in the plane of the plate, but convex in planes normal to the plate. Further enlargement of the windows will eventually complete the conversion of the plates into a lattice of bars and rods (6), some of which in turn may be transected or even completely removed, with progressive replacement of predominantly concave by predominantly convex surfaces. Although it is impossible to make serial observations in the same location, all stages in this sequence have been demonstrated directly by scanning electron microscopy (34). The architectural disruption is more severe in patients with vertebral fracture than in normal subjects of the same age (85).

Since the process occurs irregularly, the remaining structural elements are less well connected, with more isolated profiles in a two-dimensional histologic section (Fig. 10). The residual elements also slowly become thinner, but this makes a smaller contribution to the total loss of bone than the reduction in their number. The marrow spaces are increased in size as the result of complete removal of part of their walls, so that spaces that were previously separated coalesce, a process that is conceptually similar to the enlargement of alveoli in an emphysematous lung. Exactly the same mechanisms underly loss of the new trabecular bone that arises from the inner cortex (Fig. 9). The complete removal of structural elements has implications for the cellular mechanisms of bone loss (page 69), and for bone strength and fracture risk (page 76). Even more important are the consequences for therapeutic intervention (page 82), since the loss is not only permanent in the sense of being irrevocable (page 60), but cannot ever be repaired by normal bone remodeling, since there is no longer a surface on which osteoblasts can work.

Although the quantitative basis of this model of trabecular bone loss has been derived mainly from the ilium, the changes in the spine are qualitatively similar (5,6,10,40,41,148, 161). There is preferential loss of horizontally disposed structures in the spine (10,161), but the *in vivo* orientation of trabecular loss in the ilium cannot be determined by present methods. Removal of horizontal structures in the spine is widely believed to initiate compensatory thickening of the remaining vertical structures which are subject to increased mechanical strain, but this belief rests mainly on misinterpretation of the radiographic appearance of ac-

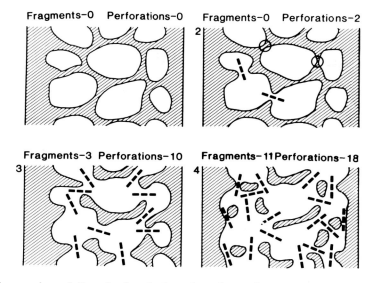

FIG. 10. Microscopic evolution of trabecular bone loss. Successive stages in the conversion of the continuous trabecular network present at skeletal maturity to the discontinuous network seen in the elderly. Fragments are isolated trabecular profiles seen in the two-dimensional section; they are connected in the third dimension rather than lying free in the marrow space. Perforations are the focal breaks in continuity postulated to initiate trabecular bone loss, that bring adjacent but separated marrow cavities into communication. The same changes occur in the new trabecular bone that arises from the inner third of the cortex as shown in Fig. 9. From Parfitt, ref. 132, with permission.

centuated vertical striation, supplemented by a few anecdotal reports, and is not supported by the only available histologic measurements (132). Local hypertrophy from callus occurs during healing of microscopic fractures of individual trabeculae (4), but the ultimate effect of this process on trabecular dimensions is conjectural. An apparent increase in mean trabecular thickness in some individuals could result from the preferential removal of thinner structures. Whether compensatory thickening of trabeculae is possible and if so, whether it can fail to occur in some individuals, are important but currently unanswered questions.

Types of Focal Remodeling Imbalance

The concept that focal remodeling imbalance is both a necessary and a sufficient condition for the occurrence of bone loss was briefly mentioned on page 60 and must now be examined in more detail. The size and shape of a resorption cavity depend on the direction and rate of advance, or velocity, and duration of activity of a team of osteoclasts, that together determine the distance which the resorption front will travel through the bone. Similarly, the total amount of bone formed within the cavity depends on the velocity and duration of activity of a corresponding team of osteoblasts, that together determine how far the formation front will travel through the bone (129). For both osteoclasts and osteoblasts, velocity, time and distance are interrelated variables. The distance traveled (a measure of the work to be completed) and the rate of advance (a measure of individual cell vigor) are independent variables, and time is the dependent variable. This is because bone cells are work-oriented rather than time-oriented, they are programmed to carry out a particular amount of work (however long it takes), rather than to work only for a particular period of time (however little has been accomplished).

Whatever its cellular basis, remodeling imbalance must be much greater on the endocortical than on the trabecular surface, at least in women, since the rate of loss is a much higher proportion of the rate of turnover in cortical than in trabecular bone. At the inner cortical surface of the metacarpal, the mean net loss of bone between the ages of 40 and 70 years in normal female subjects is about 50 μm/year (122). In the ilium, various indices of bone remodeling are very similar on the endocortical and trabecular surfaces (81,147). Mean wall thickness falls with age (Fig. 11) and from the rate at which this occurs, it can be estimated that the mean net loss of bone in a single remodeling cycle, assuming no change in cavity depth, is unlikely to exceed 10 μm. With representative values for formation period of 100 days, and for the fraction of surface covered by osteoid of 20%, the mean time interval between the beginning of successive remodeling cycles at the same location is 500 days (100/0.2). Consequently, the net annual loss of metacarpal cortical bone explainable on the basis of the observed reduction in mean wall thickness alone is only 7.3 μm/year (100 × 365/500), or about one-seventh of the observed rate of loss (132).

Clearly the remodeling imbalance that leads to cortical thinning must be mainly due to an increase in resorption cavity depth, since this is the only way in which removal of subendosteal cortrical bone at the rate of 50 μm/year could possibly occur, a conclusion already implicit in the description of its morphologic features. Most of the large subendosteal resorption cavities in the femur become lined by new lamellar bone with a wall thickness of 70 to 80 μm, which is appropriate for the age of the subject and for the location of remodeling within the cortex, but is far too small to repair the cavities (7). In normal human subjects the surface extent of osteoclastic resorption increases after menopause, but the increase is more evident on the endocortical than on the trabecular surface (Table 2). In patients with osteoporosis, the amount of bone removed by each cycle of remodeling on the endocortical surface of the rib estimated indirectly from double tetracycline labeling is significantly increased (176), and the same is evidently also true in the ilium (81). The initial increase in resorption cavity depth makes more surface available for remodeling, so that for a given degree of focal remodeling imbalance the rate of bone loss is amplified by positive geometric feedback (98).

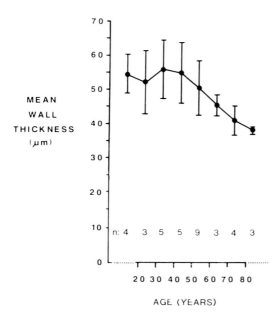

FIG. 11. Effect of age on mean wall thickness. Data from Lips et al., ref. 94. Decade-specific values (mean ± SD) estimated from the individual values depicted. Although there is a significant negative regression on age for the entire data set, it appears more likely that there is no change before age 50 and a linear fall of about 4 μm/decade after age 50.

TABLE 2. *Osteoclast surfaces in ilium—effect of menopause in normal subjects*

	Menopausal status		% change	p
	Pre	Post		
n	24	27		
Trabecular surface	0.46	0.68	+ 48	< 0.05
Endocortical surface	0.34	0.70	+ 106	< 0.05
Intracortical surface	0.41	0.69	+ 68	< 0.05
Combined total surface	0.44	0.69	+ 57	< 0.02

Data expressed as percent of total surface.

In the outer half of the cortex there is no increase in the size of resorption cavities with age (7,31,100), but there is an increase in the number of incompletely closed osteons, which contributes modestly to the increase in total porosity, more so in the femur than in the rib (7,77,100). Incomplete closure can occur in at least three ways. First, there are small resorption cavities in which formation never occurs (72); these are probably attempts at focal reconstruction that for some reason are aborted. Second, there can be a permanent deficit, in the sense explained on page 60, because of premature cessation of bone formation and reduced wall thickness (78,100). Third, radial closure can be greatly prolonged (55,117), presumably because of the same kind of age-related osteoblast defect as is found in trabecular bone. There is also an increase in the number of osteons of relatively low mineral density by microradiography (78,117), but it is unclear whether this reflects an independent defect that results in a permanent failure to complete secondary mineralization, or is a necessary consequence of the retardation of radial osteon closure. Finally, it is possible that following osteocyte death the bone adjacent to the Haversian canal of a completed osteon may crumble away like weathered stone, a possibility referred to by its proponents as delitescence (36).

The most commonly emphasized form of remodeling imbalance in trabecular bone is that osteoblasts deposit new layers of bone that are too shallow (28,94), accounting for the fall in mean wall thickness with increasing age (Fig. 11), an abnormality that is even more evident in patients with various forms of osteoporosis (32,168). Although this is most likely a genuine and important phemomenon, its occurrence and magnitude are subject to a subtle and previously unrecognized sampling bias. If, as is indicated by the usual maintenance of smooth contours on trabecular bone surfaces, the depth of new bone deposited is correlated with the depth of the resorption cavity, structures with high values for mean wall thickness would be the first to disappear, because their resorption cavities would be deeper and so more likely to cause focal perforation (Fig. 12). The apparent fall in mean wall thickness with age in a cross-sectional study (Fig. 11) might simply reflect the preferential survival of structures subject to less vigorous remodeling.

Even discounting this possibility, a reduction in wall thickness is an unlikely explanation for plate perforation. Unless repeated cycles of remodeling occurred preferentially at exactly the same location, for which there is no evidence, plate perforation by this mechanism would be preceded by a generalized reduction in thickness. A significant increase in trabecular separation occurs at an earlier age than a fall in trabecular thickness, and there is no increase with age in the accumulation of thinner than normal structural elements (169). Furthermore, mean interstitial bone thickness in-

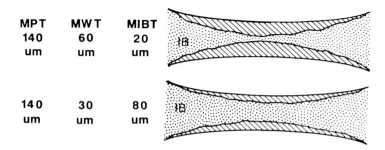

MPT	MWT	MIBT
140	60	20
um	um	um

140	30	80
um	um	um

FIG. 12. Sampling bias in apparent age-dependence of mean wall thickness (MWT). Sections through two trabeculae with similar values for mean plate thickness (MPT). If MWT is higher, mean interstitial bone thickness (MIBT) is lower and the probability of perforation is increased because of greater resorption cavity depth. Because of complete removal, the site will no longer be available for sampling.

creases with age, implying that resorption
cavities become shallower and so less likely to
cause perforation (28). Finally, if perforation
was the culmination of a progressive reduction
in thickness, the entire process would take too
long to account for the rate at which complete
structural elements are removed. From the observed regression of mean wall thickness on
age (94) the fall in the first five years after
menopause would be less than 3 μm, and with
the same assumptions about remodeling as in
the discussion of cortical thinning, trabecular
plate thickness would fall only by about 2
μm/year.

These arguments indicate that the loss of trabecular bone that is initiated by plate perforation and fenestration cannot be explained on
the basis of incomplete refilling of normal size
resorption cavities, and so must have the same
cellular basis as cortical thinning increased
depth of osteoclastic penetration. Two mechanisms for this have been proposed. Even if
mean resorption depth and formation thickness
are equal, the scatter in normal values for cavity depth and trabecular thickness is so wide
that random coincidence of deep cavities and
thin plates will lead to some minimum rate of
plate perforation (Fig. 13; 152). This may be
one reason why trabecular bone begins to be
lost as soon as it is formed by endochondral
ossification during growth (82) and why its
loss is resumed soon after attainment of peak
adult bone mass in both sexes (7,29,39,
96,154). The increase in remodeling activation
and bone turnover as a non-specific consequence of estrogen deficiency would inevitably
increase the probability of perforation by this
mechanism in the first few years after menopause.

An alternative theory attributes the acceleration of bone loss after menopause to the emergence of "killer osteoclasts" that rapidly erode
deeper than normal cavities as a specific consequence, direct or indirect, of estrogen deficiency (Fig. 14; 133). Such a mechanism can
be observed within a few days of spinal immobilization in monkeys, the earliest time of onset of a resorption cavity being indicated by

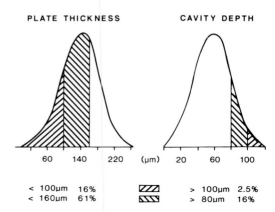

FREQUENCY DISTRIBUTION:

| PLATE THICKNESS | | CAVITY DEPTH |

| < 100μm | 16% | | > 100μm | 2.5% |
| < 160μm | 61% | | > 80μm | 16% |

FIG. 13 Plate perforation as a random process.
Predicted effect of variations in trabecular thickness
and in resorption cavity depth at different locations
on the probability of perforation. If the two variables are uncorrelated, perforation from one side
will occur with a probability of (0.16)(0.025)
= 0.4% of single activation events, and from two
sides simultaneously with a probability of
(0.61)(0.16)² = 1.56% of simultaneous activation
events on opposite sides of the plate. The probabilities will be smaller if plate thickness and cavity
depth are correlated. From Medical management of
cardiovascular, hypertensive and metabolic diseases
in the elderly, edited by J. Sowers et al. *Am.J. Med.
(Suppl)* (in press), with permission.

erosion through surfaces recently labeled with
tetracycline (101). Limited data on complete
remodeling sequence reconstruction in normal
subjects suggest an increase in resorption cavity depth in females but not males between the
ages of 50 and 60 years (45), but such a process remains to be directly demonstrated in trabecular bone in human subjects. Nevertheless
it seems likely that the cellular mechanism is
the same as on the endocortical surface, but re-
moves less bone because reduction of surface
available for remodeling diminishes the rate of
bone loss, an example of negative geometric
feedback (98). It is important to decide which
of the two theories is correct, because as will
be discussed on page 86, they have quite different implications for therapeutic intervention.

The decline in mean wall thickness with age

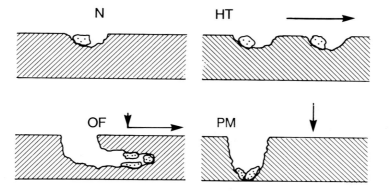

FIG. 14. Three morphologically different types of increased bone resorption. In normal state (N) a resorption cavity containing an osteoclast is depicted. In HT (hyperthyroidism) there is an increased number of resorption cavities each of normal size and shape. The predominant direction of osteoclast movement is parallel to the bone surface. In OF (osteitis fibrosa) the osteoclasts have eroded more deeply into the bone and then changed direction to undermine the surface by dissecting intratrabecular resorption. In PM (post-menopausal state) the osteoclasts have eroded a deeper than normal cavity on the way to complete perforation of the trabecular plate. The predominant direction of osteoclast movement is perpendicular to the surface. These three types of increased resorption cannot be distinguished by any combination of noninvasive diagnostic procedures. Modified from Parfitt, ref. 133, with permission.

can be demonstrated directly, at least in some locations in cortical bone, and is only partly explainable by differential survival in trabecular bone, since the frequency distribution does not become substantially more skewed with increasing age (44,94). The decline in wall thickness is accompanied by a parallel decline in the rate of radial osteon closure (55,166) and the corresponding index in trabecular bone of osteoid apposition rate (142). As a result the formation period is prolonged with corresponding increases in osteoid surface, mineralization lag time and osteoid volume (Fig. 15). These changes indicate a generalized age related impairment of the activity of teams of osteoblasts, both in the rate and in the total amount of matrix synthesis (Fig. 16). The defect accounts for the progressive decline in mean trabecular thickness throughout life and the decline in cortical thickness at locations where cancellization of the inner third is less evident. The defect would also be expected to compromise the compensatory thickening of trabeculae in response to biomechanical stimuli, if such a process is possible.

Two independent explanations can be proposed. First, the number of osteoblasts that are assembled on the cement line probably falls with age. This could reflect a defect in one or more of the coupling signals mentioned earlier (125), or a decline in the availability of precursor cells. The age-related decline in the proportion of hematopoietic marrow relative to fatty marrow is well-known (39,108), but whether the marrow stromal stem cells that are the ultimate cells of origin of osteoblasts are also involved is unclear. An extreme example of osteoblast recruitment failure occurs when attempts at focal reconstruction are aborted, as in cortical bone, a phenomenon that underlies the age-related increase in the extent of eroded surface lacking osteoclasts but covered by flat lining cells (13,129). Secondly, there is probably an age-related decline in the total amount of bone matrix that one osteoblast is able to make, analogous to the age related decline in the function of other collagen synthesizing cells such as skin fibroblasts (120,125). The relative importance of these two possible mechanisms is unknown, because separate measurements of cell number and individual cell activity are unavailable.

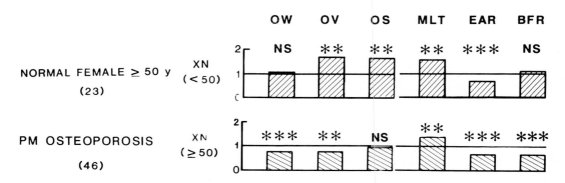

FIG. 15. Formation indices in iliac trabecular bone, effect of age and osteoporosis. The upper panel compares normal women over age 50 with normal women under age 50. The lower panel compares patients with vertebral compression fractures due to postmenopausal osteoporosis with normal women of comparable age. Data are expressed as the ratios of the mean values between groups compared. OW = osteoid width; OV = osteoid volume; OS = osteoid surface; MLT = mineralization lag time; EAR = effective apposition rate; BFR = bone formation rate/unit of bone surface. Each of the three static indices is dependent on a different pair of kinetic indices: OW depends on MLT and EAR, OV on MLT and BFR, and OS on EAR and BFR (131). *p < 0.05, **p < 0.01, ***p < 0.001.

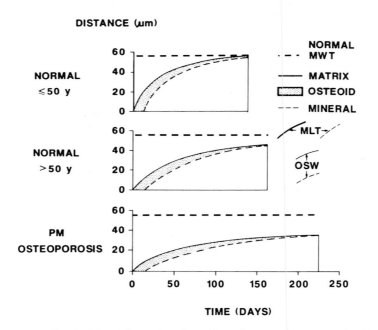

FIG. 16. Time course of typical bone formation site, effect of age and osteoporosis. The curves depict the outer boundaries of movement of total bone matrix and mineralized bone matrix away from the cement line as functions of time (44,129,146). The slopes of these lines at any point indicate the instantaneous rates of matrix apposition and mineral apposition. When the two curves meet, the new structural unit is completed. At this point the vertical distance from the baseline indicates the wall thickness of the new BSU and the horizontal distance from the origin indicates the formation period. The vertical distance between the curved lines indicates the osteoid seam width at any time from the commencement of bone formation and the horizontal difference between the curved lines indicates the mineralization lag time at any distance from the cement line. Note that the effect of age is to reduce wall thickness and prolong the formation period, and that these age-related changes are more pronounced in patients with compression fracture.

Rapid and Slow Bone Loss—The Two Stage Concept

The general concept that emerges from the preceding discussion is of two fundamentally distinct mechanisms of bone loss that have different cellular defects, remodeling mechanisms, morphologic features, structural effects and biomechanical consequences (Table 3; 132). One type of bone loss is the result of excessive depth of osteoclastic resorption leading in trabecular bone to perforation of structural elements (Fig. 17), increased size of marrow cavities and discontinuity of the bone structure, and in cortical bone to subendosteal cavitation and conversion of the inner third of the cortex to a trabecular-like structure which then undergoes the same changes as the trabecular bone originally present. These structural characteristics reduce the strength of the bones to a greater extent than the reduction in the amount of bone by itself would suggest. A second type of bone loss results from incomplete refilling by osteoblasts of resorption cavities of normal or reduced size, leading to simple thinning of residual structural elements in both trabecular and cortical bone and a proportionate reduction in bone strength (Fig. 17).

The two types of bone loss differ also in timing, rate, and magnitude (Table 3). In part, these additional differences could be predicted from the cellular and morphologic features, but they also reflect the interaction between the type of focal remodeling imbalance and the frequency of remodeling activation which, as

explained on page 60, is the main determinant of the rate of bone loss. The osteoclast-dependent type of bone loss is often accompanied by an *increase* in remodeling activation, whereas the osteoblast dependent type of bone loss is more often accompanied by a *decrease* in remodeling activation. Although these associations are by no means invariable, they exemplify the important general principle that activation as an event, and cell activity as a process, frequently change in the same direction. Proliferation and differentiation of precursor cells and the function of the resultant differentiated cells evidently have some control factors in common as well as other control factors that are separate. Further examples are the increases in both remodeling activation and initial matrix apposition rate in renal osteitis fibrosa (146), and the depression of both remodeling activation and osteoclast function by calcitonin (130).

A sustained increase in total body bone resorption is always associated with an increase in remodeling activation, but there may or may not also be an increase in the size and a change in the shape of resorption cavities because of an increase in the vigor and/or lifetime work capacity of individual osteoclasts, qualitative abnormalities in osteoclast function that do not usually occur in isolation. For example, in hyperthyroidism teams of osteoclasts and osteoblasts work more rapidly (46), another example of the phenomenon just mentioned. Nevertheless, resorption cavities are morphologically normal (Figure 14) and any irrevers-

TABLE 3. *Comparison of two morphologic types of bone loss*

Characteristic	Osteoclast-mediated	Osteoblast-mediated
Cellular defect	Lack of restraint	Lack of number
Remodeling mechanism	Deeper resorption	Shallower formation
Structure		
trabecular	Perforation and disconnection	Simple thinning
cortical	Subendosteal cavitation	Simple thinning
Reduction in strength	More than predicted[a]	As predicted[a]
Timing	Early	Late
Rate	Rapid	Slow
Magnitude	Usually greater	Usually less
Activation	Often increased	Often decreased

[a]From reduction in mass or mineral content. Modified from Parfitt, ref. 132, with permission.

RAPID LOSS   **SLOW LOSS**

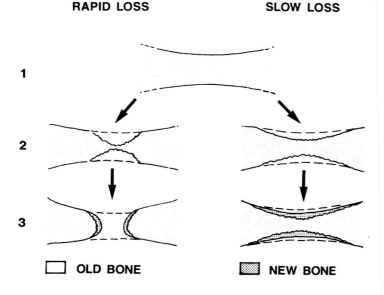

FIG. 17. Rapid and slow loss of trabecular bone. Rapid loss is osteoclast-dependent with increased resorption cavity depth and plate perforation leading to reduction in plate density. Slow loss is osteoblast-dependent with reduced wall thickness and plate thickness (compare with Fig. 4). Modified from Parfitt, ref. 124, with permission.

☐ OLD BONE   ▨ NEW BONE

ible bone loss results from the amplification of existing remodeling imbalance together with the stochastic mechanism described earlier (152). Similarly, mild hyperparathyroidism does not increase mean resorption cavity depth on the trabecular surface (47) except when secondary to calcium malabsorption (143). When hyperparathyroidism is severe enough to cause osteitis fibrosa, the osteoclasts travel further than normal but dissect *within* rather than perforating *through* the trabeculae (156), so that the original structure is usually preserved (Fig. 14).

The combination of increased remodeling activation together with increased rate and depth of bone resorption by individual osteoclast teams occurs most commonly in the first few years after menopause, accounting not only for the accelerated loss of bone during this period but for the architectural disruption that is of greatest biomechanical significance, and giving rise to the focal defects in vertebral trabecular bone that can be detected by quantitated computed tomography within two years of oophorectomy (20). The stage is now set for the development in some individuals of a significant increase in bone fragility and fracture risk. In most women, the rates of remodeling

activation and bone loss both decline after the first few years, and the balance gradually shifts away from osteoclast-dependent rapid bone loss towards osteoblast-dependent slow bone loss, a shift that is usually earlier and more pronounced in trabecular than in cortical bone (154). In animal models increased resorption cavity depth is found soon after high dose corticosteroid administration (138), extremity immobilization (71), and spinal immobilization probably combined with autonomic and adrenal stimulation (101), and it is likely that all clinically significant forms of bone loss evolve through these two successive stages.

FRACTURE PATHOGENESIS: QUANTITATIVE AND QUALITATIVE ASPECTS

Any fracture results from the interplay of three factors—the energy released by the injury or fall, the proportion of this energy dissipated by soft tissue absorption and muscle contraction, and the strength of the bone. Concerning bone strength, most current discussion of osteoporosis treats the skeleton as an amorphous lump of mineral of which the only important property is its mass, with the corollary that the most important clinical problem is how to measure bone mass with the greatest accuracy and the least cost in the largest number of people. Certainly bone strength is related to bone mass. Differences in fracture frequency in groups defined by age, sex or race can partly be accounted for by corresponding differences in bone mass (106). Many facts of fracture epidemiology can be explained by a simple model in which individual fracture risk depends only on the extent by which the amount of bone falls below some fracture threshold (65). Persons with atraumatic fracture have less bone than unfractured persons of the same age, sex, and race, regardless of the means of measurement and even at skeletal sites remote from the site of fracture (1,30,141). But there is always a considerable overlap between fracture and non-fracture groups, so that factors other than bone mass must contribute to fracture risk.

It would be astonishing if bones were the only weight bearing structures whose failure under load could be explained solely in terms of the amount of structural material present. In accordance with standard engineering principles (see Chapter 4, *this volume*), how bone is distributed and connected in three-dimensional space is likely to have some bearing on the strength of the bones. All structural materials subjected to frequently repeated cyclical loading are liable to fatigue failure (22). Bone is no exception, but differs from other structural materials in being able to repair itself. Because of the remodeling mechanism, bone that has undergone fatigue damage is removed and replaced by new bone before microscopic and ultimately macroscopic fracture can occur. Consequently, a fault in the repair mechanism is likely to be an important independent risk factor for overt fracture (54). Because a reduction in the amount of bone augments strain-dependent fatigue damage, more demands are made on the repair mechanism at a time when its efficiency is likely to be reduced.

A major impediment to the investigation of fracture pathogenesis is that individual risk is low. A large number of subjects is needed for a prospective study, and bone biopsy is unlikely ever to be included among the baseline observations. Bone remodeling can be examined histologically only after a fracture has occurred, and with the assumption that the changes observed preceded the fracture and were not caused by it. A rise in lower forearm (or Colles) fracture incidence occurs at an earlier age than can be accounted for by the fall in local bone mass; the effect of the menopausal increase in bone remodeling on cortical porosity is a plausible qualitative factor (135) but this theory lacks direct confirmation. Bone structural data in patients with hip fracture suggest that relative losses of cortical and trabecular bone are similar but absolute losses are somewhat more than expected for age and sex (30,74,95,132,141). Remodeling data are few and are difficult to interpret because of varying periods of immobilization, the stress of injury and major surgery, an increased prevalence of alcoholism, diabetes and many other diseases, and wide variation in the apparent frequency of subclinical vitamin D deficiency, with or without osteomalacia (30,93,127). Consequently, detailed discussion is possible only for vertebral fracture, although some of the important conclusions probably apply also to hip fracture.

Vertebral Fracture—Amount and Structure of Bone

For the understanding of pathogenesis the study should be restricted to patients with significant compression (or crush) fracture with visible reduction in posterior as well as anterior vertebral height. For the conduct of clinical trials it may be convenient to redefine a fracture as a measureable change in vertebral body shape regardless of symptoms (83), but subjects with wedge deformity (reduction in anterior height alone) and no compression fracture usually do not differ significantly from control subjects (66). Wedge deformities can be developmental in origin or associated with ankylosing vertebral hyperostosis (138), and when due to fracture may represent defects too subtle to survive the large sampling variation that is inevitable with bone biopsy.

Unlike patients with hip fracture, patients with vertebral fracture have a relatively greater deficit of trabecular bone than of cortical bone (132). This difference is more consistent and unambiguous when trabecular bone is examined directly by histology than when it is examined indirectly by non-invasive procedures (1,74,155). For example, trabecular bone volume (Tb.BV), which is the proportion of bone in iliac trabecular tissue, is reduced by about 35% (16,132,141), but iliac cortical thickness is reduced only by about 10% (16,85). There is less overlap between fracture cases and controls for trabecular density (page 67) than for Tb.BV (141). More importantly, plate density is significantly lower in fracture than in non-fracture cases, even when they are matched for Tb.BV and for various indices of cortical bone mass as well as for age, sex, race, and menopausal status (85). As a consequence of the method of selection, plate thickness was also significantly higher in the fracture group, but for whatever reason this had occurred, it had failed to compensate for the disproportionate loss of compressive strength brought about by loss of a larger number of structural elements and consequent greater loss of three-dimensional connectivity.

Patients with compression fractures have either accumulated less trabecular bone during growth and consolidation or have lost more trabecular bone as a result of aging and menopause, but are they *losing* trabecular bone faster than normal? Serial measurements by dual photon absorptiometry of the spine have shown greater fractional bone loss in patients with osteoporosis than in normal women (89). But if initial bone mass is reduced, the fractional rate of loss would be increased even if the absolute rate of loss was normal. Furthermore, the difference could have been mainly in the cortical rather than in the trabecular bone of the spine. Limited data from metabolic balance studies in the untreated state suggest that absolute whole body bone loss is about 25% higher than expected for age or for years past menopause (42,150), but it is likely that most of the excess loss is in cortical rather than in trabecular bone. In cross-sectional studies in compression fracture patients, axial trabecular bone does not change with age regardless of the site or method of measurement (21,111, 141,155), but the rate of appendicular cortical bone is faster than expected for age (42). Serial measurements of vertebral trabecular bone by quantitated computed tomography in untreated patients with compression fracture will be needed to settle the issue with certainty, but the weight of present evidence indicates that in most patients with compression fracture, the rate of trabecular bone loss is not increased at the time of diagnostic evaluation.

Vertebral Fracture—Bone Remodeling

In contrast to the period immediately after the menopause, when a combination of increased activation and increased resorption cavity depth is the major remodeling abnormality, in patients with compression fracture reduced activation and impaired function of osteoblast teams are the major findings, together with increased variance of all histologic indices (140,142). In iliac trabecular bone, osteoid appositional rate (142) and mean wall thickness (32,168) are reduced compared to age and sex matched controls and the formation period prolonged, as was previously found in rib cortical bone (166). These abnormalities represent an exaggeration of the normal age-related decline in the rate and amount of matrix synthesis by teams of osteoblasts (Figures 15 and 16) but whether the defect is mainly in cell recruitment or mainly in cell activity is not known. In either case the age-related fall in thickness of residual structural elements is enhanced, and compensatory thickening, to the extent that it is possible, would be retarded. The severity of the osteoblast defect is the major determinant of the current rate of whole body bone loss (3). Possibly of even greater importance, bone that has undergone fatigue damage would take longer to replace, increasing the likelihood that the damaged bone would accumulate and predispose to overt fracture (54).

Reduced activation is manifested by low values for mineralized bone formation rate, (Figs. 15 and 18) whether expressed in relation to a unit of bone surface (appropriate for the response to humoral agents), a unit of bone volume (appropriate for the estimation of bone turnover), or a unit of tissue volume (appropriate for the relationship to kinetic and biochemical indices). Because of the fall in osteoid appositional rate and consequent prolongation of formation period, osteoid surface is no longer a useful index of formation rate, as it is in young normal subjects (Fig. 18). In contrast to impaired function of individual teams of osteoblasts, which seems to affect the entire skeleton, reduced activation is most evident on the trabecular surface, at least in the ilium; individual values are markedly skewed downwards (Fig. 19) with only about 10% above normal (139). On the endocortical and intracortical surfaces mean bone formation rate is normal, but the total formation rate for the entire biopsy sample is still reduced (147). As a result of

lower bone turnover, iliac trabecular bone age is increased about twofold and exceeds 10 years, the highest value found in normal subjects, in almost one-third of fracture patients (136).

Bone age is rarely mentioned in current discussion of either normal or abnormal skeletal physiology, but in all structural materials age is a major determinant of the risk of fatigue failure (54). An even more important consequence of excessive age in bone is death of osteocytes leading to micropetrosis, hypermineralization of perilacunar bone, filling of canaliculae with mineralized connective tissue, and increased brittleness (51). Osteocyte death probably also impairs the detection of fatigue damage, of which the repair would consequently be delayed in onset as well as retarded in rate (54). In patients with vertebral compression fractures osteocyte death and micropetrosis in cortical bone are more extensive than in normal subjects (162). Osteocyte death has not been studied systematically in trabecu-

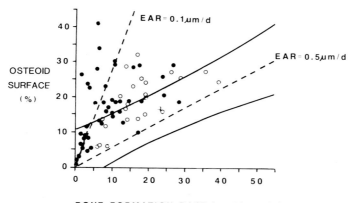

FIG. 18. Relationship between osteoid surface and bone formation rate. The solid curved lines are 95% confidence limits for individual values based on the regression in normal female subjects under age 50 (r = 0.84). Open circles are individual values for normal female subjects over age 50 years (r = 0.63). Closed circles are individual values for patients with compression fracture due to postmenopausal osteoporosis (r = 0.51). Interrupted lines radiating from the origin connect points of equal value for effective apposition rate (EAR). With increasing age osteoid surface becomes more dependent on effective apposition rate and less dependent on formation rate, with almost half of the values above the confidence limits established in the young normal subjects. This trend is further accentuated in the patients with compression fracture; in those with the lowest values for EAR, use of the regression in young normal subjects to predict bone formation rate from osteoid surface would overestimate the true value more than ten-fold.

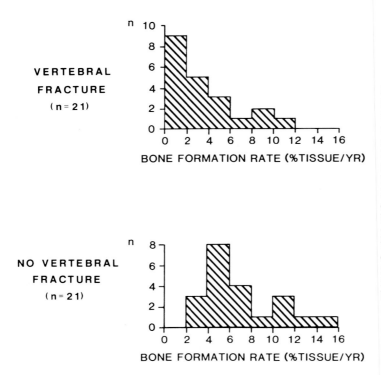

FIG. 19. Bone formation rate in patients with and without vertebral fracture. Subjects were matched for age, sex, race, menopausal status and for histologic and photon absorptiometric indices of both cortical and trabecular bone mass (85,136). Formation rates were measured on iliac bone biopsies after double tetracycline labeling. In this particular study none of the vertebral fracture patients had increased bone formation rate, but in previous studies we found this in up to 10% of the total vertebral fracture population.

lar bone, but increases with age in the femoral head (173) and probably contributes to the pathogenesis of hip fracture. The life span of osteocytes in trabecular bone is unknown, but a mean bone age greater than 10 years is probably long enough to significantly increase the risk of osteocyte death, particularly since trabecular bone turnover is lower in the vertebral bodies than in the ilium (129), and the bone correspondingly older.

In normal subjects there are good correlations between eroded surface, osteoclast surface and various biochemical indices of bone remodeling, all increasing after menopause (13,26,86,142,159), but in patients with compression fracture these correlations are lost and there is a disproportionate increase in eroded surface on the trabecular surface without a corresponding increase in osteoclasts (86,147). Most likely this reflects an exaggeration of the same abnormalities that give rise to the small increase in porosity in the outer half of the cortex—a delay in onset of bone formation within each resorption cavity, and accumulation of

small cavities that remain permanently unrefilled because remodeling has been aborted (13,72,129). Resorption rates on the trabecular surface, estimated from the deficit in bone volume relative to age and the measured formation rate, are reduced in most patients (128,142). By contrast, on the endocortical surface and its subendosteal extensions, the osteoclast surface is increased compared to normal subjects of the same age and menopausal status (Table 4). These surface differences are consistent with the other evidence that cortical bone loss remains faster than normal, but that the rate of trabecular bone loss has declined to the level expected for the patient's age.

Vertebral Fracture—Heterogeneity and the Two-Stage Concept

The most frequently emphasized characteristic of bone remodeling in patients with compression fracture is histologic heterogeneity (110,171). Geographic differences in remodeling patterns probably reflect etiologic differ-

TABLE 4. *Resorption indices in ilium in postmenopausal osteoporosis*

	ES	p	OClS	p
Trabecular surface	+ 75	< 0.05	− 14	NS
Endocortical surface	+ 41	< 0.05	+ 86	< 0.05
Intracortical surface	+ 25	NS	+ 21	< 0.05
Combined total surface	+ 59	< 0.05	+ 9	NS

Data expressed as percent difference from age matched control subjects.
ES = eroded surface; OClS = osteoclast surface.

ences. For example, increased bone turnover seems to be substantially more common in France (>30%, 19,75,107) than in Michigan (<10%; 139) and the most likely explanation is an increased prevalence of subclinical vitamin D deficiency and secondary hyperparathyroidism in France, where dairy products are not fortified with vitamin D (25). But before concluding that histologic heterogeneity within the same center implies etiologic heterogeneity, several reservations are in order. First, greater sampling variation has not been excluded, although virtually all measurements appear to have greater variance in osteoporotic patients than in normal subjects. Second, there is probably greater spontaneous variation with time than in normal subjects (35). Third, the variability is no greater than in primary hyperparathyroidism or in hypovitaminosis D osteopathy (140), and so is not inconsistent with a widely varying individual response to a single major etiologic factor. Finally, heterogeneity could result because a single disease process is intercepted at different stages of its evolution.

Many investigators believe that the state of bone remodeling at the time of vertebral fracture indicates the cellular mechanisms that were responsible for the patient's current level of bone mass, but this can be so only in a minority of cases. Rapid bone loss occurs in all women, but only for a few years after menopause, so that the aggressive osteoclastic resorption responsible for the most rapid and most biomechanically disruptive bone loss subsided in most patients 5 to 10 years before the first fracture! But the cellular abnormalities

found at the time of diagnosis, although not usually responsible for the earlier accelerated loss of bone, are some of the factors that select, from among the totality of women placed at risk, those in whom a fracture will occur. The minority of patients in whom trabecular bone turnover is increased are probably those in whom the cellular and remodeling effects of estrogen deficiency and consequent acceleration of bone loss have persisted much longer than usual, although there may be other causes of high turnover awaiting discovery. Patients in whom trabecular bone turnover is normal for their age are probably those in whom fracture occurs because structural defects already established at the time of skeletal maturity, either too little bone or, more likely, suboptimal three-dimensional connectivity, are intensified by the normal effects of menopause.

The remaining patients have some combination of depressed remodeling activation and defective osteoblast function in differing degrees. In this subgroup, there is some qualitative abnormality that cannot be accounted for, as can the features of the other two subgroups, by known genetic and hormonal influences on the skeleton. In both the high and normal turnover groups the patients' structural and remodeling state at the time of study after fracture are consistent with the wide variation found among normal subjects in peak adult bone mass, rate and duration of postmenopausal bone loss, and magnitude of age-related changes in bone remodeling. But in the low turnover group, the patients' current low rate of bone formation and impaired osteoblast function could not be representative of the entire period since menopause or else an impossibly large amount of trabecular bone would have been lost and the bone remaining would in some cases be older than the patient! Subsequent to the period of accelerated bone loss after menopause, these patients have, for unknown reasons, developed cellular defects that contributed to fracture risk by the mechanisms previously described.

According to this view all women undergo a morphologically specific form of accelerated bone loss after menopause in the absence of estrogen replacement therapy, a necessary but not a sufficient condition for susceptibility to osteoporotic fracture. From among the population thus placed in potential jeopardy, those with normal turnover developed clinical osteoporosis because they had too little bone or the wrong architectural type of bone at skeletal maturity, those with high turnover because they continued to lose bone too rapidly for too long after menopause, and those with low turnover because of specific defects in bone cell function. In this manner the histologic heterogeneity observed among patients with compression fracture can be reconciled with an integrated concept of histopathogenesis. The same general concept probably applies not only to postmenopausal osteoporosis but also to bone loss and fractures after corticosteroid administration (18,33,38), in traumatic and immobilization osteodystrophy (71,114,115), and in patients with non-osteomalacic intestinal bone disease with or without secondary hyperparathyroidism (143). In each of these four disorders the major unsolved problems are the pathogenesis of the remodeling suppression and defective osteoblast function. The similarity of the cellular defects found in such diverse circumstances raises the possibility of an undiscovered common etiologic factor in addition to individual factors that may be specific to each clinical setting.

BONE REMODELING AND FRACTURE PREVENTION—OPPORTUNITIES AND LIMITATIONS

It is conventional to distinguish between the prevention of bone loss, and the treatment of established osteoporosis. The aim in both cases is the prevention of fracture, but prevention of the first fracture and prevention of subsequent fractures may require different strategies. Before the first fracture it is likely that a critical reduction in bone strength has not yet occurred; prevention of further bone loss may be all that is needed, but because bone loss is irreparable, prevention should begin as early as possible. After the first fracture a critical re-

duction in bone mass has already occurred and prevention of further fracture may require at least partial restoration of normal bone structure, a task that is much more difficult than the prevention of bone loss and which may be impossible. Although a useful general principle, the change in emphasis is gradual rather than abrupt, and therapeutic intervention should be guided by what is happening throughout the skeleton and not just at the actual or expected site of fracture.

Suppression of Remodeling Activation and Its Consequences

Most therapeutic agents currently used for the prevention of bone loss and fractures have as their most important effect a fall in the frequency of remodeling activation, and for many agents this is the only effect. Such agents are commonly described as inhibitors of bone resorption, but this usage obscures the crucial distinction between the recruitment of new teams of osteoclasts and the effectiveness of each team in resorbing bone. This distinction is important *in vitro* as well as *in vivo:* among the bisphosphonates clinical efficacy correlates better with inhibition of the accession of new osteoclasts to the bone surface, a component of activation, than with inhibition of resorbing osteoclasts already present (14). Calcitonin reversibly inhibits osteoclasts *in vitro* at relatively low dose (24) and there is indirect evidence that estrogen in some manner reduces the aggressiveness of osteoclasts *in vivo,* but much of the effect of these agents and all of the effect of other agents on bone resorption *in vivo* is brought about by suppression of activation. In accordance with the discussion on pages 58–65, this will reduce whole body rates of resorption and formation, reduce the rate of irreversible bone loss and reduce the magnitude of the reversible mineral deficit, all in the same proportion as the fall in activation.

Regardless of the site or method of measurement, the respone of bone mass to suppression of activation is dominated in the short term by the fall in reversible mineral deficit (121). For example, a fall in the rate of irreversible bone loss from 2% to 1% per year will produce a difference in total body calcium between treated and control groups of about 5.0 g after six months. Over the same period, the fall in reversal mineral deficit of 7.5 g resulting from a reduction by 50% in remodeling activation will convert a loss of 5.0 g to a gain of 2.5 g and will represent 60% of the total effect of treatment. If the same fall in activation is maintained for 5 years, the difference in rates of irreversible bone loss between treated and control groups will result in a difference in total body calcium of 50 g and the same fall in reversible mineral deficit will represent only 13% of the total treatment effect. The initial increase in bone mass of 2 to 3% provides important information on the mechanism of action of the therapeutic agent and may be of modest therapeutic benefit, because a reduction in cortical porosity will protect slightly against certain kinds of fracture, but even if measured with infinite precision, it provides no information on either the magnitude or the direction of change after the first six months.

Because of the short-term dominance of the fall in reversible mineral deficit, serial measurements of bone mass usually show the gradual attainment of a plateau response (121). The total response is characterized by two parameters, the time taken to reach the plateau, which is 2 to 3 times the formation period determined at a single location (page 62), and the difference between the plateau and the pretreatment level, which reflects the magnitude of change in reversible mineral deficit. The existence of the plateau is an inevitable and predictable consequences of quantal remodeling and does not indicate resistance to or loss of effectiveness of the therapeutic agent, any more than the return of increased urinary sodium excretion to the baseline level after attainment of dry weight indicates resistance to the action of a diuretic. The nature of the remodeling system imposes an absolute requirement concerning the proper duration of any therapeutic study using bone mass as an index of response. The minimum duration is three years, one year to

ensure completion of the transient response and two years to measure the slope of the steady state response with acceptable precision, and to differentiate between a reduction in the rate of irreversible bone loss alone and an additional effect to reduce the magnitude of focal remodeling imbalance (121).

A further consequence of a fall in remodeling activation is a reduction in the rate of bone turnover and a consequent increase in mean bone age. Could this, by increasing the likelihood of osteocyte death, impair the detection of fatigue microdamage and increase fracture risk by the mechanism discussed in the previous section, so that any gain in bone quantity as a result of reduced activation would be more than offset by a loss of bone quality? Although a conclusive answer to this question is not yet available, a harmful effect seems unlikely for several reasons. First, maintenance of bone mass will minimize strain-related microdamage (54); so that the qualitative factors previously discussed will be less important than if bone loss is allowed to occur. Second, osteocyte death and consequent impaired detection of microdamage probably requires a greater prolongation of bone age than can be produced by pharmacologic depression of remodeling activation alone, in the absence of additional effects such as inhibition of mineralization (49). Finally, from evolutionary considerations, basal rates of remodeling activation close to the lower limit of normal should not inhibit the focal increase in activation needed for microdamage repair. Consequently, in most subjects the benefits of conserving bone mass probably outweigh the hypothetical risk of increasing bone age.

Prevention of the First Fracture

Increased peak adult bone mass and attenuation of early age-related bone loss between the ages of 35 and 50 years are both potentially important goals, but how to accomplish them is unknown. At present the only therapeutic intervention that has been demonstrated not only to retard bone loss but to reduce fracture risk is long-term estrogen replacement therapy (130), begun as soon as possible after menopause for maximum protection against the most biomechanically significant component of bone loss. Many possible substitutes for estrogen have been tested, but so far all have been ineffective (26,27). The apparent specificity of estrogen-replacement in the prevention of estrogen-dependent bone loss is not surprising and probably relates to the alternative mechanisms discussed on page 72. If increased plate perforation is a nonspecific consequence of increased remodeling activation, any suppressor of activation should be equally effective in preventing the acceleration of bone loss that follows menopause, but this is evidently not the case. Although incomplete, the therapeutic data support the concept that estrogen deficiency induces, directly or indirectly, a specific disorder of osteoclast function as well as an increase in activation (137).

This conclusion has several implications for the direction of future research. First, the mechanism of action of estrogen is not only a fundamental question of bone cell biology, but is of immediate practical importance. Second, effective substitutes for estrogen as currently used are unlikely to come from among the many nonspecific suppressors of remodeling activation; success is more likely with alternative routes of administration, with other agents that could mediate the effect of estrogen on bone, with modification of the estrogen molecule in the hope of reducing the risks but retaining the benefits, or with the synthesis of new compounds that can elicit similar responses in the estrogen-sensitive cells that initiate the effects on bone, whatever these cells turn out to be. Third, the many nonspecific suppressors of remodeling activation are more likely to be effective at earlier and at later times in a woman's life, when estrogen deficiency is not the dominant factor in bone loss and when estrogen administration is of no value. The concept that the effectiveness of therapeutic agents may be specific to particular times of life is also important in the management of patients who have sustained their first osteoporotic fracture.

Prevention of Subsequent Fractures

Osteosarcoma cells can make bone *de novo* in the connective tissue of the bone marrow, but net bone gain ordinarily occurs only by the addition of bone to an existing surface. How effective this can be in restoring normal biomechanical competence will depend on how much surface remains and how wide are the gaps between the surviving structural elements. The net addition of 50 μm of new bone over the entire surface, a more favorable effect than has so far been accomplished by any treatment in any study, would increase trabecular bone volume by 60 to 70%, for example, from 12% to 20% of trabecular tissue volume, because the structural elements that remain will increase in thickness. But there would be only a modest increase in structural connectivity, since only small perforations could be repaired, and the majority of trabecular windows are more than 100 μm across (137). Cortical thickness would increase by 5 to 10% in the ilium in the average patient, but would increase only by about 1% in the femur, which is hardly likely to be of biomechanical significance. Any therapeutic intervention that is delayed until after the first fracture is subject to such limitations, and a radical new approach is likely to be needed in the most severe cases. For example, the direct instillation of bone morphogenetic protein (163) into the marrow cavity might accomplish in a controlled manner what osteosarcoma cells do in an uncontrolled manner, stimulate the formation of new bone without reference to an existing surface (80).

Three mechanisms for the net addition of bone to an existing surface are currently under investigation (Fig. 20). As explained on page 59, sodium fluoride shifts the balance of focal remodeling so much in favor of formation that much of the new bone is deposited on a previously smooth surface, thus effectively bypassing the normal sequence of remodeling (109,126). Bone formed in response to fluoride has many of the histologic features of woven bone, such as more numerous osteocytes, larger than normal osteocyte lacunae, and irregular collagen fiber orientation (14,165).

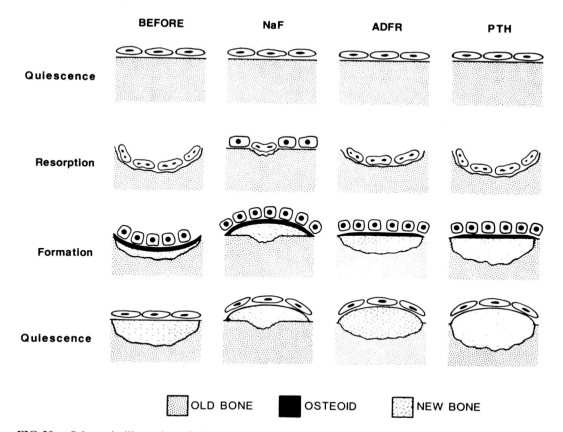

FIG. 20. Schematic illustration of three strategies for increasing trabecular thickness. In the first column successive stages in a remodeling cycle are indicated, as in Fig. 2. In the second column, sodium fluoride (NaF) causes some lining cells to transform directly to osteoblasts; exposure of a small area of bone surface initiates a small resorption cavity, but much of the new bone extends beyond its boundary. In the third column, with ADFR the resorption cavity is shallower than normal and is overfilled by a normal amount of bone. In the fourth column, parathyroid hormone (PTH) stimulates osteoblasts to make a larger than normal amount of bone in a normal size resorption cavity. For further details see text.

These histologic features may become less evident with time as the abnormal bone undergoes normal remodeling (109), but some investigators continue to find significant amounts of qualitatively abnormal bone, frequently accompanied by suggestive evidence of osteoblast toxicity (165). Nevertheless, sodium fluoride remains the only therapeutic agent consistently found to augment trabecular bone mass, and its ability to prevent fracture is currently undergoing controlled clinical trial. In individual patients classified as unresponsive to sodium fluoride because of continued vertebral fracture (153), it is unclear whether trabecular bone mass fails to increase, or whether bone mass increases without restoring three-dimensional connectivity or improving bone strength.

A second mechanism for increasing the thickness of existing trabeculae was conceived to exploit rather than to bypass the normal remodeling sequence (52,53). An agent known to activate bone remodeling is given in high dose for a short period of time in the hope of initiating many new cycles of bone remodeling more or less simultaneously. A depressant agent is then given in the hope of constraining the recently recruited osteoclasts into resorbing a shallower cavity. The depressant agent is then withdrawn in the hope that the subsequently appearing osteoblasts will lay down an amount of bone appropriate to a normal size cavity. The net result will be that more bone will be formed locally than was resorbed (Fig. 20). The concept is known by the acronym ADFR for Activate, Depress, Free and Repeat, and also referred to as coherence therapy, the normal skeleton being temporally incoherent with the remodeling cycles distributed at random in different stages of their life history, but becoming temporally coherent after a pulse of activation initiates a large number of cycles beginning at the same time. This novel idea has given rise to a great deal of discussion and to several clinical trials, but unfortunately the experiments needed to find out whether it will work have not yet been performed.

Remodeling activation can be increased by thyroxine, by parathyroid hormone, by induction of secondary hyperparathyroidism with phosphate administration and by short-term high dose administration of calcitriol, but whether the next two steps are possible remains speculative. All known depressors of bone resorption act mainly by depressing activation, and so would negate the first step if the time interval was too short. Whether any agent is able to limit the focal extent of osteoclastic resorption *in vivo* has not been demonstrated. Even if such an agent had been identified, it is not known whether the doses or time relationships of an activator followed by the putative depressor could be adjusted to result in shallower resorption cavities. Also unproven is whether osteoblasts can be deceived into laying down more bone than is needed to refill the cavity, which is the limit of their normal task. Indeed, if the number of osteoblasts that are assembled within a resorption cavity is related to the amount of some mitogenic stimulant released from resorbed bone, which is a likely component of the coupling mechanism, reducing the size of the resorption cavity would inevitably reduce also the number of new osteoblasts, unless an additional stimulus to osteoblast recruitment was given.

Not only have two of the three necessary steps not yet been validated, but in certain circumstances coherence therapy might have an adverse rather than a beneficial effect, because of the subnormal mean wall thickness in many patients with vertebral compression fractures (137). If remodeling activation was reduced to about one-third normal, a fairly large focal imbalance with the loss of 20 μm of bone thickness in each cycle could correspond to a relatively modest rate of whole body bone loss (Table 5). If activation were increased threefold to a normal level, and resorption cavity depth reduced by 60% to 20 μm, there could be a net gain of bone in each cycle, and an increase in whole body bone mass of 3%/year. But if the same increase in remodeling activation were accompanied only by a 20% reduction in cavity depth, although the net loss of bone thickness in each cycle would have been reduced from 20 μm to 10 μm thickness, the rate of loss by the whole body would have been increased from 2%/year to 3%/year! All these issues could be resolved in suitable animal models with currently available methods, and it is deplorable that seven years after its formulation the first new idea in the treatment of osteoporosis in 25 years has still not received the experimental attention it deserves and needs to be translated into a safe and effective regimen that can predictably realize its great potential for benefit.

A third mechanism for increasing trabecular thickness is based on the old observation that

TABLE 5. *Possible outcomes of coherence therapy*

Frequency of remodeling activation	Cavity depth (μm)	Mean wall thickness (μm)	Change /cycle (μm)	Total change (%)
One-third × normal	50	30	− 20	− 2
Normal	20[a]	30	+ 10	+ 3
Normal	40[b]	30	− 10	− 3

It is assumed that initially the rate of remodeling activation is reduced to one-third of normal, that mean wall thickness is reduced to a level observed in 5 to 10% of patients with low turnover osteoporosis, and that total body bone mass is declining about twice as fast as normal. Possible consequences of a three-fold increase in rate of remodeling activation to normal, and at the same time reducing resorption cavity depth either: [a]by 60%; or [b]by 20% are indicated. For further details, see text. From Parfitt, ref. 137, with permission.

parathyroid hormone (PTH) causes osteosclerosis in rats (119,151). There are some features in common with ADFR, of which the most important aspect may be that intermittent and continuous administration of the same agent often have different effects on bone rather than the details of any particular therapeutic regimen (55). In the adult skeleton PTH is an activator, as mentioned earlier, but in certain circumstances it has an additional independent effect of stimulating osteoblast teams to make more bone. A high level of endogenous PTH in the presence of a high plasma phosphate is a major etiologic factor in the osteoblast hyperfunction and osteosclerosis of chronic renal failure (119). A much lower level of exogenous PTH appears to have a similar effect, provided that the increase in plasma concentration is intermittent rather than continuous (151). Intermittent administration of PTH alone, like continuous hypersecretion of PTH, can increase cortical bone loss, but this may be preventable by alternating PTH with calcitriol (116). Robbing the appendicular skeleton to rebuild the axial skeleton could also be a problem with sodium fluoride and with ADFR.

Although restoring normal trabecular bone structure would be ideal, when osteoclastic resorption on the endocortical surface is persistently increased (Table 4) prevention of further cortical bone loss may be necessary to protect against hip and other long bone fractures. Suppression of remodeling activation in such patients may be rational therapy, even if trabecular bone turnover is already reduced. However, it is not possible in the present state of knowledge to reduce activation on one surface and to increase activation on another surface at the same time. Such patients may be better served by concentrating on a limited but attainable goal and giving up the hypothetical benefits of coherence therapy, or even the likely but uncertain benefits of fluoride therapy. How best to inhibit activation in a 60 to 70-year-old woman with compression fractures and increased endocortical resorption may depend on the etiologic importance of age-related secondary hyperparathyroidism, but agents of no value in early menopause could be effective in patients no longer suffering from the acute effects of estrogen deprivation (137). But if prevention of further cortical bone loss is worthwhile, monitoring of appendicular cortical bone, which constitutes more than half of the total skeleton (144), must continue to be included in the design of therapeutic trials, and the current trend to shift all investigative and clinical attention to the spine must be halted.

REFERENCES

1. Aloia, J.F., Vaswani, A., Ellis, K., Yuen, K., and Cohn, S.H. (1985): A model for involutional bone loss. *J. Lab. Clin. Med.*, 106:630–637.
2. Amstutz, H.C., and Sissons, H.A. (1967): The structure of the vertebral spongiosa. *J. Bone Joint Surg.*, 51B:540–550.
3. Arlot, M., Edouard, C., Meunier, P.J., Neer, R.M., and Reeve, J. (1984): Impaired osteoblast function in osteoporosis: comparison between calcium balance and dynamic histomorphometry. *Br. Med. J.*, 289:517–520.
4. Arnold, J.S. (1968) External and trabecular morphologic changes in lumbar vertebrae in aging. In: *Progress in Methods of Bone Mineral Measurement*, edited by G.D. Whedon and J.R. Cameron. U.S. Dept of Health Education and Welfare, Washington,D.C.
5. Arnold, J.S.(1970): Focal excessive endosteal resorption in aging and senile osteoporosis. In: *Osteoporosis*, edited by U.S. Barzel. pp. 80–100. Grune and Stratton, New York.
6. Arnold, J.S. (1980) Trabecular pattern and shapes in aging and osteoporosis. In: *Bone Histomorphometry. Third International Workshop*, edited by W.S.S. Jee and A.M. Parfitt, pp. 297–380. Armour Montagu, Paris.
7. Arnold, J.S., Bartley, M.H., Tont, S.A., and Jenkins, D.P. (1966): Skeletal changes in aging and disease. *Clin Orthop. Relat. Res.*, 49:17–38.
8. Arnold, J.S., and Wei, L.T. (1972): Quantitative morphology of vertebral trabecular bone. In: *Radiobiology of Plutonium*, edited by B. Stover and W.S.S. Jee, pp. 333–354. The J.W. Press, Salt Lake City.
9. Atkinson, P.J. (1965): Changes in resorption spaces in femoral cortical bone with age. *J. Pathol. Bacteriol.*, 89:173–178.
10. Atkinson, P.J., and Woodhead, C. (1973): The development of osteoporosis. A hypothesis based on a study of human bone structure. *Clin. Orthop. Rel. Res*, 90:217–228.
11. Baron, R., Neff, L., Van, P.T., Nefussi, J-R., and Vignery A. (1986): Kinetic and cytochemical identification of osteoclast precursors and their differentiation into multinucleated osteoclasts. *Am. J. Pathol.*, 122:363–378.

12. Baron, R., Vignery, A., and Horowtiz, M. (1984): Lymphocytes, macrophages and the regulation of bone remodeling. *Bone & Mineral Research 2,* edited by W. Peck, pp. 175–245. Elsevier, Amsterdam.

13. Baron, R. Vignery, A., and Lang R., (1981): Reversal phase and osteopenia: Defective coupling of resorption to formation in the pathogenesis of osteoporosis. In: *Osteoporosis: Recent Advances in Pathogenesis and Treatment,* edited by H.F. DeLuca, H. Frost, W. Jee, C. Johnston, and A.M. Parfitt, pp. 311–320. University Park Press, Baltimore.

14. Baylink, D.J., and Bernstein, D.S. (1967): The effects of fluoride therapy on metabolic bone disease. A histologic study. *Clin. Orthop.,* 55:51–85.

15. Boonekamp, P.M., van der Wee-Pals, L.J.A., van Wijk-van Lennep, M.M.L., Thesing. C.W., and Bijvoet, O.L.M. (1986): Two modes of action of bisphosphonates on osteoclastic resorption of mineralized matrix. *Bone and Mineral,* 1:27–39.

16. Boyce, B.F., Courpron. P., and Meunier, P.J. (1978): Amount of bone in osteoporosis and physiological osteopenia. Comparison of two histomorphometric parameters. *Metab. Bone. Dis. Rel. Res.,* 1:35–38.

17. Boyde, A. (1972): Scanning electron microscope studies of bone. In: *The Biochemistry and Physiology of Bone, 2nd ed, Vol. 1,* edited by G.H. Bourne. New York, Academic Press.

18. Bressot C., Meunier, P.J., Chapuy, M.C., LeJeune, E., Edouard, C., and Darby, A.J. (1979): Histomorphometric profile, pathophysiology and reversibility of corticosteroid-induced osteoporosis. *Metab. Bone. Dis. Rel. Res.,* 1:303–311.

19. Brown, J.P., Delmas, P.D., Malaval, L., Edouard, C., Chapuy, M.C., and Meunier, P.J. (1984): Serum bone Gla-protein: A specific marker for bone formation in postmenopausal women. *Lancet,* i:1091–1093.

20. Cann, C.E., and Genant, H.K. (1980): Precise measurement of vertebral mineral content using computed tomography. *J. Comput. Assist. Tomog.,* 4:493–500.

21. Cann, C.E., Genant, H.K., Kolb, F.O., and Ettinger B. (1985): Quantitative computed tomography for prediction of vertebral fracture risk. *Bone,* 6:1–8.

22. Carter, D.R. (1984): Mechanical loading histories and cortical bone remodeling. *Calcif. Tissue. Int.,* 36 Suppl:519–524.

23. Chambers, T.J., Darby, J.A., and Fuller, K. (1985): Mammalian collagenase predisposes bone surfaces to osteoclastic resorption. *Cell Tissue Res.,* 241:671–675.

24. Chambers, T.J., Fuller, K., McSheehy, P.M.J., and Pringle, J.A.S. (1985): The effects of calcium regulating hormones on bone resorption by isolated human osteoclastoma cells. *J. Pathol.,* 145:297–305.

25. Chapuy, M-C., Durr, F., and Chapuy, P. (1983): Age-related changes in parathyroid hormone and 25 hydroxycholecalciferol levels. *J. Gerontol,* 38:19–22.

26. Christiansen, C. (1984) Prophylactic treatment for age-related bone loss in women. In: *Osteoporosis. Proceedings of Copenhagen International Symposium on Osteoporosis,* June 3–8, edited by C. Christiansen, C.D. Arnaud, B.E.C. Nordin, A.M. Parfitt, W.A. Peck, and Riggs, B.L., pp. 587–593. Aalborg Stiftsbortrykkeri, Copenhagen.

27. Christiansen, C., Christensen, M.S., McNair, P., Hagen, C., Stacklund, K.E., and Transbol I. (1980): Prevention of early postmenopausal bone loss: controlled 2 year study in 315 normal females. *Eur. J. Clin. Invest.,* 10:273–279.

28. Courpron, P. (1981): Bone tissue mechanisms underlying osteoporoses. *Orthop. Clin. North Am.,* 12:513–543.

29. Courpron, P., Meunier, P., Bressot, C., and Giroux JM. (1976): Amount of bone in iliac crest biopsy. Significance of the trabecular bone volume. Its values in normal and in pathological conditions. In: *Bone Histomorphometry. Second International Workshop,* edited by P.J. Meunier, pp. 39–43. Armour Montagu, Paris.

30. Cummings, S.R., Kelsey, J.L., Nevitt, M.C., and O'Dowd K.J. (1985): Epidemiology of osteoporosis and osteoporotic fractures. *Epidemiol. Rev.,* 7:178–208.

31. Currey, J.D. (1964): Some effects of ageing in human Haversian systems. *J. Anat. Lond.,* 98:69–75.

32. Darby, A.J., and Meunier, P.J. (1981): Mean wall thickness and formation periods of trabecular bone packets in idiopathic osteoporosis. *Calcif. Tissue Int.,* 33:199–204.

33. Dempster, D.W., Arlot, M.D., and Meunier, P.J. (1982): Effect of corticosteroid (CS) therapy on the mean wall thickness (MWT) of trabecular bone packets. *Calcif. Tissue Int.,* 34(1):S4–S5.

34. Dempster, D.W., Shane, E., Horbert, W., and Lindsay, R. (1986): A simple method for correlative light and scanning electron microscopy of human iliac crest bone biopsies: Qualitative observations in normal and osteoporotic subjects. *J. Bone and Mineral Res.,* 1:15–21.

35. de Vernejoul, M.C., Belenguer-Trieto, R., Kuntz, D., Bielakoff, J. Miravet, L., Ryckewaert, A. (1987): Bone histological heterogeneity in postmenopausal osteoporosis. A sequential histomorphometric study. *Bone* (in press).

36. Dhem, A. (1980): Etude histologique et microradiographique des manifestations biologiques propres au tissu osseux compact. *Bull. Acad. Med. Bel.,* 135:368–381.

37. Doyle, F.H. (1968): Age-related bone changes in women. A quantitative x-ray study of the distal third of the ulna in normal subjects. In: *Progress in Methods of Bone Mineral Measurement,* edited by G.D. Whedon, and J.R. Cameron. U.S. Dept of Health Education and Welfare, Washington, D.C.

38. Duncan, H., Hanson, C.A., and Curtiss, A. (1973): The different effects of soluble and crystalline hydrocortisone on bone. *Calc. Tiss. Res.,* 12:159–168.

39. Dunnill, M.S., Anderson, J.A., and Whitehead, R. (1967): Quantitative histological studies on age changes in bone. *J. Pathol. Bacteriol.,* 94:275–291.

40. Eder, M. Der Strukturumbau der Wirbelspongiosa. (1960): *Virchows Arch. Path. Anat.*, 333:509–522.
41. Eger, W., Gerner, H.J., and Kämmerer, H. (1967): Bau und Dichte der menschlichen Spongiosa in Rippe, Wirbel und Becken als Ausdruck der statischen Funktion. *Arch. Orthop. Unfall-Chir.*, 62:97–112.
42. Elias, C., Heaney, R.P., and Recker, R.R. (1985): Placebo therapy for postmenopausal osteoporosis. *Calcif. Tissue Int.*, 37:6–13.
43. Epker, B.N., and Frost, H.M. (1966): Periosteal appositional bone growth from age two to age seventy in man—a tetracycline evaluation. *Anat. Rec.*, 154:573–578.
44. Eriksen, E.F., Gundersen, H.J.G, Melsen, F., and Mosekilde, L. (1984): Reconstruction of the formative site in iliac trabecular bone in 20 normal individuals employing a kinetic model for matrix and mineral apposition. *Metab. Bone. Dis. Rel. Res.*, 5:243–252.
45. Eriksen, E.F., Melsen, F., and Mosekilde, L. (1984): Reconstruction of the resorptive site in iliac trabecular bone: a kinetic model for bone resorption in 20 normal individuals. *Metab. Bone Dis. Rel. Res.*, 5:235–242.
46. Eriksen, E.F., Mosekilde, L., and Melsen, F. (1985): Trabecular bone remodeling and bone balance in hyperthyroidism. *Bone*, 6:421–428.
47. Eriksen,E.F., Mosekilde, L., and Melsen, F. (1986): Trabecular bone remodeling and balance in primary hyperparathyroidism. *Bone*, 7:213–221.
48. Farley, J.R., Masuda, T., Wergedal, J.E., and Baylink, D.J. (1982): Human skeletal growth factor: characterization of the mitogenic effect on bone cells in vitro. *Biochemistry*, 21:3508–3513.
49. Flora, L., Hassing, G.S., Parfitt, A.M., and Villanueva, A.R. (1981): Comparative skeletal effects of two diphosphonates in dogs. In: *Bone Histomorphometry: Third International Workshop*, edited by W.S.S. Jee, and A.M. Parfitt, pp. 389–407. Armour-Montagu, Paris.
50. Fornasier, V.L. (1977): Osteoid: An ultrastructural study. *Human Pathol.*, 8:243–254.
51. Frost, H.M. (1960): Micropetrosis. *J. Bone Joint Surg.*, 42-A:138–150.
52. Frost, H.M. (1979): Treatment of osteoporoses by manipulation of coherent bone cell populations. *Clin. Orthop.*, 143:227–244.
53. Frost, H.M.(1984): The ADFR concept revisited. *Calcif. Tissue Int.*, 36:349–353.
54. Frost, H.M. (1985): The pathomechanics of osteoporoses. *Clin. Orthop. Rel. Res.*, 200:198–225.
55. Frost, H.M. (1985): The skeletal intermediary organization. A synthesis. *Bone and Mineral Research 3,*edited by W. Peck, pp. 49–107. Elsevier, Amsterdam.
56. Garn, S.M. (1970): *The Earlier Gain and the Later Loss of Cortical Bone*. CC Thomas, Springfield.
57. Garn, S.M. (1981): The phenomenon of bone formation and bone loss. In: *Osteoporosis. Recent Advances in Pathogenesis and Treatment*, edited by H.F. DeLuca, H.M. Frost, W.S.S. Jee, C.C. Johnston, Jr, and A.M. Parfitt, pp. 3–16. University Park Press, Baltimore.
58. Garn, S.M., Frisancho, A.R., Sandusky, S.T.,
and McCann, MB. (1972): Confirmation of the sex difference in continuing subperiosteal apposition. *Am. J. Phys. Anthropol.*, 36:377–380.
59. Garn, S.M., Rohmann, C.G., Wagner, B., and Ascoli W. (1967): Continuing bone growth throughout life: A general phenomenon. *Am. J. Phys. Anthropol.*, 26:313–318.
60. Genant, H.K., Cann, C.E.,Ettinger, B., and Gordan, G.S. (1982): Quantitative computed tomography of vertebral spongiosa: A sensitive method for detecting early bone loss after oophorectomy. *Ann. Intern. Med.*, 97:699–705.
61. Hancox, N.M. (1972): *The Biology of Bone*. Cambridge University Press, Cambridge.
62. Hattner, R., Epker, B.N., and Frost, H.M. (1965): Suggested sequential mode of control of changes in cell behaviour in adult bone remodelling. *Nature*, 206:489–490.
63. Hattner, R., and Frost, H.M. (1963): Mean skeletal age: Its calculation, and theoretical effects on skeletal tracer physiology and on the physical characteristics of bone. *Henry Ford Hosp. Med. Bull.*, 11:201–216.
64. Hori, M., Takahashi, H., Konno, T., Inque, J., and Haba, T. (1985): A classification of in vivo bone labels after double labeling in canine bones. *Bone*, 6:147–154.
65. Horsman, A., Marshall, D.H., and Peacock, M. (1985): A stochastic model of age-related bone loss and fractures. *Clin. Orthop.*, 195:207–215.
66. Horsman, A., Nordin, B.E.C., Aaron, J., and Marshall, D.H. (1981): Cortical and trabecular osteoporosis and their relation to fractures in the elderly. In: *Osteoporosis. Recent Advances in Pathogenesis and Treatment*, edited by H.F. DeLuca, H.M. Frost, W.S.S. Jee, C.C. Johnston, Jr., and A.M. Parfitt, pp. 175–184. University Park Press, Baltimore.
67. Hui, S.L., Wiske, P.S., Norton, J.A., and Johnston, C.C., Jr. (1982): A prospective study of change in bone mass with age in postmenopausal women. *J. Chron. Dis.*, 35:715–725.
68. Jaffe, H.L. (1972): *Metabolic, Degenerative, and Inflammatory Diseases of Bones and Joints*. Lea & Febiger, Philadelphia.
69. Jaworski, Z.F.G., Duck, B., and Sekaly. G. (1981): Kinetics of osteoclasts and their nuclei in evolving secondary haversian systems. *J.Anat.*, 133:397–05.
70. Jaworski, Z.F.G., Kimmel, D.B., and Jee, W.S.S.(1983): Cell kinetics underlying skeletal growth and bone tissue turnover. In: *Bone Histomorphometry: Techniques and Interpretation*, edited by R.R. Recker, pp. 225–239. CRC Press, Boca Raton.
71. Jaworski, Z.F.G., Liskova-Kiar, M., and Uhthoff, H.K. (1980): Effect of long-term immobilisation on the pattern of bone loss in older dogs. *J. Bone Joint Surg.*, 62-B:104–110.
72. Jaworski, Z.F.G., Meunier, P., and Frost, H.M. (1972): Observations on 2 types of resorption cavities in human lamellar cortical bone. *Clin Orthop.*, 83:279.
73. Jaworski, Z.F.G., and Wieczorek, E. (1985): Con-

stants in lamellar bone formation determined by osteoblast kinetics. *Bone,* 6:361–363.

74. Johnston, C.C., Norton, J., Khairi, M.R.A., Kernek, C., Edouard, C., Arlot, M., and Meunier,
P.J. (1985): Heterogeneity of fracture syndromes in
postmenopausal women. *J. Clin. Endocrinol.
Metab.,* 61:551–556.

75. Joly, R., Chapuy, M.C., Alexandre, C., and Meunier, P.J. (1980): Osteoporoses a haut niveau de remodelage et fonction parathyroidienne. Confrontations histobiologiques. *Path. Biol.,* 28:417–424.

76. Jones, S.J., Boyde, A., Ali, N.N., and Maconna-
chie, E. (1985): A review of bone cell and substratum interactions. An illustration of the role of scanning electron microscopy. *Scanning,* 7:5–24.

77. Jowsey, J. (1966): Studies of Haversian systems in
man and some animals. *J. Anat.,* 100:857–864.

78. Jowsey, J. (1968): Age and species differences in
bone. *Cornell Veterinarian,* 58:74–94.

79. Kahn, A.J., Fallon, M.D., and Teitelbaum, S.L.
(1984): Structure-function relationships in bone: An
examination of events at the cellular level. *Bone &
Mineral Research 2,* edited by W. Peck, pp. 125–
174. Elsevier, Amsterdam.

80. Kanis, J.A. (1985): Osteoporosis. In: *The Chemistry and Biology of Mineralized Tissues,* edited by
W.T. Butler, pp. 398–407. Ebsco Media Inc. Birmingham, Alabama.

81. Keshawarz, N.M., and R.R. Recker. (1984): Expansion of the medullary cavity at the expense of
cortex in postmenopausal osteoporosis. *Metab.
Bone Dis. Rel. Res.,* 5:223–228.

82. Kimmel, D.B. (1981): Cellular basis of bone accumulation during growth: Implications for metabolic
bone disease. In: *Osteoporosis. Recent Advances in
Pathogenesis and Treatment,* edited by H.F. De-
Luca, H.M. Frost, W.S.S. Jee, C.C.Johnston, Jr.,
and A.M. Parfitt, pp. 87–95. University Park
Press, Baltimore.

83. Kleerekoper, M., Parfitt, A.M., and Ellis, B.I.
(1984): Measurement of vertebral fracture rates in
Osteoporosis. In: *Osteoporosis. Proc. Copenhagen
Int. Symposium on Osteoporosis,* June 3–8, edited
by C. Christiansen, C.D. Arnaud, B.E.C. Nordin,
A.M. Parfitt, W.A. Peck, and B.L. Riggs, pp.
103–109. Aalborg Stiftsbogtrykkeri, Copenhagen.

84. Kleerekoper, M., Tolia, L., and Parfitt, A.M.
(1981): Nutritional, endocrine and demographic aspects of osteoporosis. *Orthop. Clin. North Am.,*
12:547–558.

85. Kleerekoper, M., Villanueva, A.R., Stanciu, J.,
Rao, D.S., and Parfitt, A.M. (1985): The role of
three dimensional trabecular microstructure in the
pathogenesis of vertebral compression fractures.
Calcif. Tissue Int., 37:594–597.

86. Kleerekoper, M., Wilson, P., Parfitt, A.M., Mc-
Kenna, M.J., and Villanueva, A.R. (1986): Dis-
cordance between histologic and biochemical evaluation of bone remodeling in osteoporosis.*J. Bone
Mineral Res.,* 1(Suppl):170. (Abstr).

87. Kolbel, R. (1978): Spontane angiogene Knochen-
neubildung in spongiosem Knochen. *Z. Orthop.,*
116:682–691.

88. Kragstrup, J., and Melsen, F.(1983): Three-dimen-

sional morphology of trabecular bone osteons re-
constructed from serial sections. *Metab. Bone Dis.
Relat. Res.,* 5:127–130.

89. Krølner, B., and Nielsen, S.P. (1982): Bone mineral content of the lumbar spine in normal and osteoporotic women: cross-sectional and longitudinal
studies. *Clin. Sci.,* 62:329–336.

90. Lakes, R., and Saha, S. (1979): Cement line motion in bone. *Science,* 204:501–503.

91. Landeros, O., Frost, H.M. (1964): A cell system
in which rate and amount of protein synthesis are
separately controlled. *Science,* 145:1323–1324.

92. Lanyon, L.E. (1984): Functional strain as a determinant for bone remodeling. *Calcif. Tissue Int.,* 36
Suppl:S56–S61.

93. Lips, P. (1982): *Metabolic Causes and Prevention
of Femoral Neck Fractures.* University of Amsterdam, Amsterdam.

94. Lips, P., Courpron, P., and Meunier, P.J. (1978):
Mean wall thickness of trabecular bone packets in
the human iliac crest: changes with age. *Calcif.
Tissue Res.,* 26:13–17.

95. Lips, P., Netelenbos, J.C., Jongen, M.J.M., van
Ginkel, F.C., Althuis, A.L., van Schaik, C.L.,
van der Vijgh, W.J.F., Vermeiden, J.P.W., and
van der Meer, C. (1982): Histomorphometric profile and vitamin D status in patients with femoral
neck fracture. *Metab. Bone Dis. Rel. Res.,* 4:85–
93.

96. Malluche, H.H., Meyer, W., Sherman, D., and
Massry, S.G. (1982): Quantitative bone histology
in 84 normal American subjects. Micromorphometric analysis and evaluation of variance in iliac
bone. *Calcif. Tissue Int.,* 34:449–455.

97. Marie, P.J., Hott, M., and Garba, M-T. (1985):
Inhibition of bone matrix apposition by (3-amino-l-
hydroxypropylidene)-1,l-bisphosphonate (AHPrBP)
in the mouse. *Bone,* 6:193–200.

98. Martin, R.B.(1972): The effects of geometric feedback in the development of osteoporosis. *J. Biomech.,* 5:447–455.

99. Martin, R.B., and Burr, D.B. (1982): A hypothetical mechanism for the stimulation of osteonal remodeling by fatigue damage. *J. Biomechanics,*
15:137–139.

100. Martin, R.B., Pickett, J.C., and Zinaich, S.
(1980): Studies of skeletal remodeling in aging
men. *Clin. Orth. Rel. Res.,* 149:268–282.

101. Mathews, C.H.E., Aswani, S.P., and Parfitt,
A.M. (1981): Hypogravitational effects of hypodynamics on bone cell function and the dynamics of
bone remodeling. In: *A 14-day Ground-Based Hy-
pokinesia Study in Nonhuman Primates—A Compi-
lation of Results.* NASA Technical Memorandum
81268, April.

102. Mathews, C.H.E., Stanciu, J., Parfitt, A.M., and
Matkovic, V. (1981): Reconstruction of an Haver-
sian canal. In: *Bone Histomorphometry. Third In-
ternational Workshop,* edited by W.S.S. Lee, and
A.M. Parfitt, pp. 497 (abstr). Armour-Montagu,
Paris.

103. Mathews, J.L. (1980): Bone structure and ultrastructure. In: *Fundamental and Clinical Bone Physiology.* J.B. Lippincott, Philadelphia.

104. Mazess, R.B. (1982): On aging bone loss. *Clin. Orthop.*, 165:239–252.
105. Meema, H.E. (1977): Recognition of cortical bone resorption in metabolic bone disease in vivo. *Skelet. Radiol.*, 2–11.
106. Melton, L.J., III, and Riggs, B.L. (1983): Epidemiology of age-related fractures. In: *The Osteoporotic Syndrome*, edited by L.V. Avioli, pp. 45–72. Grune & Stratton, Orlando.
107. Meunier, P.J. (1981): Bone biopsy in diagnosis of metabolic bone disease. In: *Hormonal Control of Calcium Metabolism*, edited by D.V.Cohn, R.V. Talmage, and J.L. Mathews, pp. 109–117. Excerpta Medica, Amsterdam.
108. Meunier, P., Aaron, J., Edouard, C., and Vignon, G. (1971): Osteoporosis and the replacement of cell populations of the marrow by adipose tissue. *Clin. Orthop. Rel. Res.*, 80:147–154.
109. Meunier, P.J., Briancon, D., Vignon, E., Arlot, M., and Charhon, S. (1981): Effects of combined therapy with sodium fluoride-Vitamin D-calcium on vertebral fracture risk and bone histology in osteoporosis. In: *Osteoporosis. Recent Advances in Pathogenesis and Treatment*, edited by H.F. DeLuca, H.M. Frost, W.S.S. Jee, C.C. Johnston, Jr., and A.M. Parfitt, pp. 449–456. University Park Press, Baltimore.
110. Meunier, P.J.,Courpron, C., Edouard, C., Alexandre, C., Bressot, C., Lips, P., and Boyce, B.F. (1980): Bone histomorphometry in osteoporotic states. In: *Osteoporosis II*, edited by U.S. Barzel, pp. 27–47. Grune & Stratton, New York.
111. Meunier, P.J., Sellami, S., Briancon, D., and Edouard, C. (1981): Histological heterogeneity of apparently idiopathic osteoporosis. In: *Osteoporosis. Recent Advances in Pathogenesis and Treatment*, edited by H.F. DeLuca, H.M. Frost, W.S.S. Jee, C.C. Johnston, Jr., and A.M. Parfitt, pp. 293–301. University Park Press, Baltimore.
112. Miller, S.C., Bowman, B.M., Smith, J.A., and W.S.S. Jee. (1980): Characterization of endosteal bone-lining cells from fatty marrow bone sites in adult beagles. *Anat. Rec.*, 198:163–173.
113. Miller, S.C., and Jee, W.S.S. (1980): The microvascular bed of fatty bone marrow in the adult beagle. *Metab. Bone Dis. Rel. Res.*, 2:239–246.
114. Minaire, P., Berard, E., Meunier, P.J., Edouard, C. Goedert, G., and Pilonchery, G. (1981): Effects of disodium dichloromethylene disphosphonate on bone loss in paraplegic patients. *J. Clin. Invest.*, 68:1086–1092.
115. Minaire, P., Meunier, P., Edouard, C., Bernard, J., Courpron, P, and Bourret, J. (1974): Quantitative histological data on disuse osteoporosis: Comparison with biological data. *Calcif. Tissue Res.*, 17:57–73.
116. Neer, R.M., Slovik, D.M., Daly, M.A., Doppelt. S.H., Potts, J.T., Jr., and Rosenthal D.I. (1986): Increases in spinal bone density of osteoporotic men and women after treatment with hPTH-(1–4) + 1,25-(OH)$_2$D$_3$: Interim report. *Program and Abstracts, Endocrine Society 68th Annual Meeting.*
117. Ortner, D.J. (1975): Aging effects on osteon remodeling. *Calcif. Tissue Res.*, 18:27–36.
118. Pankovich, A.M., Simmons, D.J., and Kulkarni, V.V. (1974): Zonal osteons in cortical bone. *Clin. Orthop.*, 100:356–363.
119. Parfitt, A.M. (1976): The actions of parathyroid hormone on bone. Relation to bone remodelling and turnover, calcium homeostasis and metabolic bone disease. IV. The state of the bones in uremic hyperparathyroidism. The mechanisms of skeletal resistance to PTH in renal failure and pseudohypoparathyroidism and the role of PTH in osteoporosis, osteopetrosis and osteofluorosis. *Metabolism*, 25:1157–1187.
120. Parfitt, A.M. (1979): The quantum concept of bone remodeling and turnover. Implications for the pathogenesis of osteoporosis. *Editorial, Calc. Tissue Int.*, 28:1–5.
121. Parfitt, A.M. (1980): The morphologic basis of bone mineral measurements. Transient and steady state effects of treatment is osteoporosis. *Editorial, Mineral Electrolyte Metab.*, 4:273–287.
122. Parfitt, A.M. (1980): Richmond Smith as a Clinical Investigator: His work on adult periosteal bone expansion, and on nutritional and endocrine aspects of osteoporosis, in the light of current concepts. *HFH Med. J.*, 28:95–107.
123. Parfitt, A.M. (1981): Integration of skeletal and mineral hemeostasis. In: *Osteoporosis: Recent Advances in Pathogenesis and Treatment*, edited by H.F. DeLuca, H.M. Frost, W.S.S. Jee, C.C. Johnston, Jr., and A.M. Parfitt, pp. 115–126. University Park Press, Baltimore.
124. Parfitt, A.M. (1981): Bone remodeling in the pathogenesis of osteoporosis. *Medical Times*, 109:80–92.
125. Parfitt, A.M. (1982): The coupling of bone resorption to bone formation: A critical analysis of the concept and of its relevance to the pathogenesis of osteoporosis. *Metab. Bone Dis. Rel. Res.*, 4:1–6.
126. Parfitt, A.M. (1982): Treatment of osteoporosis: theoretical possibilities. *Program in Human Nutrition, University of Toronto, Recent Advances in Osteoporosis, Clin. & Investigative Med.* 5(2/3):181–185.
127. Parfitt, A.M., Gallagher J.C., Heaney R.P., Johnston C.C., Neer R., and Whedon, G.D., (1982): Vitamin D and bone health in the elderly. *Am. J. Clin. Nutr.*, 36:1014–1031.
128. Parfitt, A.M. (1982): Bone histomorphometry as a research tool. In: *Bone Histomorphometry for the Non-Histomorphometrist: Methods, Utility and Interpretation*, edited by P. Neunier. ASBMR Workshop.
129. Parfitt, A.M. (1983): The physiological and clinical significance of bone histomorphometric data. In: *Bone Histomorphometry. Techniques and Interpretations*, edited by R. Recker, pp. 143–223. CRC Press, Boca Raton.
130. Parfitt, A.M. (1983): Calcitonin in the pathogenesis and treatment of osteoporosis. *Triangle*, 22(2/3):91–102.
131. Parfitt, A.M. (1984): The cellular basis of bone remodeling. The quantum concept re-examined in light of recent advances in cell biology of bone. *Calcif. Tissue Int.*, 36 Supp.:S37–S45.

132. Parfitt, A.M. (1984): Age-related structural changes in trabecular and cortical bone: cellular mechanism and biomechanical consequences. a) Differences between rapid and slow bone loss. b) Localized bone gain. *Calcif. Tissue Int.*, 36 Supp.:S123–S128.

133. Parfitt, A.M. (1984): Effects of calcitonin on bone remodeling and bone loss. In: *Calcitonin: Das therapeutische Potential bei Osteoporose,* edited by L.V. Avioli, and M.A. Dambacher, pp. 59–62. Stuttgart, FK Schattauer Verlag.

134. Parfitt, A.M. (1987): Accelerated cortical bone loss in primary and secondary hyperparathyroidism. In: *Bone Fragility in Orthopaedics and Medicine,* edited by H. Uhthoff and Z.F.G. Jaworski, pp. 279–285. Springer-Verlag.

135. Parfitt, A.M. (1987): Cortical porosity in the pathogenesis of postmenopausal and adolescent wrist factures. In: *Bone Fragility in Orthopaedics and Medicine,* edited by H. Uhthoff and Z.F.G. Jaworski, pp. 167–172. Springer-Velag.

136. Parfitt, A.M.(1987): Pathogenesis of vertebral fracture: Qualitative abnormalities in bone architecture and bone age. In: *Osteoporosis: Current Concepts. Report of the Seventh Ross Conference on Medical Research,* edited by A.F. Roche. Ross Laboratories, Columbus, Ohio.

137. Parfitt, A.M., Vagenakis, A., Soucaeos, P., Avramides, A., Segre, G., and Deftos, L. (1986): Remodeling and microstructure of bone: Relation to prevention of age related fractures. In: *Proceedings of Second Conference on Osteoporosis: Social and Clinical Aspects,* pp. 197–209. Masson Italia Editori SIA, Milan.

138. Parfitt, A.M., and Duncan, H. (1982): Metabolic bone disease affecting the spine. In: *The Spine, 2nd ed,* edited by R. Rothman and F. Simeone, pp. 775–905. W.B. Saunders, Philadelphia.

139. Parfitt, A.M., and Kleerekoper, M. (1984): Diagnostic value of bone histomorphometry and comparison of histologic measurements and biochemical indices of bone remodeling. In: *Osteoporosis. Proceedings of Copenhagen International Symposium on Osteoporosis,* June 3–8, edited by C. Christiansen, C.D. Arnaud, B.E.C. Nordin, A.M. Parfitt, W.A. Peck, and B.L. Riggs, pp. 111–120. Aalborg Stiftsbogtrykkeri, Copenhagen.

140. Parfitt, A.M., Mathews, C., Rao, D., Frame, B., Kleerekoper M., and Villanueva, A.R. (1981): Impaired osteoblast function in metabolic bone disease. In: *Osteoporosis. Recent Advances in Pathogenesis and Treatment,* edited by H.F. DeLuca, H.M. Frost, W.S.S. Jee, C.C. Johnston, Jr., and A.M. Parfitt, pp. 321–330. University Park Press, Baltimore.

141. Parfitt, A.M., Mathews, C.H.E., Villanueva, A.R., Kleerekoper, M., Frame, B., and Rao, D.S., (1983): Relationship between surface, volume and thickness of iliac trabecular bone in aging and in osteoporosis. Implications for the microanatomic and cellular mechanism of bone loss. *J. Clin. Invest.,* 72:1396–1409.

142. Parfitt, A.M., Mathews, C.H.E., Villanueva, A.R., Rao, D.S., Rogers, M., Kleerekoper, M., and Frame, B. (1983): Microstructural and cellular basis of age related bone loss and osteoporosis. In: *Clinical Disorders of Bone and Mineral Metabolism,* edited by B. Frame and J.T. Potts, Jr., pp. 328–332. Excerpta Medica, Amsterdam.

143. Parfitt, A.M. Pødenphant, J., Villanueva, A.R., and Frame, B. (1985): Metabolic bone disease with and without osteomalacia after intestinal bypass surgery: A bone histomorphometric study. *Bone,* 6:211–220.

144. Parfitt, A.M., Rao, D.S., Stanciu, J., Villanueva, A.R., Kleerekoper, M., and Frame, B. (1985): Irreversible bone loss in osteomalacia: Comparison of radial photon absorptiometry with iliac bone histomorphometry during treatment. *J. Clin. Invest.,* 76:2403–2412.

145. Parfitt, A.M., Villanueva, A.R., Crouch, M.M., Mathews, C.H.E., and Duncan, H. (1977): Classification of osteoid seams by combined use of cell morphology and tetracycline labelling. Evidence for intermittency of mineralization. In: *Bone Histomorphometry: Second International Workshop,* edited by P.J. Meunier, pp. 299–310. Armour Montagu, Paris.

146. Parfitt, A.M., Villanueva, A.R., Mathews, C.H.E., and Aswani, J.A., (1981): Kinetics of matrix and mineral apposition in osteoporosis and renal osteodystrophy: Relationship to rate of turnover and to cell morphology. In: *Bone Histomorphometry: Third International Workshop,* edited by W.S.S. Jee and A.M. Parfitt, pp. 213–219. Armour Montagu, Paris.

147. Parfitt, A.M., Villanueva, A.R., Stanciu, J., and Rao, D.S. (1984): Bone formation and resorption in postmenopausal osteoporosis. Differences between intracortical, subcortical and trabecular surfaces. *Clin. Res.,* 32:764A.

148. Pesch, H-J., Scharf, H-P., Lauer, G., and Seibold, H. (1980): Der altersabhängige Vernbundbau der Lendenwirbelköper. Eine Struktur- und Formanalyse. *Virchows Arch. A. Pathol. Anat. Histol.,* 386:21–41.

149. Pritchard, J.J. (1972): General histology of bone. In: *The Biochemistry and Physiology of Bone, 2nd ed,* Vol. 1, edited by G.H. Bourne. Academic Press, New York.

150. Recker, R.R., Gallagher, J.C., and Heaney, R.P. (1984): The rapid decline in bone mass beginning at menopause and its implications. In: *Osteoporosis. Proc Copenhagen Int Symposium on Osteoporosis,* June 3–8, edited by C. Christiansen, C.C. Arnaud, B.E.C. Nordin, A.M. Parfitt, W.A. Peck, and B.L. Riggs, pp. 73–80. Aalborg Stiftsbogtrykkeri, Copenhagen.

151. Reeve, J., Meunier, P.J., Parsons, J.A., Bernat, M., Bijvoet, O.L.M., Courpon, P., Edouard, C., Klenerman, L., Neer, R.M., Renier, J.C., Slovik, D., Vismans, F.J.F.E., and Potts, J. (1980): Anabolic effect of human parathyroid hormone fragment on trabecular bone in involutional osteoporosis. *Br. Med. J.,* 280:1340–1344.

152. Reeve, J. (1986): A stochastic analysis of iliac trabecular bone dynamics. *Clin. Orthop.,* 213:264–278.

153. Riggs, B.L. (1984): Treatment of osteoporosis with sodium fluoride: an appraisal. In: *Bone and Mineral Research Annual 2*, edited by W.A. Peck, pp. 366–393. Elsevier, Amsterdam.

154. Riggs, B.L., Wahner, H.W., Melton, L.J., III, Richelson, L.S., Judd, H.L., Offord, K.P. (1986): Rates of bone loss in the appendicular and axial skeletons of women. *J. Clin. Invest.*, 77:1487–1491.

155. Riggs, B.L., Wahner, H.W., Seeman, E., et al. (1982): Changes in bone mineral density of the proximal femur and spine with aging. Differences between the postmenopausal and senile osteoporosis syndromes. *J. Clin. Invest.*, 70:716–723.

156. Sato, K., and Byers P.D. (1981): Quantitative study of tunneling and hook resorption in metabolic bone disease. *Calcif. Tissue Int.*, 33:459–466.

157. Schenk, R.K., Olah, A.J., and Herrmann, W. (1984): Preparation of calcified tissues for light microscopy. In: *Methods of Calcified Tissue Preparation*, edited by G.R. Dickson, pp. 1–56. Elsevier, Amsterdam.

158. Singh, I. (1978): The architecture of cancellous bone. *J. Anat.*, 127:305–310.

159. Stepan, J.J., Pospichal, J., Presl, J., and Pacovsky, V. (1984): Plasma tartrate resistant acid phosphatase, bone isoenzyme of serum alkaline phosphatase and urinary hydroxyproline for early identification of the patients at risk for developing osteoporosis. In: *Osteoporosis. Proceedings of Copenhagen International Symposium on Osteoporosis,* June 3–8, edited by C. Christiansen, C.C. Arnaud, B.E.C. Nordin, A.M. Parfitt, W.A. Peck, and B.L. Riggs, pp. 139–143. Aalborg Stiftsbogtrykkeri, Copenhagen.

160. Tappen, N.C. (1977): Three-dimensional studies of resorption spaces and developing osteons. *Am. J. Anat.*, 149:301–332.

161. Twomey, L., Taylor, J., Furniss, B. (1983): Age changes in the bone density and structure of the lumbar vertebral column. *J. Anat.*, 136:15–25.

162. Urist, M.R. (1964): Accelerated aging and premature death of bone cells in osteoporosis. In: *Dynamic Studies of Metabolic Bone Disease*, edited by O.H. Pearson, and G.F. Joplin. London, Blackwell.

163. Urist, M.R., Hudak, R., Huo, Y-K., Rasmussen, J., Hirota, W., Lietze, A. (1985): Bone morphogenetic protein (BMP) and anti-BMP immunoassay in patients with osteoporosis. In: *The Chemistry and Biology of Mineralized Tissues,* edited by W.T. Butler, pp. 62–69. Ebsco Media Inc., Birmingham, Alabama.

164. Vanderwiel, C.J. (1980): An ultrastructural study of the components which make up the resting surface of bone. In: *Bone Histomorphometry. 3rd International Workshop,* edited by W.S.S. Jee and A.M. Parfitt, p. 109. Armour Montagu, Paris.

165. Vigorita, V.J., and Suda, M.K. (1983): The microscopic morphology of fluoride-induced bone. *Clin. Orthop.*, 177:274–282.

166. Villanueva, A., Frost, H., Ilnicki, L., Frame, B., Smith, R., and Arnstein, R. (1966): Cortical bone dynamics measured by means of tetracycline labeling in 21 cases of osteoporosis. *J. Lab. Clin. Med.*, 68:599–616.

167. Villanueva, A.R., Kujawa, M., Mathews, C.H.E., and Parfitt, A.M. (1983): Identification of the mineralization front: Comparison of a modified toluidine blue stain with tetracycline fluorescence. *Metab. Bone Dis. Rel. Res.*, 5:41–45.

168. Villanueva, A.R., Qui, M-C., and Parfitt, A.M. (1985): Mean wall thickness in gallocyanine stained sections: Comparison with ultraviolet light (UVL) and polarized light (PL) microscopy. *Bone*, 6:412. (Abstr.).

169. Wakamatsu, E., and Sissons, H.A. (1969): The cancellous bone of the iliac crest. *Calcif. Tissue Res.*, 4:147–161.

170. Whitehouse, W.J.(1977): Cancellous bone in the anterior part of the iliac crest. *Calcif. Tissue Res.* 23:67–76.

171. Whyte, M.P., Bergfeld, M.A., Murphy, W.A., Avioli, L.V., and Teitelbaum, S.L. (1982): Postmenopausal osteoporosis: A heterogeneous disorder as assessed by histomorphometric analysis of iliac crest bone from untreated patients. *Am. J. Med.*, 72:193–202.

172. Wilson, J.S., and Genant, H.K. (1979): In vivo assessment of bone metabolism using the cortical striation index. *Invest. Radiol.*, 14:131–136.

173. Wong, S.Y.P., Kariks, J., Evans, R.A., Dunstan, C.R., Hills, E. (1985): The effect of age on bone composition and viability in the femoral head. *J. Bone Joint Surg.*, 67-A:274–283.

174. Woods, C.G. (1980): The relationship of osteoclasts to collagen fibre orientation. In: *Bone Histomorphometry: Third International Workshop,* edited by W.S.S. Jee, A.M. Parfitt, pp. 41–45. Armour Montagu, Paris.

175. Wronski, T.J., Smith, J.M., and Jee, W.S.S., (1980): The microdistribution and retention of [239]Pu on the trabecular bone surfaces of the beagle: implications for the induction of osteosarcoma. *Radiol. Res.*, 83:74–89.

176. Wu, K., Jett, S., and Frost, H.M. (1967): Bone resorption rates in rib in physiological, senile, and postmenopausal osteoporoses. *J. Lab. Clin. Med.*, 69:810–818.

Osteoporosis: Etiology, Diagnosis, and Management, edited by B. Lawrence Riggs and L. Joseph Melton, III. Raven Press, New York © 1988.

3

The Biochemistry of Bone

Pamela Gehron Robey, Larry W. Fisher, Marian F. Young and John D. Termine

Bone Research Branch, The National Institute of Dental Research, The National Institutes of Health, Bethesda, Maryland 20892

The bone-forming cells, osteoblasts, synthesize, assemble and mineralize the extracellular matrix of bone. Because of the unique role of the skeleton in mineral ion homeostasis, osteoblasts are target cells for the many hormones and growth factors that regulate bone turnover. The regulation of bone cell metabolism can be divided into three events: (1) the interaction of the cell with regulatory factors either by receptor-mediated phenomena or by direct membrane permeabilization; (2) intracellular events (e.g., cytoskeletal changes, calcium movement); and (3) a secretory response of the cell, encompassing production of the extracellular matrix and/or secretion of specific factors. Calcium regulating hormones such as parathyroid hormone and $1,25-(OH)_2 D_3$ have been shown to directly affect osteoblasts through receptor-mediated events. In addition, many cytokines also appear to alter osteoblastic metabolism. The secretory capacity of the cell is either stimulated or depressed accordingly (48).

The organic matrices of bone, tendon and ligament are predominantly type I collagen (approximately 90%). Since under physiological conditions, formation of hydroxyapatite crystals occurs only in bone, it is likely that noncollagenous proteins that are specific to, or enriched in bone, play an important role in the initiation of the mineralization process.

COLLAGEN

The most abundant class of extracellular matrix proteins, the collagens, play an important role in the normal structure and function of all vertebrate connective tissue. Collagen is defined as a protein in which the amino acid sequence is characterized by a repeating triplet amino acid sequence, Glycine-X-Y, where X and Y are often the amino acids proline and hydroxyproline, respectively. This repetitive sequence allows three collagenous polypeptides (termed α chains) to form a semi-rigid and extremely stable, triple helical molecule, which can be homopolymeric (three identical α chains) or heteropolymeric (two or three different α chains). These triple helical collagen molecules, usually measuring approximately 300 nm in length, associate laterally and longitudinally to form fibrillar or network structures providing the structural support appropriate for each connective tissue (36).

The last decade of research in connective tissue biochemistry has expanded the list of collagen types to include at least 10 genetically distinct triple helical molecules (for review, see

32). Of these, the interstitial (fibrillar) collagens are the best characterized. With the exception of cartilage and basement membranes, type I collagen is the predominant type of collagen in connective tissues, and is a heteropolymer composed of two α1(I) chains and one α2(I) chain. Type II collagen is found in cartilage, and to a lesser extent in other specialized tissues such as vitreous humor in some species. Type III collagen is generally codistributed with type I, except in bone and tendon. Somewhat higher levels of type III collagen in relationship to type I collagen are found in fetal tissues. Type V collagen may also form fibrillar structures that are codistributed along with types I and III, and has been localized to the pericellular spaces of smooth muscle cells.

The nonfibrillar types of collagen, with the exception of type IV collagen, are less well characterized with regards to their assembly and matrix deposition. Type IV collagen is found in basement membranes, which are thin structures formed underneath epithelial and endothelial cells, and which surround muscle and nerve fibers. Unlike the fibrillar collgen, type IV α chains contain noncollagenous amino acid domains (i.e., not Gly-X-Y-) at the amino (N) and carboxy (C) terminals, and throughout the molecule which confer flexibility to the resultant tissue matrix. The type IV collagen triple helical molecules form end-to-end associations to form a matrix network. Type VI collagen α chains, like type IV, contain large noncollagenous domains at the N and C terminals. These triple helical molecules form dimers and tetramers that give rise to microfibrillar components found in most interstitial tissues. Type VII collagen may comprise the structural component of small fibrils that appear to anchor basement membranes to the underlying connective tissue stroma. This collagen type is unusual in that the triple helical domain is 1.5 times longer than that found in type I collagen, and the resultant molecules associate in an antiparallel array with a 60 nm overlap region. Type VIII collagen has as yet only been identified as a biosynthetic product of certain endothelial cells *in vitro* and appears

to be composed of short triple helical stretches interspersed with domains of noncollagenous sequence. Cartilage, in addition to type II collagen contains low amounts of other collagenous proteins (types IX and X). Although the structure of the native protein is not yet known, type IX collagen appears to have two triple helical stretches, one large and one short, and also contains a glycosaminoglycan side chain composed of chondroitin sulfate. Calcifying cartilage and certain cultured chondrocytes synthesize type X collagen, which is composed of helices that are 1/2 the length of the interstitial collagen.

Taking into account the current list of collagen types, there are at least 18 different genes that encode for the different α chains. The amino acid and nucleotide sequences for many of these α chains are now known (8). The collagen genes have a high number of intervening sequences which do not code for protein (introns), 51 in the case of α1(I). The genes, therefore, are considerably larger than expected considering the size of the expressed protein (see Fig. 1). Another notable feature is that many of the transcribed portions of the gene (exons) are 54 and 108 base pairs (bp) which encode for exactly 6 and 12 (GLY-X-Y) triplets, respectively (62). It has been proposed that the 54 bp exon may represent a primordial collagen gene. However, the gene for α1(IX) does not contain 54 bp exons (32).

Like many other messenger RNAs (mRNA), there are nucleotide sequences in the collagen mRNAs that code for a signal peptide which affords attachment of the mRNA-ribosome complex to the cytosolic surface of the endoplasmic reticulum (ER). As the mRNA is further translated, the protein is translocated into the ER and the signal peptide is cleaved. In general, the initial product of translation, a pro α chain, contains noncollagenous amino acid sequences at both its N and C terminals (see Fig. 1).

Collagenous polypeptides undergo a number of post-translational modifications (for review, see 14). Certain prolyl and lysyl residues are hydroxylated within the endoplasmic reticulum

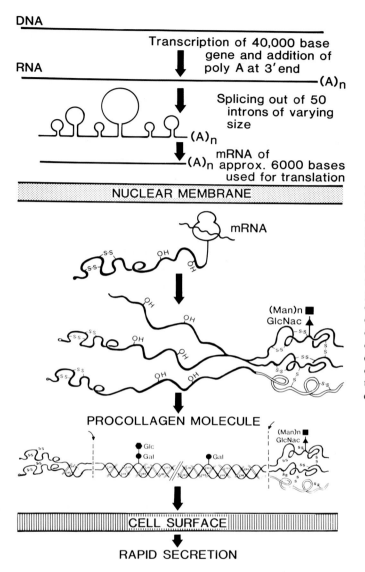

DNA

RNA

Transcription of 40,000 base
gene and addition of
poly A at 3′ end

$(A)_n$

Splicing out of 50
introns of varying
size

$(A)_n$

$(A)_n$ mRNA of
approx. 6000 bases
used for translation

NUCLEAR MEMBRANE

mRNA

$(Man)_n$
GlcNac

PROCOLLAGEN MOLECULE

Glc
Gal
Gal
$(Man)_n$
GlcNac

CELL SURFACE

RAPID SECRETION

FIG. 1. Intracellular pathways of type I collagen metabolism. Precursor mRNA is translated from the gene and polyadenylated. The introns (non-coding sequences) are spliced and the mature mRNA is transported to the cytoplasm and translated by ribosomes. Certain prolyl and lysyl residues are hydroxylated and hydroxylysyl residues are glycosylated. Two pro α1(I) and one pro α2(I) chains are disulfide bonded at their C-terminal ends and triple helix formation proceeds. The completed molecule is then rapidly secreted into the extracellular environment.

(ER). There are two forms of prolyl hydroxylase which hydroxylate proline at different ring positions (C-3 or C-4). In addition, certain hydroxylysyl residues are glycosylated by specific sugar transferases to form galactosyl-hydroxylysyl or glucosyl-galactosyl-hydroxylysyl residues. N-linked glycosylation of the C terminal noncollagenous extensions also occurs in many, if not all, collagen types. Association of three nascent α chains is initiated by interchain disulfide bond formation at their C termi-

nal noncollagenous extension peptides. The processes of hydroxylation and glycosylation continue in the ER until three α chains have associated to form a stable triple helical molecule (Fig. 1).

Triple helix formation is completed within the ER and the molecule is transported to the Golgi where the cellular products are packaged for secretion. The secretory vesicles are then transported to the cell surface where the procollagen molecules are extruded into the extracellular space. At this point, the noncollagenous N and C terminal domains of the interstial (fibrillar) collagens, types I, II, III and V, are removed by specific N- and C-peptidases which may regulate fibril formation (Fig. 2). Fibers are formed by aggregation of triple helical molecules in a parallel, but longitudinally staggered fashion, which gives rise to the typical banding pattern of 67 nm seen by electron microscopy (Fig. 2). The noncollagenous extension peptides of other collagen types (nonfibrillar), most notably type IV, do not appear to be removed and it is perhaps for this reason that these collagens do not form banded, fibrillar structures, but form other types of networks (see 32 for review).

Once deposited in the tissue, the collagen fibers formed are further stabilized by the formation of covalent crosslinks. These crosslinks are initiated by the conversion of lysyl or hydroxylysyl residues to the aldehydic derivatives (allysine and hydroxyallysine) of these two amino acids by the enzyme, lysyl oxidase. These two altered amino acids condense with lysyl or hydroxylysyl residues to form intra- and intermolecular crosslinks. Multichain complex crosslinks (pyrodinolines) may also form. The main site of crosslinking of the fibrils appears to be in short telopeptide regions at the N and C terminals, although crosslinks within the triple helical portion of the molecule are also found (13).

Collagen composes at least 90% of the organic matrix of bone, and the mineralized matrix is composed exclusively of the type I collagen, $[\alpha 1(I)_2\alpha 2(I)]$. Type III and V collagens are generally associated with blood vessels found within the bone. Compared to type I col-

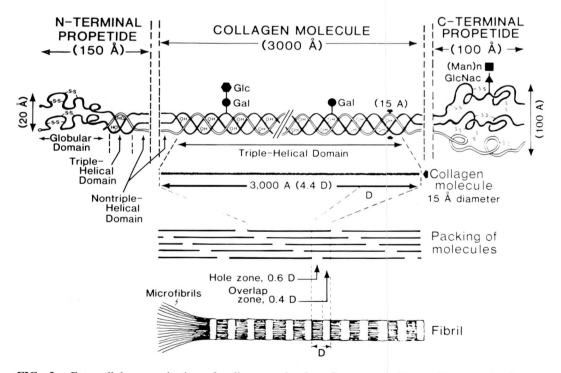

FIG. 2. Extracellular organization of collagen molecules. Once secreted, procollagen molecules are trimmed by specific enzymes to remove the N- and C-terminal domains. The collagen molecules then associate in a staggered array that generates a characteristic striation pattern ("D"). So called "hole" regions represent the space in between collagen molecules, and are typically the site of initial hydroxyapatite deposition.

lagen isolated from other sources, bone collagen contains more hydroxylysine, which in turn is more frequently glycosylated. In addition, cross-linking found in bone type I collagen differs from that of soft tissue colagens. The predominant crosslinks in bone originate from the hydroxyallysine pathway. The maturation of these crosslinks from borohydride reducible to nonreducible (13) appears to be much slower in bone, most likely due to the deposition of hydroxyapatite along the type I collagen fibril. In bone, type I collagen may associate with noncollagenous proteins such as fibronectin, osteonectin, bone proteoglycan and bone sialoprotein. The formation of supramolecular, heteropolymeric, complexes containing these proteins conveys the resultant matrix with the structural and functional properties that are unique to bone.

NONCOLLAGENOUS PROTEINS OF BONE

The noncollagenous proteins (NCP) of bone constitute a wide spectrum of molecules that become entrapped within the mineralized bone compartment. These range from true matrix assembly proteins (osteoid components) to adsorbed blood proteins with an inherent affinity for the bone mineral crystals. Questions about the roles of the NCPs in bone have been asked since the turn of the century, but only in the last decade has sufficient progress been made in the protein biochemistry of these molecules to begin to shed some light on this topic. While no NCP has yet been assigned a completely unambiguous role in bone, a considerable amount of information is known about a few of these proteins.

Osteocalcin, or the bone gla protein (BGP), is the best chemically characterized noncollagenous protein in bone. Comparison of the amino acid sequences of osteocalcins from a wide variety of vertebrates has shown this molecule to be highly conserved. This evidence alone suggests that osteocalcin plays a critical, if as yet unknown, role in vertebrates. This molecule is first synthesized by the osteoblast

as a 99 amino acid protein that includes: (1) a hydrophobic signal peptide (see above), (2) a stretch of basic amino acids hypothesized to encode the recognition site for the γ-carboxyglutamate enzyme complex, and (3) the 50 amino acid (5800 dalton) sequence actually secreted from the cell (35). Following cleavage of the signal peptide, three of the glutamyl amino acid residues are carboxylated at their γ positions by a vitamin K-dependent enzyme. Following γ carboxylation, cleavage of the putative signal peptide occurs and the native form of osteocalcin is then secreted into the extracellular space.

Osteocalcin may comprise as much as 10 to 20% of the total NCPs in bone although considerable interspecies and developmental variation exists. Rat bone, for example, contains about ten times as much of this protein as does human bone (45). In the developing chicken, osteocalcin synthesis appears correlated with the onset of mineralization (25,26), but no such correlation could be found for the rat. Fully γ-carboxylated osteocalcin binds both ionic calcium (Kd approximately 10^{-3} M) (45) and hydroxyapatite (Kd approximately 10^{-7} M) (39) and has been reported both to block the transition of precursor mineral phase to hydroxyapatite (24), and to inhibit the precipitation of hydroxyapatite from saturated solutions of calcium and phosphate ions (38). In fact, it is this strong association with the mineral phase of bone that is responsible for the retention of osteocalcin in bone.

Osteosarcoma cells, intact rat calvaria and human bone cell cultures produce osteocalcin at an accelerated rate when stimulated by 1,25 $(OH)_2$ D_3 (3,9,43). Interestingly in rat bone and bone cell culture systems, similar levels of this sterol decrease the production of collagen (23). This ability to dissociate the synthesis of osteocalcin from that of collagen has led some investigators to call into question the role of osteocalcin in bone matrix synthesis, maturation and mineralization.

Serum has been shown to contain significant levels of osteocalcin-like proteins (42). The best evidence to date suggests that the serum osteocalcin arises from new protein synthesis, probably due to molecules that diffuse away from areas of new bone formation. The circulatory osteocalcin immunoactivity appears to turnover rapidly at a rate similar to that of other small proteins such as RNase. Serum osteocalcin levels are found elevated in metabolic diseases involving increased bone turnover such as Paget's disease, renal osteodystrophy and primary hyperparathyroidism (40). While it is accepted that it is generally useful to measure circulating levels of osteocalcin-like molecules in metabolic bone disease, the exact significance of these measurements in most clinical bone disorders has yet to be established. Undoubtedly part of the present confusion results from the use of radioimmunoassays (RIA) based on different antisera, some of which may bind to a different spectrum of circulating osteocalcin-like molecules.

Other γ-carboxyglutamate-containing proteins may also occur in bone. Non-osteocalcin gla-containing proteins have been suggested to account for 50% of the total gla content of adult bone and over 90% of embryonic bone. The most thoroughly characterized of these is the matrix gla protein (MGP), a 10,000 dalton protein found tightly associated with the bone morphogenic protein (BMP) preparations described by Urist (45). MGP contains five γ-carboxyglutamate residues and has sufficient sequence homology with osteocalcin to suggest that the two proteins derive from a common ancestor. Accumulation of MGP in bone appears to be less dependent on γ-carboxylation reactions than is the case for osteocalcin (41). This is illustrated by the finding that about one fourth of the normal levels of MGP are retained in the bones of warfarin-treated rats while less than 2% of the normal levels of osteocalcin are retained under these conditions. (Warfarin, acting through the vitamin K pathway, blocks γ-carboxylation of glutamyl residues but does not affect total synthesis and secretion of proteins.)

Phosphoproteins and glycoproteins have been known to be present in bone for a number of years. The phosphate is covalently bound to the protein backbone through serine and/or threonine amino acid residues. Both N- (asparagine) and O- (serine) linked oligosaccharides with varying amounts of constituent sialic acid (see below) are found in glycoproteins. Probably the best characterized of these types of

TABLE 1. *Phosphoproteins and glycoproteins*

Protein	Molecular weight	Comments
Proteoglycan I (PG-I)	250,000 (SDS gels) 120,000 (actual)	45,000 Mr core protein, two chondroitin sulfate chains, high in leucine
Proteoglycan II (PG-II)	200,000 (SDS gels) 85,000 (actual)	45,000 Mr core protein, one chondroitin sulfate chain
Type I collagen $\alpha^3 1(I)_2 \alpha^3 2(I)$	120,000 (SDS gels) 95,000 (actual) ^{3} chains	high hydroxylysine, high glucosyl-galactosyl-hydroxylysine hydroxyallysine pathway of cross-link formation
Bone sialoprotein (BSP I)	75,000 (cow and man)	contains sialic acid, stains with Coomassie Blue
Bone sialoprotein (BSP II)	75,000 (cow) 60,000 (rat)	rich in sialic acid, stains with Alcian Blue, 50% carbohydrate
75 Kd phosphoprotein	75,000	phosphorylated and glycosylated
α^3_2HS Glycoprotein	72,000 (bovine) 60,000 (man)	concentrated from blood by hydroxyapatite surfaces
Serum albumin	67,000	mildly concentrated from blood by hydroxyapatite surfaces
Osteonectin	38,000 (pre-pro) 32,000 (secreted)	binds to both collagen and hydroxyapatite, initiates mineral formation *in vitro*
24 Kd Phosphoprotein	24,000	phosphorylated, contains hydroxyproline
Matrix Gla protein	10,000	contains 5 γ-carboxy-glutamic acid residues, found associated with the bone morphogenetic protein
Osteocalcin	9,000 (pre-pro) 5,800 (secreted)	contains 3 γ-carboxy-glutamic acid residues, binds to hydroxyapatite

bone protein is osteonectin. This phosphory-lated bone glycoprotein has a molecular weight of 32,000 on guanidine hydrochloride gel filtration chromatography, a Mr = 40 to 46,000 on sodium dodecyl sulfate polyacrylamide gel electrophoresis, and a molecular weight of 29,000 on sedimentation equilibrium (57,58). Osteonectin is found in bone from a variety of species including man, cow, rat, dog, chicken, rabbit, pig, monkey, sheep and mouse. The amount of osteonectin in developing bone ranges from only small amounts in the rat to about 15% of the total NCPs in cow and man. In general, the amount of osteonectin in bone appears to reflect the relative amounts of lamellar bone present (10). For example, young rat bone and early fetal bovine bone are highly woven in character and contain relatively little osteonectin, while later fetal bovine bone and structural bone from animals such as the chicken with a high lamellar or osteonal bone content, contain substantial amounts of osteonectin. Osteonectin exhibits saturable and exchangable binding to both collagen and hydroxyapatite, the dissociation constant for the latter being 8×10^{-8} M. On a molar basis, this acidic protein (isoelectric point, pI = 5.5) is 5 times more effective than osteocalcin in inhibiting seeded crystal growth of hydroxyapatite crystals in vitro (49). Osteonectin has been shown to have separate binding domains for collagen and mineral and to promote mineral deposition onto type I collagen films in vitro (58). Thus, it is possible that this protein, after binding to collagen fibrils, may present a fixed oriented field of calcium binding sites to nucleate hydroxyapatite crystals in a highly controlled manner. Areas in woven bone, primarily interfibrillar regions appear to nucleate apatite crystals by other mechanisms (e.g., matrix vesicles).

Although bone and dentin contain by far the highest percentages of osteonectin in the body, other tissues such as periodontal ligament (65) and tendon (22) contain small amounts of osteonectin. In addition, platelets also appear to contain osteonectin and are induced to secrete it after thrombin stimulation (56). Osteonectin is synthesized and secreted by bovine, human, sheep, dog and rat bone cells in culture. The mRNA for osteonectin appears to encode for a protein about 6,000 daltons larger than the secreted form (31). It is not known whether the additional amino acids are due to a larger than normal signal peptide or represent an extended portion of a pro-osteonectin molecule. In culture, many cell types other than the osteoblast appear to make an osteonectin-like protein (J.N. Beresford, P. Gehron Robey, and J.D. Termine, unpublished data, and 65). Recent unpublished data from our laboratory using monoclonal antisera, however, suggest that the non-bone cell osteonectin-like proteins may differ from the bone osteonectin protein. The role of these osteonectin-like proteins in culture, if any, is not known.

Bone contains at least three other phosphoproteins not yet fully characterized, and known only as the 75,000 dalton, 62,000 dalton and 24,000 dalton bone phosphoproteins. All contain large amounts of aspartic and glutamic acids and are relatively acidic. The 24,000 Mr protein is particularly interesting with its hydroxyproline content of six residues per molecule, an amino acid relatively rare for a non-collagenous protein (57). It is not known whether this bone protein represents a segment of a collagenous protein (e.g., the N propeptide of type I collagen chains) or a distinct, low molecular weight bone cell product. Like osteonectin, the 75,000 (A. Butler, unpublished data) and 62,000 (57 Mr proteins are glycosylated while the 24,000 Mr protein is not. The functions of these three phosphoproteins in bone are not known.

Proteoglycans are composed of a protein core to which are attached one or more long acidic polysaccharide chains called glycosaminoglycans. It is the presence of these very acidic, sulfated carbohydrate chains (previously called mucopolysaccharides) in the bone matrix which binds the majority of acid-seeking histochemical stains such as Alcian blue, Toluidine blue, Ruthenium red and Saffronin O.

In bone, the proteoglycans consist of small protein cores (Mr of approximately 45,000 on SDS gels) to which are attached either one or two chondroitin-4-sulfate chains (Mr of approximately 40,000 each) (15,18). Very similar proteoglycans have been found in the developing bone of all species investigated to date. They constitute about 10% of the noncollagenous proteins in the mineralized compartment of bone. There reports are conflicting in the literature concerning the fate of the matrix proteoglycans as the bone osteoid becomes mineralized. These levels have been reported to 1) increase (4), 2) not to change (46) and 3) to be completely lost (2). Two factors may account for these divergent observations: (1) histochemical stains are not specific for the proteoglycans, and (2) the small proteoglycans of bone are easily lost during demineralization of fixed sections. (The extremely large proteoglycans in calcified cartilage, Mr = 1–10 × 10^6 are less likely to diffuse away during demineralization.) The most convincing biochemical data indicate that there are no major changes in the two predominant proteoglycans in the osteoid as matrix mineralizes. This does not rule out the possibility that small but biologically significant changes are made or that significant changes in some minor species of proteoglycan do occur as osteoid matures and mineralizes. Recent results in ours and other laboratories (28) indicate that related but not completely identical small proteoglycan species are found in other, nonmineralizing tissues such as cartilage, tendon, skin and placenta. This would strongly suggest that the functions of these proteoglycans are performed during the secretion, assembly and/or maturation of collagen-based matrices.

Small proteoglycans have long been known to interact in a periodic manner with collagen fibrils (52,53) and recent *in vitro* experiments have shown that they may be involved in control of the rate and extent of fibril formation (7,64). The subtle differences between these otherwise similar proteoglycans from the different connective tissues may reflect a fine tuning of their assembly and maturation for specific matrix functions (Fig. 3).

The mineralized bone compartment is rich in sialoproteins (7.5% of the total NCP). The nine carbon acidic sugar, sialic acid, (N-acetyl-neuraminic acid) is attached in noncollagenous proteins to short oligosaccharide chains. In developing bovine bone, the predominant bone sialoprotein (BSP) is 50% protein, 12% sialic acid, 7% glucosamine, 6% galactosamine, the rest being neutral sugars, water of hydration and counterion salts (16). This 70-80,000 Mr glycoprotein stains with Alcian blue but not with the more commonly used protein stain, Coomassie blue, unless pretreated with neuraminadase to remove sialic acid groups. Bone sialoprotein was originally described in the late 1960s in steer bone as a protein of approximately 25,000 daltons (27), a species that is certainly the naturally occuring breakdown product of the higher molecular weight synthesized sialoprotein. A second bone sialoprotein was also found in developing bovine bone (17). This glycoprotein has the same apparent molecular weight (70 to 80,000) on SDS polyacrylamide electrophoresis gels but could be stained with Coomassie blue without prior neuraminidase treatment. This Coomassie-staining BSP contains fewer glutamic acid and glycine residues but more leucine and isoleucine than the Alcian blue-staining BSP. (The Coomassie blue binding BSP in rat bone appears to be of lower Mr (60,000) (21), while rat bone Alcian blue staining BSP is both identical in size and is immunologically cross-reactive with its bovine analogue (17).) Neither of the BSP molecules can be detected in tissues other than bone (with a lower limit of detection being 1/1000 the amount in bone) (21). The original work in the 1960s showed the sialoproteins to be calcium-binding glycoproteins, but their exact function in bone is not known at this time. Several highly acidic sialic acid-rich proteins in other tissues have been hypothesized as having roles in cell adhesion and in the processing of cell secretion products; whether or not osteoblasts may use their BSPs in similar ways is as yet unclear.

Perhaps, the largest group of NCPs present in bone is represented by the serum proteins. Serum albumin (34), α^3_2HS glycoprotein (60), transferrin and some classes of immunoglobu-

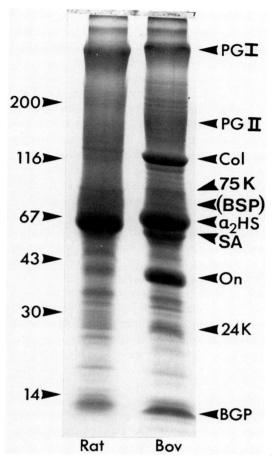

200►

116►

67►

43►

30►

14►

◄PGI

◄PG II

◄Col

◄75K

◄(BSP)

◄α₂HS

◄SA

◄On

◄24K

◄BGP

Rat   Bov

FIG. 3. Sodium dodecyl sulfate polyacrylamide gradient (4 to 20%) gel electrophoresis of bone matrix proteins. Rat or bovine bone were initially extracted with 4M guanidine hydrochloride containing protease inhibitors (G solution) to remove cellular proteins, and proteins not bound to the mineralized matrix. Subsequently, the bones were extracted with G solution containing 0.5 M ethylenediaminetetraacetic acid (E solution) to remove proteins tightly bound to the mineral phase. These E extracts were electrophoresed using a modified Laemmli polyacrylamide gel system. Bone matrix proteins were identified by staining with Coomassie blue and Alcian blue: Proteoglycan-I (PG-I), proteoglycan-II (PG-II), type I collagen (Col), 75,000 Mr phosphoprotein (75K), bone sialoprotein (BSP), α^3_2 HS serum glycoprotein ($^3_2$ HS), albumin (SA), osteonectin (On), 24,000 Mr protein (24K), and osteocalcin (BGP). Molecular weight standards are indicated in the left panel: myosin (200K), β-galactosidase (116K), albumin (67K), ovalbumin (43K), carbonic anhydrase (30K) and ^{3}-lactalbumin (14K).

lins (1) have all been reported to be contained within the calcified bone matrix. The most abundant serum proteins in bone, serum albumin and the α^3_2HS glycoprotein, may be enriched in bone to levels up to 50 to 100 times those found in serum depending on the animal species under study. Presumably these proteins bind to the growing hydroxyapatite crystals of bone through simple ionic interactions and then become entombed in the matrix as the mineralization is completed. A reasonable estimate of the amount of serum derived NCPs entrapped within the bone mineral compartment is about 25% of the total NCP. The functions of these proteins in bone. if any, are unknown.

MINERALIZATION OF THE BONE EXTRACELLULAR MATRIX

The mineral phase of bone is composed of so called ''impure'' hydroxyapatite (small crystals of carbonate-containing apatite). However, hydroxyapatite deposition may be preceded by fleeting precursor form(s). Although not conclusively identified *in vivo,* amorphous calcium phosphates may be the initial precursor in the formation of hydroxyapatite. Due to its greater instability, amorphous calcium phosphates rapidly transform into crystalline hydroxyapatite with either octacalcium phosphate or brushite as intermediates (5,19).

Although the precise pathway(s) by which bone matrix becomes calcified are not yet defined, it is clear that the spatial and temporal relationship between osteoblastic cells and the mineralization front are highly regulated. Mineralization begins between 2 to 10 μm away from the osteoblast cell surface and occurs between 24 hr and 10 days after the deposition of non-mineralized, newly synthesized osteoid (depending on the age and metabolic state of the animal) (50). Deposition of hydroxyapatite appears to occur by matrix vesicles or by deposition along collagen fibrils. In woven bone, found primarily in early embryonic fetal bone or in normal and pathological situations of rapid growth, the osteoid layer is relatively thin (2 to 3 μm) and is composed of a meshwork of relatively unoriented collagen fibrils. This type of bone appears to be initially mineralized primarily via matrix vesicles, which are trilamellar structures formed by budding of cell processes. Initial mineralization is rapid (24 to 72 hr) and occurs by the formation of hydroxyapatite crystals in close approximation to the matrix vesicle which may serve as a nucleation site for continued deposition. Lamellar bone, dominant in growing adult bone, contains a thick osteoid layer ($\sim$ 10 μm), with relatively few matrix vesicles. Calcification appears to proceed via deposition directly on to collagen fibrils in the ''hole'' regions (spaces between collagen triple helices, see Fig. 2), which initially highlights the striation pattern of collagen fibrils noted at the electron microscopic level. As deposition proceeds, the striation pattern is obliterated due to the increased number of hydroxyapatite crystals (50). The mechanism by which collagen acts as a nucleation site is controversial (47). It has been suggested that collagen in bone is phosphorylated and that this may serve as a Ca^{2+} binding site, thereby acting as a nucleator. The binding of non-collagenous proteins to collagen fibrils may also act as nucleators for the deposition of hydroxyapatite (47,58).

MOLECULAR BIOLOGY OF BONE

The most crucial questions in bone molecular biology center on how the expression of bone protein is regulated. That is to say, if the DNA in all cells is for the most part constant, why are bone genes differentially expressed in bone tissue? To answer these questions one must consider the intricacy of gene expression and all the steps that take place from gene to protein.

The genetic information for all proteins is located in the nucleus. Genes are encoded in discrete segments and are first transcribed through the action of RNA polymerase into precursor RNA called Hn RNA (heterogeneous nuclear RNA). The Hn RNA is processed from a large precursor to a smaller functional RNA (sometimes 1/10 the size) that is transported to the cytoplasm. The specific processing of the RNA message encoding for protein includes splicing out introns (non-coding regions), cap addition (a modified guanine at the 5' end) and covalent addition of a long string of adenines at the 3' end commonly referred to as a poly A tail. Mature messages (mRNA) are finally transported to the cytoplasm and then translated into protein using ribosomal machinery and tRNA previously linked to specific amino acids. Following cleavage of the signal peptide, matrix proteins are modified in the ER and Golgi apparatus (oligosaccharide addition, etc.) and secreted from the cell.

One approach to investigating the precise mechanisms controlling bone gene expression is to isolate recombinant DNA clones (cDNA) encoding these proteins. Rapid advances have been made in molecular cloning technology and, given specific antibody or a substantial stretch of amino acid protein sequence, the gene for almost any well-characterized protein can now be cloned. By using suitable cDNA as probes, one can begin to study the mechanisms which regulate bone gene expression at the nucleic acid level.

By far, the most rapid advances in structural bone protein molecular biology have been made using type I collagen DNA probes. As early as 1978, both chick $\alpha1(I)$ and $\alpha2(I)$ cDNA were isolated and definitively identified (54,63). Since then, cDNA probes have become available for human, rat and chick type I, II and III collagen genes (for review see 8). Only recently, cDNA encoding osteocalcin (35), osteonectin (66) and the small bone proteoglycan (11) have been isolated and characterized.

The regulation of type I collagen appears to be controlled at both transcriptional and translational levels. Type I collagen protein synthesis was measured in a variety of tissues (20), with tendon exhibiting maximal production (normalized to equal 100%), with less in skin (65%) and still less in muscle (25%). When RNA was extracted from the tissue, electrophoresed and transferred to solid support and analyzed by Northern analysis (RNA–DNA hybridization) using radiolabeled type I collagen cDNA, equivalent levels of hybridization were found in skin, muscle and tendon. Some hybridization was also found in cartilage (25% of tendon level), a tissue previously shown to produce no type I collagen protein. Thus, because much more type I collagen message was present than actual protein synthesized, the expression of this protein in skin, muscle and cartilage appears to be regulated at translational levels. The levels of type II collagen protein synthesized correlated precisely with type II collagen mRNA levels in all tissues (this protein is predominantly found in cartilage, see above). The type II collagen gene then, by this analysis, appears regulated mostly at transcriptional levels. Similar transcriptional control has been observed in cells forced to dedifferentiate in the presence of the thymidine analogue, bromodeoxyuridine (Budr). When chondrocytes are treated for 48 hr in the presence of Budr, the cells alter dramatically in morphology, changing to a more elongated, fibroblastic shape. In conjunction with these changes, the cells cease production of type II collagen and begin to synthesize type I collagen. Cell free translation of mRNA from such affected cells as well indicated that expression of both genes was regulated at transcriptional levels (37). Thus, the type I collagen gene in connective tissue cells can be regulated both transcriptionally and translationally. It is interesting to note that a detailed analysis of the collagen $\alpha2(I)$ gene promoters from chick and mouse showed an extremely conserved region around the start of translation that, by its sequence, is predicted to form a stem loop structure (51). Conversely, detailed sequence analysis of the type II collagen promoter from rat showed no such structure at the corresponding start of translation (30). It has been suggested that this conserved sequence in the type I collagen genes could contain a translational regulatory sequence specific for the type I protein.

The regulation of collagen synthesis has also been studied extensively during transformation. When chick embryo fibroblasts are transformed with the retrovirus, Rous sarcoma virus

(RSV), or treated with the tumor promoter, phorbol ester, production of type I collagen is drastically decreased (12). Following transformation, measurements of type I collagen mRNA showed an equally dramatic decrease indicating a transcriptional level of regulation (55). Northern analysis of similar RNA preparations using osteonectin cDNA as probes also showed a dramatic decrease in response to transformation (66). Thus, osteonectin, like type I collagen, appears transcriptionally regulated in transformed cells. Myeloblastosis associated virus (MAV.2–0) is a retrovirus which causes extended bone formation and osteoblastic hyperplasia (6). In contrast to RSV, this virus causes an increase in type I collagen synthesis in infected fibroblasts (61). Analysis of the mRNA from the infected cells showed an increase for both the $\alpha1(I)$ and $\alpha2(I)$ collagen genes.

Detailed studies of the type I and type II collagen promoters have revealed possible regulatory regions within these genes. A comparison of the chick and mouse type I promoter revealed several highly conserved regions upstream from the start of transcription that were interspersed between several nonconserved areas (51). The type II collagen promoter, on the other hand, contains three repeated hexanucleotides (5'GGGCGG3') that are identical to a hexanucleotide found within the thymidine kinase (tk) promoter (30). In the tk system, mutations within this hexanucleotide sequence were shown to reduce transcriptional efficiency to 5 to 15% of the wild type levels (33). It has been speculated that the conserved regions within the type I promoter region and the unique repeated sequences around the type II gene could play a role in the regulation of their expression.

The ultimate test of determining how the location of a matrix protein promoter regulates tissue specific expression requires transgenic expression during development. Only recently have such experiments been performed for the collagen genes (29). In these experiments, a 2000 bp sequence of the mouse $\alpha2(I)$ promoter was fused to the bacterial chloramphenicol acetyltransferase (CAT) gene and then injected into male pronuclei from fertilized mouse eggs. Transgenic embryos containing the foreign DNA were placed back into the uterus and allowed to develop to term. Southern analysis (DNA–DNA hybridization) of DNA from the transgenic mouse showed it to contain the chimeric $\alpha2$(I) promoter-CAT gene integrated into the mouse genome. When CAT enzymatic activity (a reflection of $\alpha2$(I) promoter activity) was measured in various tissues of the mouse, it was found (29) that the greatest activity was located in the tail, a tissue known to contain the highest levels of collagen in the mouse. Furthermore, expression of the chimeric gene was detected in the embryo after 8 1/2 days of gestation, about the same time that endogenous type I collagen genes become active. This experiment demonstrated that all the information necessary to direct tissue-specific expression of collagen DNA is located in a 2000 bp sequence upstream from the start of transcription. Future studies will undoubtedly involve systematic deletion and substitution of putative promoter regions to determine the exact base sequences which confer differential expression of the collagen genes, and further, to determine their relationship to other factors involved in this process.

As molecular probes encoding more bone protein genes become available, it will be possible to study the coordinated expression of structural bone matrix proteins. Such experiments will in turn provide important information about the mechanisms regulating normal bone development. Once these processes are understood for normal tissue, it will be possible to examine how these mechanisms are perturbed in bone disease states.

MATRIX VARIATION IN BONE DISEASE

Determination of quantitative and qualitative changes in the extracellular matrix components of bone associated with age and disease has only recently become possible with the development of new techniques to chemically dissect mineralized matrices via demineralizing and dissociative reagents. As of yet, matrix changes in brittle bone diseases have only been described in very few instances such as in some but not all forms of osteogenesis imperfecta (OI). Several genetic defects (either deletions or insertions) have been identified in genes encoding for the $\alpha1$(I) and $\alpha2$(I) chains of type I collagen. In these defects, it is apparent that mutations which produce $\alpha1$(I) or $\alpha2$(I) chains that still can be incorporated into the collagen triple helix and transported to the extracellular space result in more severe forms of the disease (i.e., OI–II, perinatal lethal) compared to mutations that do not allow defective chains to become incorporated into triple helices. The latter situation is that found in type I OI, (mildly deforming) which is characterized biochemically by a reduced type I collagen content in connective tissues, with the collagen that is present in the matrix being normal (8).

Recently, two bovine variants of OI have been identified where collagen defects are not yet apparent based on present technology. Interestingly, however, several NCPs were found to be deficient in the affected bones. The Australian variant (BOI–A) contained reduced levels (25% of normal) of bone proteoglycan (17), whereas the Texan variant (BOI–T) contained reduced levels of osteonectin (1% of normal, bone proteoglycan (10%) and bone sialoprotein (60%) (59). However, when bone cells from the affected animals were cultured *in vitro*, the proteins previously deficient in bone tissue were found to be produced by the cells in culture, although their incorporation into the bone matrix-rich cell layer was reduced compared to normal (unpublished data) (Fig. 4). The reason for this discrepancy is not yet clear but points to a possible defect in the formation of a supramolecular matrix complex arising from a mutation in any one of the constitutive bone matrix proteins. Also of interest is the finding that in bovine and rodent (OP/OP) osteopetrosis, a brittle bone disease attributed to impaired osteoclastic function, decreased levels of bone osteonectin and/or bone sialoprotein were

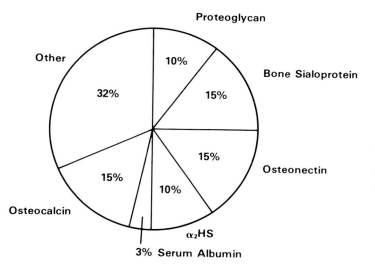

FIG. 4. Approximate percentages of noncollagenous bone matrix proteins extracted from fetal bovine subperiosteal bone. Similar amounts are also obtained from human bone specimens.

found with little change in other proteins (unpublished data). Thus, estimations of NCP variance may be important to many bone disease states.

In osteoporosis, the observed decrease in mass or mineralized bone may arise from either increased resorption or decreased osteoblastic function, or some combination of the two processes. Increased resorption could be related to: (1) humoral factors that stimulate osteoclastic function, or (2) changes in the extracellular matrix that allow osteoclasts to become unbalanced in their cytogenesis or modality of action. Since osteoblasts are also influenced by humoral factors, it is clear that continued study of osteoblastic metabolism will eventually elucidate mechanisms by which increased local output of a mineralized extracellular matrix can be achieved to restore normal balance between bone formation and resorption in affected individuals.

REFERENCES

1. Ashton, B.A., Triffitt, J.T., and Herring, G.M. (1974): The isolation and partial characterization of two glycoproteins from bovine cortical bone. *Eur. J. Biochem.*, 45:525–533.
2. Baylink, D., Wergedal, J., and Thompson, E. (1972): Loss of protein polysaccaride at sites where bone mineralization is initiated. *J. Histochem. Cytochem.*, 20:279–292.
3. Berseford, J.N., Gallanger, J.A., Poser, J.W., and Russell, R.G.G. (1984): Effects of 1,25-dihydroxyvitamin D_3, 24,25-dihydroxyvitamin D_3, PTH and glucocorticoids. *Metab. Bone Dis. Relat. Res.*, 5:229–234.
4. Bevelander, G., and Johnson, P.L. (1950): A histochemical study of the development of membrane bone. *Anat. Rec.*, 108:1–13.
5. Boskey, A.L. (1981): Current concepts of the physiology and biochemistry of calcification. *Clin. Orthop.*, 157:225–257.
6. Boyde, A., Banes, A.J., Dullamans R.M., and Mechanic, G.L.(1978): A morphological study of an avian bone disorder caused by myeloblastosis-associated virus. *Metab. Bone Dis. Rel. Res.*, 1:235–242.
7. Chandrasekhar, S., Kleinman, H.K., Hassell, J.R., Martin, G.R., Termine, J.D., and Trelstad, R.L.(1984): Regulation of type I collagen fibril assembly by link protein and proteoglycans. *Coll. Rel. Res.*, 4:323–338.
8. Cheah, K.S.E. (1985): Collagen genes and inherited connective tissue disease. *Biochem. J.*, 229:287–303.
9. Chen, P.V., Hauschka, P.V., and Feldman, D. (1984): 1,25(OH)₂D₃ stimulation of osteocalcin and inhibition of collagen synthesis in rat osteoblasts. Potentiation by glucocorticoids which up-regulate 1,25(OH)₂D₃ receptors. *Am. Soc. Bone Min. Res.*, 63(A).
10. Conn, K.M., and Termine, J.D. (1985): Matrix protein profiles in calf bone development. *Bone*, 6:33–36.
11. Day, A.A., Ramis, C.I., Fisher, L.W., Gehron Robey, P., Termine, J.D., and Young, M.F. (1986): Characterization of bone PG 11 cDNA and its relationship to PG II mRNA from other connective tissues. *Nucl. Acids Res.*, 14:9861–9876.
12. Delclos K.B., and Blumberg P.M. (1979): Decrease in collagen production in normal and Rous sarcoma virus transformed chick embryo fibroblasts induced

by phorbol myristate acetate. *Cancer Res., 39*:1667–1672.

13. Eyre, D.R., Paz, M.A., and Gallop, P.M. (1984): Cross-linking in collagen and elastin. *Ann. Rev. Biochem., 53*:717–748.

14. Fessler, J.H., and Fessler, L.I. (1978): Biosynthesis of procollagen. *Ann Rev. Biochem., 47*:129–169.

15. Fisher, L.W., Termine, J.D., Dejter, S.W., Whitson, S.W., Yanagishita, M., Kimura, J.H., Hascall, V.C., Kleinman, H.K., Hassell, J.R., and Nilsson, B. (1983): Proteoglycans of developing bone. *J. Biol. Chem., 258*:6588–6504.

16. Fisher, L.W., Whitson, S.W., Avioli, L.V., and Termine, J.D.(1983): Matrix sialoprotein of developing bone. *J. Biol. Chem., 258*:12723–12727.

17. Fisher, L.W. and Termine, J.D. (1985): Noncollagenous proteins influencing the local mechanisms of calcification. *Clin. Orth. Rel. Res., 200*:362–385.

18. Fisher, L.W. (1985): The nature of the proteoglycans of bone. In: *The Chemistry and Biology of Mineralized Tissues.* edited by W.T. Butler, pp. 186–196. Ebsco Media, Birmingham, Alabama.

19. Fleisch, H. (1982): Mechanisms of normal mineralization in bone and cartilage. In: *Biological Mineralization and Demineralization.* edited by G.H. Noncollas, pp. 233–241. Springer Verlag, New York.

20. Focht, R.J., and Adams, S.L. (1984): Tissue specificity of type I collagen gene expression is determined at both transcriptional and post transcriptional levels. *Mol. Cell. Biol., 4*:1843–1852.

21. Franzen, A., and Heinegard, D. (1985): Proteoglycans and proteins of rat bone. Purification and biosynthesis of major noncollagenous macromolecules In: *The Chemistry and Biology of Mineralized Tissues.* edited by W.T. Butler, pp. 132–141. Ebsco Media, Birmingham, Alabama.

22. Gehron Robey, P., Fisher, L.W., Stubbs, J.T., and Termine, J.D. (1986): Biosynthesis of osteonectin and a small proteoglycan (PG II) by connective tissue *in vitro.* In: Development and Diseases of Cartilage and Bone Matrix. edited by A. Sen, and T. Thornhill, pp. 115–125. Alan R. Liss, Inc., New York.

23. Genovese, C., Rowe, D., and Kream. B.E. (1984): Construciton of DNA sequences complimentary to rat α1 and α2 collagen mRNA and their use in studying the regulation of type 1 collagen synthesis by 1,25(OH)$_2$D$_3$. *Biochemistry, 23*:6210–6216.

24. Hauschka, P.V., and Gallop, P.M. (1977): In: Purification and calcium-binding properties of osteocalcin, in γ-carboxyglutamate-containing protein of bone. *Calcium Binding Proteins and Calcium Functions.* edited by R.H. Wasserman, R.A. Corradino, E. Carafoli, R.H. Kretsinger, D.H. MacLennan, and F.L. Seigel, pp. 338–347. North Holland Associated Press, New York.

25. Hauschka, P.V., and Reid, M.L. (1978): Timed appearance of a calcium-binding protein containing γ-carboxyglutamic acid in developing chick bone. *Dev. Biol., 65*:42–43.

26. Hauschka, P.V., Frenkel, J., DeMuth, R., and Gundberg, C.M. (1983): Presence of osteocalcin and related higher molecular weight γ-carboxyglutamic

acid-containing proteins in developing bone. *J. Biol. Chem., 258*:176–182.

27. Herring, G.M. (1972): The organic matrix of bone. In: *The Biochemistry and Physiology of Bone. Vol. 1.* edited by G.H. Bourne, pp. 127–189. Academic Press, New York.

28. Heinegarde, D., Bjorne-Persson, Coster, L., Franzen, A., Gardell, S., Malstrom, A., and Paulsson, M.(1985): The core proteins of large and small interstitial proteoglycans from various connective tissues from distinct subgroups. *Biochem. J., 230*:181–194.

29. Khillan, J.S., Schmidt, A., Overbeck, P.A., de-Crombrugghe, B, and Westphal, H. (1986): Developmental and tissue specific expression directed by the α2 type I collagen promoter in transgenic mice *Proc. Nat'l Acad. Sci., 83*:725–729.

30. Kohno, K., Sullivan, M., and Yamada Y. (1985): Structure of the promoter of the rat type II procollagen bone. *J. Biol. Chem., 260*:4441–4447.

31. Kuwata, F., Yao, K.-L., Sodek, J., Ives, S., and Pulleyblank, D. (1985): Identification of pre-osteonectin produced by cell-free translation of fetal porcine calvarial mRNA. *J. Biol. Chem., 260*:6993–6998.

32. Martin, G.R., Timpl R., Miller, P.K., and Kuhn, K. (1985): The genetically distinct collagens. *Trends Biochem. Sci.,* July: 285–287.

33. McKnight, S.L., Kingsbury, R.C., Spence, A., and Smith, M. (1984): The distal transcription signals of the Herpes virus tk gene share a common hexanucleotide control sequence. *Cell,* 37:253–262.

34. Owen, M., Triffitt, J.T., and Melick, R.A.: (1973) Albumin in bone. Ciba Foundation Symp. No. 11 (New series). In: *Hard Tissue Growth, Repair and Remineralization,* pp. 263–293. Elsevier Excerpta Medica North Holland Associated Science Publishers, Amsterdam.

35. Pan, L.C., and Price, P.A. (1975): The propeptide of rat bone carboxyglutamic acid protein shares homology with other vitamin K-dependent-protein precursors. *Proc. Natl Acad. Sci.* (USA), 82:6109–6113.

36. Piez, K.A., and Reddi, A.H.(1984): In: *Extracellular Matrix Biochemistry,* edited by K.A. Piez and A.H. Reddi, pp. 1–39. Elsevier, Amsterdam.

37. Powlowski, P.J., Brierley, G.T., and Lukens, L. (1981): Changes in the type II and type I collagen messenger RNA population during growth of Chondrocytes in 5-bromo-2-diosyuridine. *J. Biol. Chem.,* 256:7695–7698.

38. Price, P.A., Otsuka, A.S., Poser, J.W., Kristaponis, J., and Raman, N. (1976): Characterization of γ-carboxyglutamic acid-containing protein from bone. *Proc. Natl. Acad. Sci.* (USA), 73:1447–1451.

39. Price, P.A., Epstein, D.J., Lothringer, J.W., Nishimoto, S.K., Poser, J.W., and Williamson, M.K. (1979): Structure and function of the vitamin K-dependent protein of bone. In: *Vitamin K Metabolism and Vitamin K-dependent Proteins.* edited by J.W. Suttie, pp. 219–230. University Park Press, Baltimore.

40. Price, P.A., Parthemore, J.G., and Deftos, L.J. (1980): A new biochemical marker for bone metabolism. *J. Clin. Invest.,* 66:878–883.

41. Price, P.A., Lothringer, J.W., and Nishimoto, S.K. (1980): Absence of the vitamin K-dependent bone protein in fetal rat mineral. Evidence for another γ-carboxyglutamic acid-containing component in bone. *J. Biol. Chem.*, 255:928–935.

42. Price, P.A., and Nishimoto, S.K. (1980): Radioimmunoassay for the vitamin K-dependent proteins of bone and its discovery in plasma. *Proc. Natl. Acad. Sci.* (USA), 77:2234–2238.

43. Price, P.A., and Baukol, S.A. (1980): 1,25 dihydroxyvitamin D_3 increases synthesis of the vitamin-K dependent bone protein by osteosarcoma cells. *J. Biol. Chem.*, 255:11660–11663.

44. Price, P.A., Williamson, M.K., and Otawara, Y. (1985): Characterization of matrix gla protein. A new vitamin K-dependent protein associated with the organic matrix of bone. In: *The Chemistry and Biology of Mineralized Tissues*. edited by W.T. Butler, pp.159–163. Ebsco Media, Birmingham Alabama.

45. Price, P. Osteocalcin. (1983) In: *Bone and Mineral Research Annual 1*, edited by W.A. Peck, pp. 157–190. Exceprta Medica, Amsterdam.

46. Pritchard, J.J. (1952): A cytological and histochemical study of bone and cartilage formation in the rat. *J. Anat.*, 86:259–277.

47. Prockop, D.J., and Williams, C.J. (1982): Structure of the organic matrix: collagen structure (chemical). In: *Biological Mineralization and Demineralization*. edited by G.H. Nancollas, pp. 161–177. Springer-Verlag, New York.

48. Rodan, G.A., and Rodan, S.B. (1983): Expression of the osteoblastic phenotype. In: *Bone and Mineral Research Vol. 2*, edited by W.A. Peck, pp. 244–284. Elsevier Science Publishers, New York.

49. Romberg, R.W., Werness, P.G., Lollar, P., Riggs, B.L., and Mann, K.G. (1985): Isolation and characterization of native osteonectin. *J. Biol. Chem.*, 260:2728–2736.

50. Schenck, R.K., Humziker, E., and Hermann, W. (1982): Structure properties of cells related to tissue mineralization. In: *Biological Mineralization and Demineralization*.edited by G.H. Nancollas, pp. 143–160. Springer-Verlag, New York.

51. Schmidt, A., Yamada, Y., and deCrombrugghe, B. (1984): DNA sequence comparison of the regulatory signals at the 5' end of the mouse and chick α2 Type I collagen genes. *J. Biol. Chem.*, 259:7411–7415.

52. Scott, J.E., Orford, C.R., and Hughes, E.W. (1981): Proteoglycan-collagen arrangements in developing rat tail tendon. *Biochem. J.*, 195:573–581.

53. Scott, J.E., and Orford, C.R. (1981): Dermatan sulphate-rich proteoglycan associates with rat tail tendon collagen at the D band in the gap region. *Biochem. J.*, 197:213.

54. Sobel, M.E., Yamamoto, T., Adams, S.L., DiLauro, R., Enrico, V., Avvedimento, V., de Crombrugghe, B., and Pastan, I. (1978): Construction of a recombinant bacterial plasmid containing a chick pro α2 collagen gene sequence. *Proc. Nat. Acad. Sci.* (USA), 75:5846–5850.

55. Sobel, M.E., Yamamoto, T., de Crombrugghe, B., and Paston I. (1981): Regulation of Procollagen messenger ribonucleic acid levels in Rous sarcoma virus transformed chick embryo fibroblasts. *Biochemistry*, 20:2678–2684.

56. Stenner, D.D., Tracy, R.P., Riggs, B.L., and Mann, K.G. (1986): Human platelets contain and secrete osteonectin, a major protein of mineralized bone. *Proc. Nat. Acad. Sci.* (USA), 83:6892–6896.

57. Termine, J.D., Belcourt, A.B., Conn K.M., and Kleinman, H.K. (1981): Mineral and collagen-binding proteins of fetal calf bone. *J. Biol. Chem.*, 256:10403–10408.

58. Termine, J.D., Kleinman, H.K., Whitson, S.W., Conn, K.M., McGarvey, M.L., and Martin, G.R. (1981): Osteonectin, a bone-specific protein linking mineral to collagen. *Cell*, 26:99–105.

59. Termine, J.D., Gehron Robey, P. Fisher, L.W., Shimokawa, H. Drum, M.A. Conn, K.M., Hawkins, G.R., Cruz, J.B., and Thompson, K.G. (1984): Osteonectin, bone proteoglycan, and phosphophoryn defects in a form of bovine osteogenesis imperfecta. *Proc. Natl. Acad. Sci.* (USA), 81:2213–2217.

60. Triffitt, J.T., Owen, M.E., Ashton, B.A., and Wilson, J.M. (1978): Plasma disappearance of rabbit α_2HS-glycoprotein and its uptake by bone tissue. *Calcif. Tissue Res.*, 26:155–161.

61. Tuderman, L., and Franklin, R.M.(1985): Effect of avian osteopetrosis virus infection on cells and their collagen synthesis *in vitro*. *Eur. J. Biochem.*, 148:169–175.

62. Yamada, Y., Avvedimento, V.E., Mudryi, M., Onkubo, H., Vogeli, G., Irani, M., Pastan, I., and de Crombrugghe, B. (1980): The collagen gene: evidence for its evolutionary assembly by amplification of DNA segment containing an exon of 54 bp. *Cell*, 22:887–892.

63. Yamamoto, T., Sobel, M.E., Adams S.L., Avvedimento, B., DiLauro, R., Pastan, I., deCrombrugghe, B., Showalter, A., Pesciotta, D., Fritzek, P., and Olsen, B.(1980): Construction of a recombinant bacterial plasmid containing pro α1 (I) Collagen DNA Sequences *J. Biol. Chem.*, 255:2612–2615.

64. Vogel, K.G., and Heinegard, D. (1983): Proteoglycans of bovine fibrous tendon and their interaction with tendon collagen in vitro. In: *Proceedings Seventh International Symposium Glycoconjugates*. edited by M.A. Chester, D. Heinegard, A. Lundblad, and S. Svenssen, pp. 830–831. Rahms, Lund.

65. Wasi, S., Otsuka, K., Yao, K.L., Tung, P.S., Aubin, J.E., Sodek, J., and Termine, J.D. (1984): An osteonectin-like protein in porcine periodontal ligament and its synthesis by periodontal ligament fibroblasts. *Can. J. Biochem. Cell Biol.*, 62:470–478.

66. Young, M.F., Bolander, M.E., Day, A.A., Ramis, C.I., Gehron Robey, P., Yamada, Y., and Termine, J.D. (1986): Osteonectin mRNA: Distribution in normal and transformed cells. *Nucl. Acids Res.*, 14:4483–4497.

Osteoporosis: Etiology, Diagnosis, and Management, edited by B. Lawrence Riggs and L. Joseph Melton, III. Raven Press, New York © 1988.

4

Biomechanical Aspects of Fractures

*L. Joseph Melton, III, **Edmund Y. S. Chao, and †Joseph Lane

*Department of Medical Statistics and Epidemiology, and the **Biomechanics Laboratory, Department of Orthopedics, Mayo Clinic and Mayo Foundation, Rochester, Minnesota 55905; †Department of Orthopaedic Surgery, The Hospital for Special Surgery, New York, New York 10021*

Osteoporosis might be of academic interest alone were it not for the associated fractures. Since these fractures exact a staggering burden of morbidity, mortality, and social costs (Chapter 5, *this volume*), the biomechanical aspects of osteoporosis assume exceptional practical importance. This chapter will summarize the structural (whole bone) and material (bone tissue) changes due to osteoporosis. Basic biomechanical principles relating to bone strength will be reviewed, and the occurrence of fractures at specific anatomical sites will be discussed in terms of the mechanical and material principles involved. This understanding of the structural consequences of osteoporosis should lead to a better appreciation of the fracture syndromes commonly seen with aging.

GENERAL PRINCIPLES

Loss of Bone with Aging

After peaking in young adulthood, bone mass begins to decline with advancing age and reaches lower levels among women than men. Details are presented in Chapter 2. While both cortical and trabecular bone are affected, patterns of loss may vary by site (106). Peak cortical bone mass, for example, is achieved by the mid- to late 30s (54). These levels are generally maintained until around the time of menopause in women and about the same age in men, although slow loss begins earlier (82). Trabecular (cancellous) bone reaches peak mass in the early 30s and begins to decline in some, but not all, individuals soon afterwards (82). The proportion of women experiencing significant premenopausal trabecular bone loss is somewhat controversial but may be substantial (117).

Bone loss is proportionately greater in women than men (82), in part because a period of accelerated bone loss accompanying menopause is superimposed upon the underlying age-related loss in women. The ultimate result is that by age 90 years, women have lost one-fifth of their original peak cortical bone mass (midradius), compared to less than 5% in men (115). By age 90 years, women have lost 40 to 50% of their peak trabecular bone mass, while men have lost 10 to 25% (89,115).

Cortical bone is lost from endosteal surfaces at a more rapid rate than it is gained periosteally, leading to a net reduction of as much as 30 to 50% in the thickness of cortical bones in women. Endosteal resorption and the resulting loss of cortical thickness is less dramatic in men (84,121). Bone diameter slowly increases, however; and, when endosteal loss slows among the very old, cortical thickness may actually increase somewhat. Such changes are much greater in the lower extremity (121) than in the upper (84). Moreover, there is evidence that cortical thickness may be preferentially maintained in bone segments subjected to high bending and torsional stresses, i.e., the diaphyseal regions, while metaphyseal bone becomes progressively weaker (121). Thus, cortical thickness may vary by age, sex, and skeletal site. Porosity of cortical bone also increases with aging, and porosity may be enhanced during the perimenopausal phase of bone loss in women (107) as it is transiently during adolescence (108).

Cancellous bone loss, on the other hand, leads to perforation of trabecular plates, to thinning of plates and, ultimately, to the loss of some plates entirely (107). There is some evidence that the early postmenopausal phase of bone loss is marked by rapid perforation and loss of plates, while the slower thinning process continues with aging (105). These changes in cortical and trabecular bone have structural sequelae that degrade the biomechanical integrity of the skeleton. To relate these changes to bone fragility, however, a review of the material and structural behavior of bone is necessary.

Material Behavior of Bone

Material properties vary according to type of bone, geometry, anatomic location, age, species, and pathologic condition (153). While the geometries of whole bones are complex, the important mechanical properties of bone can be determined by subjecting small specimens of regular geometry to specific loading conditions. Loading changes the configuration of deformable objects, through the development of internal forces (or pressure) within the object.

Such internal force per unit area is defined as *stress*. When the internal force is perpendicular to a particular plane within the bone, it is called *normal stress;* and, when parallel to the plane, it is defined as *shear stress*. Deformation resulting from the stress may involve a percentage change in length, defined as *normal strain,* or a relative change in shape, termed *shear strain*. The strain corresponding to a given load depends on the type of material involved. Hence, the relationship between stress and strain can be regarded as a fundamental physical characteristic of any material, including bone, and represents the key parameter describing the mechanical behavior of the material. Under test conditions with a standardized specimen, stress and strain can be recorded continuously under increasing load until failure occurs, resulting in an idealized stress-strain curve (Fig. 1).

Stress-strain curves and the material properties derived from them vary according to the type of loading (normal versus shear). Material properties within an intact bone may also differ depending on the location of the bone specimen (material *inhomogeneity*) or when test specimens are taken from the same location but at different orientations (material *anisotropy*). The strength (ultimate stress before fracture) and stiffness (modulus) of bone, for example, are usually greater in the direction of customary loading. Bone also demonstrates different mechanical characteristics under different rates of loading and is, therefore, viscoelastic.

Mean values of key material parameters of human cortical and trabecular bone are summarized in Table 1. The anisotropic nature of cortical bone is immediately apparent, as strength and modulus are greater with longitudinal loading. Irreversible (or plastic) deformation is less with transverse loading (114) and, thus, bone appears to be more brittle in that direction (63). Cortical bone is stronger in compression than in tension (63). Strength also varies with the strain rate (20), being greater with more rapid rates of loading. Tensile strength and modulus of cortical bone in the femur decrease about 2% per decade after maturation in both tension and compression (19).

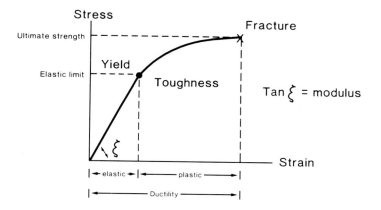

FIG. 1. Key material properties of bone under uniaxial loading. Stress and strain rise with increasing force. When resulting strain changes proportionally with the stress, the material is linearly elastic. The linear portion of the curve is thus the *elastic region,* while the nonlinear portion is the *plastic region.* The junction of these two is the *yield point,* where the corresponding stress is defined as the *elastic limit.* Loading beyond the yield point will result in permanent deformation of the material, even after the load is removed. The slope of the normal stress-strain curve in the elastic region is defined as the *modulus of elasticity* (E, Young modulus) of the material, or material stiffness. [When shear stress and strain are plotted, the slope is defined as the *shear moduls* (G)]. The maximum stress and strain at failure are the *ultimate tensile strength* and *ductility,* respectively. The area under the curve is defined as the *strain energy,* and the total strain energy stored at the point of fracture is call the *toughness* of the material.

In trabecular bone, ultimate compressive strength is related to the square of apparent density so that a decline in bone density with aging to one-third of the value in normal young adults could be associated with a reduction in compressive strength to one-ninth of normal (20). Trabecular bone is also anisotropic: compressive strength is greatest along the vertical axis of trabeculae in the lumbar vertebrae (52,94) and parallel to trabecular systems in the femoral neck (16,81). Compressive strength and tensile strength are equivalent in trabecular bone (22,63,97), as is the elastic modulus under both loading directions. The elastic modulus for trabecular bone is much less than that for cortical bone, however, as stiffness is correlated with the cube of apparent density (20). Although less stiff, trabecular bone can withstand greater strain, fracturing at about 7% of original length when cortical bone fails at 2% (102).

Overall, 75 to 85% of variance in the ultimate strength of bone tissue is accounted for changing bone mineral density with age (131).

TABLE 1. *Mean values of human bone material parameters (114)*

Bone type	Loading direction	Apparent density (g/cm^3)	Ultimate strength (10^6 MPa)	Elastic modulus (10^6 MPa)
Cortical[a] bone	Longitudinal tension	1.85	133	17,000
	Longitudinal compression	1.85	193	17,000
	Longitudinal shear	1.85	68	3,300
	Transverse tension	1.85	51	11,500
	Transverse compression	1.85	133	11,500
Cancellous[b]	Compression	0.31	6	76

[a]Obtained from human midfemoral diaphysis, ages 19 to 80 years.
[b]Obtained from human vertebral body, ages 41 to 71 years.

The remainder may be due to qualitative changes associated with altered composition of mineral or matrix (104). Collagen, which apparently remains stable with aging when expressed per unit weight of bone and does not vary with sex, may change qualitatively (36); but this appears to be without effect on the elastic modulus of bone. Increased mineralization is seen in osteoporosis (37,104), however, and may be associated with the formation of occasional large apatite crystals (23,74). Geometric defects—such as large crystals, small holes, notches (areas of enhanced resorption), and sudden thinning of cortex and/or trabeculae—cause significantly higher local bone stress *(stress risers)*. Even under normal loading, these high stresses may initiate localized bone failure through crack formation, although this is not believed to be the primary determinant of bone strength (132). Nonetheless, such factors may lead to decreased energy absorption and reduced plastic deformation before failure (32), reflected by microfractures (104).

Structural Behavior of Bone

Material parameters describe the relative mechanical properties of different types of bone tissue in the skeletal system. However, fracture represents failure of the whole bone; and, consequently, a set of biomechanical parameters that specify the behavior of the entire bone is required. These parameters are structural stiffness (or rigidities) and structural load capacity(or failure load). Such properties depend on the type of load applied to bone and represent a combination of geometric and material characteristics.

The major types of bone loading commonly experienced in the human body are axial compression or tension, bending, and torsion. When intact bone is loaded under each mode, load-deformation curves (Fig. 2) can be recorded in a fashion similar to the stress-strain curves. The slope of the linear portion of each load-deformation curve is defined as the structural stiffness (or rigidity) of the bone. Hence, under axial load, bending, and torsion, respectively, the load-deformation curves will provide the values for axial rigidity (AE), flexural rigidity (EI), and torsional rigidity (GJ). These parameters describe the stiffness of the structure under specific loading conditions and are dependent upon both the geometric parameters (area, A; area moment of inertia, I; and polar area moment of inertia, J, see below) and the intrinsic material parameters (elastic modulus, E; shear modulus, G). As load is increased until fracture, the maximum force (bending moment or torque) is defined as the ultimate failure moment or torque. The structural behavior of bone can thus be quantified using the stiffness characteristics and failure loads without delineating the underlying geometric and material properties. Although the problems of inhomogeneity and anisotropy are then obscured, it is important to realize that the overall structural response is a combination of both material properties of bone tissue and its geometric arrangement.

Axial loading can be in tension or compression (Fig. 2). Tension is important in fractures due to excessive loads on tendons (102) and with some fractures of the posterior elements of the vertebrae that occur with severe trauma (72). However, vertebral bodies and other short bones fracture primarily under compressive loads. Unexpectedly, perhaps, the mechanism of fracture usually involves bending rather than compression per se (33). This is especially pertinent to vertebral fractures because trabeculae are thin relative to their length. Age-related bone loss may reduce the cross-sectional area but, more importantly, increases the effective length of vertical trabeculae by removing the horizontal trabeculae that act as lateral supports or cross-ties (94). Trabeculae thus behave somewhat like columns, and the main parameter used to describe the structural behavior of a column is the critical buckling load. Engineering principles indicate that a 50% reduction in cross-sectional area is associated with a reduction in load carrying capacity to 25% of the original figure (55). A doubling in effective length, by the loss of alternate horizontal trabeculae, for example, also leads to a

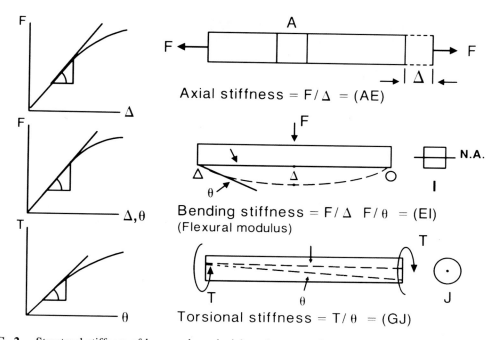

Axial stiffness = F / Δ = (AE)

Bending stiffness = F / Δ F / θ = (EI)
(Flexural modulus)

Torsional stiffness = T / θ = (GJ)

FIG. 2. Structural stiffness of bone under uniaxial tension—top; three-point bending force—middle; and torsion—bottom. As illustrated by a cylindrical bar of bone of a given length (L) and cross-sectional area (A), axial stress is defined by the tension force (F) divided by the area (F/A). Strain is defined by change in length (Δ/L). This change is directly proportional to applied force and bone length and inversely proportional to cross-sectional area and E, the material modulus (Δ = FL/AE). This relationship can be rewritten (AE = FL/Δ). If bone length (L) is constant, the axial stiffness (AE) or rigidity will be proportional to F/Δ. The change in length (Δ) with the force (F) defines the load deformation curve. During three-point bending, the applied force (F) and the beam deflection (Δ) or rotation (Θ) can be plotted. The slope of the linear portion of this is defined as the flexural rigidity (EI) or bending stiffness (EI = F/Δ or F/Θ). In three-point bending, the deflection can be calculated from $\Delta = \frac{FL}{EI}$. If the length of the bone (L) is constant, $\frac{F}{\Theta}$ is proportional to EI, where E is the elastic modulus and I is the area moment of inertia around the neutral axis (N.A.). In torsion (T), the angular rotation of the bone(Θ) can be plotted. The slope of the linear portion of the curve is defined as the torsional stiffness (GJ) or rigidity (GJ = T/Θ). The rotation (Θ) can be calculated from the formula $\Theta = \frac{TL}{GJ}$. If bone length (L) is constant, the torsional stiffness T/Θ can be expressed in terms of the product GJ, where G is the shear modulus and J is the polar area moment of inertia.

reduction in the critical buckling load to one-fourth of the original value.

Long bones usually fail under a combination of axial compression, bending and torsion. Bending occurs because long bones are slightly curved and subjected to longitudinal compression at the joint surfaces. Since this compressive force is eccentric to the centroid of the bone cross-section, bending and longitudinal compression are combined. As described by the three point loading configuration (Fig. 2), bending can subject one side of the cortex to tension and the opposite side to compression. The rigidity of bone under these conditions depends on the cross-sectional shape of the bone, its length, and its material properties, as well as how the ends of the bone column are fixed. With bending or torsion, however, the bone cross-sectional area is less important than its distribution with respect to the axis of loading. In bending, it would be ideal for the bone tissue to be distributed as far as possible away from the axis of bending (the neutral axis). The geometric parameter used to describe this property is the area moment of inertia (I). In torsion, it would be more efficient to resist deformation if the bone were distributed further away from the torsional axis (Fig. 2). This geometric parameter is defined as the polar area moment of inertia (J). With aging, the outer cortical diameter increases while the inner cortical wall diameter is also expanding. Although the net result is cortical wall thinning, the increased average diameter of the bone improves its resistance to bending and torsional loads, through its area moment properties, and may be sufficient to offset any bone loss. Thus, cortical bone fractures are not especially common in osteoporotic patients.

Bone is subjected to forces from gravitational effects and from muscle contraction and limb movement (inertial effects). Even with normal daily activity, large forces are produced. This fact has often been ignored, since such activity does not generally involve heavy lifting or exercise. When a force is applied away from a point of support (fulcrum) on an object, it tends to rotate the object. Such mechanical action is defined as the *moment* of a force and is equal to the force times the distance from the fulcrum to the force application point (moment arm). The human musculoskeletal system is rather inefficient in resisting external loads, including gravitational force exerted on limb segments and torso, because the muscles that counteract gravity are attached close to the joints and have relatively small moment arms. Hence, they must exert forces many times higher than those applied externally, simply to maintain posture in the face of gravitational loads. When abducting an outstretched arm or bending the trunk, for example, the shoulder and lumbar intervertebral joints can be subjected to forces exceeding body weight (127,146). This joint reaction force is transmitted to bone.

Under normal conditions, the skeleton can sustain these loads with a sufficient margin of safety to avoid fracture. However, bone that has undergone pathologic change may not be able to resist nominal loading, especially of a repetitive nature. When loads are applied to bone in a repetitive manner, fracture can occur even if the stress is substantially below the ultimate strength of the bone. This phenomenon is described as stress or fatigue fracture. By inducing microdamage that shifts the load to the remaining intact bone (21), fatigue loading can greatly magnify the deleterious effects of structural and material weakness. Ultimate strength is reduced significantly and fatigue failure may become prominent as local stresses in the affected region become higher. Under normal conditions, biological remodeling can repair the microfractures caused by fatigue loading (50). In osteoporotic patients, however, the normal repair mechanisms required to prevent or reverse such damage may be inhibited, causing the accumulation of microfractures (50) and perhaps resulting in bone failure even under low loading conditions.

FRACTURE PATTERN AND LOCATION IN OSTEOPOROTIC BONE

Although bone loss appears to be systemic to some degree, fractures secondary to osteoporosis occur predominantly at specific anatomic sites. Fractures in the neck and intertrochanteric regions of the proximal femur, Colles' fractures of the distal radius, and vertebral body fractures are most notable. Though composed largely of trabecular bone, these anatomic regions have distinctly different skeletal shapes and loading configurations. The biomechanical factors previously discussed may thus help explain the pattern and location of such fractures in osteoporotic individuals.

Long Bone Fractures

Long bones, like the shaft of the femur, undergo an age-related increase in diameter (121,135). At the mid-femur, for example, the outer diameter increased by about 20% from age 45 to 49 to age 75+ years in one study of ambulatory women (135). However, the width of the medullary cavity, or endosteal diameter, increased to an even greater degree because of endosteal bone resorption so that cortical thickness declined somewhat as a result. Nonetheless, bone loss is compensated for by this modeling, which relocates the remaining bone further from the centroid of the bone cross-sectional area and thus increases both the area moment of inertia and the polar area moment of inertia (Fig. 3). As noted above, this tends to maintain bone strength for bending and torsional loads.

Traumatic forces sufficient to break such bone could, and do, cause fractures in anyone (27,76,93). Consequently, a peculiar association of diaphyseal fractures with old age or female sex is not commonly recognized. Instead, age- and sex-specific incidence rates for diaphyseal fractures tend to reflect the patterns of occupational or behavioral exposure to severe trauma: fractures of this sort are more common among the young and are more frequent in men than women (2,17,120). The question of impaired bone strength rarely arises.

Distal Forearm Fractures

The midradius, comprised almost entirely of cortical bone (115), has the biomechanical properties of other long bones. Even the distal radius, at some sites traditionally used for single photon absorptiometry scanning, is mostly cortical bone. The cortical shell diminishes distally, however, and the proportion of trabecular bone increases, reaching 38 to 50 percent at the 5 mm site (7,40) and up to 75% at the ultradistal radius site (40,126). Trabecular bone serves to protect joint surfaces, through compliance (68), and to transmit loads from the joint surface to the diaphysis. The metaphyseal regions of the radius and ulna also become wider distally in order to enhance joint stability and to provide the greater surface area needed to transmit forces across the joints without damaging synovial cartilage or subchondral bone (33).

With aging, trabecular bone is lost from this area, although at a lower rate than in the spine

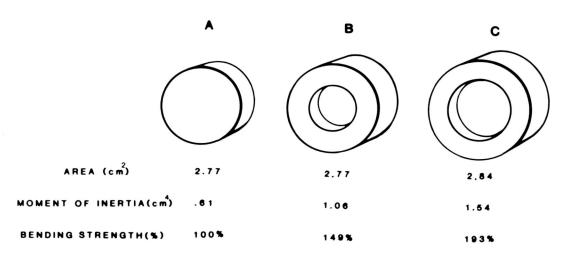

	A	B	C
AREA (cm^2)	2.77	2.77	2.84
MOMENT OF INERTIA(cm^4)	.61	1.06	1.54
BENDING STRENGTH(%)	100%	149%	193%

FIG. 3. Effect of changes in distribution of cross-sectional area on the area, moments of inertia and bending strength of some regular cylindrical geometries. These idealized geometries reflect the approximate dimensions of the femoral midshaft of the Pecos Pueblo population. The changes between **B** and **C** are thus comparable to the geometric remodeling that occurred with aging in that population. From Hayes and Gerhart, ref. 63, with permission.

(108). However, there is increasing endosteal trabeculation of cortical bone with age (107) so that the volume of trabecular bone may actually increase somewhat (126). The metaphyseal shell, already thin, is further compromised by the increasing cortical porosity (10,108). The decline in bone mass is correlated with a reduction in strength (68). There is no compensatory increase in the diameter of the radius with age (84,133) comparable to that seen in the femur shaft, perhaps through lack of the mechanical stimulation for subperiosteal bone apposition that is associated with weight-bearing (121,135). Consequently, the area moment of the distal radius is not readjusted as much as in the femur, and the net bone loss is not compensated for as well biomechanically. The result is low stiffness and strength of the metaphysis (63,68) and a reduced capacity for load resistance and energy absorption (33,68).

Despite these changes, the radius and ulna are able to withstand the stresses of daily living because the distal forearm is not usually a site of heavy loading during normal activities. "Spontaneous" fractures of the forearm are not seen. Instead, forearm fractures are almost always due to a specific episode of trauma. Direct blows to the arm or falls from heights, for example, may result in fractures of the shaft of the radius and/or ulna (4). The more usual event, however, is a fall on the outstretched hand. If the wrist is not dorsiflexed, a proximal forearm fracture may result (51), but this is uncommon. If dorsiflexion is extreme ($> 90°$), on the other hand, carpal bone fractures may occur (38,51). With a lesser degree of dorsiflexion, falls exert a large impact force on the wrist. Up to half of this energy is absorbed by skin and subcutaneous tissue and another third by muscles and tendons, but that remaining is transmitted to the radius (99). Additionally, the distal radius is subjected to a bending load accentuated by the wedging effect of the carpal bones and ligamentous constraints at the wrist joint. As summarized by Frykman, the process proceeds as follows:

> . . . at the moment of fracture, the hand stays put on the surface of impact; the kinetic energy

causes the forward movement of the body to continue, the wrist becomes hyperextended and the patient falls over the hand; this loads the volar ligament and the radius is pressed against the carpal articular surface, the force being stopped by the scaphoid and lunate bones; it is then transmitted to the radius, which fractures at its weakest point in the same manner as a beam that is loaded beyond the limit of its elasticity. (51).

Thus, in Colles' fracture, the usual clinical pattern of a sharp fracture line through the palmar surface with compression of trabecular bone and comminution of the cortex dorsally (78) indicates that bending forces initially fracture the volar aspect of the radius in tension (38). Propagation of the fracture then causes compression forces to be concentrated along the dorsum. Fracture of the distal radius can result in either Colles' fracture (metaphyseal fracture through the distal radius with dorsal displacement of the hand), Smith's fracture (fracture of the distal radius with volar displacement of the hand), or Barton's fracture (distal radius fracture with intraarticular involvement). The specific fracture seen is determined by the position of hand and arm on impact (38,51), although Colles' fractures are by far the most frequent (138).

Because most Colles' fractures are due to falls and because the forces delivered in falls may be sufficient to cause fractures over a wide range of bone mass values (69), bone mineral density may be a relatively insensitive risk factor. Nonetheless, radial bone mass is generally somewhat reduced in women with Colles' fractures. Differences are modest, however, with substantial overlap between fracture patients and controls (62,65,75,100), although there may be a somewhat greater discrepancy in trabecular than in cortical bone (62,65). More importantly, bone mass in women with Colles' fractures is much less than in young normal women (75). As with fractures of the vertebrae and proximal femur (see below), the risk of Colles' fracture in women appears to rise as bone density falls (R. Eastell, unpublished data).

One would thus expect Colles' fracture incidence rates to be greater in women than men at any given age, since bone mass is less in adult women than men. Indeed, the amount of force *in vitro* required to produce Colles' fractures in women is only 70%, on average, of that in men (51). Also rates should rise with age as bone mass falls. Both expectations are borne out (Chapter 5, *this volume*). However, a most distinctive feature is the plateau in Colles' fracture incidence among women after age 60 years. This is especially striking in contrast to the continued exponential rise in hip fracture incidence with age. A variety of explanations have been proposed, including a reduction in trauma due to inability of elderly individuals to put out a hand to break the impact of a fall (42). This would not appear to account, however, for the appearance of the plateau in rates at an age when such reflexes should be relatively unimpaired or for the lower fracture incidence among men. Variations in bone mass provide a more general explanation. The plateau in incidence rates, for example, may be due to a decline in the population at risk because of stabilizing bone mass later in life (98). A number of studies have suggested, on both theoretical (69) and empirical (70) grounds, that net bone loss in the distal forearm ultimately slows, or perhaps even reverses because of continued periosteal apposition with reduced endosteal absorption (70). It has also been suggested that the postmenopausal accentuation of bone loss (and fracture risk) could be accounted for by increased endosteal trabeculation or by transiently increased cortical porosity in the perimenopausal period (107), thus accounting for the association of Colles' fracture with type I osteoporosis (108,116).

Vertebral Fractures

The vertebral fractures seen in conjunction with osteoporosis involve the vertebral body and are usually classified into three forms, although a single vertebra may have characteristics of more than one (137). Crush (collapse, compression) fractures involve compression of the entire vertebral body, including the poste-

rior aspect. In wedge fractures, posterior height is relatively maintained but there is collapse anteriorly. Concave (ballooning, biconcave, codfish) vertebrae feature collapse of the superior or inferior endplates, or both, with relative maintenance of anterior and posterior heights. All of these changes indicate fracturing (104). Many other varieties of vertebral fractures occur in association with severe trauma (35).

Vertebral bodies are primarily subjected to compression, with superimposed bending in the midsagittal plane and torsion about the long axis of the spine. In the standing position, about half of the compressive load is due to ligament and muscle tension needed to keep the spinal column erect (80). The other half is due to the body weight carried above the level of each vertebrae, increasing to over one-half body weight at the lumbosacral joint (43). Compressive loads may be increased manyfold by lifting, depending on the distance of the object from the center of motion in the spine, the degree of flexion of the spine, and other factors (80,96). Lifting a given load in a forward bending position, for example, can produce pressure on the lumber vertebrae that is 10 to 20 times greater than the weight lifted (110), although these forces may be reduced somewhat by increased intraabdominal pressure (80,127). Even coughing and laughing are associated with compression loads 50 to 70 percent greater than quiet standing, figures similar to that seen for jumping (96).

Compression forces are resisted through a variety of mechanisms. The intervertebral disc functions hydrostatically to cushion shocks, to distribute loads evenly over the surface, and to transfer compressive loads across the joint. The nucleus pulposus is relatively imcompressible (118), however, and continued loading causes the cartilaginous endplate and underlying vertebral body to deform (149). Lumbar vertebrae can be compressed to 16% of their height (111) or more (59) before fracture occurs. This deformation forces blood out of the vertebral body into the perivertebral sinus (118) and "results in load damping quite similar to that of an automobile shock absorber'' (72). Moreover, the marrow under pressure may exert hydraulic effects (73,149), perhaps accounting for the fact that vertebrae can tolerate higher loads at greater strain rates (110,149), as in a fall (43).

The thin boney endplate is less strong than the intact intervertebral disc (110,118) and may be weakened further by age-related bone loss. It will thus collapse under smaller loads in older individuals than in younger ones. Perey (110) showed that the endplates in subjects over 60 years of age bore little more than half the pressure tolerated in subjects under 40 years old, the lowest value of which was greater than the mean in older subjects. This problem may be accentuated by the preferential loss of trabeculae from the center of the vertebral body with age (6). It is said that the superior surface typically fractures before the inferior surface (72,141) but both defects may occur, leading to the appearance of biconcave vertebrae. The shape of the deformity reflects the condition of the disc, with normal discs producing more or less spherical depressions (61,72). Biconcave fractures may be relatively more frequent in the lumbar vertebrae (39,137) due to the extension that occurs on loading the lordotic curve of the spine and the central loading associated with a more posterior center of gravity (35).

Within the vertebral body, most of the strength is provided by trabecular bone (11). In normal elderly individuals, the cortex contributes only about 10% of vertebral strength in compression (83), and the resistance to crushing of the entire vertebral body is similar to that of samples of vertebral trabecular bone (9). Vertebral body strength declines with aging, however, and is lower in women than men (9), coinciding with the loss of trabecular bone (59). Some trabecular plates are lost completely (107), especially the horizontal trabeculae which act as column crossties (6,105,141, 142). As noted under structural principles, the consequent reduction in strength is disproportionately greater than the reduction in mass (11,149). Vertical trabeculae are also lost, but those that remain are thicker, accounting for the radiographic appearance of accentuated vertical trabeculae in the osteoporotic spine (see Chapter 7, Fig. 2, *this volume*). This may come about through compensatory thickening of remaining trabeculae (6,104,141) or, alternatively, selective removal of the thinner vertical trabeculae (Chapter 2, *this volume*). Ultimately, however, few vertical trabeculae and only sparse, irregular horizontal trabeculae may remain (Fig. 4).

Loss of trabeculae increases the load on those remaining (50,88). This, and local factors such as increased brittleness (104), encourage the development of microfractures (50,58). Because microdamage repair is impaired in osteoporosis, these increase in number (60,143) and may coalesce and propagate. However, it has been noted that vertebrae can maintain 60 to 70% of load-bearing capacity even after fracture and, after compression to one-half original height, may again approach their original load-bearing capacity, although this capability may vary by age and sex (149). Also seen *in vitro* (79), this phenomenon may be associated with pore closure after trabecular

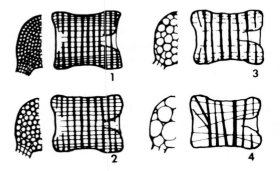

FIG. 4. Radiographic trabecular patterns in the vertebral body illustrated schematically: type 1, checker pattern in Plane A and small uniform ring pattern in Plane B. Type 2, slight distended ring pattern in Plane B and slight decrease in trabecular density in plane A. Type 3, widened ring pattern in Plane B and partly disappeared horizontal trabeculae in Plane A. Type 4, extremely distended ring pattern in Plane B and significant decrease in trabecular density in Plane A. From Tanaka, ref. 141, with permission.

collapse (20). Crush fractures may also be influenced by disc pathology. Older discs are flatter, less elastic, and unable to distribute stresses evenly over the surface (80,110). Compressive loads are then transmitted more through the peripheral annulus fibrosa (110), causing buckling of the lateral cortex and consequent collapse of the entire vertebral body (43,118).

Anterior wedging fractures, on the other hand, are associated with forward flexion of the spine. While the lesser anterior height of midthoracic vertebral bodies relative to posterior height (149) contributes to the impression of anterior wedging, and may account in part for reports of wedge fractures clustering in the midthoracic area (53), wedge fractures are more frequent in the lower thoracic and upper lumbar areas. As a result of the residual curvature of the spinal column, the center of gravity passes anteriorly to the vertebral bodies in this area and loading of the kyphotic curve of the spine leads to flexion. The spine has less resistance to loads applied eccentrically in flexion (73,80). The reason for this is shown in Fig. 5. The axis of movement of the intervertebral joint is through the nucleus pulposus. Thus, the distance from the axis to the spinous process posteriorly is three times (thoracic spine) to four times (lumbar spine) greater than the distance to the anterior margin of the vertebral body (72). As a consequence, when forward flexion is resisted by the erector spinae muscles and posterior ligaments, the compressive load on the vertebral body is three to four times greater than the tensile load on the posterior elements, perhaps exceeding the capacity of the vertebral endplate (118). Moreover, the weight-bearing surface area is effectively reduced and compressive stress is concentrated anteriorly (149). Under such conditions the anterior cortex may collapse but the posterior cortex, under tension, is not usually affected, hence the wedge-shaped appearance. Anterior wedging may increase the curvature, in turn producing more bending of the spine and additional compression of the vertebral bodies. This mechanism constitutes a vicious cycle ob-

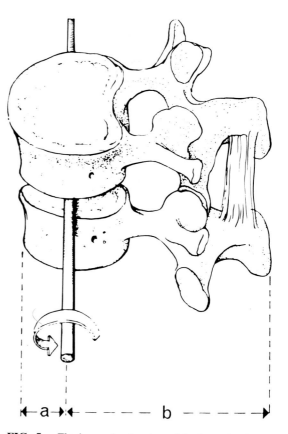

FIG. 5. Flexion and extension of the intact lumbar spine normally occur around an axis which passes through the center of the nucleus pulposus. The distance from this axis to the anterior margin of the body (**a**) is one-fourth the distance from the axis to the tip of the spinous process (**b**). During flexion, the anterior part of the vertebral body will be subjected to compression force four times as great as the tension force which is generated in the interspinous ligaments. From Smith, W.S., and Kaufer, H. (1969): Patterns and mechanisms of lumbar injuries associated with lap seat belts. *J. Bone Joint Surg.*, 51A:239–254, with permission.

served in postmenopausal osteoporosis patients with severely kyphotic spines. That wedge fractures typically involve multiple vertebrae stems from the fact that vertebrae do not move independently but rather in groups, or motion segments (80), so that forces sufficient to cause fractures may be acting on several vertebrae simultaneously.

Lateral wedge fractures may occur with lateral bending but they are uncommon (72). This is because, in the absence of scoliosis, much lower loads are incurred. The spine cannot bend as far laterally as anteriorly, so that the moment is not as large, and lateral bending is resisted more by lateral abdominal wall muscles than by spinal musculature (127). The lateral abdominal musculature acts through a larger moment arm and, thus, produces less compressive load on the lumbar vertebrae than do the erector spinae muscles, which contract strongly through short moment arms to resist forward flexion of the spine (127). Moreover, lateral mobility of the spine may be reduced up to 40% with aging in women, with an equal reduction in extension (90). Mobility in anterior flexion is much less impaired with aging. Because the spine is mostly loaded in flexion during the activities of daily living and because the posterior elements of the vertebrae may bear up to 30% of the compressive load in extension (80), vertebral body fractures due to hyperextension are uncommon in the absence of severe trauma (72).

Because activities of daily living can generate forces sufficient to fracture vertebrae weakened by osteoporosis (110,128), falls are not prominent in etiology, and fracture risk is more closely associated with bone mass than is the case with Colles' fracture. Women with vertebral fracture generally have lower spinal bone mass than controls (45,75) and histologic (14) and radiographic (6,141) studies show reduced trabecular bone in the vertebral bodies of such women. Ninety percent of women with vertebral fractures have spinal bone mineral density values less than 0.97 g/cm^2, a figure 2.3 standard deviations below the mean for normal 30-year olds (115). Newton-John and Morgan (98) hypothesized that a *fracture threshold* would be reached when bone mass fell 2.5 standard deviations below the mean for normal young women.

However, as discussed in Chapter 5, the fracture threshold approach to fracture risk is not very sensitive. A *gradient-of-risk* approach, associating fracture prevalence with specific levels of bone mass, may be more use-

ful (117). About 60% of a random sample of Rochester, Minnesota, women 35 years old and over had spinal BMD$\geq$ 1.0 g/cm^2, and the prevalence of one or more vertebral fractures in this group was 4%. Forty percent had BMD < 1.0 g/cm^2, with a fracture prevalence of 32%, and vertebral fracture prevalence increased as spinal BMD declined. Only about 10% of Rochester women had spinal BMD <0.80 g/cm^2 but nearly half had fractures (L.J. Melton and B.L. Riggs, unpublished data, 1986). This close relationship between spinal bone mass and vertebral fracture prevalence has been observed by others (103,136,148). Since bone mass is less in adult women than men at any given age, fracture rates are greater in women. Since spinal bone mass declines with age, fracture risk increases with age (Chapter 5, *this volume*).

Proximal Femur Fractures

The proximal femur is also a heavily loaded region. The neck of the femur is said to be loaded normally in compression (47,95) produced by body weight and muscle action. In standing, about one-third of body weight is supported by each hip (101,123). When weight is shifted to one leg, increased muscle forces are added to body weight so that the joint reaction force is 2.5 to 3 times body weight (101,124,146). Although women have lower body weight on average than men, their broader pelvis reduces mechanical advantage and increases forces around the joint (18). During walking, the joint reaction force in the hip rises to over six times body weight in men and over four times body weight in women (101), increasing with more rapid movement and impact loading (119).

The proximal femur is constructed to meet these loads (46). The elliptical shape of the femoral neck enhances its capability to sustain the superior-inferior bending moment normally encountered (122), and the cortical shell is reinforced by internal trabecular systems. The medial trabecular system counteracts the joint reaction force, while the lateral trabecular system resists resultant compressive forces produced on the cortical shell by the abductor musculature (101). The arcuate system bears tensile loads along the femoral neck. The thinness of the cortical shell superiorly reflects the fact that under normal conditions there is little tension on the femoral neck (8,15,46). Instead, the direction of loading at the femoral head, combined with the curvature of the proximal femur, tends to produce large bending and torsional loads at the femoral neck base and trochanteric region, and the strong contraction of the abductor musculature further aggravates the loading condition in this anatomic region. Consequently, the elliptical shape of the femur neck increases laterally (8), where bending forces are greater; and the cortical shell gradually increases in thickness anteriorly, posteriorly and especially inferiorly and at the *calcar femorale* (8), where maximum compression forces are concentrated and transmitted to the femoral shaft (46). Normally, cortical bone makes up 75% of the femoral neck and 50% of the intertrochanteric area (115) and accounts for 50 to 70% of the strength of the femoral neck (66,81).

Although there is little conpensatory increase in the diameter of the femoral neck to offset cortical bone loss with aging (121,135), the cortex is relatively spared, especially medially, compared to trabecular bone loss (13, Chapter 9, Fig. 1, *this volume*). According to Singh (129), the trabecular systems that bear the smallest loads are lost first (Fig. 6).The thin trabeculae in Ward's triangle disappear on roentgenograms, followed by secondary compressive and tensile trabeculae, the primary tensile (arcuate) system, and finally the primary compressive (medial) system. This order of loss is inversely correlated with the initial thickness of trabeculae in the various regions (44). As a consequence, however, there is relative preservation of the medial trabecular system, which supports most of the compressive load from the head of the femur, until late in the course of osteoporosis. Between the ages of 20 and 90, bone mineral density of the femoral neck falls an estimated 58% in women and 39% in men, while intertrochanteric BMD falls 53% and 35%, respectively (115). This decline in femoral neck bone mass is correlated with decreased bone strength (34,56,77,90,144).

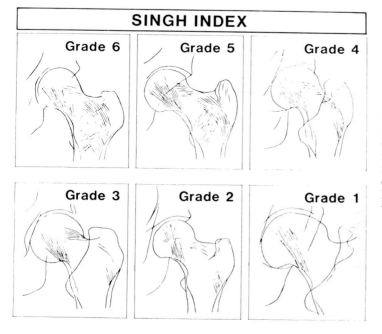

SINGH INDEX

Grade 6   Grade 5   Grade 4

Grade 3   Grade 2   Grade 1

FIG. 6. The proximal femoral trabecular (Singh) index based on changes in the trabecular pattern of the upper end of the femur: Grades 4 and under indicate significant osteoporosis. From Singh, et al., ref. 129, with permission.

Consequently, femoral neck strength is less in women than men (46) and declines with age in both sexes (47).

The proximal femur may fail *in vitro* under loads of a magnitude encountered in everyday life (111). Unaccustomed cyclical loading can even produce *fatigue fractures* in young individuals with normal bones (42,109). Similar fractures seen in the elderly and resulting from physiologic loading of abnormal bone (57) are deemed *insufficiency fractures*. Changes in material and structural characteristics of bone in osteoporosis and the diminished repair capacity lead to an increased prevalence of microfractures in femoral neck trabeculae (48), which may coalesce to produce clinical fractures. Microfractures have been observed to be concentrated in areas of increased stress (48). Other than this, however, there is little more than anecdotal evidence to show that falls are the result of essentially spontaneous hip fractures rather than the cause (48,130,134). For example, a patient often reports that his or her leg gave way prior to the fall (113). However, this history is noted in nearly 10% of all falls among the elderly, even in the absence of hip fracture (112). Most elderly women have low bone mass levels, and the relatively low risk of hip fracture (1 to 2% per year in women with very low femoral bone mineral density, Table 2) in this group also argues against this being the primary mechanism of femoral neck fractures generally. Moreover, proximal humerus and other upper limb fractures display similar increases in incidence with age; are associated with falls; and cannot be explained on the basis of spontaneously occurring fractures. Thus, while isolated cases may be due to spontaneous fracture (3,24), the more conservative explanation is that falls produce the majority of hip fractures (8,147).

Others have suggested that femoral neck fractures are caused by muscle contraction alone. Especially vigorous muscle contraction may be sufficient to avulse portions of the greater or lesser trochanter (28,95), and neck fractures are sometimes seen with seizures even in young people without osteoporosis (93). The more typical case is said to result

TABLE 2. *Estimated incidence of cervical and intertrochanteric femur fractures by bone mineral density level (BMD as assessed by dual photon absorptiometry) among Rochester, Minnesota, women ≥ 35 years of age.*

Cervical BMD (g/cm^2)	Cervical femur fractures		
	Number of fractures	Person-years of observation	Incidence[a]
≥ 1.30	~ 0	4322.0	~ 0
1.20–1.29	0.2	6175.5	~ 0
1.10–1.19	1.1	9253.0	0.1
1.00–1.09	4.5	10,642.5	0.4
0.90–0.99	12.4	10,150.0	1.2
0.80–0.89	24.9	8577.5	2.9
0.70–0.79	34.7	6428.0	5.4
0.60–0.69	31.2	4005.0	7.8
< 0.60	23.5	2816.0	8.3
Total	132.5	62,370.0	

Intertrochanteric BMD (g/cm^2)	Intertrochanteric femur fractures		
	Number of fractures	Person-years of observation	Incidence[a]
≥ 1.30	~ 0	1946.0	~ 0
1.20–1.29	~ 0	4043.5	~ 0
1.10–1.19	0.1	7776.0	~ 0
1.00–1.09	0.9	10,920.5	0.1
0.90–0.99	4.4	11,750.5	0.4
0.80–0.89	13.9	10,275.5	1.4
0.70–0.79	28.4	7592.0	3.7
0.60–0.69	37.4	4676.5	8.0
< 0.60	56.3	3389.5	16.6
Total	141.4	62,370.0	

[a]Incidence of hip fracture per 1,000 person-years, by type.

from attempting to externally rotate the femur when the foot is fixed on the ground (134). Backman (8) pointed out conceptual flaws in this argument, however, and demonstrated empirically that insufficient muscle force could be generated to regularly produce fractures in this way. Muscle forces resulting from a stumble or slip have also been blamed (47,95). One of the earliest observers (29) and one of the most recent (24) contend that the commonest cause of intracapsular fractures is a misstep, with abrupt perpendicular forces resulting from a drop of several inches. However, the shearing and bending forces thus produced are more likely to give rise to a basal or intertrochanteric fracture (28).

Even those patients said to have spontaneous fractures normally fall on the affected hip (130), and the majority of investigators attribute femoral neck fractures to the fall (8,64,150). Falls are capable of generating sufficient forces to induce fracture (47), and the femoral neck is less strong in the directions that loading occurs during falls (8). Moreover, in a fall, rotation of the femoral head in the acetabulum may be hampered, inducing torsional forces along the axis of the femoral neck; these were shown to be important in the production of cervical fractures resembling those seen clinically (8). A typical pattern is failure of the anterior cortex of the neck in tension and the posterior cortex in compression (125). Since the femoral neck is convexly curved anteriorly, it has been suggested that forces applied laterally by muscle action or a fall on the greater trochanter cause compression, bending then failure of the neck (125). However, both bending and compression must be taken into account to accurately predict the strength of the femoral neck (56). If bending is the predominant force, a transcervical fracture is more likely, while a subcapital fracture results from a relatively greater compression component (46).

The biomechanical basis of intertrochanteric fractures is less well established. Typical intertrochanteric fractures may be produced by forces transmitted upward through the shaft of the femur (28). The compensatory increase in femoral shaft diameter with age described above renders it less able to flex or to absorb energy (135), and more energy is then transmitted to the metaphysis. However, trochanteric fractures can also be produced by a blow to the greater trochanter (139), and most intertrochanteric fractures are said to be due to falls (24,26). These fractures occur in areas of trabecular bone loss, and poorly-mineralized bone breaks with only half the force needed to fracture well-mineralized bone (139). Osteoporosis is also associated with a relatively greater proportion of comminuted intetrochanteric fractures (154).

Most hip fractures occur indoors (25), possibly contributing to injury since hard surfaces do not dissipate energy well (147). However, the actual amount of force generated by a fall may vary with sex or age, as the potential energy in a fall is quite large:

> In a standing position, the body possesses a considerable amount of potential energy. In falling, the potential energy changes to kinetic energy which, upon impact with the floor, must be absorbed by the structures of the body if a fracture is not to occur. There is sufficient potential energy in the standing body which, if unabsorbed on falling, could break any bone in the body. In an average-sized woman, the amount of potential energy to be absorbed in a fall would be approximately 4000 kg cm, and the energy absorbing capacity of the upper end of the femur is only 60 kg cm approximately. Thus if a boney injury is not to occur, energy absorbing mechanisms must operate. (95).

Since the majority of falls do not result in significant injury (85), these energy absorbing mechanisms must be extremely effective, although there may be some impairment among the elderly. Coordination, for example, may be reduced in this group (71) so that elderly individuals might not be as able to break the impact of a fall (42). If muscular reaction were slowed, either neurologically (140,151) or muscularly (5), bone loading might be increased because muscle action is the major component of energy dissipation (47,95). Reduced muscle strength in the elderly (151) could contribute to this problem. Reduced muscle mass, along with the reduction in adipose tissue often seen in the aged, may also reduce the effectiveness of energy absorption by soft tissue (31,99).

The large potential forces involved in falls, and the relatively modest reductions in femoral bone mass seen in hip fracture patients compared to age- and sex-matched controls (12,67,115,145), have led some to question the role of bone fragility in the etiology of hip fractures (1,30). As with vertebral fractures, however, hip fractures are uncommon in those with bone mass above the "fracture threshold" (115,145). Also like vertebral fractures, hip fracture risk increases as bone mineral density continues to fall (Table 2). Cervical or intertrochanteric fractures are rare among Rochester,

Minnesota, women with femoral bone mineral density ≥ 1.0 g/cm^2. Among those with cervical bone density less than 1.0 g/cm^2, the overall cervical fracture incidence rate was 4.0 per 1000 person-years, while intertrochanteric fracture incidence was a comparable 3.7 per 1000 person-years in women with intertrochanteric bone density less than 1.0 g/cm^2. Hip fracture incidence rates increased as femoral bone mass declined, reaching levels of 8.3 and 16.6 per 1000 person-years, respectively, among the relatively few women with cervical or intertrochanteric bone density levels less than 0.6 g/cm^2 (86).

These data indicate that bone fragility, reflected *in vivo* by bone mineral density, is an important determinant of the age-related pattern of hip fracture incidence. However, osteoporosis alone may not be sufficient to produce such fractures, since many individuals remain fracture-free even within the subgroups of lowest bone density. Nonetheless, because hip fracture risk is associated with absolute bone mass (not that relative to ones' age- and sex-matched peers), it is to be expected that hip fractures will be more frequent among women than men and that incidence rates will rise with age as bone mass falls. Because of the greater contribution of falls, however, bone mass does not have as close a relationship to hip fracture risk (87) as it does to vertebral fracture risk.

SUMMARY

Bone has essential mechanical properties in addition to its metabolic functions. As the framework for attachment of muscles and ligaments, bone permits the movements necessary for living. Since bone is also a unique biological tissue that remodels and repairs itself throughout life (Chapter 2, *this volume*), it is able to undergo changes of property and geometric configuration in accordance with imposed physical demands (49,152). Under certain circumstances, however, the compensatory mechanisms may fail, resulting in an imbalance of biomechanical integrity and biological demands that could lead to fracture in the absence of major trauma. Osteoporosis is one of the entities that can effect such an imbalance. Since osteoporosis is more pronounced in trabecular bone and because the metaphyseal regions are more sensitive to structural weakness, the frequency of fracture is expected to be higher at these anatomic sites. However, additional factors, such as bone geometry and loading pattern, as well as changes in bone quality and structure, must also be considered in evaluating the mechanisms that lead to fracture.

ACKNOWLEDGMENTS

The authors would like to thank Miss Mary Ramaker for help in preparing the manuscript.

This work was supported in part by research grants AM-27065 and AM-30582 from the National Institutes of Health.

REFERENCES

1. Aitken, J.M. (1984): Relevance of osteoporosis in women with fractures of the femoral neck. *Br. Med. J.*, 288:597–601.
2. Alffram, P.-A., and Bauer, G.C.H. (1962): Epidemiology of fractures of the forearm. *J. Bone Joint Surg.*, 44A:105–114.
3. Alffram, P.-A. (1964): An epidemiologic study of cervical and trochanteric fractures of the femur in an urban population: Analysis of 1,664 cases with special reference to etiologic factors. *Acta Orthop. Scand.* (Suppl.), 65:1–109.
4. Anderson, L.D. (1975): Fractures of the shafts of the radius and ulna. Chapter 9. In: *Fractures*, Vol. 1, edited by C.A. Rockwood, Jr., and D.P. Green, pp. 441–485. J.B. Lippincott Company, Philadelphia.
5. Aniansson, A., Zetterberg, C., Hedberg, M., and Henriksson, K.G. (1984): Impaired muscle function with aging: A background factor in the incidence of fractures of the proximal end of the femur. *Clin. Orthop.*, 191:193–201.
6. Atkinson, P.J. (1967): Variation in trabecular structure of vertebrae with age. *Calcif. Tissue Res.*, 1:24–32.
7. Awbrey, B.J., Jacobson, P.C., Grubb, S.A., McCartney, W.H., Vincent, L.M., and Talmage, R.V. (1984): Bone density in women: A modified procedure for measurement of distal radial density. *J. Orthop. Res.*, 2:314–321.
8. Backman, S. (1957): The proximal end of the femur. *Acta Radiologica* (Suppl.), 146:10–166.
9. Bartley, M.H., Arnold, J.S., Haslam, R.K., and Jee, W.S.S. (1966): The relationship of bone

strength and bone quantity in health, disease, and aging. *J. Gerontol.*, 21:517–521.

10. Batra, H.C., Smith, D.A., Waddell, G.F., and Anderson, J.B. (1975): Colles' fracture and bone density. *J. Bone Joint Surg.*, 57-B:247.

11. Bell, G.H., Dunbar, O., and Beck, J.S.(1967): Variations in strength of vertebrae with age and their relation to osteoporosis. *Calcif. Tissue Res.*, 1:75–86.

12. Bohr, H., and Schaadt, O. (1983): Bone mineral content of femoral bone and the lumbar spine measured in women with fracture of the femoral neck by dual photon absorptiometry. *Clin. Orthop.*, 179:240–245.

13. Bohr, H., and Schaadt, O. (1985): Bone mineral content of the femoral neck and shaft: Relation between cortical and trabecular bone. *Calcif. Tissue Int.*, 37:340–344.

14. Bromley, R.G., Dockum, N.L., Arnold, J.S., and Jee, W.S.S. (1966): Quantitative histological study of human lumbar vertebrae. *J. Gerontol.*, 21:537–543.

15. Brown, T.D., and Ferguson, A.B., Jr. (1978): The development of a computational stress analysis of the femoral head. *J. Bone Joint Surg.*, 60-A:619–629.

16. Brown, T.D., and Ferguson, A.B., Jr. (1980): Mechanical property distributions in the cancellous bone of the human proximal femur. *Acta Orthop. Scand.*, 51:429–437.

17. Buhr, A.J., and Cooke, A.M. (1959): Fracture patterns. *Lancet*, 1:531–536.

18. Burr, D.B., Van Gerven, D.P., and Gustav, B.L. (1977): Sexual dimorphism and mechanics of the human hip: A multivariate assessment. *Am. J. Phys. Anthrop.*, 47:273–278.

19. Burstein, A.H., Reilly, D.T., and Martens, M. (1976): Aging of bone tissue: Mechanical properties. *J. Bone Joint Surg.*, 58-A:82–86.

20. Carter, D.R., and Hayes, W.C. (1977): The compressive behavior of bone as a two-phase porous structure. *J. Bone Joint Surg.*, 59-A:954–962.

21. Carter, D.R., and Hayes, W.C. (1977): Compact bone fatigue damage—I. Residual strength and stiffness. *J. Biomech.*, 10:325–337.

22. Carter, D.R., Schwab, G.H., and Spengler, D.M. (1980): Tensile fracture of cancellous bone. *Acta Orthop. Scand.*, 51:733–741.

23. Chatterji, S., Wall, J.C., and Jeffrey, J.W. (1981): Age-related changes in the orientation and particle size of the mineral phase in human femoral cortical bone. *Calcif. Tissue Int.*, 33:567–574.

24. Citron, N. (1985): Femoral neck fractures: Are some preventable? *Ergonomics*, 28:993–997.

25. Clark, A.N.G. (1968): Factors in fracture of the female femur: A clinical study of the environment, physical, medical and preventative aspects of this injury. *Geront. Clin.*, 10:257–270.

26. Clawson, D.K., and Melcher, P.J. (1975): Fractures and dislocations of the hip. In: *Fractures*, Volume 2, edited by C.A. Rockwood, Jr. and D.P. Green, pp. 1012–1074. J.B. Lippincott Company, Philadelphia.

27. Conwell, H.E., and Reynolds, F.C. (1961): Frac-

tures of shaft of femur. Chapter 19. In: *Key and Conwell's Management of Fractures, Dislocations, and Sprains*, 7th Edition, pp. 851–861. C.V. Mosby Company, St. Louis.

28. Conwell, H.E., and Reynolds, F.C. (1961): Fractures of upper end of femur. In: *Key and Conwell's Management of Fractures, Dislocations, and Sprains*. 7th Edition, pp. 782–803. C.V. Mosby Company, St. Louis.

29. Cooper, Sir Astley (1842): *A Treatise on Dislocations and Fractures of the Joints*, edited by F.R.S. Cooper, and B. Bransby. John Churchill, London.

30. Cummings, S.R. (1985): Are patients with hip fractures more osteoporotic? Review of the evidence. *Am. J. Med.*, 78:487–494.

31. Currey, J.D. (1968): The effect of protection on the impact strength of rabbits' bones. *Acta Anat.*, 71:87–93.

32. Currey, J.D. (1979): Changes in the impact energy absorption of bone with age. *J. Biomech.*, 12:459–469.

33. Currey, J.D. (1984): *The Mechanical Adaptations of Bones*, Princeton University Press, Princeton, New Jersey.

34. Dalén, N., Hellström, L.-G., and Jacobson, B. (1976): Bone mineral content and mechanical strength of the femoral neck. *Acta Orthop. Scand.*, 47:503–508.

35. Denis, F. (1983): The three column spine and its significance in the classification of acute thoracolumbar spinal injuries. *Spine*, 8:817–831.

36. Dequeker, J., and Merlevede, W. (1971): Collagen content and collagen extractability pattern of adult human trabecular bone according to age, sex and amount of bone mass. *Biochim. Biophys. Acta*, 244:410–420.

37. Dickenson, R.P., Hutton, W.C., and Stott, J.R.R. (1981): The mechanical properties of bone in osteoporosis. *J. Bone Joint Surg.*, 63-B:233–238.

38. Dobyns, J.H., and Linscheid, R.L. (1975): Fractures and dislocations of the wrist. Chapter 7. In: *Fractures* edited by C.A. Rockwood, Jr., and D.P. Green, pp. 345–440. J.B. Lippincott Company, Philadelphia.

39. Doyle, F.H., Gutteridge, D.H., Joplin, G.F., and Fraser, R. (1967): An assessment of radiological criteria used in the study of spinal osteoporosis. *Br. J. Radiol.*, 40:241–250.

40. Eastell, R., Wahner, H.W., Melton, L.J., O'Fallon, W.M., and Riggs, B.L. (1986): Comparison of bone mineral density of the lumbar spine and ultradistal radius in women with vertebral fractures. (Abstr.) *J. Bone Min.*, 1(Suppl. 1):271A.

41. Erne, P., and Burckhardt, A. (1980): Femoral neck fatigue fracture. *Arch. Orthop. Traumat. Surg.*, 97:213–220.

42. Evans, J.G. (1982): Epidemiology of proximal femoral fractures. Chapter 12. In: *Recent Advances in Geriatric Medicine*, 2:201–204.

43. Farfan, H.F. (1973): *Mechanical Disorders of the Low Back*. Lea & Febiger, Philadelphia.

44. Fazzalari, N.L., Darracott, J., and Vernon-Roberts, B. (1983): A quantitative description of selected stress regions of cancellous bone in the head

of the femur using automatic image analysis. *Metab. Bone Dis. Rel. Res.,* 5:119–125.

45. Firooznia, H., Golimbu, C., Rafii, M., Schwartz, M.S., and Alterman, E.R. (1984): Quantitative computed tomography assessment of spinal trabecular bone. II. In osteoporotic women with and without vertebral fractures. *CT: Comput. Tomogr.,* 8:99–103.

46. Frankel, V.H. (1960): *The Femoral Neck,* edited by C.W. Goff. Charles C. Thomas, Springfield, Illinois.

47. Frankel, V.H., and Pugh, J.W. (1984): Biomechanics of the hip. Chapter 5. In: *Surgery of the Hip Joint,* edited by R.F. Tronzo, pp. 115–131. Springer-Verlag, New York.

48. Freeman, M.A.R., Todd, R.C., and Pirie, C.J. (1974): The role of fatigue in the pathogenesis of senile femoral neck fractures. *J. Bone Joint Surg.,* 56-B:698–702.

49. Frost, H.M. (1982): Mechanical determinants of bone modeling. *Metab. Bone Dis. Rel. Res.,* 4:217–229.

50. Frost, H.M. (1985): The pathomechanics of osteoporoses. *Clin. Orthop.,* 200:198–225.

51. Frykman, G. (1967): Fracture of the distal radius including sequelae—shoulder-hand-finger syndrome, disturbance in the distal radio-ulnar joint and impairment of nerve function. *Acta Orthop. Scand.,* Supplementum No. 108:1–155.

52. Galante, J., Rostoker, W., and Ray, R.D. (1970): Physical properties of trabecular bone. *Calcif. Tissue Res.,* 5:236–246.

53. Gallagher, J.C., Aaron, J., Horsman, A., Marshall, D.H., Wilkinson, R., and Nordin, B.E.C. (1973): The crush fracture syndrome in post-menopausal women. *Clin. Endocrinol.,* 2:293–315.

54. Garn, S.M. (1981): The phenomenon of bone formation and bone loss. In: *Osteoporosis: Recent Advances in Pathogenesis and Treatment,* edited by H.F. DeLuca, H.M. Frost, W.S.S. Jee, C.C. Johnston, Jr., and A.M. Parfitt, pp. 3–16. University Park Press, Baltimore.

55. Gibb, A. (1967): Appendix to Bell, G.H., Dunbar, O., Beck, J.S., and Gibb, A. Strength of vertebrae in osteoporosis. *Calcif. Tissue Res.,* 1:83–86.

56. Gies, A., Carter, D.R., Sartoris, D.J., and Sommer, F.G. (1985): Femoral neck strength predicted from dual energy projected radiography. Transactions of the 31st Annual ORS, Las Vegas, Nevada, Jan. 21–24, 1985, p. 357.

57. Griffiths, W.E.G., Swanson, S.A.V., and Freeman, M.A.R. (1971): Experimental fatigue fracture of the human cadaveric femoral neck. *J. Bone Joint Surg.,* 53-B:136–143.

58. Hansson, T. (1977): *The Bone Mineral Content and Biomechanical Properties of Lumbar Vertebrae: An In Vitro Study Based on Dual Photon Absorptiometry.* Uno Lundgren Tryckeri AB, Göteborg.

59. Hansson, T., Roos, B., and Nachemson, A. (1980): The bone mineral content and ultimate compressive strength of lumbar vertebrae. *Spine,* 5:46–55.

60. Hansson, T., and Roos, B. (1981): Microcalluses of the trabeculae in lumbar vertebrae and their relation to the bone mineral content. *Spine,* 6:375–380.

61. Hansson, T., and Roos, B. (1981): The relation between bone mineral content, experimental compression fractures, and disc degeneration in lumbar vertebrae. *Spine,* 6:147–153.

62. Härmä, M., and Karjalainen, P. (1986): Trabecular osteopenia in Colles' fracture. *Acta. Orthop. Scand.,* 57:38–40.

63. Hayes, W.C., and Gerhart, T.N. (1985): Biomechanics of bone: Applications for assessment of bone strength. Chapter 9. In: *Bone and Mineral Research/3,* edited by W.A. Peck, pp. 259–294. Elsevier Science Publishers B.V., Amsterdam.

64. Hedlund, R.(1985): *Incidence and Cause of Femur Fractures.* Kongl Carolinska Medico Chirurgiska Institutet, Stockholm.

65. Hesp, R., Klenerman, L., and Page, L. (.984): Decreased radial bone mass in Colles' fracture. *Acta Orthop. Scand.,* 55:573–575.

66. Hirsch, C., and Brodetti, A. (1956): The weight-bearing capacity of structural elements in femoral necks. *Acta Orthop. Scand.,* 26:15–24.

67. Horsman, A., Nordin C., Simpson, M., and Speed, R. (1982): Cortical and trabecular bone status in elderly women with femoral neck fracture. *Clin. Orthop.,* 166:143–151.

68. Horsman, A., and Currey, J.D. (1983): Estimation of mechanical properties of the distal radius from bone mineral content and cortical width. *Clin. Orthop.,* 176:298–304.

69. Horsman, A., Marshall, D.H., and Peacock, M. (1985): A stochastic model of age-related bone loss and fractures. *Clin. Orthop.,* 195:207–215.

70. Hui, S.L., Wiske, P.S., Norton, J.A., and Johnston, C.C., Jr. (1982): A prospective study of change in bone mass with age in post-menopausal women. *J. Chron. Dis.,* 35:715–725.

71. Isaacs, B. (1978): Are falls a manifestation of brain failure? *Age Ageing,* 7(Supplement):97–105.

72. Kaufer, H. (1975): The thoracolumbar spine. Part 2 of Chapter 12 Fractures and dislocations of the spine. In: *Fractures,* Vol. 2, edited by C.A. Rockwood, Jr., and D.P. Green, pp. 861–903. J.B. Lippincott Company, Philadelphia.

73. Kazarian, L., and Graves, G.A., Jr. (1977): Compressive strength characteristics of the human vertebral centrum. *Spine,* 2:1–14.

74. Kent, G.N., Dodds, R.A., Klenerman, L., Watts, R.W.E., Bitensky, L., and Chayen, J. (1983): Changes in crystal size and orientation of acidic glycosaminoglycans at the fracture site in fractured necks of femur. *J. Bone Joint Surg.,* 65-B:189–194.

75. Krølner, B., Tøndevold, E., Toft, B., Berthelsen, B., and Nielsen, S.P. (1982): Bone mass of the axial and the appendicular skeleton in women with Colles' fracture: Its relation to physical activity. *Clin. Physiol.,* 2:147–157.

76. Kulowski, J. (1964): Fractures of the shaft of the femur resulting from automobile accidents. *J. Int. Coll. Surg.,* 42:412–420.

77. Leichter, I, Margulies, J.Y., Weinreb, A., Mizrahi, J, Robin, G.C., Conforty, B., Makin, M., and Bloch, B. (1982): The relationship between bone density, mineral content, and mechanical

strength in the femoral neck. *Clin. Orthop.*, 163:272–281.

78. Lewis, R.M. (1950): Colles fracture—causative mechanism. Surgery 27:427–436.

79. Lindahl, O. (1976): Mechanical properties of dried defatted spongy bone. *Acta Orthop. Scand.*, 47:11–19.

80. Lindh, M. (1980): Biomechanics of the lumbar spine. In: *Basic Biomechanics of the Skeletal System*, edited by V.H. Frankel, and M. Nordin, pp. 255–290. Lea and Febiger, Philadelphia.

81. Martens, M., Van Audekercke, R., Delport, P., De Meester, P., and Mulier, J.C. (1983): The mechanical characteristics of cancellous bone at the upper femoral region. *J. Biomech.*, 16:971–983.

82. Mazess, R.B. (1982): On aging bone loss. *Clin. Orthop.*, 165:239–252.

83. McBroom,R.J., Hayes, W.C., Edwards, W.T., Goldberg, R.P., and White, A.A., III (1985): Prediction of vertebral body compressive fracture using quantitative computed tomography. *J. Bone Joint Surg.*, 67-A:1206–1214.

84. Meema, H.E., and Meema, S. (1978): Compact bone mineral density of the normal human radius. *Acta Radiol. Oncol.*, 17:342–352.

85. Melton, L.J., and Riggs, B.L. (1985): Risk factors for injury after a fall. Symposium on Falls in the Elderly: Biological and Behavioral Aspects. *Clin. Geriatr. Med.*, 1:525–539.

86. Melton, L.J., Wahner, H.W., Richelson, L.S., O'Fallon W.M., and Riggs, B.L. (1986): Osteoporosis and the risk of hip fracture. *Am. J. Epidemiol.*, 124:254–261.

87. Melton, L.J., and Riggs, B.L. (1986): Impaired bone strength and fracture patterns at different skeletal sites. In: *Current Concepts of Bone Fragility*, edited by H.K. Unthoff, and E. Stahl, pp. 149–157. Springer-Verlag, Berlin.

88. Merz, W.A., and Schenk, R.K. (1970): Quantitative structural analysis of human cancellous bone. *Acta Anat.*, 75:54–66.

89. Meunier, P., Courpron, P., Edouard, C., Bernard, J., Bringuier, J., and Vignon, G. (1973): Physiological senile involution and pathological rarefaction of bone. *Clin. Endocrinol. Metab.*, 2:239–256.

90. Mizrahi, J, Margulies, J.Y., Leichter, I., and Deutsch, D. (1984): Fracture of the human femoral neck: Effect of density of the cancellous core. *J. Biomed. Eng.*, 6:56–62.

91. Moll, J.M.H., and Wright, V. (1971): Normal range of spinal mobility: An objective clinical study. *Ann. Rheum. Dis.*, 30:381–386.

92. Mooney, V. (1975): Fractures of the shaft of the femur. Chapter 15. In: *Fractures*, Volume 2, edited by C.A. Rockwood, Jr., and D.P. Green, pp. 1075–1129, J.B. Lippincott Company, Philadelphia.

93. Morrey, B.F., and O'Brien, E.T. (1977): Femoral neck fractures following water-soluble myelography induced spinal seizures. *J. Bone Joint Surg.*, 59-A:1099–1100.

94. Mosekilde, Li., Viidik, A., and Mosekilde, Le. (1985): Correlation between the compressive strength of iliac and vertebral trabecular bone in normal individuals. *Bone*, 6:291–295.

95. Muckle, D.S., Bentley, G., Deane, G., and Kemp, F.H. (1978): Basic sciences of the hip. In: *Femoral Neck Fractures and Hip Joint Injuries*, edited by D.S. Muckle. John Wiley and Sons, New York.

96. Nachemson, A. (1975): Towards a better understanding of low-back pain: A review of the mechanics of the lumbar disc. *Rheum. Rehab.*, 14:129–143.

97. Neill, J.L., Demos, T.C., Stone, J.L., and Hayes, W.C. (1983): Tensile and compressive properties of vertebral trabecular bone. *Transactions of the 29th Annual ORS*, Anaheim, CA, March 8–10, 1983, Abstract, p. 344.

98. Newton-John, H.F., and Morgan, D.B. (1970): The loss of bone with age, osteoporosis, and fractures. *Clin. Orthop.*, 71:229–252.

99. Nikolić, V. Hančević, J, Hudec, M., and Banović, B. (1975): Absorption of the impact energy in the palmar soft tissues. *Anat. Embryol.*, 148:215–221.

100. Nilsson, B.E., and Westlin, N.E. (1974): The bone mineral content in the forearm of women with Colles' fracture. *Acta Orthop. Scand.*, 45:836–844.

101. Nordin, M., and Frankel, V.H. (1980): Biomechanics of the hip. Chapter 5. In: *Basic Biomechanics of the Skeletal System*, by V.H. Frankel, and M. Nordin, edited by L. Glass, pp. 149–177, Lea and Febiger, Philadelphia.

102. Nordin, M., and Frankel, V.H. (1980): Biomechanics of whole bones and bone tissue. Chapter 1. In: *Basic Biomechanics of the Skeletal System*, by V.H. Frankel, and M. Nordin, edited by L. Glass, pp. 15–60. Lea and Febiger, Philadelphia.

103. Odvina, C.V., Wergedal, J.E., Libanati, C., Schulz, E.E., and Baylink, D.J. (1984): Relationship between quantitative computerized tomography scan values and vertebral fractures in osteoporotics. In: *1984 Program and Abstracts of the Sixth Annual Scientific Meeting of the American Society for Bone and Mineral Research*. June 26–29, 1984, Hartford, Connecticut. A47.

104. Parfitt, A.M., and Duncan, H. (1982): Metabolic bone disease affecting the spine. Chapter 13. In: *The Spine*, edited by R.H. Rothman, and F.A. Simeone, pp. 775–905. W.B. Saunders Company, Philadelphia.

105. Parfitt, A.M., Mathews, C.H.E., Villanueva, A.R., Kleerekoper, M., Frame, B., and Rao, D.S. (1983): Relationships between surface, volume, and thickness of iliac trabecular bone in aging and in osteoporosis. *J. Clin. Invest.*, 72:1396–1409.

106. Parfitt, A.M. (1984): Definition of osteoporosis: Age-related loss of bone and its relationship to increased fracture risk. In: *Osteoporosis.*, pp. 15–19. National Institutes of Health Consensus Development Conference. April 2–4, Bethesda, Maryland.

107. Parfitt, A.M. (1984): Age-related structural changes in trabecular and cortical bone: Cellular mechanisms and biomechanical consequences. *Calcif. Tissue Int.*, 36:S123–S128.

108. Parfitt, A.M. (1986): Cortical porosity in postmenopausal and adolescent wrist fractures. In: *Current Concepts of Bone Fragility*, edited by H. Unthoff, and E. Stahl, pp. 168–172. Springer-Verlag, Berlin.

109. Pentecost, R.L., Murray, R.A., and Brindley, H.H. (1964): Fatigue, insufficiency, and pathologic fractures. *JAMA*, 187:1001–1004.

110. Perey, O. (1957): Fracture of the vertebral end-plate in the lumbar spine: An experimental biomechanical investigation. *Acta Orthop. Scand.* (Suppl.) 25:3–101.

111. Phillips, J.R., Williams, J.F., and Melick, R.A. (1975): Prediction of the strength of the neck of femur from its radiological appearance. *Biomed. Engineering*, 10:367–372.

112. Prudham, D., and Evans, J.G. (1981): Factors associated with falls in the elderly: A community study. *Age Ageing*, 10:141–146.

113. Reeves, B. (1977): What comes first, the fracture or the fall? A study of subcapital fractures. *J. Bone Joint Surg.*, 59-B:375.

114. Reilly, D.T., and Burstein, A.H. (1975): The elastic and ultimate properties of compact bone tissue. *J. Biomech.*, 8:393–405.

115. Riggs, B.L., Wahner, H.W., Seeman, E., Offord, K.P., Dunn, W.L., Mazess, R.B., Johnson, K.A., and Melton, L.J. (1982): Changes in bone mineral density of the proximal femur and spine with aging: Differences between the postmenopausal and senile osteoporosis syndromes. *J. Clin. Invest.*, 70:716–723.

116. Riggs, B.L., and Melton, L.J. (1983): Evidence for two distinct syndromes of involutional osteoporosis. *Am. J. Med.*, 75:899–901.

117. Riggs, B.L., and Melton, L.J. (1986): Medical Progress: Involutional osteoporosis. *N. Engl. J. Med.*, 314:1676–1686.

118. Roaf, R. (1960): A study of the mechanics of spinal injuries. *J. Bone Joint Surg.*, 42-B:810–823.

119. Röhrle, H., Scholten, R., Sigolotto, C., and Sollbach, W. (1984): Joint forces in human pelvis-leg skeleton during walking. *J. Biomech.*, 17:409–424.

120. Rose, S.H., Melton, L.J. III, Morrey, B.F., Ilstrup, D.M., and Riggs, B.L. (1982): Epidemiologic features of humeral fractures. *Clin. Orthop.*, 168:24–30.

121. Ruff, C.B., and Hayes, W.C. (1982): Subperiosteal expansion and cortical remodeling of the human femur and tibia with aging. *Science*, 217:945–948.

122. Ruff, C.B., and Hayes, W.C. (1983): Cross-sectional geometry of Pecos Pueblo femora and tibiae—A biomechanical investigation: I. Method and general patterns of variation. *Am. J. Phys. Anthropol.*, 60:359–381.

123. Rydell, N.W. (1966): Forces acting on the femoral-head prosthesis. *Acta Orthop. Scand.*, 37(Suppl. 88):1–132.

124. Rydell, N. (1973): Biomechanics of the hip-joint. *Clin. Orthrop.*, 92:6–15.

125. Scheck, M. (1959): Intracapsular fractures of the femoral neck: Comminution of the posterior neck cortex as a cause of unstable fixation. *J. Bone Joint Surg.*, 41-A:1187–1200.

126. Schlenker, R.A., and VonSeggen, W.W. (1976): The distribution of cortical and trabecular bone mass along the lengths of the radius and ulna and the implications for in vivo bone mass measurements. *Calcif. Tissue Res.*, 20:41–2.

127. Schultz, A.B., Andersson, G.B.J., Haderspeck, K, Ortengren, R., Nordin, M., and Björk R. (1982): Analysis and measurement of lumbar trunk loads in tasks involving bends and twists. *J. Biomech.*, 15:9:669–675.

128. Scott, W.W., Jr. (1984): Osteoporosis-related fracture syndromes. In: *Osteoporosis*, pp. 20–24. Proceedings of the NIH Consensus Development Conference, April 2–4, 1984, Bethesda, Maryland.

129. Singh, M., Nagrath, A.R., Maini, P.S., and Haryana, R. (1970): Changes in trabecular pattern of the upper end of the femur as an index of osteoporosis. *J. Bone Joint Surg.*, 52-A:457–467.

130. Sloan, J., and Holloway, G. (1981): Fractured neck of the femur: The cause of the fall? *Injury*, 13:230–232.

131. Smith, C.B., and Smith, D.A. (1976): Relations between age, mineral density and mechanical properties of human femoral compacta. *Acta Orthop. Scand.*, 47:496–502.

132. Smith, C.B., and Smith, D.A. (1978): Structural role of bone apatite in human femoral compacta. *Acta Orthop. Scand.*, 49:440–444.

133. Smith, D.M., Khairi, M.R.A., and Johnston, C.C., Jr. (1975): The loss of bone mineral with aging and its relationship to risk of fracture. *J. Clin. Invest.*, 56:311–318.

134. Smith, L.D. (1953): Hip fractures: The role of muscle contraction or intrinsic forces in the causation of fractures of the femoral neck. *J. Bone Joint Surg.*, 35-A:367–383.

135. Smith, R.W. Jr., and Walker, R.R. (1964): Femoral expansion in aging women: Implications for osteoporosis and fractures. *Science*, 145:156–157.

136. Smith,R.W. Jr., and Rizek, J. (1966): Epidemiologic studies of osteoporosis in women of Puerto Rico and southeastern Michigan with special reference to age, race, national origin and to other related or associated findings. *Clin. Orthop.*, 45:31–48.

137. Smith, R.W., Jr., and Taft, P.M. (1967): Relationship of vertebral size to fracture in osteoporotic spines. *Henry Ford Hosp. Med. J.*, 15:101–106.

138. Solgaard, S., and Petersen, V.S. (1985): Epidemiology of distal radius fractures. *Acta Orthop. Scand.*, 56:391–393.

139. Spears, G.N., and Owen, J.T. (1949): The etiology of trochanteric fractures of the femur. *J. Bone Joint Surg.*, 31-A:548–552.

140. Stelmach, G.E., and Worringham, C.J. (1985): Sensorimotor deficits related to postural stability: Implications for falling in the elderly. *Clin. Geriatr. Med.*, 1:679–694.

141. Tanaka, Y. (1975): A radiographic analysis on human lumbar vertebrae in the aged. *Virchows Arch. A Path. Anat. Histol.*, 366:187–201.

142. Twomey, L., Taylor, J., and Furniss, B. (1983): Age changes in the bone density and structure of the lumbar vertebral columnn. *J. Anat.*, 136:15–25.

143. Vernon-Roberts, B., and Pirie, C.J. (1973): Healing trabecular microfractures in the bodies of lumbar vertebrae. *Ann. Rheum. Dis.*, 32:406–412.

144. Vose, G.P., and Mack, P.B. (1963): Roentgenologic assessment of femoral neck density as related to fracturing. *Am. J. Roentgenol.*, 89:1296–1301.

145. Vose G.P., and Lockwood R.M. (1965): Femoral neck fracturing—Its relationship to radiographic bone density. *J. Gerontol.*, 20:300–305.

146. Walker, P.S. (1977): *Human Joints and their Artificial Replacements.* Charles C. Thomas, Springfield, Illinois.

147. Waller, J.A. (1978): Falls among the elderly—Human and environmental factors. *Accid. Anal. Prev.*, 10:21–33.

148. Wasnich, R.R., Ross, P.D., Heilbrun, L.K., and Vogel, J.M. (1985): Prediction of postmenopausal fracture risk with use of bone mineral measurements. *Am. J. Obstet. Gynecol.*, 153:745–751.

149. White, A.A., III, and Panjabi, M.M. (1978): *Clinical Biomechanics of the Spine*, pp. 115–190. J.B. Lippincott Company, Philadelphia.

150. Wicks, M., Garrett, R., Vernon-Roberts, B., and Fazzalari, N. (1982): Absence of metabolic bone disease in the proximal femur in patients with fracture of the femoral neck. *J. Bone Joint Surg.*, 64-B:319–332.

151. Wolfson, L.I., Whipple, R., Amerman, P., Kaplan, J., and Kleinberg, A. (1985): Gait and balance in the elderly: Two functional capacities that link sensory and motor ability to falls. *Clin. Geriatr. Med.*, 1:649–659.

152. Woo, S.L.-Y., Kuei, S.C., Amiel, D., Gomez, M.A., Hayes, W.C., White, F.C., and Akeson, W.H. (1981): The effect of prolonged physical training on the properties of long bone: A study of Wolff's law. *J. Bone Joint Surg.*, 63-A:780–787.

153. Yamada, H. (1970): *Strength of Biological Materials*, edited by F.G. Evans. Williams and Wilkins Company, Baltimore.

154. Zain Elabdien, B.S., Olerud, S., and Karlstrom, G. (1984): The influence of age on the morphology of trochanteric fracture. *Arch. Orthop. Trauma Surg.*, 103:156–161.

Osteoporosis: Etiology, Diagnosis, and Management, edited by B. Lawrence Riggs and L. Joseph Melton, III. Raven Press, New York © 1988.

5

Epidemiology of Fractures

L. Joseph Melton, III

Department of Medical Statistics and Epidemiology, Mayo Clinic and Mayo Foundation, Rochester, Minnesota 55905

This chapter covers epidemiologic contributions to osteoporosis research in the area of skeletal fractures. The general patterns of fracture occurrence in the population are described, and the fracture syndromes which are age-related, and thus possibly associated with osteoporosis, are defined. Specific characteristics peculiar to each fracture type are then presented, as this information may be of use in formulating etiologic hypotheses and developing prophylactic measures. Finally, the impact of age-related fractures is documented to help determine the need for intervention on a societal level and to aid in judging the potential benefits of prevention programs. These data provide a link between the osteoporosis manifest in the community and that seen by clinicians treating individual patients or by investigators focused on particular aspects of pathophysiology.

EPIDEMIOLOGIC PATTERNS OF FRACTURES

Nonosteoporotic Fractures

Overall fracture incidence is bimodal, with peaks in the young and the old (Fig. 1). Fractures responsible for the early peak occur in four general varieties. The first is represented by skull fractures, where incidence rates are very high among infants but decline to relatively low levels by one year of age and remain at that frequency throughout life (76). A second type, prewage-earner's fractures (15), are characterized by high incidence rates among adolescents and young adults, which also decline with advancing age. Such fractures are more common among men than women and usually result from significant trauma. Fractures of the shafts of the long bones best display this pattern of occurrence. Fractures of the shaft and distal humerus, for example, are five times more frequent among those less than 35 years of age than among older individuals; incidence rates are higher in men; and the most common causes are motor vehicle accidents and falls from heights (88). Other fractures, such as Colles' fracture of the distal forearm, comprise the composite type (15), which occur among adolescents as well as the elderly. Below age 25 years, Colles' fractures are more frequent among males than females, and usually occur in association with significant, often sprots-related, trauma. They are also very common, with a peak incidence of nearly 1% per year in the age-group 10 to 14 years. Wage-earner's fractures (15), on the other hand, are most common in young and

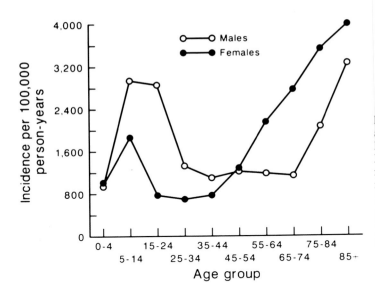

FIG. 1. Average annual age- and sex-specific incidence of all limb fractures among Rochester, Minnesota, residents. From Garraway et al., ref. 34, with permission.

middle-aged adults. More frequent in men than women, these fractures are also due to significant trauma, often of an occupational nature. Examples are fractures of the feet and toes and hands and fingers. The incidence of hand and finger fractures, for example, is nearly three times greater among men than women in Rochester, Minnesota, and is almost twice as high among those less than 35 years old compared to those over that age. Over a third of these fractures are incurred during recreation and sports, while about one-fifth are related to crush injuries.

None of these fractures seems to have any relationship with involutional osteoporosis. Because the forces involved in the production of such fractures are generally substantial, the question of underlying bone strength rarely arises. The overall pattern of incidence is, thus, largely determined by the occurrence of significant trauma. We have designated these as "type C" fractures (85), to distinguish them from the type A (distal forearm and postmenopausal vertebral fractures) and type B (hip, pelvis, proximal humerus, and proximal tibia) fractures that are responsible for the late peak in fracture incidence (Fig. 1).

Age-related Fractures

General Features

Emphasis in this chapter will be on the fractures related to aging and, by extension, to osteoporosis. The classical example is proximal femur (hip) fractures. Fractures of the vertebrae and distal forearm in middle-aged and elderly persons are also traditionally included, especially when they occur with only minimal or moderate trauma. Recent detailed studies have revealed, however, that fractures of the proximal humerus (88) and most pelvic fractures (68) should definitely be included in this category and that the risk of some other limb fractures increases with advancing age as well. These fractures are distinguished epidemiologically by three distinctive characteristics, namely, (1) incidence rates that increase greatly with age, (2) rates that are higher among women than men, and (3) association with moderate trauma at sites containing substantial amounts of trabecular bone. Although these general features were recognized over a century ago (2), additional data are now available concerning the etiologic factors mainly responsible.

Incidence rates for the age-related fractures are from 2 to 100 times greater among adults over 35 years of age than for younger individuals (Table 1). The only exception is for distal forearm fractures, where the figures include the previously mentioned adolescent Colles' fractures. All age-related sites reveal at least a two-fold excess of incidence among women, even after age-adjustment of the sex-specific rates. Because there are proportionately more elderly women than men, the female excess in actual numbers of cases is even greater (Table 1). The ratio of moderate to severe trauma is also notably higher for age-related fracture sites than for limb fractures in general. This is not to say that a person with osteoporosis cannot experience a fracture with severe trauma like anyone else, but the incidence of fractures due to severe trauma does not rise substantially with age and rates are not greater for women than men (68,72,79,88). Because the risk of fracture rises with the level of trauma and with reduction in the ability of bone to withstand the loads imposed (71), these general epidemiologic patterns have been explained on the basis of age- and sex-related differences in trauma or, alternatively, on the basis of age- and sex-related reductions in bone strength.

Role of Trauma

Osteoporotic fractures are typically associated with a fall to the floor. The frequency of falls increases with age and is greater among women than men (41). A third or more of all elderly individuals may experience a fall each year. The causes of these falls are complex. In terms of host factors, half or more of the falls among elderly persons are associated with definable organic dysfunction, and the proportion increases with advancing age (61,77,104). Most victims have a variety of deficits (100), including diminished postural control, gait changes, muscular weakness, decreased reflexes, poor vision, postural hypotension, vestibular problems, confusion, or dementia. Specific diseases, such as parkinsonism, hemi-

plegia, cardiac arrhythmias, arthritis, and alcoholism, may predispose to falls in some patients (60). Iatrogenic problems include excessive use of sedatives leading to falls at night and overtreatment of hypertension with resulting orthostatic hypotension (63). So-called drop attacks, postulated to result from disturbances in blood flow to brainstem postural centers (92), may account for 10 to 20% of falls among elderly people (13). Environmental hazards are directly responsible for about a third of falls (61), although the aforementioned factors may contribute. The leading hazards are slippery surfaces and loose rugs, but steps, curbs, light cords, and other obstacles also lead to falls. About three-fourths of all falls in the elderly occur indoors, and many are associated with merely getting in or out of a chair or bed. Falls seem to be somewhat more common during the active hours of daylight than at night, and perhaps more common in winter than in other seasons. Both environmental and seasonal variation in falls are minimized among nursing home residents and other institutionalized individuals.

However, the incidence of falls does not appear to increase 30-fold as does, for example, the incidence of hip fractures between the ages of 50 and 80 years. One possible explanation for this discrepancy could be a declining capacity for energy absorption with age, leading to an age-related increase in the degree of trauma actually experienced in a fall (see Chapter 4, *this volume*). However, documentation of this is lacking. In any event, trauma cannot by itself account for the age-related pattern of fracture incidence. Most falls do not result in a fracture, even among the elderly (5,41), and vertebral fractures are not closely associated with falls at all (30,90).

Influence of Bone Strength

Since falls alone are not sufficient to cause all age-related fractures, attention has turned to factors that reduce bone strength. While it is generally presumed that osteoporosis is the

TABLE 1. *Ratios of numbers of cases and of incidence rates by sex, age, and severity of trauma for selected fractures sites among Rochester, Minnesota residents*

| | ≥ 35 yr:< 35 yr | | For residents ≥ 35 years only | | | |
| | | | Female:male | | Moderate:severe | |
Fracture Site	Numbers	Rates[a]	Numbers	Rates[a]	Numbers	Rates[a]
Distal forearm	0.4:1	0.5:1	6.3:1	4.8:1	11.9:1	11.7:1
Proximal humerus	4.8:1	6.4:1	3.9:1	2.7:1	4.4:1	4.3:1
Vertebrae	—	—	—	—	—	—
Pelvis	1.8:1	2.4:1	4.0:1	2.4:1	2.6:1	2.4:1
Cervical femur	76:1	102:1	4.8:1	2.5:1	6.3:1	6.5:1
Intertrochanteric femur	70:1	90:1	3.9:1	2.1:1	6.7:1	7.0:1
All other limb fractures	0.4:1	0.6:1	1.3:1	1.0:1	0.7:1	0.7:1

[a]Incidence per 100,000 person-years age-adjusted (for sex comparison) or age- and sex-adjusted (for age and severity comparison) to the population structure of United States whites in 1985.

main cause of reduced bone strength (see Chapter 2, *this volume*), there is no clear bimodality in the distribution of bone mineral density in the population, and values overlap widely for age- and sex-matched individuals with and without the fractures of interest (84). This has led some to question the etiologic importance of osteoporosis in age-related fractures (3,21), but epidemiologic data show that the risk of fracture varies with bone mineral density at the fracture site (Fig. 2). As noted in Chapter 4, this helps account for the relationship of fractures with increasing age and female sex, insofar as women have a lower peak bone mass than men and lose bone at a more rapid rate, although men lose substantial bone with aging as well.

Variation in bone mass may also explain racial differences in fracture risk. Age-related fractures have long been thought uncommon among blacks in the United States, and epidemiologic documentation is now available. Farmer et al. (29) show that hip fracture incidence rates, adjusted for age, are twice as great in white as in nonwhite women in the District of Columbia and in the United States generally; little difference is seen between white and black men. These findings confirm those of earlier, more limited studies (11). Rates are also similar for nonwhite men and nonwhite women in the United States (29), as they are in underdeveloped countries. The absence of a consistent effect of sex within races and the lack of a racial difference in men seems at first to be at variance with the reported genetic determination of bone mass (93). However, anatomic studies show that bone mass is greater in white and black men (101) and black women (18,101) than in white women, and *in vivo* studies indicate that black women have greater axial (94) and peripheral (38,64) bone density and fewer fractures than their white counterparts. Multifactorial models of osteoporosis indicate that the greater initial bone mass of blacks should offer relative protection against fractures throughout life (87), although there is also evidence that blacks may lose bone more slowly (7,33). The South African Bantu seem anomalous in this regard. They have very low hip fracture incidence rates but are reported to have values for metacarpal bone density lower than those of Johannesburg whites (97), who display the usual Western pattern of fracture incidence.

Correlation of Age-related Fractures

It is commonly recognized that patients with one type of age-related fracture often have another. Patients with hip fracture are about twice as likely as expected to have had a prior fracture of the proximal humerus (31) or distal forearm (4) and 3 to 10 times more likely (depending on age) to have had a prior vertebral

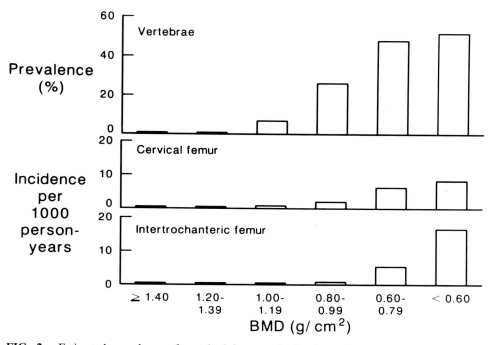

FIG. 2. Estimated prevalence of vertebral fractures by lumbar spine bone mineral density (BMD) and estimated incidence of cervical and intertrochanteric hip fractures by cervical and intertrochanteric BMD, respectively, among Rochester, Minnesota women ≥ 35 years of age. From Riggs, and Melton, ref. 87, with permission.

fracture (82). Similarly, patients with a Colles' fracture seem to be at about twice the usual risk for a subsequent hip fracture (80), while those with vertebral osteopenia may have a five-fold increase in hip fracture risk compared to those with more normal vertebrae (57). Nonetheless, the correspondence between different fractures is less than one would expect if all were related to exactly the same underlying disorder. Thus, even though the risk is increased significantly, the practical result is that most patients with Colles' fracture will not have a subsequent hip fracture and most patients with hip fracture will not have had a prior Colles' fracture. It has been suggested that, because Colles' fractures become common 15 to 20 years before hip fractures do, they could be used as a predictor of hip fracture risk (6). This is an example of the "ecologic fallacy," the assumption that relationships seen in populations apply to individuals within the population. In fact, the ability of a

Colles' fracture to predict which patients will sustain subsequent hip fractures is small (80).

Given the similarities alluded to previously, it is perhaps surprising that the various age-related fractures are not more closely correlated with each other. When age- and sex-specific incidence rates for the major fractures are plotted on a semilogarithmic grid to emphasize the rate of change in incidence with aging (Fig. 3), considerable variability is apparent. The age- and sex-specific incidence rates for cervical and intertrochanteric hip fractures (which are combined in the figure) are essentially identical in Rochester, although the cervical region is composed predominantly of cortical bone (75% cortical and 25% trabecular) and the intertrochanteric region is composed of about 50% of each bone type. The former approximates the composition of the distal radius at the usual absorptiometry scanning sites, but age- and sex-specific incidence patterns for hip and Colles' fractures are quite different. Al-

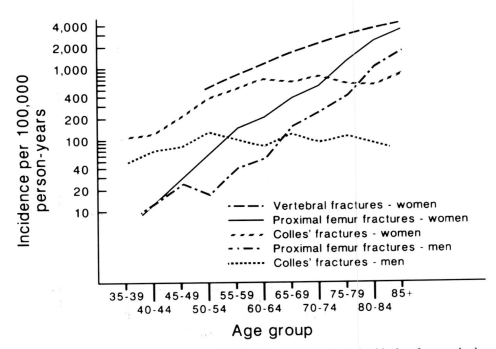

FIG. 3. Age- and sex-specific incidence of Colles' fractures contrasted with that for vertebral and hip fractures among Rochester, Minnesota, residents. From Melton, et al. *Bone and Mineral,* 2:321–331, 1987, with permission from Elsevier Science Publishers, Inc.

though rates at both sites begin to increase steeply prior to the usual age of menopause, the incidence of hip fractures rises exponentially throughout life for both men and women, while the rapid rise in Colles' fracture incidence is not sustained in either sex. This observation alone provides sufficient evidence to discount any simplistic view of age-related fractures as solely due to the effects of menopause on the bone density of middle-aged women.

One important reason for the poor correlation among the various fractures is that, to some degree, they represent the consequences of difference syndromes of osteoporosis (see Chapter 6, *this volume*). Distal forearm fracture and postmenopaual vertebral crush fractures seem to be most closely related to type I (or postmenopausal) osteoporosis, and we have designated them type A fractures to reflect this (85). Hip fractures, on the other hand, are associated with type II (or senile) osteoporosis, as are fractures of the pelvis, proximal hu-

merus, proximal tibia, and the vertebral wedge fractures seen in the elderly. We group these together as type B fractures. The age-specific incidence curve for vertebral fractures shown in Fig. 3 represents a composite of the vertebral fractures associated with type I and type II osteoporosis.

SPECIFIC FRACTURE SYNDROMES

Within the general pattern of higher incidence rates with advancing age, female sex, and white race, and, to a lesser degree within the type A and type B designations, each individual fracture site has its own peculiar epidemiologic features.

Proximal Femur

The apparent incidence of hip fractures varies enormously from one geographic area to another (Table 2). Some differences may be due to methodologic problems, such as incom-

TABLE 2. *Age-adjusted[a] incidence (per 100,000 per year) of various limb fractures in different populations among persons 35 years of age or older.*

Geographic locality	Proximal femur		Distal forearm or Colles'		Proximal humerus	
	Women	Men	Women	Men	Women	Men
USA, Rochester	319.7	177.0	409.7	84.6	163.2	60.8
USA, District of Columbia						
whites	231.8	82.0				
blacks	118.8	109.7				
Finland	212.8	136.1				
Norway, Oslo	421.0	230.5	767.3	201.5		
Sweden, Malmö	237.2	101.4	731.5	177.5	136.4	76.6
Holland	187.2	107.9				
United Kingdom, Oxford-Dundee	142.2	69.2	309.4	73.1	58.4	39.6
Yugoslavia						
high calcium area	43.5	44.5	227.6	94.8		
low calcium area	105.3	93.9	195.5	110.5		
Israel, Jerusalem						
American/European-born	201.8	113.9				
Native-born	168.0	107.5				
Asian/African-born	141.7	109.2				
Hong Kong	87.1	73.0				
Singapore (total)	42.1	73.1	58.7	63.3	12.2	9.7
Indian	312.9	131.4				
Chinese	59.0	106.1				
Malay	24.2	35.4				
New Zealand						
whites	220.4	98.6				
Maori	104.4	84.0				
South Africa, Johannesburg						
whites	256.5	98.8				
Bantu	14.0	14.3				

[a]Age-adjusted to the population structure of United States whites ≥ 35 years old in 1985 (both sexes combined).

plete case ascertainment. Others may be due to the timing of the study, insofar as dramatic increases in hip fracture incidence rates have been reported from many regions of the world (72). For example, the rates for Oxford-Dundee from 1954–58 (54), are only about 40% of those for Rochester, Minnesota, residents in 1968–82. Newer data (12) show, however, that the age-adjusted incidence of hip fracture in Oxford residents was about 75% greater in 1983 than it was in 1954–58 (259.9 per 100,000 person-years in women and 125.2 in men). Likewise, the hip fracture data shown for Malmö, Sweden, in Table 2 are from the classic study of Alffram (4). More recent reports do not include sufficiently detailed age-

and sex-specific incidence rates to use here but clearly indicate that the incidence of hip fractures has risen substantially among Malmö residents (50). Current rates in Malmö appear to be greater even than those in Rochester. The explanation for the secular increase in hip fracture incidence is unknown (72).

Hip fracture rates seem to be higher among whites than nonwhites regardless of the geographic area involved. Rochester, Minnesota, for example, is populated largely by persons of northern European extraction; and incidence rates are high for similar ethnic groups in Scandinavia, New Zealand, and South Africa (Table 2). Conversely, the incidence of hip fractures is very low for the Maori people in

New Zealand (99) and the Bantu in South Africa (96), while rates are relatively high among Indians in Singapore (106), an otherwise low incidence area. There are sex and age differences as well. Among the Maori in New Zealand, men and women have similar hip fracture incidence rates (99), while rates are higher in men among South African Bantu (96) and the Chinese and Malay residents of Singapore (106). Moreover, none of the above populations displays the dramatic rise in incidence with aging that is seen in all communities in developed countries. In Singapore, 26% of men and 11% of women are under age 50 years at the time of hip fracture (108). This is unusual in the West. In Rochester, Minnesota, for example, only 4% of patients with hip fracture are less then 50 years old. The explanation for these discrepancies is unknown, although speculation has centered on differences in physical activity and diet (16).

In Rochester, the incidence of proximal femur fractures among women rises exponentially from 9 per 100,000 person-years (p-y) at 35–44 years to 3,317 per 100,000 p-y (or 3.3% per year) for women 85 years old and over (71). The incidence among 35–44 year-old men is similar, 10 per 100,000 p-y, but the peak reached among men aged 85 years or older, 1,833 per 100,000 person-years, is only about half as great (Fig. 4). Although Rochester rates (based almost entirely on whites) are greater than those reported for whites in the District of Columbia (29), they may be fairly representative of the United States as a whole where such detailed rates are not available. For example, when the Rochester rates for 1978–1982 are extrapolated to the white population of the United States in 1980, 216,000 hip fractures are predicted. This corresponds reasonably well with the 237,000 hospital discharges reported nationally for neck of femur fractures in 1980 (75), considering that only about 95% of these patients would be white (29) and that some cases would not represent new fractures. The Rochester rates thus seem closer to national data than those for District of Columbia whites, which predict only 139,500 hospital discharges nationally in 1980.

Hip fracture incidence rates for women in Rochester are substantially greater than those for men at all ages beyond 50 years. Overall, about 98% of all fractures of the proximal femur occur among persons age 35 years or older, and 80% or so occur in women. The predominance of older women, along with the effects of menopause on bone metabolism and the influence of estrogen therapy in preventing fractures (see Chapter 11, *this volume*), suggests a close relationship with the menopause; it has thus been considered curious that no sharp postmenopausal increase in hip fracture incidence rates can be seen (14,43). However, hip fracture risk depends on a substantial reduction in bone mass (see Chapter 4, *this volume*), and postmenopausal bone loss alone may be insufficient in this regard. When combined with age-related bone loss (see Chapter 6, *this volume*), however, postmenopausal bone loss has an important additive effect, although this may not be reflected in fracture rates until late in life.

Proximal femur fractures typically occur through the neck of the femur (cervical, intracapsular) or in the region between the greater and lesser trochanters (intertrochanteric, extracapsular). Age- and sex-specific incidence rates for cervical and intertrochanteric hip fractures are similar in Rochester, except for the suggestion of a somewhat more rapid increase in the incidence of intertrochanteric fractures among the very elderly (32). This general similarity occurs despite the fact that trabecular bone makes up only about 25% of the femoral neck compared to 50% of the intertrochanteric region of the proximal femur (84). Patients with hip fractures do seem to have both trabecular and cortical osteoporosis, as is characteristic of type II osteoporosis (see Chapter 6, *this volume*). Patients with intertrochanteric hip fractures, however, are much more likely to have a recurrent fracture in the intertrochanteric region of the opposite hip (25,70), and they are more likely than patients with cervical femur fractures to have had a previous vertebral fracture (10,31,82,98) or evidence of trabecular osteoporosis (55,59,98). Patients with cervical fractures, on the other hand, are more

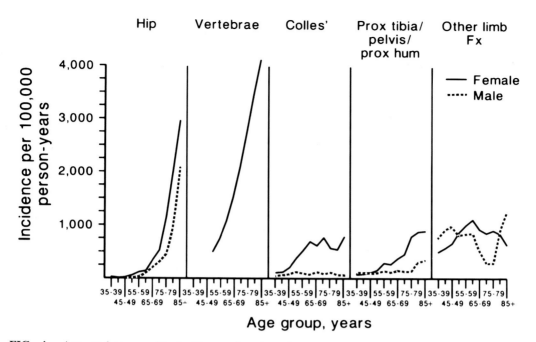

FIG. 4. Age- and sex-specific incidence of various fractures among Rochester, Minnesota, residents. From Melton, et al. *Bone and Mineral*, 2:321–331, 1987, with permission from Elsevier Science Publishers, Inc.

likely to have a recurrent fracture in the cervical region of the opposite hip (25,70).

The uncommon hip fractures among young people are likely to be associated with severe trauma, such as motor vehicle accidents, and the incidence of hip fractures associated with severe trauma does not rise with age (72). However, most hip fractures occur among older persons, and nearly 90 percent of these occur as a result of only moderate trauma (69). A few of these fractures seem to be spontaneous (see Chapter 4, *this volume*), and another small group are associated with specific pathological lesions, such as metastatic malignant tumors or bone cysts. Most of the hip fractures associated with moderate trauma, however, are due to falls, typically a "simple" fall to the floor. Reasons for the falls vary from study to study, depending on whether the authors emphasize the external circumstances or the patients' underlying deficits. In general, however, a third to a half are due to tripping or slipping, another fifth are secondary to syncope or a drop attack, a fifth to a third are due to a loss of balance, and the remainder are the re-

sult of miscellaneous factors such as collisions with others or seizures (13,17). Trips and slips may be somewhat more frequent causes of falls among the less elderly patients with hip fracture, whereas the very elderly are more likely to fall because of loss of balance or drop attacks (13).

Vertebrae

The falls that are so conspicuous with hip fractures do not play a prominent role in the etiology of vertebral fractures, which are rarely associated with a specific episode of external trauma (36,90). They are due instead to the compressive loading associated with lifting, changing positions, etc. (37,89). Many are discovered only incidentally, particularly in the very elderly. As Riggs (86) has noted, vertebral fractures occurring in the first 15 to 20 years after menopause often involve high-grade compression or collapse and severe pain. Vertebral fractures diagnosed after age 75 years, on the other hand, are more likely to have gradual onset and often are painless. Characteristically, the latter are wedge and balloon fractures, often of minimal degree, which may involve multiple vertebrae. Of 70-year-old Danish women with vertebral fractures, for example, 20% had collapse fractures, while 80% had vertebral wedging (47).

Due to the gradual and often painless onset of many vertebral fractures, it has proven difficult to measure their incidence in the general population. An additional serious problem is that no general agreement exists as to what constitutes a vertebral fracture (53). For example, one study in Oxford-Dundee reported vertebral fracture incidence rates that were only 8% as great as rates for distal radius fractures and were only 15% of rates for hip fractures (54). This does not correspond to the clinical impression that vertebral fractures are a very common manifestation of osteoporosis. These incidence rates for vertebral fracture were generally greater in men than women and did not rise markedly with aging; moreover, most of the vertebral fractures were due to a recognized accident (54). Thus, the study appears to describe traumatic vertebral fractures rather than the more typical atraumatic variety common in the general population.

That the true incidence is much greater is revealed by the high prevalence rates found in most studies. Data from a radiographic survey of an age-stratified random sample of adult Rochester, Minnesota, women show a rapid rise in the prevalence of vertebral fractures with age, affecting over one-half of white women over the age of 85 years (73). Correcting for the different age-specific sampling fractions and using smoothed prevalence figures, it is estimated that almost a third of women 65 years of age and over in the general population of Rochester have one or more vertebral fractures, counting crushed, wedged or ballooned vertebrae. Nontraumatic vertebral fractures are uncommon prior to age 50 years. The Rochester prevalence rates, extrapolated to the population structure of United States whites 50 years old or over in 1985, suggest that over 5 million white women nationally might have one or more vertebral fractures as defined above. Only a fraction of these, an estimated 83,000 with vertebral fractures, are medically attended each year, however (44).

The high prevalence rates for vertebral fractures found in Rochester are, however, very close to estimates from a random sample of 70-year-old Danish women (47) and selected nursing home residents (36). Other nonpopulation-based estimates are generally compatible as well (62,65). Smith and Rizek's age-specific estimates are much lower (94), but these were based on women attending a general medical clinic and, thus, cannot be representative of the population in general. Also, women were excluded from their study who had any condition that might be related to osteoporosis. The prevalence of vertebral compression fractures was much lower in a random sample of Israelis assessed with roentgenograms, reaching only 6.8% in women 75–84 years old (82); but hip fracture incidence rates were also low in that population compared to Rochester.

Although it is generally agreed that vertebral fractures are much more common in women than men (19,62), reliable epidemiologic data on this point are few. Among randomly sampled Jerusalem residents 45 to 84 years of age (82), the prevalence of vertebral compression fractures was seven times greater among women (2.7%) than men (0.4%) overall and in the oldest age-group studied (75–84 years, 6.8% versus 0.9%). A female:male ratio of only 2:1 was found in a study using miniature roentgenograms of the abdomen, and sex-specific prevalence rates (1.2% versus 0.6%) were much lower as well (39). That study could not have been expected to identify all spinal fractures, however, due to insensitivity of the method and because only lumbar vertebrae were assessed. Among patients with vertebral fractures referred to a Metabolic Bone Disease Clinic, the female:male ratio was 4:1 (85).

Prevalence rates were higher in two surveys of clinic outpatients in North Dakota—about 10% in women over 65 years of age in a high-fluoride area and almost 35% in those from an area with low fluoride levels in drinking water

(9). Rates in men, however, were much greater, from about 20% in those 45–54 years old to nearly 50% in men 65 years of age and over. These figures are much higher than anticipated and may reflect occupationally-related vertebral fractures, insofar as the primary occupation in these rural areas was farming. This conjecture is supported by the similar prevalence of collapsed vetebrae in men from the high- and low-fluoride regions.

The influence of race is also poorly documented. There appear to be no studies assessing the influence of race on vertebral fracture prevalence in unselected individuals from the general community. Smith and Rizek (94) found vertebral fractures in about 5% of selected white women 45 years old and over but in none of 137 black women studied. They also found that black women had more dense vertebrae, as have others (38).

Since it was not feasible to determine the incidence of vertebral fractures directly, incidence rates were estimated from the Rochester prevalence data using the method of Leske (56). As shown in Fig. 4, the estimated incidence of vertebral fractures in women is already rising around the time of menopause. In contrast to Colles' fractures, which increase until age 65 years and then plateau, the estimated incidence of vertebral fractures continues to rise. Most of the early postmenopausal increase in vertebral fracture incidence seems to be related to the crush fractures associated with type I osteoporosis (87), whereas most of the increase late in life represents the multiple wedge deformations (47) of type II osteoporosis (87). Thus, as noted earlier, the overall vertebral fracture curve appears to represent a summation of the two different types of vertebral fractures. Interestingly, if incidence rates for Colles' fractures (a type I fracture) and hip fractures (a type II fracture) are added together, the result is a curve that closely resembles the age-specific incidence of vertebral fractures in women.

Based on the estimated incidence rates among women 50 years of age and over, vertebral fractures are nearly three times as frequent as hip fractures when patients are counted. If individual vertebrae were counted, of course, this difference would be greatly magnified. The overall age- and sex-adjusted incidence of vertebral fractures, 1,540 per 100,000 person-years among white women 50 years old and over, is also much higher than the estimated incidence of vertebral fractures nationally, 130 per 100,000 per year (44). However, the latter rate was averaged over blacks as well as whites and over men as well as women, and no rise in incidence between 45–64 and 65+ years was seen. Moreover, the national estimate was restricted to fractures that led to a physician visit or restricted activity and were more likely of the collapse type. The Rochester figures, on the other hand, include wedged and ballooned vertebrae, which are usually not medically attended.

Distal Forearm

Almost all fractures of the distal forearm are of the Colles' type (95), and the two terms are used interchangeably here. The incidence of distal forearm fracture varies from one geographic area to another (Table 2), generally in parallel with hip fracture incidence rates. Exceptions are noted in rural Yugoslavia (66), especially in a high calcium area, where the incidence of hip fracture is proportionately lower, compared to Western Europe, than is the incidence of distal forearm fractures. This anomaly is exaggerated if the higher wrist fracture incidence rates for the urban population of Zagreb are considered (67).

As noted for hip fracture, some of these differences may be methodological (34). Case ascertainment, specifically, is much more difficult since less than 20% of forearm fracture patients are hospitalized (35). The inability to rely on hospital-based record systems in this instance probably accounts for the small number of population-based studies of Colles' fracture that have been done. In addition, rising Colles' fracture incidence rates have been reported from Malmö, Sweden (8), and widespread increases could cause variation associated with the time of study as seen for hip fracture. Age- and sex-adjusted incidence rates for Colles' fracture in Rochester did not increase significantly between 1945 and 1974 (79), however, and the influence of secular trends is uncertain at present.

In comparison with other types of age-related fractures, Colles' fractures display a somewhat different pattern of incidence. As shown in Fig. 4, the steep rise in incidence begins at an earlier age, even discounting the forearm fractures in adolescents. Among Rochester, Minnesota, residents, distal forearm fractures are somewhat more common in women than men in the 35–44 year age-group, 112 versus 56 per 100,000 p-y, respectively. Instead of continuing to increase exponentially with age, however, the incidence rates plateau after about age 60 years. Incidence rates among men show little tendency to rise after age 50. By age 80 years and over, the rates are 593 per 100,000 p-y in women and only 78 per 100,000 p-y in men (71). This plateau in Colles' fracture incidence may be due to reversal of the cortical porosity that develops in the distal forearm around the time of menopause or to cessation of the bone loss associated with type I osteoporosis (see Chapter 2, *this volume*). Alternatively, it has been suggested that the plateau (79) or even decline (28) in incidence after mid-life results from the loss of protective reflexes, with a resulting reduction in the tendency to break falls with an outstretched arm (27). It seems unlikely that this could account for a leveling of fracture risk beginning as early as age 60 years, but the actual explanation for the plateau is not known.

Overall, Colles' fractures that occur at age 35 years or after are as common as hip fractures (based on age- and sex-adjusted incidence rates), and about 85% of them occur in women. There is some evidence of variation in distal forearm fracture incidence by race, with Malays and Chinese in Singapore having distal forearm fracture rates that are as high among men as among women (107). Moreover, Chinese and Malay residents of Singapore have lower rates than Singapore women of Indian heritage (largely Caucasoid), who have rates

virtually superimposable on those for adults in Malmö, Sweden.

The distal forearm contains a substantial amount of trabecular bone (84), and 92% of the fractures at that site are associated with only moderate trauma, again, typically a fall from standing height or less (79). While the falls leading to Colles' fractures have not been studied in as much detail as those associated with hip fractures, a greater proportion of them seem to occur outside of the home (54). This finding is supported by the seasonal pattern of Colles' fracture (Fig. 5), that reveals an increased incidence in winter. Although an epidemic of limb fractures following an ice storm has been reported (83), less than 8% of falls leading to limb fractures in Rochester over a three-year period occurred on icy or snowy surfaces. An alternative suggestion for the seasonality of Colles' fracture is a seasonal decline in bone mass of the radius (2), although others have not confirmed this (102). A related hypothesis is that a seasonal increase in osteomalacia is responsible for an excess of hip fractures in the winter, at least in the United Kingdom (1). Osteomalacia may be less frequent among hip fracture patients in the United States (see Chapter 14, *this volume*), however, and the seasonal pattern of hip fracture incidence in Rochester is not as marked as for Colles' fracture (Fig. 5). Nonetheless, environmental factors may play some role in the different influence of season on distal forearm and hip fracture incidence.

Proximal Humerus

Among women aged 35 years and over, incidence rates for fractures of the proximal humerus, pelvis, and proximal tibia resemble the pattern seen for proximal femur (Fig. 4). Among men, however, the incidence of fractures at those sites does not appear to increase as rapidly with advancing age as in the case of hip fractures. In Rochester, Minnesota, the incidence of proximal humerus fractures is approximately equal for men and women aged 35–44 years, at 41 and 36 per 100,000 p-y. Rates then increase with advancing age to 439

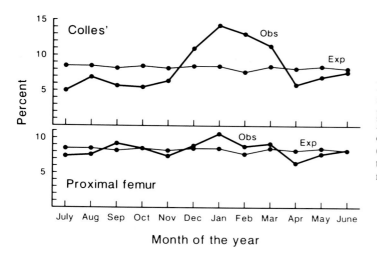

FIG. 5. Observed (OBS) seasonal distribution of Colles' and proximal femur fractures among Rochester, Minnesota residents compared with that expected (EXP) if the fractures were distributed evenly from month to month.

per 100,000 p-y in women and only 112 per 100,000 p-y in men aged 80 years and over (88). Overall, 83% of proximal humerus fractures occur in individuals 35 years old and over, and 74% occur in women. The same general picture is seen in population-based studies from Malmö, Sweden (45) and Oxford-Dundee, United Kingdom (54). The Oxford-Dundee rates are much lower, as they are for most other skeletal sites, in comparison to Rochester figures (34). In Rochester, fractures of the proximal humerus are common, occurring at about 70% of the age-adjusted rate for hip fractures when all ages are considered.

Nearly three-fourths of all proximal humerus fractures are due to moderate trauma, typically a fall from standing height or less (88). By contrast, no notable increase with age is seen for fractures of the shaft or distal humerus, which are comprised almost exclusively of cortical bone; and incidence rates at the latter sites are not greater in women. Severe trauma accounts for about two-thirds of these: Fractures of the humeral shaft are most commonly caused by motor vehicle accidents (35%) and falls from heights (23%); those of the distal humerus are most often associated with falls from heights (64 percent), especially falls from playground equipment in children (88).

In Rochester, about one-third of the fractures of the proximal humerus involve the greater tuberosity. Estimates from other studies

of the proportion of this type of proximal humerus fracture are lower (45,108). There is more general agreement, however, that the incidence of fractures involving the greater tuberosity does not increase with aging to the degree seen for those proximal fractures not involving the greater tuberosity. This finding has been attributed to weaker rotator cuff musculature among elderly persons or to a reduced tendency to tense shoulder muscles to break a fall (45).

Pelvis

Incidence rates for pelvic fractures are low and not too dissimilar among 35 to 44-year-old Rochester men and women (14 and 31 per 100,000 p-y, respectively), but they rise subsequently to 220 and 446 per 100,000 p-y among those aged 85 years and over (71). Overall, 64% of all pelvic fractures occur among persons aged 35 years or older, and 69% occur in women (68). The only other population-based study of pelvic fractures, in the United Kingdom (54), failed to show a substantial female excess in incidence and also appeared to underestimate the effect of age. These results may have been due to incomplete case ascertainment, inasmuch as comparable age-adjusted rates in Rochester are three times greater for men and eight times greater for women (68). When fractures at all ages are considered, pelvic fractures occur at about one-third of the age- and sex-adjusted rate of hip fractures.

Multiple pelvic fractures and acetabular fractures are closely associated with severe trauma, occur in men more than women, and are proportionately more common in the young. The overall increase in incidence with age and the excess risk among women, on the other hand, are largely due to pelvic fractures resulting from moderate trauma, usually falls (54). Moderate trauma accounts for nearly two-thirds of all fractures of isolated pelvic bones and single breaks in the pelvic ring; these, in turn, comprise about 80% of all pelvic fractures in the community (68). Although trabecular bone is found throughout the pelvis, most pelvic fractures involve the pubic rami or sacrum. The rami fractures are most closely associated with advancing age, as nearly 60% occur in patients 65 years of age and over. Moreover in the Rochester study, 40% of men and 70% of women aged 35 years and over at the time of pelvic fracture exhibited some stigmata of osteoporosis, namely prior osteoporotic fractures or a previous radiologic diagnosis of osteoporosis (68). This must be a conservative estimate, however, because patients were not evaluated in a consistent manner in this retrospective study and because assessment predated the availability of more sensitive methods like dual photon absorptiometry. Based on these epidemiologic features, however, a portion of pelvic fractures appear to be osteoporosis-related.

Other Sites

In addition to the skeletal sites covered above, Buhr (15) identified the ankle as an age-related fracture site. However, ankle fracture incidence rates among women rise during the postmenopausal period but then fall (24,78). This is also the pattern seen for all other limb fractures in Rochester, Minnesota (Fig. 4). Ankle fractures are one of the largest components of this group, being more common than hip fractures on a per capita basis. In Rochester, the overall incidence of ankle frac-

tures is about 20% greater in men than women. Among those 35 years old and over, however, age-adjusted rates are 50% greater in women, and fractures due to moderate trauma are proportionately more common (24). The decline in incidence among women after a postmenopausal peak is not typical of osteoporotic fractures but could be related to postmenopausal porosity of cortical bone as described by Parfitt (81).

Fractures of the proximal tibia, proximal radius, and femoral shaft have been classified as composite fractures, with bimodal peaks in incidence among the young and the old (15). In Rochester, age-specific incidence rates for proximal tibia fractures are highest in those 10 to 19 years old and, in that age-group, are more common in boys. However, proximal tibia fractures in women outnumber those in men by 2:1 after the age of 50, and age-adjusted incidence rates are 30% greater in women. Over 40% of proximal tibia fractures are due to severe trauma, especially motor vehicle accidents. About 28% are sport-related, and only one-fourth are associated with falls.

Others have found that distal femur fractures occurring after childhood also have some of the characteristics of an age-related fracture. Hedlund (42) has shown that the incidence of diaphyseal femur fractures in Stockholm is greater in women than men after age 65 years, that the majority of such fractures in the middle-aged and elderly are due to falls, and that the incidence of fractures due to moderate trauma increases exponentially with age in both sexes. In Oxford-Dundee, rates also rose with age in both sexes but were greater in men after age 75 years in Dundee, Scotland but not in Oxford, England (54). These latter figures were based on very few cases, however, and such inconsistency is not surprising.

IMPACT OF AGE-RELATED FRACTURES

The medical and social consequences of these fractures make osteoporosis an enormous public health problem.

Morbidity

At least 1.3 million fractures in the United States each year are attributable to the disease (51), presuming that 70% of all fractures in persons aged 45 years or over are due to osteoporosis (46). Detailed estimates suggest that the age-related increase in fracture incidence accounts for over half of all limb fractures in white adults (Table 3), including nearly 230,000 hip fractures and over 170,000 Colles' fractures. As many as 500,000 white women may be newly affected by vertebral fractures each year (73). The prevalence of vertebral fractures among 70-year-old Danish women is reported to be 21% (47). Overall, almost a third of women aged 65 years and over will have one or more vertebral fractures (73). The prevalence of limb fractures in the general population is undocumented but, as estimated by cumulative incidence, is substantial: Up to 33% of women and more than 17% of men who survive to age 90 years will experience a hip fracture, while 24% of women and 5% of

men will have a Colles' fracture (71). Not everyone lives 90 years, of course, and the lifetime risk of a hip fracture is less, 15% in women and 5% in men, when the average life expectancy for each sex is taken into account (22). These figures are equivalent, respectively, to the combined lifetime risk of developing breast, uterine, or ovarian cancer in white women and about the same as the lifetime risk of prostate cancer in white men (91). The lifetime risk of a Colles' fracture from age 50 years onward is also 15% in white women and a little over 2% in white men (22). Other osteoporosis-related fractures are less common. The cumulative incidence to age 90 years for proximal humerus fractures is 12% in women and 4% in men; for pelvic fractures, the rates are 9% and 2.5%, respectively (71).

Mortality

Age-related fractures also have a significant impact on mortality. Hip fractures are by far the most serious, of course, and are associated

TABLE 3. *Excess (estimated minus expected) limb fractures among United States whites age 40 years or over in 1985*

Fracture site	Number of fractures			
	Estimated in those ≥ 40 yr old[a]	Expected at 35–39 yr old rates[a]	Annual excess	Excess as % of total
WOMEN				
Proximal femur	184,947	7,155	177,792	96.1
Proximal humerus	85,382	11,954	73,428	86.0
Distal forearm	202,828	46,467	156,361	77.1
Pelvis	42,286	14,647	27,639	65.4
All other limb fractures	373,754	210,155	163,599	43.8
Subtotal	889,197		598,819	67.3
MEN				
Proximal femur	58,455	8,790	49,665	85.0
Proximal humerus	22,091	14,685	7,406	33.5
Distal forearm	32,532	16,556	15,976	49.1
Pelvis	13,448	2,330	11,118	82.7
All other limb fractures	285,040	287,633	0	0
Subtotal	411,566		84,165	20.4
All sites both sexes	1,300,763		682,984	52.5

[a]Age- and sex-specific fracture incidence rates used in these calculations are from the population of Rochester, Minnesota.

with an overall 12 to 20% reduction in expected survival (22). The excess mortality may be evident for up to six months following fracture and varies with age and sex (Fig. 6). Weiss et al. (105) reported a reduction in expected survival at one year of only about 4% among women 50 to 74 years old, but institutionalized individuals were not studied. When unselected hip fracture patients from an entire community were evaluated, 90% of those under 75 years of age were still alive at one year (92% of expected), compared to only 73% (83% of expected) of those aged 75 years and over at the time of fracture. Survival was better among women, 83% of whom were still alive one year after the fracture (91% of expected), compared to only 63% of men (70% of expected). Although subsequent survival is generally poor for these typically elderly patients, it is not consistently less than expected for persons of comparable age and sex in the general population. Hip fractures are nonetheless associated with many deaths and are largely responsible for the observation that falls are the leading cause of accidental death among men and women aged 75 years or older in the United States and the second leading cause among those aged 45 to 74 years (71).

The relative contribution to mortality of poor health and predisposing medical conditions versus the sequelae of fracture and surgery is uncertain. Hip fracture patients have a variety of concomitant chronic diseases, and survival is directly related to the number of conditions present (23,52), as well as to preoperative mobility (40) and functional status (49). In this context, hip fracture is an indicator of poor health, and survival in such a group might be less than expected even without a fracture. However, the occurrence of a fracture often precipitates additional adverse events. Emergency surgery on these elderly individuals may be associated with increased mortality (52), while complications of surgery and hospitalization sometimes prove fatal (49). The falls leading to hip fracture do not seem to contribute directly to overall mortality (105). Other age-related fractures rarely result in death, except when the patient has substantial associated injuries with severe trauma. Colles' fractures, for example, are also associated with falls; but 98% of Rochester, Minnesota, residents with a Colles' fracture are still alive after one year and 90% after five years. These figures represent 100% of expected values for these generally younger individuals. Others have also reported unimpaired survival among those with Colles' fracture (105).

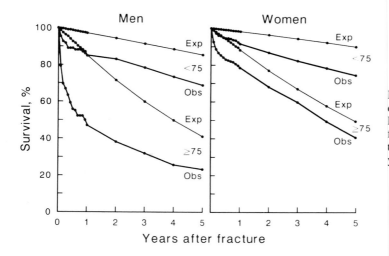

FIG. 6. Observed (OBS) and expected (EXP) survival for Rochester, Minnesota, residents following proximal femur fracture at ages under 75 years or 75 years and over.

Disability

Death is not the only adverse outcome of an age-related fracture. Many patients develop chronic complications, such as pressure sores (103); and rehabilitation is often unsuccessful, especially among elderly patients with lower limb fractures. At least half of those able to walk before sustaining a hip fracture, for example, cannot walk independently afterward (74). The ability of such patients to get about and care for themselves is greatly compromised, and their quality of life is considerably reduced. Half of all hip fracture victims may experience social deterioration, and a third may be totally dependent (48). Hip fracture is often the event that precipitates institutionalization, and as many as 8% of all nursing home residents have had a hip fracture (44).

Cost

The economic burden of age-related fractures is huge because of the large number of people affected and because of the expensive and protracted care that is often required. A fourth of all patients with limb fractures require hospitalization (ranging from one-fifth of forearm fractures to nearly all hip fractures), and the mean hospital stay increases with age up to 32.6 days among those over 65 years old (35). Fractures of the proximal femur account for as many as half of all days of hospitalization for limb fractures (26,35). Hip fractures also lead to over 7 million restricted activity days (62.5 days per episode among noninstitutionalized individuals) in the United States annually, while vertebral fractures account for over 5 million and forearm fractures for 6 million restricted activity days annually (44). Hip, vertebral, and forearm fractures are the primary reasons, respectively, for 122,000, 161,000, and 422,000 physician office visits annually by persons 45 years old or over in the United States (44). Of the total direct and indirect costs associated with all musculoskeletal diseases in the United States annually, 62 percent ($18 billion) is due to fractures; almost half of

this ($7 billion) is due to hip fractures alone (Table 4).

PROSPECTS

While the expenses associated with osteoporosis and its attendant fractures impose a formidable burden on the medical care system and on society at large, these costs will increase further as the number of elderly people grows. It is estimated that people aged 65 years and over will increase from 11% of the population in 1980 to 22% in 2050, while the proportion over 85 will rise from 1% of United States residents to 5% (22). The actual number of people 65 years old and over will increase from 25 to 67 million during the interval. Because hip fracture incidence rates rise exponentially with age, the annual number of fractures could double or triple by the year 2050 (22) solely on the basis of these demographic changes.

To make matters worse, however, recent reports from Great Britain, Scandinavia, and other areas suggest that age- and sex-specific hip fracture incidence rates are also rising (72). Long-term studies over a 55-year period in Rochester, Minnesota, confirm the increase in age-adjusted rates for men, but adjusted hip fracture incidence rates for women in Rochester have been level for almost three decades (Fig. 7). The reason for this discrepancy is not known. Rochester rates for Colles' fracture in adults have also been stable (79) in contrast to findings from Malmö, Sweden (8), where there were substantial increases in age- and sex-specific incidence rates at all ages above 25 years. Hospital discharges for vertebral fractures have risen 40% between 1970 and 1980 (58); but, since relatively few patients are hospitalized for age-related vertebral fractures, the relationship of this finding to actual secular changes in vertebral fracture incidence is unclear.

Nonetheless, with continued aging of the population and with increases in age- and sex-specific incidence rates in some regions of the world, the annual number of hip fractures is expected to rise dramatically in the coming de-

TABLE 4. *Annual cost of fractures in the United States[a]*

	All fractures	Hip fractures alone
Direct costs		
Hospital inpatient services	$4,467,440,000	$1,136,030,000
Outpatient and emergency room institutional services	88,410,000	2,530,000
Outpatient diagnostic and therapeutic services	3,200,400,000	24,650,000
Physician inpatient services	1,570,340,000	739,310,000
Physician office, outpatient and emergency room services	356,850,000	10,220,000
Other practitioner services	211,990,000	82,450,000
Drugs	120,020,000	3,440,000
Nursing home services	4,534,520,000	4,001,930,000
Prepayments and administration	654,750,000	270,030,000
Non-health sector goods and services	2,182,500,000	900,080,000
Total direct costs	$17,387,220,000	$7,170,670,000
Indirect costs		
Lost earnings–wage earners	425,960,000	9,240,000
Lost earnings–homemakers	330,870,000	83,400,000
Total indirect costs	$756,830,000	$92,640,000
Total costs	$18,144,050,000	$7,263,310,000

[a]From Holbrook et al., ref. 44, reproduced with permission of the author and the American Academy of Orthopedic Surgeons.

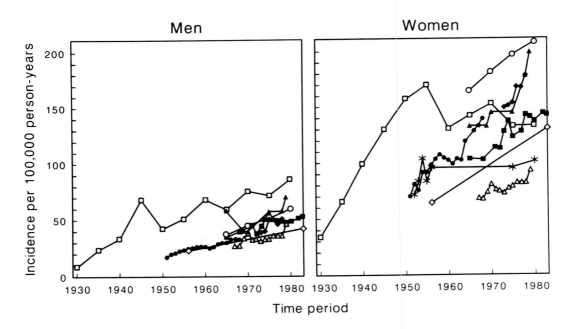

FIG. 7. Incidence of hip fractures over time as reported from various studies: □—□ Rochester, Minnesota; ■—■ United States; ◇—◇ Oxford, England; ◆—◆ Funen County, Denmark; △—△ Holland; ▲—▲ Göteborg, Sweden; ○—○ Uppsala, Sweden; ●—● New Zealand; *—* Dundee, Scotland. From Melton, et al., ref. 72, with permission.

cades. Other osteoporosis-related fractures should increase concomitantly. One note of optimism is provided by the suggestion that osteoporosis need not be prevented completely but only delayed in onset by five to six years to realize a 50% reduction in the number of hip fractures otherwise expected (14). Unless therapeutic or, preferably, prophylactic interventions are implemented on a large scale, however, the economic and social costs of osteoporosis will continue their alarming growth.

ACKNOWLEDGMENTS

The author would like to thank Miss Mary Ramaker for help in preparing the manuscript.

This work was supported in part by research grants AM-27065 and AM-30582 from the National Institutes of Health.

REFERENCES

1. Aaron, J.E., Gallagher, J.C., Anderson, J., Stasiak, L., Longton, E.B., Nordin, B.E.C., and Nicholson, M. (1974): Frequency of osteomalacia and osteoporosis in fractures of the proximal femur. *Lancet*, 1:229–233.
2. Aitken, J.M., Anderson, J.B., and Horton, P.W. (1973): Seasonal variations in bone mineral content after the menopause. *Nature*, 241:59–60.
3. Aitken, J.M. (1984): Relevance of osteoporosis in women with fracture of the femoral neck. *Br. Med. J.*, 288:597–601.
4. Alffram, P.-A. (1964): An epidemiologic study of cervical and trochanteric fractures of the femur in an urban population. *Acta Orthop. Scand. (Suppl.)*, 65:9–109.
5. Baker, S.P., and Harvey, A.H. (1985): Fall injuries in the elderly. Symposium on falls in the elderly: Biological and behavioral aspects. *Clinics Geriatr. Med.*, 1:501–508.
6. Bauer, G.C.H. (1960): Epidemiology of fracture in aged persons: A preliminary investigation in fracture etiology. *Clin. Orthop.*, 17:219–225.
7. Bell, N.H., Greene A., Epstein, S., Oexmann, M.J., Shaw, S., and Shary, J. (1985): Evidence for alteration of the vitamin D-endocrine system in blacks. *J. Clin. Invest.*, 76:470–473.
8. Bengnér, U., and Jonnell, O. (1985): Increasing incidence of forearm fractures: A comparison of epidemiologic patterns 25 years apart. *Acta Orthop. Scand.*, 56:158–160.
9. Bernstein, D.S., Sadowsky, N., Hegsted, D.M., Guri, C.D., and Stare, F.J. (1966): Prevalence of osteoporosis in high- and low-fluoride areas in North Dakota. *J.A.M.A.*, 198:499–504.
10. Bohr, H., and Schaadt, O. (1983): Bone mineral content of femoral bone and the lumbar spine measured in women with fracture of the femoral neck by dual photon absorptiometry. *Clin. Orthop.*, 179:240–245.
11. Bollett, A.J., Engh, G., and Parson, W. (1965): Epidemiology of osteoporosis: Sex and race incidence of hip fractures. *Arch. Intern. Med.*, 116:191–194.
12. Boyce, W.J., and Vessey, M.P. (1985): Rising incidence of fracture of the proximal femur. *Lancet*, 1:150–151.
13. Brocklehurst, J.C., Exton-Smith, A.N., Lempert Barber, S.M., Hunt, L.P., and Palmer, M.K. (1978): Fracture of the femur in old age: A two-centre study of associated clinical factors and the cause of the fall. *Age Ageing*, 7:7–15.
14. Brody, J.A., Farmer, M.E., and White, L.R. (1984): Absence of menopausal effect on hip fracture occurrence with white females. *Am. J. Public Health*, 74:1397–1398.
15. Buhr, A.J., and Cooke, A.M. (1959): Fracture patterns. *Lancet*, 1:531–536.
16. Chalmers, J., and Ho, K.C. (1970): Geographical variations in senile osteoporosis: The association with physical activity. *J. Bone Joint Surg.*, 52-B:667–675.
17. Clark, A.N.G. (1968): Factors in fracture of the female femur: A clinical study of the environment, physical, medical and preventative aspects of this injury. *Geront. Clin.*, 10:257–270.
18. Cohn, S.H., Abesamis, C., Yasumura, S., Aloia, J.F., Zanzi, I., and Ellis, K.J. (1977): Comparative skeletal mass and radial bone mineral content in black and white women. *Metabolism*, 26:171–178.
19. Consensus Conference (1984): Osteoporosis. *J.A.M.A.*, 252:799–802.
20. Cooper, A.P. (1842): *A Treatise on Dislocations and Fractures of the Joints*, edited by B.B. Cooper. John Churchill, London.
21. Cummings, S.R. (1985): Are patients with hip fractures more osteoporotic? Review of the evidence. *Am. J. Med.*, 78:487–494.
22. Cummings, S.R., Kelsey, J.L., Nevitt, M.C., and O'Dowd, K.J. (1985): Epidemiology of osteoporosis and osteoporotic fractures. *Epidemiol. Rev.*, 7:178–208.
23. Dahl, E. (1980): Mortality and life expectancy after hip fractures. *Acata Orthop. Scand.*, 51:163–170.
24. Daly, P.J., Fitzgerald, R.H., Melton, L.J., III, and Ilstrup, D.M. (1987): Ankle fracture in Rochester, Minnesota, 1979–1981. *Acta Orthop. Scand.* (in press).
25.. Dretakis, E., Kritsikis, N., Economou, K., and Christodoulou, N. (1981): Bilateral non-contemporary fractures of the proximal femur. *Acta Orthop. Scand.*, 52:227–229.
26. Engesaeter, L.B., and Sreide, O. (1985): Consumption of hospital resources for hip fracture: Discharge rates for fracture in Norway. *Acta Orthop. Scand.*, 56:17–20.
27. Evans, J.G. (1982): Epidemiology of proximal femoral fractures. Chapter 12. *Rec. Adv. Geriatr. Med.*, 2:201–214.

28. Falch, J.A. (1983): Epidemiology of fractures of the distal forearm in Oslo, Norway. *Acta Orthop. Scand.,* 54:291–295.

29. Farmer, M.E., White, L.R., Brody, J.A., and Bailey, K.R. (1984): Race and sex differences in hip fracture incidence. *Am. J. Public Health,* 74:1374–1380.

30. Frost, H.M. (1981): Clinical management of the symptomatic osteoporotic patient. *Orthop. Clin. North Am.,* 12:671–681.

31. Gallagher, J.C., Melton, L.J., and Riggs, B.L. (1980): Examination of prevalence rates of possible risk factors in a population with a fracture of the proximal femur. *Clin. Orthop.,* 153:158–165.

32. Gallagher, J.C., Melton, L.J., Riggs, B.L., and Bergstralh, E. (1980): Epidemiology of fractures of the proximal femur in Rochester, Minnesota. *Clin. Orthop.,* 150:163–171.

33. Garn, S.M., and Shaw, H.A. (1977): Extending the Trotter model of bone gain and bone loss. *1976 Yearbook of Physical Anthropology,* 20:45–56.

34. Garraway, W.M., Stauffer, R.N., Kurland, L.T., and O'Fallon, W.M. (1979): Limb fractures in a defined population. I. Frequency and distribution. *Mayo Clin. Proc.,* 54:701–707.

35. Garraway, W.M., Stauffer, R.N., Kurland, L.T., and O'Fallon, W.M. (1979): Limb fractures in a defined population. II. Orthopedic treatment and utilization of health care. *Mayo Clin. Proc.,* 54:708–713.

36. Gershon-Cohen, J., Rechtman, A.M., and Schraer, H. (1953): Asymtomatic fractures in osteoporotic spines of the aged. *J.A.M.A.,* 153:625–627.

37. Goldring, S.R., and Krane, S.M. (1981): Metabolic bone disease: Osteoporosis and osteomalacia. *DM Disease-a-Month,* 27(7):1–103.

38. Goldsmith, N.F., and Johnston, J.O. (1973): Mineralization of the bone in an insured population: Correlation with reported fractures and other measures of osteoporosis. *Int. J,. Epidemiol.,* 2:311–327.

39. Goldsmith, N.F., Johnston, J.O., Picetti, G., and Garcia, C. (1973): Bone mineral in the radius and vertebral osteoporosis in an insured population. *J. Bone Joint Surg.,* 55-A:1276–1293.

40. Gordon, P.C. (1971): The probability of death following a fracture of the hip. *Can. Med. Assoc. J.,* 105:47–51,62.

41. Gryfe, C.I., Amies, A., and Ashley, M.J. (1977): A longitudinal study of falls in an elderly population: I. Incidence and morbidity. *Age Ageing,* 6:201–210.

42. Hedlund, R., and Lindgren, U. (1987): The epidemiology of fractures of the diaphyseal femur. *Acta Orthop. Scand.* (in press).

43. Hedlund, R., Lindgren, U., and Ahlbom, A. (1987): Age- and sex-specific incidence rates of femoral neck and trochanteric fractures. *Clin. Orthop.* (in press).

44. Holbrook, T.L., Grazier, K., Kelsey, J.L., and Stauffer, R.N. (1984): *The Frequency of Occurrence, Impact and Cost of Selected Musculoskeletal Conditions in the United States.* American Academy of Orthopedic Surgeons, Chicago.

45. Horak, J., and Nilsson, B.E. (1975): Epidemiology of fracture of the upper end of the humerus. *Clin. Orthop.,* 112:250–253.

46. Iskrant, A.P., and Smith, R.W., Jr. (1969): Osteoporosis in women 45 years and over related to subsequent fractures. *Public Health Rep.,* 84:33–38.

47. Jensen, G.F., Christiansen, C., Boesen, J., Hegedüs, V., and Transbøl, I. (1982): Epidemiology of postmenopausal spinal and long bone fractures: A unifying approach to postmenopausal osteoporosis. *Clin. Orthop.,* 166:75–81.

48. Jensen, J.S., and Bagger, J. (1982): Long-term social prognosis after hip fractures. *Acta Orthop. Scand.,* 53:97–101.

49. Jensen, J.S. (1984): Determining factors for the mortality following hip fractures. *Injury,* 15:411–414.

50. Johnell, O., Nilsson, B., Obrant, K., and Sernbo, I. (1984): Age and sex patterns of hip fracture—changes in 30 years. *Acta Orthop. Scand.,* 55:290–292.

51. Kelsey, J.L. (1984): Osteoporosis: Prevalence and incidence. In: *Osteoporosis,* Proceedings of the NIH Consensus Development Conference, April 2–4, 1984, Bethesda, Maryland pp. 25–28.

52. Kenzora, J.E., McCarthy, R.E., Lowell, J.D., and Sledge, C.B. (1984): Hip fracture mortality: Relation to age, treatment, preoperative illness, time of surgery, and complications. *Clin. Orthop.,* 186:45–56.

53. Kleerekoper, M., Parfitt, A.M., and Ellis, B.I. (1984): Measurement of vertebral fracture rates in osteoporosis. In: *Osteoporosis,* Proceedings of the Copenhagen International Symposium on Osteoporosis, June 3–8, 1984, edited by C. Christiansen, C.D. Arnaud, B.E.C. Nordin, A.M. Parfitt, W.A. Peck, B.L. Riggs, pp. 103–109. Alborg, Copenhagen.

54. Knowelden, J., Buhr, A.J., and Dunbar, O. (1964): Incidence of fractures in persons over 35 years of age: A report to the M.R.C. Working Party on fractures in the elderly. *Brit. J. Prev. Soc. Med.,* 18:130–141.

55. Krølner, B., and Nielsen, S.P. (1982): Bone mineral content of the lumbar spine in normal and osteoporotic women: Cross-sectional and longitudinal studies. *Clin. Sci.,* 62:329–336.

56. Leske, M.C., Ederer, F., and Podgor, M. (1981): Estimating incidence from age-specific prevalence in glaucoma. *Am. J. Epidemiol.,* 113:606–613.

57. Lewinnek, G.E., Kelsey, J., White, A.A., III, and Kreiger, N.J. (1980): The significance and a comparative analysis of the epidemiology of hip fractures. *Clin. Orthop.,* 152:35–43.

58. Lindsay, R., Dempster, D.W., Clemens, T., Herrington, B.S., and Wilt, S. (1984): Incidence, cost, and risk factors of fracture of the proximal femur in the U.S.A. In: *Osteoporosis.* Proceedings of the Copenhagen International Symposium on Osteoporosis. June 3–8, 1984, edited by C. Christiansen, C.D. Arnaud, B.E.C. Nordin, A.M. Parfitt, W.A. Peck, B.L. Riggs, pp. 311–315. Alborg, Copenhagen.

59. Lips, P., Netelenbos, J.C., Jongen, M.J.M., van

Ginkel, FC., Althuis, A.L., van Schaik, C.L., van der Vijgh, W.J.F., Vermeiden, J.P.W., and van der Meer, C. (1982): Histomorphometric profile and vitamin D status in patients with femoral neck fracture. *Metab. Bone Dis. Rel. Res.*, 4:85–93.

60. Livesley, B., Atkinson, L. (1974): Repeated falls in the elderly. *Mod. Geriatr.*, 4:458–467.

61. Lucht, U. (1971): A prospective study of accidental falls and resulting injuries in the home among elderly persons. *Acta Socio-Medica Scand.*, 2:105–120.

62. Lutwak, L., and Whedon, G.D. (1963): Osteoporosis. *DM Disease-a-Month* Apr:1–39.

63. Macdonald, J.B. (1985): The role of drugs in falls in the elderly. *Clin. Geriatr. Med.*, 1:621–636.

64. Mangaroo, J., Glasser, J.H., Roht, L.H., and Kapadia, A.S. (1985): Prevalence of bone demineralization in the United States. *Bone*, 6:135–139.

65. Marshall, D.H., Horsman A., Simpson, M., Francis, R.M., and Peacock, M. (1984): Fractures in elderly women: Prevalence of wrist, spine and femur fractures and their concurrence. In: *Osteoporosis*, Proceedings of the Copenhagen International Symposium on Osteoporosis, June 3–8, 1984, edited by C. Christiansen, C.D. Arnaud, B.E.C. Nordin, A.M. Parfitt, W.A. Peck, B.L. Riggs, pp. 361–363. Alborg, Copenhagen.

66. Matković, V., Kostial, K., Šimonović, I., Buzina, R., Brodarec, A., and Nordin, B.E.C. (1979): Bone status and fracture rates in two regions of Yugoslavia. *Am. J. Clin. Nutr.*, 32:540–549.

67. Matković, V., Ciganovic, M., Tominac, C., and Kostial, K. (1980): Osteoporosis and epidemiology of fractures in Croatia: An international comparison. *Henry Ford Hosp. Med. J.*, 28:116–126.

68. Melton, L.J., Sampson, J.M., Morrey, B.F., and Ilstrup, D.M. (1981): Epidemiologic features of pelvic fractures. *Clin. Orthop.*, 155:43–47.

69. Melton, L.J., Ilstrup, D.M., Riggs, B.L., and Beckenbaugh, R.D. (1982): Fifty-year trend in hip fracture incidence. *Clin. Orthop.*, 162:144–149.

70. Melton, L.J. III, Ilstrup, D.M., Beckenbaugh, R.D., and Riggs, B.L. (1982): Hip fracture recurrence: A population-based study. *Clin. Orthop.*, 167:131–138.

71. Melton, L.J., and Riggs, B.L. (1983): Epidemiology of age-related fractures. In: *The Osteoporotic Syndrome: Detection, Prevention, and Treatment,* edited by L.V. Avioli, pp. 45–72. Grune and Stratton, Inc., New York.

72. Melton, L.J., O'Fallon, W.M., and Riggs, B.L. (1987): Secular trends in the incidence of hip fractures. *Calcif. Tissue Int.*, 41:57–64.

73. Melton, L.J., (1987): Epidemiology of vertebral fractures. Proceedings of the International Symposium on Osteoporosis, Aalborg, Denmark, September 27–October 2, 1987.

74. Miller, C.W. (1978): Survival and ambulation following hip fracture. *J. Bone Joint Surg.*, 60-A:930–934.

75. National Center for Health Statistics, E. McCarthy: Inpatient utilization of short-stay hospitals by diagnosis, United States, 1980. Vital and Health Statistics. Series 13, No. 74. DHHS Pub. No. (PHS) 83-1735. Public Health Service. Washington. U.S. Government Printing Office, Sept. 1983.

76. Nelson, E.L., Melton, L.J. III, Annegers, J.F., Laws, E.R., and Offord, K.P. (1984): Incidence of skull fractures in Olmsted County, Minnesota. *Neurosurgery,* 15:318–324.

77. Nickens, H. (1985): Intrinsic factors in falling among the elderly. *Arch. Intern. Med.*, 145:1089–1093.

78. Nilsson, B.E.R. (1969): Age and sex incidence of ankle fractures. *Acta Orthop. Scand.*, 40:122–129.

79. Owen, R.A., Melton, L.J. III, Johnson, K.A., Ilstrup, D.M., and Riggs, B.L. (1982): Incidence of Colles' fracture in a North American community. *Am. J. Public Health*, 72:605–607.

80. Owen, R.A., Melton, L.J., III, Ilstrup, D.M., Johnson, K.A., and Riggs, B.L. (1982): Colles' fracture and subsequent hip fracture risk. *Clin. Orthop.*, 171:37–43.

81. Parfitt, A.M. (1985): Cortical porosity in the pathogenesis of wrist fractures: Similarities between adolescence and postmenopause. In: *Proceedings of the Conference on Bone Fragility in Orthopaedics and Medicine*, Ottawa, May 16–18, 1985. Springer-Verlag, New York.

82. Pogrund, H., Makin, M., Robin, G., Menczel, J., and Steinberg, R. (1977): Osteoporosis in patients with fractured femoral neck in Jerusalem. *Clin. Orthop.*, 124:165–172.

83. Ráliš, Z.A. (1981): Epidemic of fractures during period of snow and ice. *Br. Med. J.*, 282:603–605.

84. Riggs, B.L., Wahner, H.W., Seeman, E., Offord, K.P., Dunn, W.L., Mazess, R.B., Johnson, K.A., and Melton, L.J. (1982): Changes in bone mineral density of the proximal femur and spine with aging: Differences between the postmenopausal and senile osteoporosis syndromes. *J. Clin. Invest.*, 70:716–723.

85. Riggs, B.L., and Melton, L.J. (1983): Evidence for two distinct syndromes of involutional osteoporosis. *Am. J. Med.*, 75:899–901.

86. Riggs, B.L. (1987): In: *Textbook of Endocrinology*, Second Edition, edited by L.J. DeGroot. Grune and Stratton, Orlando.

87. Riggs, B.L., and Melton, L.J. III (1986): Medical Progress: Involutional osteoporosis. *N. Engl. J. Med.*, 314:1676–1684.

88. Rose, S.H., Melton, L.J. III, Morrey, B.F., Ilstrup, D.M., and Rigs, B.L. (1982): Epidemiologic features of humeral fractures. *Clin. Orthop.*, 168:24–30.

89. Saville, P.D. (1970): Observations on 80 women with osteoporotic spine fractures. In: *Osteoporosis*, edited by U.S. Barzel, pp. 38–46. Grune and Stratton, New York.

90. Scott, W.W., Jr. (1984): Osteoporosis-related fracture syndromes. In: *Osteoporosis*, Proceedings of the NIH Consensus Development Conference, April 2–4, 1984, pp. 20–24. Bethesda, Maryland.

91. Seidman, H., Silverberg, E., and Bodden, A. (1978): Probabilities of eventually developing and of dying of cancer (Risk among persons previously undiagnosed with the cancer). *CA-A Cancer J. for Clin.*, 28:33–44.

92. Sheldon, J.H. (1960): On the natural history of falls in old age. *Br. Med. J.*, 2:1685–1690.

93. Smith, D.M., Nance, W.E., Kang, K.W., Christian, J.C., and Johnston, C.C., Jr. (1973): Genetic factors in determining bone mass. *J. Clin. Invest.*, 52:2800–2808.

94. Smith, R.W. Jr., and Rizek, J. (1966): Epidemiologic studies of osteoporosis in women of Puerto Rico and southeastern Michigan with special reference to age, race, national origin and to other related or associated findings. *Clin. Orthop.*, 45:31–48.

95. Solgaard, S., and Petersen, V.S. (1985): Epidemiology of distal radius fractures. *Acta Orthop. Scand.*, 56:391–393.

96. Solomon, L. (1968): Osteoporosis and fracture of the femoral neck in the South African Bantu. *J. Bone Joint Surg.*, 50-B:2–13.

97. Solomon, L. (1979): Bone density in ageing Caucasian and African populations. *Lancet*, 2:1326–1330.

98. Stevens, J., Freeman, P.A., Nordin, B.E.C., and Barnett, E. (1962): The incidence of osteoporosis in patients with femoral neck fracture. *J. Bone Joint Surg.*, 44-B:520–527.

99. Stott, S., and Gray, D.H. (1980): The incidence of femoral neck fractures in New Zealand. *New Zealand Med. J.*, 91:6–9.

100. Tinetti, M.E., Williams, T.F., and Mayewski R. (1986): Fall risk index for elderly patients based on number of chronic disabilities. *Am. J. Med.*, 80:429–434.

101. Trotter, M., Broman, G.E., and Peterson, R.R. (1960): Densities of bones of white and Negro skeletons. *J. Bone Joint Surg.*, 42-A:50–58.

102. Tsai, K.-S., Wahner, H.W., Offord, K.P., Melton, L.J., III, Kumar, R., and Riggs, B.L. (1987): Effect of aging on vitamin D stores and bone density in women. *Calcif. Tissue Int.*, 40:241–243, 1987.

103. Versluysen, M. (1986): How elderly patients with femoral fracture develop pressure sores in hospital. *Br. Med. J.*, 292:1311–1313.

104. Waller, J.A. (1978): Falls among the elderly—Human and environmental factors. *Accid. Anal. Prev.*, 10:21–33.

105. Weiss, N.S., Liff, J.M., Ure, C.L., Ballard, J.H., Abbott, G.H., and Daling, J.R. (1983): Mortality in women following hip fracture. *J. Chron. Dis.*, 36:879–882.

106. Wong, P.C.N. (1984): Femoral neck fractures among the major racial groups in Singapore. Incidence patterns compared with non Asian communities. No. II. *Singapore Med. J.*, 5:150–157.

107. Wong, P.C.N. (1965): Epidemiology of fractures in the aged, its application in Singapore. *Singapore Med. J.*, 6:62–70.

108. Wong, P.C.N. (1966): Fracture epidemiology in a mixed Southeastern Asian community (Singapore). *Clin. Orthop.*, 45:55–61.

Osteoporosis: Etiology, Diagnosis, and Management, edited by B. Lawrence Riggs and L. Joseph Melton, III. Raven Press, New York © 1988.

6

Clinical Spectrum

L. Joseph Melton, III and B. Lawrence Riggs

Department of Medical Statistics and Epidemiology, and the Division of Endocrinology and Metabolism, Department of Internal Medicine, Mayo Clinic and Mayo Foundation, Rochester, Minnesota 55905

Bone is limited in the ways that it can respond to disease processes. A common skeletal response is bone loss. The decrease in bone mass leads to the occurrence of fractures, with resultant pain and deformity. These are the sole clinical manifestations. Thus, it is not surprising that osteoporosis is a syndrome, with many causes and a number of clinical forms. We have suggested (211) that the multiple causes of osteoporosis can be subsumed into as few as four terms: namely, factors associated with peak adult bone mass, with age-related bone loss, with menopausal or hypogonadal bone loss, and with the bone loss that may be related to numerous medical conditions and drugs. Although such an approach is a useful way to derive theoretical models for bone loss and fracture patterns in the population, the clinician needs a more practical classification based on etiology or, where this is unknown, on clinical presentation.

Table 1 provides a traditional classification of the clinical spectrum of generalized osteoporosis. Osteoporosis is categorized as primary or secondary by the absence or presence of associated medical diseases, surgical procedures, or medications known to be associated with osteoporosis. Although this categorization is useful, it is somewhat misleading because it suggests that these medical conditions are

independent of the other causes of bone loss—which is not so. Thus, vertebral fractures are more likely to occur in postmenopausal women taking corticosteroids than in premenopausal women on the same regimen. Also, a woman who breaks her hip at age 80 ordinarily would not be classified as having secondary osteopo-

TABLE 1. *Classification of generalized osteoporosis*

Primary

    Idiopathic juvenile osteoporosis
    Idiopathic osteoporosis in young adults
    Involutional osteoporosis
        type I ("postmenopausal" osteoporosis)
        type II ("senile" osteoporosis)
        type III (osteoporosis associated with increased parathyroid function)

Secondary (partial listing)

    Hypercortisolism
    Hypogonadism
    Hyperthyroidism
    Diabetes mellitus
    Hyperparathyroidism
    Seizure disorder (anticonvulsants)
    Gastrectomy
    Malabsorption syndrome
    Rheumatoid arthritis
    Connective tissue disease
    Chronic neurological disease
    Chronic obstructive lung disease
    Malignancy

rosis because she had hyperthyrodism 40 years earlier. Yet, there are some indications that hyperthyroidism in young adulthood is a risk factor for hip fractures late in life (L. J. Melton, unpublished data, 1985). In this classification, we also follow the usual practice of dividing primary osteoporosis into idiopathic osteoporosis (which consists of the uncommon forms of primary osteoporosis that are found in children and young adults) and involutional osteoporosis (the common form of osteoporosis that begins in middle life and becomes increasingly more frequent with age). The term idiopathic clearly is appropriate for the forms of osteoporosis in children and young adults for which little is known about pathogenesis. But it infers that all causes of involutional osteoporosis are known. Although the menopause and aging are important causes of involutional osteoporosis (as is discussed later in this chapter), it is not clear why only some but not all postmenopausal women develop osteoporosis, nor are the exact mechanisms by which aging produces bone loss entirely understood. Thus, in a partial sense, involutional osteoporosis is also "idiopathic". Nevertheless, this classification of osteoporosis is clinically useful, and we will employ it as the basis for discussion of the clinical spectrum.

IDIOPATHIC OSTEOPOROSIS

Idiopathic Juvenile Osteoporosis

Dent and Friedman (53) described a self-limiting form of osteoporosis in prepubertal children and clearly differentiated it from osteogenesis imperfecta and other forms of juvenile osteoporosis. Subsequently, more than 50 patients with this rare disorder have been reported (35,71,72,113,123,124,150,237,246). It occurs in previously healthy children, usually between the ages of 8 and 14 years. The disease runs an acute course, usually over a period of 2 to 4 years, during which time there is growth arrest and multiple fractures, and then remits. Both the axial and the appendicular skeleton are affected. There is a wide spectrum of severity. The osteoporosis may be relatively mild and may cause only one or two collapsed vertebrae or it may be severe, causing deformity of virtually all thoracic and lumbar vertebrae. The severe cases also may have fractures of the extremities, particularly in the metaphyseal regions; fractures of the distal tibia are especially common. The disease may be devastating in some patients, producing severe kyphoscoliosis, crippling deformities of the extremities, and even collapse of the rib cage and death from respiratory failure. It has been suggested that some patients with adolescent kyphoscoliosis diagnosed as having Scheuermann's disease, in fact, have the residua of mild idiopathic juvenile osteoporosis (26,123).

The most remarkable feature of the disease is the almost invariable spontaneous remission. Subsequently, there is resumption of normal linear and radial bone growth. In the vertebrae, the new bone formed at the endochondrial growth plate is of normal density. In the healed adult vertebrae, this gives the roentgenographic appearance of *window framing* in which normal vertebral bone encloses its osteoporotic ghost. The patients with mild or moderate disease may be left with only a mild kyphosis, short stature, and boney deformity due to fractures. Those with more severe disease, however, may be incapacitated for life.

As would be expected from the rapid bone loss, there is a large negative calcium balance. This is associated with a decrease in calcium absorption (53) and low serum levels of 1,25-dihydroxyvitamin D (1,25-[OH]$_2$D$_3$) (150). Both findings are probably secondary to the bone loss rather than a cause of it because serum immunoreactive parathyroid hormone (iPTH) levels are not increased (150). Serum calcium and phosphorus are normal but there is a slight increase in serum alkaline phosphatase and urinary hydroxyproline (124).

The bone remodeling abnormality characteristic of idiopathic juvenile osteoporosis is controversial. Only a few of the cases have had bone histological studies. Jowsey and Johnson (124) studied iliac crest biopsies in seven patients using quantitative microradiography. They found that all cases had an increase in bone resorption surfaces but normal values for bone formation surfaces. Based on this, they concluded that the bone loss was due to an absolute increase in the resorption rate. In a study of four patients, Smith (237) found a normal osteoclast count but increased resorption surface and reduced osteoblast surface. This suggested to him that the cause of bone loss was osteoblast failure and that increased resorption surfaces in both his and in Jowsey and Johnson's studies was due to impaired bone formation. Because of this, the osteoblasts did not remodel previously resorbed areas at a normal rate. In a single patient, who received double tetracycline labels to assess bone formation rate, bone formation rate was found to be normal (71). Possibly this subject, a 12-year-old boy, had achieved remission by the time the bone biopsy was taken. Clearly, it will be necessary to obtain tetracycline-based bone histomorphometric studies in patients with active disease, and to compare them with age-matched normal subjects, before this issue can be settled definitively. The clinical characteristics, however, suggest a profound uncoupling of the two components of bone turnover due to both an increase in resorption and a decrease in formation. The arrest of linear and radial growth of long bones suggests osteoblast impairment, while the rapidity with which bone is lost suggests an increase in bone resorption as well. Increased resorption is further implicated by the dramatic improvement observed in a patient with idiopathic juvenile osteoporosis treated with aminopropylidene diphosphonate (APD) (113), a drug whose effect on bone is antiresorptive.

The close relationship of the disease to puberty led Dent to suggest that hormonal factors may play a role (54). There is no direct evidence for this, however, nor have the quantitative relationships among hormonal changes, puberty, and activity of the disease been adequately quantified. Moreover, the recent report of idiopathic osteoporosis occurring in a 3-year-old girl who achieved densitometric remission by age 6 years calls into question the role of puberty in pathogenesis (72).

From the clinical standpoint, it is important to exclude other causes of osteoporosis in juveniles, especially adrenal cortical hyperfunction and acute leukemia (62). The present syndrome is distinguished from osteogenesis imperfecta by lack of blue sclera and other characteristic stigmata, by the absence of a history of fractures of long bones, and by the lack of a family history of bone disease. Cushing's syndrome should be excluded by adrenal function tests.

The basic strategy of treatment is to protect the spine until remission occurs. Sex steroids are contraindicated because of the possibility of early closure of the growth plates. Hoekman et al. (113) obtained dramatic results using the diphosphonate, APD. They were able to convert a pretreatment negative calcium balance of −280 mg/day to a positive balance of +356 mg/day after two months of treatment in a 13-year-old boy. This dramatic finding warrants further study.

Idiopathic Osteoporosis in Young Adults

Osteoporosis occurring in young adults (25,119,192,253) is more often encountered than the rarer idiopathic juvenile osteoporosis syndrome, but it still is relatively infrequent compared with involutional osteoporosis. In contrast to involutional osteoporosis, which has a female preponderance, idiopathic osteoporosis occurs with equal frequency in women and men. The condition has a wide clinical spectrum, perhaps because more than one disorder is involved. In some patients, the disease runs a mild course and is clinically manifested by a single or only a few vertebral fractures, even in the absence of treatment. The more usual clinical presentation, however, is the occurrence of multiple vertebral fractures over a period of 5 to 10 years, with an associated loss of height of up to 6 inches. Fractures of the ribs and metatarsals are also common. In severely affected patients, unilateral or bilateral hip fractures may occur. At the extreme end of the spectrum, patients may become incapacitated as the disease progresses and, rarely, may even die from respiratory failure within 10 years.

As with involutional osteoporosis, serum

values for calcium, phosphorus, and alkaline phosphatase are normal. Hypercalciuria is common, particularly in young men with idiopathic osteoporosis, and may be associated with renal lithiasis (25,192). The increased urinary calcium excretion is associated wtih normal values for serum $1,25-(OH)_2D_3$ (192). Perry et al. (192) found that hypercalciuria decreased but did not normalize when dietary calcium intake was restricted and concluded that it had both a resorptive and absorptive component.

Studies assessing bone turnover have given conflicting results. Bordier et al. (25) made iliac crest bone biopsies in 11 patients and found that bone resorption surfaces were increased in 3 and normal in 8, whereas bone formation surfaces were below the normal mean in all but one patient. Vernejoul et al. (253) found a decrease in mean wall thickness of trabecular packets on iliac crest biopsy. Both groups of investigators concluded that the major cause of the bone loss was decreased bone formation. Perry et al. (192), on the other hand, made iliac crest bone biopsies following tetracycline double labeling in 5 osteoporotic young men with hypercalciuria and found that bone turnover was increased. Very likely the high and low turnover groups represent separate clinical types which may have different proportional representation in various clinical series.

In contrast to patients with idiopathic juvenile osteoporosis, who seem to form a more homogeneous group, it is likely that idiopathic osteoporosis in young adults is etiologically heterogeneous. Patients with a mild form of the disease may simply have failed to achieve an adequate amount of bone mass during bone growth. Some of these may have a mild variant of osteogenesis imperfecta tarda (234), all forms of which may not have characteristic stigmata such as blue sclerae and otosclerosis. Other subjects may have a genetic predisposition for low initial bone mass. Even normal premenopausal women with bony density values two standard deviations below the mean are at the threshold for vertebral fractures (208). Also, it is tempting to speculate that many patients with idiopathic osteoporosis

have a primary defect in local regulation of bone cell function. Pacifici et al. (183) recently found that a male with idiopathic osteoporosis associated with high bone turnover had increased production of interleukin-I by cultured bone marrow monocytes. Interleukin-I has been shown to be a potent stimulator of bone resorption (96). Conversely, the subgroup of patients with idiopathic osteoporosis who have low bone turnover may have a primary defect in the function or regulation of osteoblasts.

Nordin and Roper (180) described a form of idiopathic osteoporosis in young women associated with pregnancy and lactation, but the evidence that this is a distinct syndrome is far from convincing. More likely the mechanical stresses on the spine associated with pregnancy precipitate vertebral fractures in women predisposed to idiopathic osteoporosis. The finding by Gruber et al. (100), however, that bone biopsies performed after parturition gave normal values for bone turnover in three young women who developed vertebral fractures during pregnancy and lactation are consistent with a self-limited acceleration of bone loss associated with pregnancy. Thus, this matter needs further study.

Pregnancy and lactation seem to make little contribution to involutional osteoporosis. While some workers have shown large bone losses among lactating adolescents (33), it has been suggested that such results are erroneous (40,98). Others find minimal (11) or no (136) net bone loss during lactation among older women. Indeed, cortical (176) and axial (144) bone mass seem to be greater and fracture risk lower in women with increasing parity (260) and with a history of breast-feeding (6,132). This may be due, in part, to an association between parity and obesity (110).

INVOLUTIONAL OSTEOPOROSIS

It is becoming increasingly clear that this common variety of osteoporosis is also heterogeneous. After examining the clinical features, hormonal changes, and relation of disease patterns to age and menopause (Table 2), Riggs

TABLE 2. *Characterization of the two main types of involutional osteoporosis*

	Type I	Type II
Age (yr)	51–75	> 70
Sex ratio (F:M)	6:1	2:1
Type of bone loss	Mainly trabecular	Trabecular and cortical
Rate of bone loss	Accelerated	Not accelerated
Fracture sites	Vertebrae (crush) and distal radius	Vertebrae (multiple wedge) and hip
Parathyroid function	Decreased	Increased
Calcium absorption	Decreased	Decreased
Metabolism of 25-OH-D to 1,25-$(OH)_2D_3$	Secondary decrease	Primary decrease
Main causes	Factors related to menopause	Factors related to aging

From Riggs, and Melton, ref. 211, with permission.

and Melton (210) postulated several distinctive syndromes of involutional osteoporosis that may prove helpful in examining pathophysiology or in evaluating therapy.

Type I ("Postmenopausal") Osteoporosis

This classic form of the disease was described in 1941 by Fuller Albright and his associates (5) and characteristically affects women within 15 to 20 years after menopause (210). Less commonly, men have a form of osteoporosis that is indistinguishable from that occurring in postmenopausal women. Vertebral fracture is the main clinical manifestation, but Colles' fracture of the distal forearm occurs frequently (210). Also, there is an increased incidence of edentulism because of excess loss of perialveolar bone (45). The vertebral body, the ultradistal radius, and the mandible contain large amounts of trabecular bone.

Patients with type I osteoporosis have a rate of trabecular bone loss that is three times greater than that in normal peers (220). Although these patients have lost substantial amounts of trabecular bone, they have lost only slightly more cortical bone than have age-matched subjects (152,208). Our analysis of the pathophysiology is as follows (Fig. 1): The accelerated bone loss leads to decreased parathyroid hormone (PTH) secretion (206,210) which, in turn, leads to decreased production of 1,25-$(OH)_2D_3$ (87). Decreased circulating serum 1,25-$(OH)_2D_3$ results in impaired calcium absorption (87), which may further increase bone loss (90). The predilection for women and the temporal proximity to menopause implicate estrogen deficiency as an etiologic agent. Yet, only a relatively small subset of postmenopausal women have this form of osteoporosis (210), even though all are deficient in estrogen. In postmenopausal women, most (48,205) but not all (38) investigators have found similar sex steroid levels in those with and without osteoporosis. Thus, some factor or factors in addition to menopause must determine individual susceptibility.

Type II ("Senile") Osteoporosis

This syndrome refers to the clinical picture of bone disease seen in men and women 75 years of age or older. The syndrome is mani-

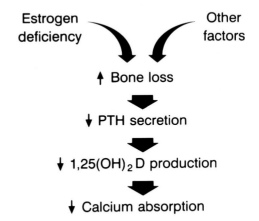

FIG. 1. Type I osteoporosis, "postmenopausal." From Riggs, B.L., Melton, L.J., III, and Wahner, H.W. (1983): Heterogeneity of involutional osteoporosis: Evidence for two distinct osteoporosis syndromes. In: *Clinical Disorders of Bone and Mineral Metabolism,* Proceedings of the Frances and Anthony D'Anna Memorial Symposium, Detroit, MI, May 9–13, 1983, edited by B. Frame, and J.T. Potts, Jr., International Congress Series No. 617, Excerpta Medica, Amsterdam, pp. 337–341, with permission.

fested mainly by hip fractures and vertebral wedge fractures, but fractures of the proximal humerus, proximal tibia, and pelvis may also occur. In patients with type II osteoporosis, individual bone densitometric values for the proximal femur, vertebrae, and bones of the appendicular skeleton are in the lower part of the age- and sex-adjusted normal range (209). Thus, type II osteoporosis is characterized by proportionate losses of both cortical and trabecular bone and a rate of loss similar to that in the general population. This syndrome, therefore, corresponds to the model proposed by Newton-John and Morgan (171): As age-related bone loss progresses, an increasing number of elderly men and women will have bone density values below the fracture threshold; those with the lowest bone mineral density values will have the greatest risk of fracture (162,211).

In our analysis of the major causes of type II osteoporosis, we detect two principal tissues—impaired bone formation per se and the skeletal consequences of secondary hyperparathyroid-

ism. First, from the fourth decade of life onward, less bone is formed than is resorbed at individual remodeling foci (145), and this imbalance increases with aging. Second, an age-related increase in parathyroid function may occur secondary to an age-related decrease in calcium absorption (Fig. 2). Although serum levels of 25(OH)D are generally normal, serum levels of $1,25\text{-}(OH)_2D_3$ decrease in the elderly and may be even lower in patients with hip fracture (87,248). These decreases may be caused by impaired conversion of 25(OH)D to $1,25\text{-}(OH)_2D_3$ (248). Recent observations (50, 67) that overall bone turnover among women may increase with aging (as assessed by measurement of serum bone Gla-protein and other biochemical markers) suggests that secondary hyperparathyroidism may increase the number of individual bone remodeling units and thus increase bone turnover at the tissue level. Because bone formation remains decreased at the level of individual remodeling units, increased bone turnover would result in increased bone loss.

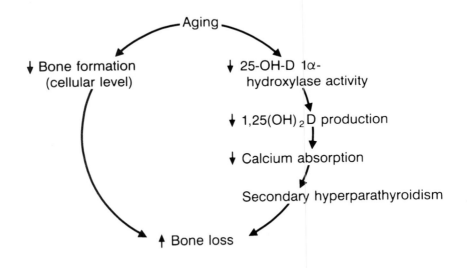

FIG. 2   Type II osteoporosis, "senile." From Riggs, B.L., Melton, L.J., III, and Wahner, H.W. (1983): Heterogeneity of involutional osteoporosis: Evidence for two distinct osteoporosis syndromes. In: *Clinical Disorders of Bone and Mineral Metabolism*, Proceedings of the Frances and Anthony D'Anna Memorial Symposium, Detroit, MI, May 9–13, 1983, edited by B. Frame, and J.T. Potts, Jr., International Congress Series No. 617, Excerpta Medica, Amsterdam. pp. 337–341, wtih permission.

Type III Osteoporosis

About 10% of osteoporotic women presenting with vertebral fractures in the first 20 years after menopause have an absolute increase in serum iPTH (89,122,206,207,245), and thus differ sharply from the remainder who have decreased levels. These patients also have increased bone turnover as assessed by bone histomorphometry (122,245). Riggs et al. (207) carried out detailed metabolic studies on three patients and found a severe impairment of calcium absorption, normal serum 25(OH)D levels, and low normal levels of serum 1,25-$(OH)_2D_3$ despite high serum iPTH; one patient had surgically proved parathyroid hyperplasia. These findings suggest an impairment of 25(OH)D 1α-hydroxylase function. At present, it is unclear whether this syndrome represents a more severe form of type II osteoporosis occurring at an earlier age or a separate entity. Although less common, type III osteoporosis is important because it is potentially remediable by treatment with 1,25-$(OH)_2D_3$.

SECONDARY OSTEOPOROSIS

As noted above, the designation "secondary" osteoporosis has traditionally been used when medical conditions are present that might be responsible for bone loss. While these conditions may be the major cause of bone loss in some patients, it is more realistic to consider them as risk factors whose impact is added to the effects of other risk factors. This model of osteoporosis is shown conceptually in Fig. 3. The main determinants of low bone mass in this scheme are: (1) the peak bone mass achieved prior to the onset of net bone loss, (2) the adverse effect of the menopause in women and hypogonadism in some men, (3) the endogenous factors responsible for age-related bone loss, and (4) the net effect of all factors that occur sporadically in the population and, when present, increase or decrease in the rate of bone loss, e.g., certain diseases and surgical procedures and the use of some drugs. These various influences on bone mass are additive and cumulative; and their relative impact, although not well quantified to date, determines individual bone mass and fracture risk (211).

This view is reinforced by the observation that the osteoporosis associated with various clinical conditions is rarely characteristic. Instead of attempting to describe specific clinical syndromes, then, most research has been directed at identifying diseases that contribute to bone loss and uncovering the pathophysiologic processes involved. However, documentation of the role of each suspected condition is still very uneven. In large part, this relates to the use of inappropriate methodology. The presence of a variety of chronic diseases and abnormal physiological states, for example, could be attributed simply to the fact that most patients with osteoporosis are elderly. Few studies have employed methods suitable for assessing the actual risk of osteoporosis associated wtih any specific factor (160). Consequently, the practical significance of some of the clinical associations noted below is uncertain.

Clinical evidence seems persuasive, for example, for a strong relationship between osteoporosis and Cushing's disease (232). However, this condition, along with a number of others prominently mentioned in the literature (Table 3), is sufficiently uncommon that its contribution to the overall problem of osteoporosis in the community may be small. Other diseases, surgical procedures, and medications associated with bone loss occur more frequently than has generally been assumed (Table 3). We found that one or more of these factors were present in about 20% of women and 40% of men presenting with vertebral or hip fractures (L. J. Melton, unpublished data, 1986). Especially common were early oophorectomy (in women), hypogonadism (in men), subtotal gastrectomy, hyperthyroidism, hemiplegia, chronic obstructive lung disease, and the use of glucocorticoid and anticonvulsant drugs. In contrast, obesity (44,233) and thiazide diuretic therapy (254) are protective against bone loss. In general, younger patients with age-related

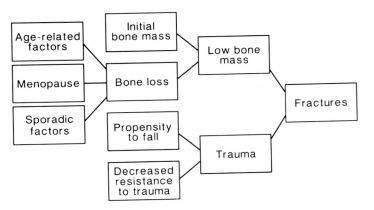

FIG. 3. Model of risk factors for osteoporotic bone loss and fractures.

fractures are more likely to have an underlying illness and, conversely, patients with secondary osteoporosis are likely to have fractures at a somewhat younger age. One would also anticipate that the influence of any specific factor would seem greater for men than women, because of the higher background level of involutional osteoporosis among women.

A final group of conditions (Table 3) are either explained by other associations or may simply be coincidentally related to bone loss and fractures. Peptic ulcer disease, for example, seems to be accounted for by its relationship with gastrectomy (L. J. Melton, unpublished data, 1986), while the effects of rheumatoid arthritis are due to disuse osteoporosis (9,114). In other instances, the primary pathophysiology is uncertain. Chronic obstructive lung disease, for example, may be associated with metabolic abnormalities, with smoking and ethanol use, with inactivity, and with corticosteroid use (see below). Further research is necessary to delineate the roles of Parkinsonism, hypertension, atherosclerosis, chronic anticoagulation therapy, pulmonary tuberculosis, chronic liver disease and other conditions that have been mentioned in connection with osteoporosis.

TABLE 3. *Relative impact of various purported causes of ''secondary'' osteoporosis*

Uncommon conditions that contribute little to osteoporosis in the community		
Acromegaly	Hyperpara-thyroidism	Osteogenesis imperfecta
Cushing's disease	Hypopituitarism	Multiple myeloma

Important risk factors for secondary osteoporosis in the community		
Hyperthyroidism	Hemiplegia	Leanness
Thyroidectomy	COLD	Inactivity
Gonadal hypo-function	↑	↑
	Dilantin therapy	Cigarette smoking
Gastrectomy	Phenobarbital therapy	Ethanol consumption

Common conditions with no increased risk for osteoporosis in the community		
Diabetes mellitus	Parkinsonism	Peripheral vascular disease
↑		Stroke (without paralysis)
Diverticulitis	Peptic ulcer disease (without gastrectomy)	
↑	↑	↑
Inguinal hernia		Thyroid adenoma
Osteoarthritis	Rheumatoid arthritis (without disability)	Urolithiasis

Specific Conditions

The more common conditions associated with secondary osteoporosis are discussed in greater detail in the following sections:

Hypercortisolism

Osteoporosis may be associated with a number of syndromes of endocrine dysfunction, such as hypercortisolism. Endogenous hypercortisolism (Cushing's syndrome) is a relatively uncommon conditon, however; and, as a consequence, it is not a prominent cause of fractures in the community (L. J. Melton, unpublished data, 1986). Corticosteroid use is much more frequent, and exogenous hypercortisolism has long been considered a risk factor for fractures, especially vertebral fractures (103). These radiologic features are covered in Chapter 7. We found a substantial increase in risk for vertebral fractures in a recent case-control study in men (233). However, preliminary data from a case-control study of hip fractures in Rochester, Minnesota, (L. J. Melton, unpublished data, 1986) as well as other epidemiologic studies (184) indicate that steroid use is not associated with a marked increase in risk for hip fractures. These observations are consistent with data showing greater trabecular than cortical bone loss with corticosteroid use (102,227), although methodologic deficiencies of various studies do raise some questions in this regard (101).

Disproportionate effects on the axial rather than the appendicular skeleton (92,103,232) and on children (14) may reflect a greater sensitivity of high turnover bone to any adverse influences of corticosteroids (64). Both endogenous and exogenous hypercortisolism are associated with decreased bone formation and increased bone resorption (Fig. 4) that leads to rapid bone loss (204). The decrease in bone formation results from inhibition of collagen biosynthesis by osteoblasts (191) and from a reduction in the change of precursor cells into functioning osteoblasts (103). The increase in bone resorption is mediated by PTH. Although there are suggestions of a direct stimulatory effect on PTH secretion (103), indirect effects are more prominent, with secondary hyperparathyroidism caused by increased renal excretion of calcium (29,242) and reduced intestinal absorption (29,128). The impaired calcium absorption can be reversed by administering vitamin D (86) or its active metabolite (128), but a direct disruption of vitamin D metabolism by steroids has not been conclusively established (104,231). The adverse effects of corticosteroids on bone are mitigated with time (92), perhaps because of reduced bone turnover in advanced cases (189).

Hypogonadism.

Hypogonadism in either sex also leads to an increased risk of osteoporosis. Hypogonadism is probably the main cause of osteoporosis associated with ovarian agenesis (Turner's syndrome), although a genetic abnormality of bone maturation may also be present (212). Bone mass is also reduced in amenorrheic women with premature ovarian failure (31), hyperprolactinemia (31,130), and anorexia nervosa (39,213). Amenorrhea associated with hypothalamic hypogonadism in female athletes leads to excessive bone loss as well (31, 60,77), and this is reversible when training distances are decreased (61).

Acquired hypogonadism more commonly results from oophorectomy, and women who have undergone oophorectomy in young adulthood have lower bone density in later life than their peers (203). Surgical menopause is associated with an increased risk of osteoporosis (3,30,41,142), vertebral deformities (142) and, less often, hip fractures (132,184,256). These effects can be prevented or slowed by estrogen replacement therapy (91,142). These phenomena are covered more thoroughly in Chapter 12.

Men do not undergo the equivalent of menopause, but gonadal function does decline in some elderly men (80). Overt male hypogonadism is often associated with abnormal calcium metabolism (83) and with vertebral fractures (233). As with women, osteoporosis in men has been reported in association with hyperprolactinemia (97,118) and anorexia nervosa (214).

Acromegaly.

Osteoporosis associated with acromegaly is rare and, when present, is the result of concomitant hypogonadism. Most patients with

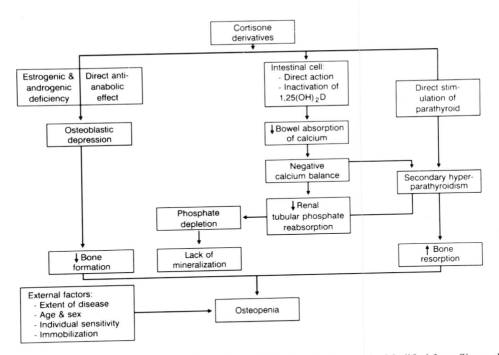

FIG. 4. Pathophysiologic mechanisms in corticosteroid-induced osteoporosis. Modified from Siame, J.L., Sebert, J.L., and Delcambre, B. (1979): L'osteoporose cortisonique. *Nouv. Presse Med.,* 8:1675–1680. Reprinted with permission of publisher and author.

acromegaly have increases in both trabecular and cortical bone mass related to the anabolic effects of growth hormone on the skeleton (232).

Hyperthyroidism.

Both thyroxine (T3) and triiodothyronine (T3) directly stimulate bone resorption, and the effect is dose-dependent (166). One consequence is an increase in bone turnover seen consistently with hyperthyroidism (69). The primary pathogenesis remains uncertain, although hypothesized mechanisms include thyroid hormone stimulated increases in osteoclast-activating factor or interleukins (13). Heightened bone resorption leads to hypercalcemia and functional hypoparathyroidism with lowered serum PTH and 1,25-$(OH)_2D_3$ levels and negative calcium balance (13). Elevated alkaline phosphatase and bone GLA protein levels provide evidence for a concomitant rise in osteoblastic activity (13). Thus, despite the increased bone turnover, bone resorption and

formation remained linked in some (106), but not all (13,69), patients with hyperthyroidism.

This is reflected in bone mass measurements (Fig. 5). Mean levels are generally reduced in patients with untreated hyperthyroidism (84 141,173,232), but some individuals have normal values. Reductions may be greater in the axial than in the appendicular skeleton (232). The defect is also generally greater in older women than it is in younger women or men (84,141). This may account, in part, for the observation that clinically significant osteoporosis generally occurs in postmenopausal women (84). However, in accordance with our model of osteoporosis (Fig. 3), it is anticipated that an additive risk factor like hyperthyroidism would have its greatest influence on fracture risk among those whose bone density levels were already reduced.

Despite these findings, symptomatic osteoporosis associated with hyperthyroidism is relatively unusual (49,82), perhaps because deficiencies in bone mass are largely reversed by

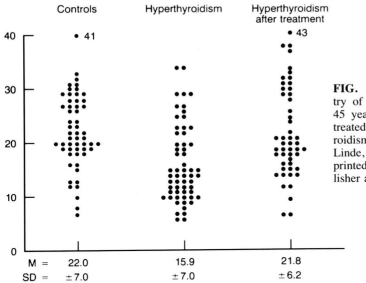

FIG. 5. Photon absorptiometry of the calcaneus in women 45 years of age and over with treated or untreated hyperthyroidism or not (controls). From Linde, and Friis, ref. 141. Reprinted with permission of publisher and author.

treatment of hyperthyroidism (133,141,173). Treatment itself, however, can cause problems in some cases. A condition functionally equivalent to hyperthyroidism results iatrogenically from excessive doses of thyroid hormone (70,73), while even customary levels of thyroid hormone replacement appear to cause bone loss in individuals with primary hypothyroidism (36,133).

Thyroidectomy.

Thyroidectomy has also been tied to bone loss and fractures. Totally thyroidectomized patients have markedly reduced plasma calcitonin levels and severely impaired responses to calcium infusion (24,247), and others have found reduced bone mineral content in these patients (155). Since most biologically active calcitonin is produced by C-cells centrally located in each lobe of the thyroid, even partial thyroidectomy might render a person relatively calcitonin-deficient. Epidemiologic data from a case-control study of hip fracture in Rochester (L. J. Melton, unpublished data, 1986) showed that thyroidectomy may be an important risk factor for hip fracture and that thyroidectomy may account for part, but not all, of the fracture risk associated with hyperthyroidism.

However, the latter study did not evaluate other modes of thyroid ablation, such as ^{131}I therapy, so the relative contribution of thyroid ablation and thyroid hyperfunction is still unsettled.

Diabetes mellitus.

Most (115,139,235,259) but not all (172) studies of insulin-dependent diabetes mellitus have revealed evidence of moderate osteopenia of cortical bone. Proposed mechanisms include hyperglycemia (156), renal loss of calcium (156,199) or phosphate (93), hypocalcemia (78), and abnormal vitamin D metabolism (85). However, other researchers have found no evidence of disturbed calcium homeostasis or vitamin D metabolism (107,241) in human diabetes mellitus or much relationship between bone loss and poor blood glucose control (115).

By contrast, recent studies indicate undiminished or even increased bone mass among patients with noninsulin-dependent diabetes (121,255). Such patients are generally obese. Obesity offers protection against osteoporosis (225) and fractures (116,132,184), perhaps as a result of enhanced conversion of testosterone to estradiol and of androstenedione to estrone in peripheral fat (18,99,129). Diabetic women do have elevated serum estrone levels (56,121), although this does not appear to completely account for the increased bone mass in this group (121).

Although some studies have reported an increased risk of fracture in elderly diabetics, these have generally had biases that tend to favor a positive association, such as inappropriate or absent controls or use of glucose tolerance tests to diagnose diabetes in patients with recent fractures. Alffram found an increased prevalence of diabetes in his classic study of hip fracture (7), but this was an artifact resulting from the spuriously low diabetes prevalence rates that he used (108). We found the prevalence of diabetes to be somewhat higher than expected in a descriptive survey of hip fractures in Rochester, Minnesota, in 1965–74, but the increase was not statistically significant (88). A three-fold increase in hip fracture risk with diabetes was reported in a case-control study conducted in a retirement community (184), but this estimate was also based on very small numbers.

The most definitive data on fracture risk are derived from a large retrospective cohort study involving all incidence cases of diabetes that were diagnosed in the population of Rochester, Minnesota (108). Both prior and subsequent fractures were assessed in comparison with an age- and sex-matched control cohort of nondiabetics from the general population. As would be anticipated, diabetic patients had no greater incidence of fracture prior to diagnosis. Unexpectedly, perhaps, the incidence of fractures after the diagnosis of diabetes was not elevated either. As shown in Table 4, the relative risk was 0.66 for diabetic men, 0.89 for diabetic women, and 0.80 overall. Fracture risk among diabetics was not significantly elevated for any site except leg and ankle fractures, where there was an excess of medial malleolar fractures. It should be noted that the risk was not elevated for age-related fractures of the vertebrae, proximal humerus and femur, or distal forearm. These data strongly affirm that diabetes mellitus is not a risk factor for skeletal fractures among the non-insulin-dependent individuals

TABLE 4. *Relative risk (RR) of fracture after date of diagnosis of diabetes mellitus among cases, as compared with risk among controls*

Fracture site	Men		Women		Both sexes	
	N^a	RR	N^a	RR	N^a	RR
Osteoporotic	30	0.52^b	96	0.73^b	126	0.66^b
Vertebrae	10	0.68	16	0.49^b	26	0.55^b
Proximal humerus	2	0.27^b	14	0.74	16	0.61^b
Distal forearm	7	0.51^b	32	0.83	39	0.74^b
Proximal femur	11	0.52^b	37	0.88	48	0.76^b
Nonosteoporotic	54	0.77^b	89	1.18	143	0.98
Skull/face	5	1.09	6	3.33	11	1.73
Chest	20	1.09	16	0.94	36	1.02
Pelvis	3	3.28	9	1.00	12	1.20
Leg/ankle	10	1.21	22	2.45^c	32	1.86
Hand/foot	14	0.39^b	26	1.00	40	0.65^b
Other	2	0.55	6	0.48^b	8	0.49^b
Overall results	84	0.66^b	185	0.89	269	0.80^b

[a]Denotes number of fractures observed among diabetic individuals.
[b]Significantly lower than control value (p < 0.05).
[c]Significantly higher than control value (p < 0.05).
Modified from Heath, Melton, and Chu, ref. 108, with permission.

who comprise almost 90% of the diabetic population in the community (161). Whether or not insulin-dependent diabetes involves a clinically significant risk of fracture remains to be determined.

Primary Hyperparathyroidism

Bone mass may be reduced in patients with hyperparathyroidism (58,202,216), especially at sites comprised largely of trabecular bone (232). While osteoitis fibrosa is the skeletal abnormality characteristically associated with hyperparathyroidism (Chapter 8, *this volume*), 5 to 10% of patients, mostly postmenopausal women, present with substantial osteopenia and vertebral compression fractures (46,135). Bone loss seems to relate to disease severity, as reflected by the degree of hypercalcemia (58), and this effect may be partly reversed by parathyroidectomy (151,232). Patients with serum calcium less than 11.0 mg/dl are relatively unaffected, however, and such individuals are increasingly recognized as making up the majority of hyperparathyroid patients in the community (109).

Secondary Hyperparathyroidism

Secondary hyperparathyroidism is much more prevalent and may result from disorders more commonly linked with osteomalacia, such as renal disease, anticonvulsant medications, and gastrectomy and malabsorption syndromes.

Secondary hyperparathyroidism may be induced in renal failure by decreased renal hydroxylation of vitamin D to its active metabolite (81,236), with a subsequent reduction in intestinal calcium absorption. This does not always result in osteopenia, however (232). Secondary hyperparathyroidism has also been associated with renal leak hypercalciuria (186). Such patients have impaired tubular reabsorption of calcium (27) that may lead to excessive mobilization of calcium from bone and reduced bone density (185). These individuals may account for reports of urolithiasis as a risk factor for osteoporosis (258). However, urolithiasis patients with hyperabsorption of dietary calcium (absorptive hypercalciuria) have normal bone density (138) and may not be at risk of osteoporotic fractures. Moreover, some forms of urolithiasis therapy result in increased serum calcium (188) or reduced bone demineralization at fracture sites (94). The practical implication of these influences has not been determined, although preliminary data from a case-control study of hip fracture in Rochester residents showed that fracture risk was not increased for urolithiasis patients in general (L. J. Melton, unpublished data, 1986).

Patients on long-term anticonvulsant therapy, especially phenobarbital and diphenylhydantoin, also may have reduced bone mass and fractures. Osteopenia (16,34,238) is traditionally associated with osteomalacia resulting from increased vitamin D degradation by hepatic enzyme systems induced by the anticonvulsants (103). However, the accentuated bone loss seen in those with greater neurological deficits, along with the observation of equal bone loss in institutionalized individuals with or without anticonvulsant therapy (16), suggests that inactivity or other factors may also be important (167). While the increased risk of fractures in these patients is due in part to seizures, the incidence of nonseizure-related fractures is increased as well (140). The concentration of these fractures in metaphyseal areas of the skeleton is also consistent with osteoporosis, which has been documented in some (125) and attributed to secondary hyperparathyroidism or altered sex hormone metabolism (43,181). The contribution of osteoporosis relative to that of osteomalacia is uncertain but may be substantial.

Gastrectomy.

A history of gastrectomy is commonly obtained from hip fracture victims, especially men (7,177), and gastrectomy patients are also overrepresented among men and women with vertebral fractures (198,233). Although some have suggested a direct association with peptic ulcer disease, a case-control study of hip fracture among Rochester, Minnesota, residents (L. J. Melton, unpublished data, 1986) showed that gastrectomy accounted for the fracture risk associated with peptic ulcer disease. In this study, the risk of hip fractures after gastrectomy was elevated 2.5-fold in men and almost twofold in women. This result was similar to the estimated threefold increase in age-related fractures among Swedish men who had undergone Billroth II procedures for peptic ulcer disease (178). However, the latter study also documented an increased risk of fractures at skeletal sites not generally associated with osteoporosis.

The increased fracture risk appears to be due to reduced cortical (215) and trabecular (153) bone mass in this group of patients. Lowered bone mass is seen both in patients with 2/3 gastric resection and Billroth II reconstruction (12,23,157) and in those with 1/3 resection and Billroth I reanastomosis (12,23,157). Selective vagotomy alone is said by some (228) to spare mineral metabolism, while others find deficits in vitamin D (79).

The mechanism whereby gastrectomy leads to osteopenia is unclear, however. One school of thought holds that osteomalacia is the primary defect (182). Gastrectomy can lead to decreased absorption of dietary vitamin D, with or without steatorrhea (81), and can be associated with achlorhydria, that may impair calcium absorption in the presence of low dietary calcium. However, therapy with vitamin D or calcium does not consistently reverse the defect (8). Others contend that these metabolic changes lead to secondary hyperparathyroidism (175) and osteoporosis or mixed osteoporosis and osteomalacia (23,198). The reduction in bone mass is modest (12,23), however, and the conditions often seen in conjunction with peptic ulcer disease, such as alcoholism (179), might also influence fracture risk after gastrectomy.

Other gastrointestinal disorders can cause osteoporosis, osteomalacia or both (147). Malabsorption syndromes impair absorption of calcium and vitamin D. This usually results in osteomalacia but, if the impairment is mild, the predominant lesion may be secondary hyperparathyroidism and osteoporosis (65). Chronic obstructive jaundice may be associated with osteoporosis (112,239) as well as osteomalacia due to impaired enterohepatic circulation of active vitamin D metabolites (134). Severe malnutrition involving both protein and calcium deficiency—as has been observed in prisoners of war and in patients with anorexia nervosa (213) may cause osteoporosis. Additional causal factors in these cases may be functional hypogonadism (in women) and decreased physical activity (213). Lactose intolerance has been found in up to a third of osteoporotic subjects (21,170); the intolerance to milk may cause a life-long low calcium intake (75).

Rheumatoid Arthritis

Many authors suggest that osteoporosis occurs with increased frequency among patients with rheumatoid arthritis (RA) (22,250) and that this results in an unusual number of proximal femur and other osteoporotic fractures (14,57,126,149,154,163,244). The pathophysiologic basis for this is unclear, however, and others contend that the risk of proximal femur fractures may actually be reduced among individuals with RA (252) and that vertebral fractures in this group may be no more common than in the general population (226). Rheumatoid arthritis does produce local changes such as bone erosion near inflamed joints (64,218); but, while fractures have been reported in conjunction with osteolytic lesions (37), most fractures occur in bone that is not eroded (14). Nor is there much evidence for an hypothesized generalized systemic effect of the disease on bone mass (10). Reid et al. (201) found reduced total body calcium among patients with rheumatoid arthritis, but the effects of inactivity and other risk factors for osteoporosis were not taken into account. Likewise, a small number of patients with classic rheumatoid arthritis displayed bone demineralization in the ribs, but these observations were not adjusted for aging or other possible contributing factors (63). Diminished bone density in the metacarpals, attributed to generalized effects of RA (229), could have been caused by decreased hand function (59).

Alternatively, rheumatoid arthritis may appear to be a risk factor for osteoporosis only through its association with other factors more directly responsible for the observed effects, such as corticosteroid use or immobilization. The role of steroid treatment in inducing osteoporosis and eventual fractures in RA patients remains controversial, in part as a result of methodologic difficulties (47,101). Thus, McConkey et al. (154) and Saville and Kharmosh (226) found no significant difference in the frequency of osteoporosis in steroid-treated versus nontreated RA patients, while Bjelle and Nilsson (22) arrived at the opposite conclusion. However, the latter researchers did note that bone density was decreased among patients with functional impairment (22).

Rheumatoid arthritis can, of course, lead to decreased activity as well as actual invalidism (14,51), and such patients have been shown to have reduced bone mass (226). Detailed studies demonstrate that disuse osteoporosis is the primary determinant of bone loss in rheumatoid arthritis (9). A recent population-based cohort study in Rochester, Minnesota, supports this position (114). While the risk of various osteoporotic fractures was increased in women with RA, the excess was most notable in those with impaired activity and ambulation (Table 5). The influence of functional disability is not surprising in light of the known effect of exercise on maintaining bone mass and the role of disuse in augmenting bone loss (see Chapter 19, *this volume*).

Other Connective Tissue Diseases

An unusually severe form of osteoporosis may occur in osteogenesis imperfecta. The most common variety of the disease is inherited as an autosomal dominant trait and is associated with blue sclera, deafness, thin skin, and impaired biosynthesis of type I collagen (194). Other varieties may have different clinical spectra and modes of inheritance (249), but all feature brittle bones. Although onset usually is in childhood, some patients present with premature spinal osteoporosis in the absence of a history of limb fractures. There are suggestions, moreover, that these or related defects may account for a portion of the cases attributed to involutional osteoporosis (234). Marfans' and Ehlers-Danlos syndromes also may be associated with spinal osteopenia but less frequently include vertebral fractures (194). Osteoporosis commonly occurs in patients with homocystinuria, an autosomal recessive disorder caused by deficiency of cystathionine synthase activity (194). The resultant increase in homocysteine and other metabolites in the circulation interferes with collagen cross-linkage.

Stroke

Stroke has long been regarded as a risk factor for osteoporosis and fractures (7), but the incidence of fractures in this group has not been accurately quantified. A case-control study of risk factors for hip fracture in Roches-

TABLE 5. *Relative risk (RR) of selected osteoporotic limb fractures by impact of rheumatoid arthritis on activity level/occupation among female residents of Rochester, Minnesota initially diagnosed with rheumatoid arthritis, 1950–74*

Fracture site	Functional class					
	I		II		III or IV	
	N^a	RR	N^a	RR	N^a	RR
Proximal fermur	9	1.07	12	1.36	8	4.21[b]
Proximal humerus	5	1.43	5	1.33	2	2.32
Pelvis	4	1.97	6	2.83[b]	2	3.67
Distal forearm	11	1.50	10	1.33	2	1.18

[a]Number of fractures observed among rheumatoid arthritis patients.
[b]Significantly higher than control value (p < 0.05).
Modified from Hooyman, Melton, Nelson, O'Fallon, and Riggs, ref. 114, with permission.

ter, Minnesota (L. J. Melton, unpublished data, 1986) revealed that the risk of hip fractures was not increased subsequent to a stroke unless hemiplegia or, to a lesser degree, hemiparesis was present. Osteoporosis develops rapidly after a stroke (95,168), and Mulley and Espley (164) found that most fractures occurred within one year of the stroke. This is almost certainly an artifact of incomplete follow-up, however, since others have found that the degree of bone loss correlates with the duration of hemiplegia (52). Hemiplegia and hemiparesis impose a degree of immobilization (127), which can be associated with dramatic bone loss (4) and disuse osteoporosis (see Chapter 19, this volume). Muscle action may be more important than weight-bearing in preserving bone (1), however, and hemiplegic patients have greater bone loss on the affected side (168,187). It has been noted that fractures also occur more frequently on the hemiplegic side (164,193,196), but the relative contributions of an ipsilateral decrease in bone density or an increased propensity for falls to the affected side have not been assessed. In addition, paralysis changes the direction of loading on the femoral neck (222), which may have an adverse effect biomechanically.

Other Chronic Neurologic Conditions

Fracture risk also seems to be elevated in patients with dementia (32,105). These patients may have disuse osteoporosis as well (66), although an association with falling is also present (146,197). Whether the increased risk of falling is primary, as in Parkinsonism (2), or the result of psychotropic drug use (148,200) is not entirely clear.

Chronic Obstructive Lung Disease

Osteoporosis is associated with chronic obstructive lung disease (233), and fracture victims are not infrequently noted to have co-existing pulmonary disease (126,174,243). However, chronic obstructive lung disease (COLD) is closely allied with other independent risk factors such as smoking (111). Smoking is associated with reduced bone mass (44,143,221), as well as hip and vertebral fractures (184,233,257), and is correlated with ethanol use, another risk factor (20,224,233). Ethanol may depress bone formation by a direct effect on osteoblasts (15,74), and tobacco consumption may exert a similar effect on bone (253). However, smoking is also associated with earlier menopause and with less obesity and perhaps lower endogenous estrogen levels as well (17,120), while excess alcohol use has been linked with nutritional deficiencies and abnormal vitamin D metabolism (55) and with an increased risk of gastrectomy (179). Smoking is correlated with reduced fitness which, in turn, is associated with lower bone mass (195), while COLD may also lead to inactivity and loss of muscle mass (28). Finally, severe pulmonary disease may necessitate corticosteroid use, a risk factor for axial osteoporosis (47) and vertebral fractures in men (233). Needless to say, these relationships are very complex and have not been well worked out.

Malignancy

Diffuse osteoporosis is present in some (212) but not all (117) patients with multiple myeloma and may be a feature in a proportion of those with other myeloproliferative disorders (217). It has been postulated that increased local production of osteoclast activating factor (a lymphokine with potent bone-resorbing properties) by bone marrow cells is responsible (165).

Pathologic fractures due to metastatic malignancies contribute little to the problem of age-related fractures in the community. In prior studies in Rochester, Minnesota, pathologic fractures comprised only 1% of all hip fractures (159), 2% of all proximal humerus fractures (219), and 0.5% of all pelvic fractures (158). The vast majority of these are due to breast cancer (251), although lung, prostate and a few other cancer sites are involved as well (19). Cancer therapy, on the other hand, may have more generalized effects on bone mass.

Therapeutic oophorectomy.

Therapeutic oophorectomy can lead to reduced bone mineral and increased fracture risk in premenopausal patients (41,137). Most cancer patients are postmenopausal, however, and are not dependent on ovarian function for endogenous estrogen production (99).

Hypophysectomy and adrenalectomy.

Hypophysectomy and adrenalectomy may also have an adverse effect on bone mass, as might the use of estrogen antagonists, such as tamoxifen. Some therapeutic regimens also include prednisone.

Chemotherapy.

Chemotherapy can suppress ovarian function in premenopausal women (76,131,223); although, again, most cancer patients are postmenopausal. Some chemotherapeutic agents also suppress bone formation and may even cause osteoporosis and fractures (169,230). The resulting fractures are not typical of age-related osteoporosis, however, and the overall impact of this phenomenon is uncertain.

Radiation therapy.

Radiation therapy may produce osteopenia in the radiation field and thus increase the risk of clavicle, rib, and proximal humerus fractures (42,68), although such complications are uncommon (190). There is little systemic effect; postirradiation fractures of the proximal femur, for example, are usually due to treatment of pelvic malignancies (240) and are rare in any event.

ACKNOWLEDGMENTS

The authors would like to thank Miss Mary Ramaker for help in preparing the manuscript.

This work was supported in part by research grants AG-04875, AM-27065, and AM-30582 from the National Institutes of Health.

REFERENCES

1. Abramson, A.S., and Delagi, E.F. (1961): Influence of weightbearing and muscle contraction on disuse osteoporosis. *Arch. Phys. Med. Rehabil.*, 42:147–151.
2. Aita, J.F. (1982): Why patients with Parkinson's disease fall. *J.A.M.A.*, 247:515–516.
3. Aitken, J.M., Hart, D.M., Anderson, J.B., Smith, D.A., and Speirs, C.F. (1973): Osteoporosis after oophorectomy for non-malignant disease in premenopausal women. *Br. Med. J.*, 2:325–328.
4. Albanese, A.A., Edelson, A.H., Lorenze, E.J., Jr., Woodhull, M.L., and Wein, E.H. (1975): Problems of bone health in elderly: Ten-year study. *N.Y. State J. Med.*, 75:326–336.
5. Albright, F., Smith, P.H., and Richardson, A.M. (1941): Postmenopausal osteoporosis. *J.A.M.A.*, 116:2465–2474.
6. Alderman, B.W., Weiss, N.S., Daling, J.R., Ure, C.L., and Ballard, J.H. (1986): Reproductive history and postmenopausal risk of hip and forearm fracture. *Am. J. Epidemiol.*, 124:262–267.
7. Alffram, P.-A (1964): An epidemiologic study of cervical and trochanteric fractures of the femur in an urban population: Analysis of 1,664 cases with special reference to etiologic factors. *Acta Orthop Scand.*, 65(Suppl.):1–109.
8. Alhava, E.M., Aukee, S., Karjalainen, P., Kettunen, K., and Juuti M. (1975): The influence of calcium and calcium + Vitamin D₂ treatment on bone mineral after partial gastrectomy. *Scand. J. Gastroenterol.*, 10:689–693.
9. Als, O.S., Gotfredsen A, Riis, B.J., and Christiansen, C. (1985): Are disease duration and degree of functional impairment determinants of bone loss in rheumatoid arthritis? *Ann. Rheum. Dis.*, 44:406–411.
10. Ansell, B.M., and Bywaters, E.G.L. (1956): Growth in Still's disease. *Ann. Rheum. Dis.*, 15:295–319.
11. Atkinson, P.J., and West, R.R. (1970): Loss of

skeletal calcium in lactating women. *J. Obstet. Gynaecol. Brit. Commonwealth*, 77:555–560.
12. Aukee, S., Alhava, E.M., and Karjalainen, P. (1975): Bone mineral after partial gastrectomy II. *Scand. J. Gastroenterol.*, 10:165–169.
13. Auwerx, J., and Bouillon, R. (1986): Mineral and bone metabolism in thyroid disease: A review. *Q.J. Med.*, New Series 60:737–752.
14. Badley, B.W.D., and Ansell, B.M. (1960): Fractures in Still's disease. *Ann. Rheum. Dis.*, 19:135–142.
15. Baran, D.T., Teitelbaum, S.L., Bergfeld, M.A., Parker, G., Cruvant, E.M., and Avioli, L.V. (1980): Effect of alcohol ingestion on bone and mineral metabolism in rats. *Am. J. Physiol.*, 238:E507–E510.
16. Barden, H.S., Mazess, R.B., Chesney, R.W., Rose, P.G., and Chun, R. (1982): Bone status of children receiving anticonvulsant therapy. *Metab. Bone Dis. Rel. Res.*, 4:43–47.
17. Baron, J.A. (1984): Smoking and estrogen-related disease. *Am. J. Epidemiol.*, 119:9–22.
18. Bates, G.W., and Whitworth, N.S. (1982): Effects of obesity on sex steroid metabolism. *J. Chronic Dis.*, 35:893–896.
19. Berrettoni, B.A., and Carter J.R. (1986): Mechanisms of cancer metastasis to bone. *J. Bone Joint Surg.*, 68-A:308–312.
20. Bikle, D.D., Genant, H.K., Cann, C., Recker, R.R., Halloran, B.P., and Strewler, G.J. (1985): Bone disease in alcohol abuse. *Ann. Intern. Med.*, 103:42–48.
21. Birge, S.J., Jr., Keutmann, H.T., Cuatrecasas, P., and Whedon, G.D. (1967): Osteoporosis, intestinal lactase deficiency and low dietary calcium intake. *N. Engl. J. Med.*, 276:445–448.
22. Bjelle, A.O., and Nilsson, B.E. (1970): Osteoporosis in rheumatoid arthritis. *Calcif. Tissue Res.*, 5:327–332.
23. Blichert-Toft, M., Beck, A., Christiansen, C., and Transbøl, I. (1979): Effects of gastric resection and vagotomy on blood and bone mineral content. *World J. Surg.*, 3:99–102.
24. Body, J.-J., and Heath, H., III (1983): Estimates of circulating monomeric calcitonin: Physiological studies in normal and thyroidectomized man. *J. Clin. Endocrinol. Metabl.*, 67:897–903.
25. Bordier, Ph.J., Miravet, L., and Hioco, D. (1973): Young adult osteoporosis. *Clin. Endocrinol. Metab.*, 2:277–292.
26. Bradford, D.S., Brown, D.M., Moe, J.H., Winter, R.B., and Jowsey, J. (1976): Scheuermann's kyphosis: A form of osteoporosis? *Clin. Orthop.*, 118:10–15.
27. Breslau, N.A., and Pak, C.Y.C. (1982): Endocrine aspects of nephrolithiasis. In: *Special Topics in Endocrinology and Metabolism*, Vol. 3, edited by M.P. Cohen, and P.P. Foà, pp. 57–86. Alan R. Liss, Inc., New York.
28. Brown, H.V., and Wasserman, K. (1981): Exercise performance in chronic obstructive pulmonary diseases. *Med. Clin. North Am.*, 65:525–547.
29. Caniggia, A., Nuti, R., Loré, F., and Vattimo, A. (1981): Pathophysiology of the adverse effects of

glucoactive corticosteroids on calcium metabolism in man. *J. Steroid Biochem.*, 15:153–161.

30. Cann, C.E., Genant, H.K., Ettinger, B., and Gordon, G.S. (1980): Spinal mineral loss in oophorectomized women. *J.A.M.A.*, 244:2056–2059.

31. Cann, C.E., Martin, M.C., Genant, H.K., and Jaffe, R.B. (1984): Decreased spinal mineral content in amenorrheic women. *J.A.M.A.*, 251:626–629.

32. Cedar, L., Elmqvist, D., Svensson, S.-E. (1981): Cardiovascular and neurologic function in elderly patients substaining a fracture of the neck of the femur. *J. Bone Joint Surg.*, 63-B:560–566.

33. Chan, G.M., Ronald, N., Slater, P., Hollis, J., and Thomas, M.R. (1982): Decreased bone mineral status in lactating adolescent mothers. *J. Pediatr.*, 101:767–770.

34. Christiansen, C., Rødbro, P., and Lund, M. (1973): Effect of vitamin D on bone mineral mass in normal subjects and in epileptic patients on anticonvulsants: A controlled therapeutic trial. *Br. Med. J.*, 2:208–209.

35. Cloutier, M.D., Hayles, A.B., Riggs, B.L., Jowsey, J., and Bickel, W.H. (1967): Juvenile osteoporosis: Report of a case including a description of some metabolic and microradiographic studies. *Pediatrics*, 40:649–655.

36. Coindre, J.-M., David, J.-P., Rivière, L., Goussot, J.-F., Roger, P., Mascarel, A. de, and Meunier, P.J. (1986): Bone loss in hypothyroidism with hormone replacement: A histomorphometric study. *Arch. Intern. Med.*, 146:48–53.

37. Coltan, C.L., and Darby, A.J. (1970): Giant granulomatous lesions of the femoral head and neck in rheumatoid arthritis. *Ann. Rheum. Dis.*, 29:626–633.

38. Crilly, R., Cawood, M., Marshall, D.H., and Nordin, B.E.C. (1978): Hormonal status in normal, osteoporotic and corticosteroid treated postmenopausal women. *J. Royal Soc. Med.*, 71:733–736.

39. Crosby, L.O., Kaplan, F.S., Pertschuk, M.J., and Mullen, J.L. (1985): The effect of anorexia nervosa on bone morphometry in young women. *Clin. Orthop. Rel. Res.*, 201:271–277.

40. Cunningham, A.S., and Mazess, R.B. (1983): Bone mineral loss in lactating adolescents. Letter. *J. Pediatr.*, 103:338–339.

41. Dalén, N., Lamke, B., and Wallgren, A. (1974): Bone-mineral losses in oophorectomized women. *J. Bone Joint Surg.*, 56-A:1235–1238.

42. Dalinka, M.K., Edeiken, J., and Finkelstein, J.B. (1974): Complications of radiation therapy: Adult bone. *Semin. Roentgenol.*, 9:29–40.

43. Dana-Haeri, J., Oxley, J., and Richens, A. (1982): Reduction of free testosterone by antiepileptic drugs. *Br. Med. J.*, 284:85–86.

44. Daniell, H.W. (1976): Osteoporosis of the slender smoker: Vertebral compression fractures and loss of metacarpal cortex in relation to postmenopausal cigarette smoking and lack of obesity. *Arch. Intern. Med.*, 136:298–304.

45. Daniell, H.W. (1983): Postmenopausal tooth loss. Contributions to edentulism by osteoporosis and cigarette smoking. *Arch. Intern. Med.*, 143: 1678–1682.

46. Dauphine, R.T., Riggs, B.L., and Scholz, D.A.

47. David, D.S., Grieco, M.H., and Cushman, P., Jr. (1970): Adrenal glucocorticoids after twenty years: A review of their clinically relevant consequences. *J. Chronic Dis.*, 22:637–711.

48. Davidson, B.J., Riggs, B.L., Wahner, H.W., and Judd, H.L. (1983): Endogenous cortisol and sex steroids in patients with osteoporotic spinal fractures. *Obstet. Gynecol.*, 61:275–278.

49. Deftos, L.J. (1977): The thyroid gland in skeletal and calcium metabolism. In: *Metabolic Bone Disease*, edited by L.V. Avioli, and S.M. Krane, pp. 447–487. Vol. 2, Academic Press, New York.

50. Delmas, P.D., Stenner, D. Wahner, H.W., Mann, K.G., and Riggs, B.L. (1983): Increase in serum bone γ-carboxyglutamic acid protein with aging in women: Implications for the mechanism of age-related bone loss. *J. Clin. Invest.*, 71:1316–1321.

51. Demartini, F., Grokoest, A.W., and Ragan, C. (1952): Pathological fractures in patients with rheumatoid arthritis treated with cortisone. *J.A.M.A.*, 149:750–752.

52. Denham, M.J. (1973): Progressive osteoporosis in hemiplegia. *Gerontol. Clin.*, 15:361–365.

53. Dent, C.E., and Friedman, M. (1965): Idiopathic juvenile osteoporosis. *Q.J. Med.*, 34:177–210.

54. Dent, C.E. (1977): Osteoporosis in childhood. *Postgrad. Med. J.*, 53:450–456.

55. Department of Health, Education, and Welfare (1971): Alcohol-related illnesses. Chapter 4. In: *First Special Report to the U.S. Congress on Alcohol and Health*, edited by M. Keller, and S.S. Rosenberg, pp. 45–59. Department of Health, Education, and Welfare, DHEW Publication No. (HSM) 72-9099, Washington, D.C.

56. Deutsch, S., and Benjamin, F. (1978): Effect of diabetic status on fractionated estrogen levels in postmenopausal women. *J. Am. Obstet. Gynecol.*, 130:105–106.

57. Devas, M.B. (1965): Stress fractures of the femoral neck. *J. Bone Joint Surg.*, 47-B:728–738.

58. Devogelaer, J.P., Huaux, J.P., and Nagant de Deuxchaisnes, C. (1984): Does mild, asymptomatic, primary hyperparathyroidism require surgery to avoid bone loss in postmenopausal females? In: *Osteoporosis*, Vol. 1, edited by C. Christiansen, C.D. Arnaud, B.E.C. Nordin, A.M. Parfitt, W.A. Peck, and B.L. Riggs, pp. 365–367, Aalborg Stiftsbogtrykkeri, Glostrup, Denmark.

59. Dickson, R.A., Paice, F., and Nicolle, F.V. (1973): The assessment of hand function. Part II: Forces and bone density, a relationship in the hand. *Hand*, 5:15–24.

60. Drinkwater, B.L., Nilson, K., Chestnut, C.H., III, Bremner, W.J., Shainholtz, S., and Southworth, M.B. (1984): Bone mineral content of amenorrheic and eumenorrheic athletes. *N. Engl. J. Med.*, 311:277–281.

61. Drinkwater, B.L., Nilson, K., Ott, S., and Chestnut, C.H., III (1986): Bone mineral density after resumption of menses in amenorrheic athletes. *J.A.M.A.*, 256:380–382.

62. Dubovsky, D., and Jacobs, P. (1975): Vertebral

rarefaction in acute lymphoblastic leukaemia. *S.A. Med. J.,* 49:241–242.

63. Duncan, H., Frost, H.M., Villanueva, A.R., and Sigler, J.W. (1965): The osteoporosis of rheumatoid arthritis. *Arthritis Rheum.,* 8:943–954.

64. Duncan, H. (1972): Osteoporosis in rheumatoid arthritis and corticosteroid induced osteoporosis. Symposium on metabolic bone disease. *Orthop. Clin. North Am.,* 3:571–583.

65. Eddy, R.L. (1971): Metabolic bone disease after gastrectomy. *Am. J. Med.,* 50:442–449.

66. Engh, G., Bollet, A.J., Hardin, G., Parson, W. (1968): Epidemiology of osteoporosis. II. Incidence of hip fractures in mental institutions. *J. Bone Joint Surg.,* 50-A:557–562.

67. Epstein, S., Poser, J., McClintock, R., Johnston, C.C.Jr., Bryce, G., and Hui, S. (1984): Differences in serum bone Gla-protein with age and sex. *Lancet,* 1:307–310.

68. Ergün, H., and Howland, W.J. (1980): Postradiation atrophy of mature bone. *CRC Crit. Rev. Diagn. Imaging,* 12:225–243.

69. Eriksen, E.F., Mosekilde, L., and Melsen, F. (1985): Trabecular bone remodeling and bone balance in hyperthyroidism. *Bone,* 6:421–428.

70. Ettinger, B., and Wingerd, J. (1982): Thyroid supplements: Effect on bone mass. *West. J. Med.,* 136:473–476.

71. Evans, R.A., Dunstan, C.R., and Hills, E. (1983): Bone metabolism in idiopathic juvenile osteoporosis: A case report. *Calcif. Tissue Int.,* 35:5–8.

72. Exner, G.U., Prader, A., Elsasser, U., and Anliker, M. (1984): Idiopathic osteoporosis in a three-year-old girl: Follow-up over a period of 6 years by computed tomography bone densitometry (CT). *Helv. Paediatr. Acta,* 39:517–528.

73. Fallon, M.D., Perry, H.M., Ill, Bergfeld, M., Droke, D., Teitelbaum, S.L., and Avioli, L.V. (1983): Exogenous hyperthyroidism with osteoporosis. *Arch. Intern. Med.,* 143:442–444.

74. Farley, J.R., Fitzsimmons, R., Taylor, A.K., Jorch, U.M., and Lau, K.-H.W. (1985): Direct effects of ethanol on bone resorption and formation in vitro. *Arch. Biochem. Biophys.,* 238:305–314.

75. Finkenstedt, G., Skrabal, F., Gasser, R.W., and Braunsteiner, H. (1986): Lactose absorption, milk consumption, and fasting blood glucose concentrations in women with idiopathic osteoporosis. *Br. Med. J.,* 292:161–162.

76. Fisher, B., Sherman, B., Rockette, H., Redmond, C., Margolese, R., and Fisher, E.R. (1979): 1-phenylalanine mustard (L-PAM) in the management of premenopausal patients with primary breast cancer: Lack of association of disease-free survival with depression of ovarian function. *Cancer,* 44:847–857.

77. Fisher, E.C., Nelson, M.E., Frontera, W.R., Turksoy, R.N., and Evans, W.J. (1986): Bone mineral content and levels of gonadotropins and estrogens in amenorrheic running women. *J. Clin. Endocrinol. Metab.,* 62:1232–1236.

78. Fogh-Andersen, N., McNair, P., Møller-Petersen, J., and Madsbad, S. (1983): Lowered serum ionized calcium in insulin treated diabetic subjects. *Scand. J. Clin. Lab. Invest.,* 43(Suppl. 165):93–97.

79. Fonseca, V., Houlder, S., Thomas, M., Kirk, R.M., and Dandona, P. (1985): Vitamin D deficiency after vagotomy. *Br. Med. J.,* 290:1946.

80. Foresta, C., Ruzza, G., Mioni, R., Guarneri, G., Gribaldo, R., Meneghello, A., and Mastrogiacomo, I. (1984): Osteoporosis and decline of gonadal function in the elderly male. *Horm. Res.,* 19:18–22.

81. Frame, B., and Parfitt, A.M. (1978): Osteomalacia: Current concepts. *Ann. Intern. Med.,* 89:966–982.

82. Francis, R.M., Barnett, M.J., Selby, P.L., and Peacock, M. (1982): Thyrotoxicosis presenting as fracture of the femoral neck. *Br. Med. J.,* 285:97–98.

83. Francis, R.M., Peacock, M., Aaron J.E., Selby, P.L., Taylor, G.A., Thompson, J., Marshall, D.H., and Horsman, A. (1986): Osteoporosis in hypogonadal men: Role of decreased plasma 1,25-dihydroxyvitamin D, calcium malabsorption, and low bone formation. *Bone,* 7:261–268.

84. Fraser, S.A., Anderson, J.B., Smith, D.A., and Wilson, G.M. (1971): Osteoporosis and fractures following thyrotoxicosis. *Lancet,* 1:981–983.

85. Fraser, T.E., White, N.H., Hough, S., Santiago, J.V., McGee, B.R., Bryce, G., Mallon J., and Avioli, L.V. (1981): Alterations in circulating vitamin D metabolites in the young insulin-dependent diabetic. *J. Clin. Endocrinol. Metabl.,* 53:1154–1159.

86. Gallagher, J.C., Aaron, J., Horsman, A., Wilkinson, R., and Nordin, B.E.C. (1973): Corticosteroid osteoporosis. *Clin. Endocrinol. Metab.,* 2:355–368.

87. Gallagher, J.C., Riggs, B.L., Eisman, J., Hamstra, A., Arnaud, S.B., and DeLuca, H.F. (1979): Intestinal calcium absorption and serum vitamin D metabolites in normal subjects and osteoporotic patients: Effect of age and dietary calcium. *J. Clin. Invest.,* 64:729–736.

88. Gallagher, J.C., Melton, L.J., and Riggs, B.L. (1980): Examination of prevalence rates of possible risk factors in a population with a fracture of the proximal femur. *Clin. Orthop.,* 153:158–165.

89. Gallagher, J.C., Riggs, B.L., Jerpbak, C.M., and Arnaud, C.D. (1980): The effect of age on serum immunoreactive parathyroid hormone in normal and osteoporotic women. *J. Lab. Clin. Med.,* 95:373–385.

90. Gallagher, J.C., Jerpbak, C.M., Jee, W.S.S., Johnson, K.A., DeLuca, H.F., and Riggs, B.L. (1982): 1,25-dihydroxyvitamin D_3: Short- and long-term effects on bone and calcium metabolism in patients with postmenopausal osteoporosis. *Proc. Natl. Acad. Sci.,* (U.S.A.), 79:3325–3329.

91. Genant, H.K., Cann, C.E., Ettinger, B., and Gordon, G.S. (1982): Quantitative computer tomography of vertebral spongiosa: A sensitive method for detecting early bone loss after oophorectomy. *Ann. Intern. Med.,* 97:699–705.

92. Gennari, C. (1985): Glucocorticoids and bone. Chapter 7. In: *Bone and Mineral Research/3,* edited by W.A. Peck, pp. 213–231. Elsevier, Amsterdam.

93. Gertner, J.M., Tamborlane, W.V. Horst, R.L., Sherwin, R.S., Felig, P., and Genel, M. (1980):

Mineral metabolism in diabetes mellitus: Changes accompanying treatment with a portable subcutaneous insulin infusion system. *J. Clin. Endocrinol. Metab.*, 50:862–866.

94. Goldsmith, R.S., Woodhouse, C.F., Inglsar, S.H., and Segal, D. (1967): Effect of phosphate supplements in patients with fracture. *Lancet*, 1:687–690.

95. Goodman, C.R. (1971): Osteoporosis as early complication of hemiplegia. *N.Y. State J. Med.*, 71:1943–1945.

96. Gowen, M., Wood, D.D., Ihrie, E.J., McGuire, M.K.B., and Russel, R.G.G. (1983): An interleukin 1-like factor stimulates bone resorption in vitro. *Nature*, 306:378–380.

97. Greenspan, S.L., Neer, R.M., Ridgway, E.C., and Klibanski, A. (1986): Osteoporosis in men with hyperprolactinemic hypogonadism. *Ann. Intern. Med.*, 104:777–782.

98. Greer, F.R., and Garn S.M. (1982): Loss of bone mineral content in lactating adolescents. *J. Pediatr.*, 101:718–719.

99. Grodin, J.M., Siiteri, P.K., and MacDonald, P.C. (1973): Source of estrogen production in postmenopausal women. *J. Clin. Endocrinol. Metab.*, 36:207–214.

100. Gruber, H.E., Gutteridge, D.H., and Baylink, D.J. (1984): Osteoporosis associated with pregnancy and lactation: Bone biopsy and skeletal features in three patients. *Metab. Bone Dis. Rel. Res.*, 5:159–165.

101. Guyatt, G.H., Webber, C.E., Mewa, A.A., and Sackett, D.L. (1984): Determining causation—a case study: Adrenocorticosteroids and osteoporosis. *J. Chronic Dis.*, 37:343–352.

102. Hahn, T.J. (1978): Corticosteroid-induced osteopenia. *Arch. Intern. Med.*, 138:882–885.

103. Hahn, T.J. (1980): Drug induced disorders of vitamin D and mineral metabolism. *Clin. Endocrinol. Metab.*, 9:107–129.

104. Hahn, T.J., Halstead, L.R., and Baran, D.T. (1981): Effects of short term glucocorticoid administration on intestinal calcium absorption and circulating vitamin D metabolite concentrations in man. *J. Clin. Endocrinol. Metab.*, 52:111–115.

105. Hansson, L.I., Cedar, L., Svensson, K., and Thorngren, K.-G. (1982): Incidence of fractures of the distal radius and proximal femur: Comparison of patients in a mental hospital and the general population. *Acta Orthop. Scand.*, 53:721–726.

106. Harris, W.H., and Heaney, R.P. (1969): Skeletal renewal and metabolic bone disease. *N. Engl. J. Med.*, 280:253–259.

107. Heath, H., III, Lambert, P.W., Service, F.J., and Arnaud, S.B. (1979): Calcium homeostasis in diabetes mellitus. *J. Clin. Endocrinol. Metab.*, 49:462–466.

108. Heath, H., Melton, L.J., and Chu, C.-P. (1980): Diabetes mellitus and risk of skeletal fracture. *N. Engl. J. Med.*, 303:567–570.

109. Heath, H., III, Hodgson, S.F., and Kennedy, M.A. (1980): Primary hyperparathyroidism: Incidence, morbidity, and potential economic impact in a community. *N. Engl. J. Med.*, 302:189–193.

110. Heliövaara, M., and Aromaa, A. (1981): Parity and obesity. *J. Epidemiol. Community Health*, 35:197–199.

111. Higgins, M.W., Keller, J.B., and Metzner, H.L. (1977): Smoking, socioeconomic status, and chronic respiratory disease. *Am. Rev. Resp. Dis.*, 116:403–410.

112. Hodgson, S.F., Dickson, E.R., Wahner, H.W., Mann, K.G., and Riggs, B.L. (1984): Impaired osteoblast function in primary biliary cirrhosis. (Abstr.) *Clin. Res.*, 32:490A.

113. Hoekman, K., Papapoulos, S.E., Peters, A.C.B., and Bijvoet, O.L.M. (1985): Characteristics and biphosphonate treatment of a patient with juvenile osteoporosis. *J. Clin. Endocrinol. Metab.*, 61:952–956.

114. Hooyman, J.R., Melton, L.J., Nelson, A.M., O'Fallon, W.M., and Riggs, B.L. (1984): Fractures after rheumatoid arthritis: A population-based study. *Arth. Rheum.*, 27:1353–1361.

115. Hui, S.L., Epstein, S., and Johnston, C.C., Jr. (1985): A prospective study of bone mass in patients with Type I diabetes. *J. Clin. Endocrinol. Metab.*, 60:74–80.

116. Hutchinson, T.A., Polansky, S.M., and Feinstein, A.R. (1979): Postmenopausal oestrogens protect against fractures of hip and distal radius: A case-control study. *Lancet*, 2:705–709.

117. Ingeberg, S., Deding, A., and Jensen, M.K. (1982): Bone mineral content in myelomatosis. *Acta Med. Scand.* 211:19–21.

118. Jackson, J.A., Kleerekoper, M., and Parfitt, A.M. (1986): Symptomatic osteoporosis in a man with hyperprolactinemic hypogonadism. *Ann. Intern. Med.*, 105:543–545.

119. Jackson, W.P.U. (1958): Osteoporosis of unknown cause in younger people: Idiopathic osteoporosis. *J. Bone Joint Surg.*, 40-B:420–441.

120. Jensen, J., Christiansen C., and Rødbro, P. (1985): Cigarette smoking, serum estrogens, and bone loss during hormone-replacement therapy early after menopause. *N. Engl. J. Med.*, 313:973–975.

121. Johnston, C.C., Jr., Hui, S.L., and Longcope, C. (1985): Bone mass and sex steroid concentrations in postmenopausal Caucasian diabetics. *Metabolism*, 34:544–550.

122. Joly, R., Chapuy, M.C., Alexandre, C., and Meunier, P.J. (1980): Ostéoporoses a haut niveau de remodelage et fonction parathyröidienne: Confrontations histo-biologiques. *Pathol. Biol.*, 28:417–424.

123. Jones, E.T., and Hensinger, R.N. (1981): Spinal deformity in idiopathic juvenile osteoporosis. *Spine*, 6:1–4.

124. Jowsey, J., and Johnson, K.A. (1972): Juvenile osteoporosis: Bone findings in seven patients. *J. Pediatr.*, 81:511–517.

125. Jowsey, J., Arnaud, S.B., Hodgson, S.F., Johnson, K.A., Beabout, J.W., and Wahner, H.W. (1978): The frequency of bone abnormality in patients on anticonvulsant therapy. *Electroencephalogr. Clin. Neurophysiol.*, 45:341–347.

126. Julkunen, H., Honkonen, K., and Tarkkanen, L. (1971): Medical aspects in the treatment of femoral neck fracture. *Acta Med. Scand.*, 189:167–171.

127. Keenan, M.A., Perry, J, and Jordan, C. (1984): Factors affecting balance and ambulation following stroke. *Clin. Orthop.*, 182:165–171.

128. Klein, R.G., Arnaud, S.B., Gallagher, J.C., DeLuca, H.F., and Riggs, B.L. (1977): Intestinal cal-

cium absorption in exogenous hypercortisonism: Role of 25-hydroxyvitamin D and corticosteroid dose. *J. Clin. Invest.*, 60:253–259.

129. Kley, H.K., Deselaers, T., Peerenboom, H., and Kruskemper, H.L. (1980): Enhanced conversion of androstenedione to estrogens in obese males. *J. Clin. Endocrinol. Metab.*, 51:1128–1132.

130. Klibanski, A., Neer, R.M., Beitins, I.Z., Ridgway, E.C., Zervas, N.T., and McArthur, J.W. (1980): Decreased bone density in hyperprolactinemic women. *N. Engl. J. Med.*, 303:1511–1514.

131. Koyama, H., Wada, T., Nishizawa, Y., Iwanaga, T., Aoki, Y., Terasawa, T., Kosaki, G., Yamamoto, T., and Wade, A. (1977): Cyclophosphamide-induced ovarian failure and its therapeutic significance in patients with breast cancer. *Cancer*, 39:1403–1409.

132. Kreiger, N., Kelsey, J.L., Holford, T.R., and O'Connor, T. (1982): An epidemiologic study of hip fracture in postmenopausal women. *Am. J. Epidemiol.*, 116:141–148.

133. Krølner, B., Jørgensen, J.V., and Pors Nielsen, S.P. (1983): Spinal bone mineral content in myxoedema and thyrotoxicosis. Effects of thyroid hormone(s) and antithyroid treatment. *Clin. Endocrinol.*, 18:439–446.

134. Kumar, R. (1980): The metabolism of 1,25-dihydroxyvitamin D_3. *Endocrine Rev.*, 1:258–267.

135. Lalor, B.C., Lumb, G., Mawer, E.B., and Adams, P.H. (1986): Determinants of serum calcitriol in primary hyperparathyroidism. (Abstract) *Bone*, 7:310.

136. Lamke, B., Brundin, J., and Mobert, P. (1977): Changes of bone mineral content during pregnancy and lactation. *Acta Obstet. Gynecol. Scand.*, 56:217–219.

137. Lamke, B., and Björkholm, E. (1981): Postmenopausal bone mineral loss after treatment for malignant gynaecologic tumours. *Acta Radiologica Oncol.*, 20:109–111.

138. Lawoyin, S., Sismilich, S., Browne, R., and Pak, C.Y.C. (1979): Bone mineral content in patients with calcium urolithiasis. *Metabolism*, 28:1250–1254.

139. Levin, M.E., Boisseau, V.C., and Avioli, L.V. (1976): Effects of diabetes mellitus on bone mass in juvenile and adult-onset diabetes. *N. Engl. J. Med.*, 294:241–245.

140. Lidgren, A., and Wallöe, A. (1977): Incidence of fracture in epileptics. *Acta Orthop. Scand.*, 48:356–361.

141. Linde, J., and Friis, Th. (1979): Osteoporosis in hyperthyroidism estimated by photon absorptiometry. *Acta Endocrinol.*, 91:437–448.

142. Lindsay, R., Hart, D.M., Forrest, C., and Baird, C. (1980): Prevention of spinal osteoporosis in oophorectomised women. *Lancet*, 2:1151–1154.

143. Lindsay, R. (1981): The influence of cigarette smoking on bone mass and bone loss. (Abstract) In: *Osteoporosis: Recent Advances in Pathogenesis and Treatment*. Edited by H.F. DeLuca, H.M. Frost, W.S.S. Jee, C.C. Johnston, Jr., and A.M. Parfitt, p. 481. University Park Press, Baltimore.

144. Lindsay, R., Herrington, B.S., and Tohme, J. (1986): Reproductive history and bone mass in women. *J. Bone Min. Res.*, 1(Suppl. 1):248.

145. Lips, P., Courpron, P., and Meunier, P.J. (1978): Mean wall thickness of trabecular bone packets in human iliac crest: Changes with age. *Calcif. Tissue Res.*, 26:13–17.

146. Livesley, B., and Atkinson, L. (1974): Repeated falls in the elderly. *Modern Geriatr.*, 4:458–467.

147. Long, R.G., Meinhard, E., Skinner, R.K., Varghese, Z., Wills, M.R., and Sherlock, S. (1978): Clinical, biochemical, and histological studies of osteomalacia, osteoporosis, and parathyroid function in chronic liver disease. *Gut*, 19:85–90.

148. Macdonald, J.B. (1985): The role of drugs in falls in the elderly. *Clin. Geriatr. Med.*, 1:621–636.

149. Maddison, P.J., and Bacon, P.A. (1974): Vitamin D deficiency, spontaneous fractures, and osteopenia in rheumatoid arthritis. *Br. Med. J.*, 4:433–435.

150. Marder, H.K., Tsang, R.C., Hug, G., and Crawford, A.C. (1982): Calcitriol deficiency in idiopathic juvenile osteoporosis. *Am. J. Dis. Child.*, 136:914–917.

151. Mautalen, C., Reyes, H.R., Ghiringhelli, G., and Fromm, G. (1986): Cortical bone mineral content in primary hyperparathyroidism. Changes after parathyroidectomy. *Acta Endocrinol.*, 111:494–497.

152. Mazess, R.B. (1982): On aging bone loss. *Clin. Orthop.*, 165:239–252.

153. McClung, M., Lieberman, D., Klein, K., Parfitt, A.M., and Orwoll, E. (1983): Marked trabecular osteopenia in healthy postgastrectomized men. (Abstract). Fifth Annual Scientific Meeting, American Society for Bone and Mineral Research, San Antonio, Texas, June 5–7, 1983.

154. McConkey, B., Fraser, G.M., and Bligh, A.S. (1962): Osteoporosis and purpura in rheumatoid disease: Prevalence and relation to treatment with corticosteroids. *Q. J. Med.*, 31:419–427.

155. McDermott, M.T., Kidd, G.S., Blue, P., Ghaed, V., and Hofeldt, F.D. (1983): Reduced bone mineral content in totally thyroidectomized patients. Possible effect of calcitonin deficiency. *J. Clin. Endocrinol. Metab.*, 56:936–939.

156. McNair, P., Madsbad, S., Christensen, M.S., Christiansen, C., Faber, O.K., Binder, C., and Transbøl, I. (1979): Bone mineral loss in insulin-treated diabetes mellitus: Studies on pathogenesis. *Acta Endocrinol.*, 90:463–472.

157. Mellström, D., and Rundgren, Å. (1982): Long-term effects after partial gastrectomy in elderly men: A longitudinal population study of men between 70 and 75 years of age. *Scand. J. Gastroenterol.*, 17:433–439.

158. Melton, L.J., III, Sampson, J.M., Morrey, B.F., and Ilstrup, D.M. (1981): Epidemiologic features of pelvic fractures. *Clin. Orthop.*, 155:43–47.

159. Melton, L.J., III, Ilstrup, D.M., Riggs, B.L., and Beckenbaugh, R.D. (1982): Fifty-year trend in hip fracture incidence. *Clin. Orthop.*, 162:144–149.

160. Melton, L.J., III, and Riggs, B.L. (1983): Epidemiology of age-related fractures. In: *The Osteoporotic Syndrome: Detection, Prevention, and Treatment*, edited by L.V. Avioli, pp. 45–72. Grune and Stratton, New York.

161. Melton, L.J., III, Ochi, J.W., Palumbo, P.J., and Chu, C.-P. (1983): Sources of disparity in the spectrum of diabetes mellitus at incidence and prevalence. *Diabetes Care*, 6:427–431.

162. Melton, L.J., III, Wahner, H.W., Richelson, L.S., O'Fallon, W.M., and Riggs, B.L. (1986): Osteoporosis and the risk of hip fracture. *Am. J. Epidemiol.*, 124:254–261.

163. Miller, B., Markheim, H.R., and Towbin, M.N. (1967): Multiple stress fractures in rheumatoid arthritis: A case report. *J. Bone Joint Surg.*, 49-A:1408–1414.

164. Mulley, G., and Espley, A.J. (1979): Hip fracture after hemiplegia. *Postgrad. Med. J.*, 55:264–265.

165. Mundy, G.R., Raisz, L.G., Cooper, R.A., Schechter, G.P., and Salmon, S.E. (1974): Evidence for the secretion of an osteoclast stimulating factor in myeloma. *N. Engl. J. Med.*, 291:1041–1046.

166. Mundy, G.R., Shapiro, J.L., Bandelin, J.G., Canalis, E.M., and Raisz, L.G. (1976): Direct stimulation of bone resorption by thyroid hormones. *J. Clin. Invest.*, 58:529–534.

167. Murchison, L.E., Bewsher, P.D., Chesters, M., Gilbert, J., Catto, G., Law, E., McKay, E., and Ross, H.S. (1975): Effects of anticonvulsants and inactivity on bone disease in epileptics. *Postgrad. Med. J.*, 51:18–21.

168. Naftchi, N.E., Viau, A.T., Marshall, C.H., David, W.S., and Lowman, E.W. (1975): Bone mineralization in the distal forearm of hemiplegic patients. *Arch. Phys. Med. Rehabil.*, 56:487–492.

169. Nesbit, M., Krivit, W., Heyn, R., and Sharp, H. (1976): Acute and chronic effects of methotrexate on hepatic, pulmonary, and skeletal systems. *Cancer*, 37(Suppl.):1048–1057.

170. Newcomer, A.D., Hodgson, S.F., McGill, D.B., and Thomas P.J. (1978): Lactase deficiency: Prevalence in osteoporosis. *Ann. Intern. Med.*, 89:218–220.

171. Newton-John, H.F., and Morgan, D.B. (1968): Osteoporosis: Disease or senescence? *Lancet*, 1:232–233.

172. Nielsen, C.T., Ibsen, K.K., Christiansen, J.S., Peitersen, B., and Uhrenholdt, A. (1978): Diabetes mellitus, skeletal age and bone mineral content in children. *Acta Endocrinol.*, 88:58.

173. Nielsen, H.E., Mosekilde, L., and Charles, P. (1979): Bone mineral content in hyperthyroid patients after combined medical and surgical treatment. *Acta Radiol. Oncol.*, 18:122–128.

174. Niemann, K.M.W., and Mankin, H.J. (1968): Fractures about the hip in the elderly indigent patient. I. Epidemiology. *Geriatrics*, 23:150–158.

175. Nilas, L., and Christiansen, C. (1985): Influence of PTH and 1,25(OH)$_2$D on calcium homeostasis and bone mineral content after gastric surgery. *Calcif. Tissue Int.*, 37:461–466.

176. Nilsson, B.E. (1969): Parity and osteoporosis. *Surg. Gynecol. Obstet.*, 129:27–28.

177. Nilsson, B.E. (1970): Conditions contributing to fracture of the femoral neck. *Acta Chir. Scand.*, 136:383–384.

178. Nilsson, B.E., and Westlin, N.E. (1971): The fracture incidence after gastrectomy. *Acta Chir. Scand.*, 137:533–534.

179. Nilsson, B.E., and Westlin, N.E. (1972): Femur density in alcoholism and after gastrectomy. *Calcif. Tissue Res.*, 10:167–170.

180. Nordin, B.E.C., and Roper, A. (1955): Post-pregnancy osteoporosis: A syndrome? *Lancet*, 1:431–434.

181. Notelovitz, M., Tjapkes, J., and Ware, M. (1981): Interaction between estrogen and Dilantin in a menopausal woman. *N. Engl. J. Med.*, 304:788–789.

182. Osteomalacia after gastrectomy. (1986): *Lancet*, 1:77–78.

183. Pacifici, R., Rifas, W., Shen, V., Miller, R., Teitelbaum, S., Levy, J., Peck, W.A., and Avioli, L.V. (1986): Elevated IL-1 secretion and OAF-like activity in a case of primary osteoporosis. *J. Bone Min. Res.*, 1(Suppl. 1), Abstract 53.

184. Paganini-Hill, A., Ross, R.K., Gerkins, V.R., Henderson, B.E., Arthur, M., and Mack, T.M. (1981): Menopausal estrogen therapy and hip fractures. *Ann. Intern. Med.*, 95:28–31.

185. Pak, C.Y.C., Ohata, M., Lawrence, E.C., and Synder, W. (1974): The hypercalciurias: Causes, parathyroid functions and diagnostic criteria. *J. Clin. Invest.*, 54:387–400.

186. Pak, C.Y.C., Britton, F., Peterson, R. Ward, D., Northcutt, C., Breslau, N.A., McGuire, J., Sakhaee, K., Bush, S., Nicar, M., Norman, D.A., and Peters, P. (1980): Ambulatory evaluation of nephrolithiasis: Classification, clinical presentation and diagnostic criteria. *Am. J. Med.*, 69:19–30.

187. Panin, N., Gorday, W.J., and Paul, B.J. (1971): Osteoporosis in hemiplegia. *Stroke*, 2:41–47.

188. Parfitt, A.M. (1969): Chlorothiazide-induced hypercalcemia in juvenile osteoporosis and hyperparathyroidism. *N. Engl. J. Med.*, 281:55–59.

189. Parfitt, A.M., and Duncan, H. (1982): Metabolic bone disease affecting the spine. Chapter 13. In: *The Spine*, edited by R.H. Rothman, and F.A. Simeone, pp. 839–885. W.B. Saunders Company, Philadelphia.

190. Parker, R.G., and Berry, H.C. (1976): Late effects of therapeutic irradiation on the skeleton and bone marrow. *Cancer*, 37(Suppl.):1162–1171.

191. Peck, W.A., Brandt, J., and Miller, I. (1967): Hydrocortisone-induced inhibition of protein synthesis and uridine incorporation in isolated bone cells in vitro. *Proc. Natl. Acad. Sci. (U.S.A.)*, 57:1599–1606.

192. Perry, H.M., III, Fallon, M.D., Bergfeld, M., Teitelbaum, S.L., and Avioli, L.V. (1982): Osteoporosis in young men: A syndrome of hypercalciuria and accelerated bone turnover. *Arch. Intern. Med.*, 142:1295–1298.

193. Peszczynski, M. (1956): Prevention of falls in the hemiplegic patient. *Geriatrics*, 11:306–311.

194. Pinnell, S.R., and Murad, S. (1983): Disorders of collagen. In: *The Metabolic Basis of Inherited Disease*, Fifth Edition, edited by J.B. Stanbury, J.B. Wyngaarden, D.S. Fredrickson, J.L. Goldstein, M.S. Brown, pp. 1425–1433. McGraw-Hill Book Co., New York.

195. Pocock, N.A., Eisman, J.A., Yeates, M.G., Sambrook, P.N., and Eberl, S. (1986): Physical fitness is a major determinant of femoral neck and lumbar spine bone mineral density. *J. Clin. Invest.*, 78:618–621.

196. Poplingher, A.-R., and Pillar, T. (1985): Hip frac-

ture in stroke patients. *Acta Orthop. Scand.*, 56:226–227.

197. Prudham, D., and Evans, J.G. (1981): Factors associated with falls in the elderly: A community study. *Age Ageing*, 10:141–146.

198. Rao, S.D., Kleerekoper, M., Rogers, M., Frame, B., and Parfitt, A.M. (1984): Is gastrectomy a risk factor for osteoporosis? In: *Osteoporosis*, edited by C. Christiansen, C.D. Arnaud, B.E.C. Nordin, A.M. Parfitt, W.A. Peck, and B.L. Riggs, pp. 775–777. Aalborg Stiftsbogtrykkeri, Glostrup, Denmark.

199. Raskin, P., Stevenson, M.R.M., Barilla, D.E., and Pak, C.Y.C. (1978): The hypercalciuria of diabetes mellitus; Its amelioration with insulin. *Clin. Endocrinol.*, 9:329–335.

200. Ray, W.A., Griffin, M.R., Schaffner, W., Baugh, D.K., and Melton, L.J., III (1987): Psychotropic drug use and the risk of hip fracture. *N. Engl. J. Med.*, 316:363–369.

201. Reid, D.M., Kennedy, N.S.J., Smith, M.A., Tothill P., and Nuki, G. (1982): Total body calcium in rheumatoid arthritis: Effects of disease activity and corticosteroid treatment. *Br. Med. J.*, 285:330–332.

202. Richardson, M.L., Pozzi-Mucelli, R.S., Kanter, A.S., Kolb, F.O., Ettinger, B., and Genant, H.K. (1986): Bone mineral changes in primary hyperparathyroidism. *Skeletal Radiol.*, 15:85–95.

203. Richelson, L.S., Wahner, H.W., Melton, L.J. III, and Riggs, B.L. (1984): Relative contributions of aging and estrogen deficiency to postmenopausal bone loss. *N. Engl. J. Med.*, 311:1273–1275.

204. Riggs, B.L., Jowsey, J., and Kelly, P.J. (1966): Quantitative microradiographic study of bone remodeling in Cushing's syndrome. *Metabolism*, 15:773–780.

205. Riggs, B.L., Arnaud, C.D., Jowsey, J., Goldsmith, R.S., and Kelly, P.J. (1973): Parathyroid function in primary osteoporosis. *J. Clin. Invest.*, 52:181–184.

206. Riggs, B.L., Ryan, R.J., Wahner, W.H., Jiang, N.-S., and Mattox, V.R. (1973): Serum concentrations of estrogen, testosterone and gonadotropins in osteoporotic and nonosteoporotic postmenopausal women. *J. Clin. Endocrinol. Metab.*, 36:1097–1099.

207. Riggs, B.L. Gallagher, J.C., DeLuca, H.F., Edis, A.J., Lambert, P.W., and Arnaud, C.D. (1978): A syndrome of osteoporosis, increased serum immunoreactive parathyroid hormone and inappropriately low serum 1,25-dihydroxyvitamin D. *Mayo Clin. Proc.*, 53:701–706.

208. Riggs, B.L., Wahner H.W., Dunn, W.L., Mazess, R.B., Oxford, K.P., and Melton, L.J., III (1981): Differential changes in bone mineral density of the appendicular and axial skeleton with aging: Relationship to spinal osteoporosis. *J. Clin. Invest.*, 67:328–335.

209. Riggs, B.L., Wahner, H.W., Seeman, E., Offord, K.P., Dunn, W.L., Mazess, R.B., Johnson, K.A., and Melton, L.J., III (1982): Changes in bone mineral density of the proximal femur with aging: Differences between the postmenopausal and senile osteoporosis syndromes. *J. Clin. Invest.*, 70:716–723.

210. Riggs, B.L., and Melton, L.J. III (1983): Evidence for two distinct syndromes of involutional osteoporosis. *Am. J. Med.*, 75:899–901.

211. Riggs, B.L., and Melton, L.J., III (1986): Involutional osteoporosis. *N. Engl. J. Med.*, 314:1676–1686.

212. Riggs, B.L. (1987): Osteoporosis. In: *Textbook of Endocrinology*, Second Edition, edited by L.J DeGroot. Grune and Stratton, Orlando.

213. Rigotti, N.A., Nussbaum, S.R., Herzog, D.B., and Neer, R.M. (1984): Osteoporosis in women with anorexia nervosa. *N. Engl. J. Med.*, 311:1601–1606.

214. Rigotti, N.A., Neer, R.M., and Jameson, L. (1986): Osteopenia and bone fractures in a man with anorexia nervosa and hypogonadism. *J.A.M.A.*, 256:385–388.

215. Ringe, J.-D. (1985): Value of single photon absorptiometry as a screening method for osteopenia in different gastrointestinal disorders. *J. Comput. Assist. Tomogr.*, 9:627.

216. Robinson, B.G., Wagstaffe, C., Delbridge, L., Roche, J., and Posen, S. (1985): Bone mineral content in parathyroid disorders. (Abstract) Proceedings of the Seventh Annual Scientific Meeting of the American Society for Bone and Mineral Research, June 15–18, 1985, Washington, D.C.

217. Rogalsky, R.J., Black, G.B., and Reed, M.H. (1986): Orthopaedic manifestations of leukemia in children. *J. Bone Joint Surg.*, 68-A:494–501.

218. Ropes, M.W., Bennett, G.A., Cobb, S., Jacox, R., and Jessar, R.A. (1958): 1958 revision of diagnostic criteria for rheumatoid arthritis. *Bull. Rheum. Dis.*, 9:175–176.

219. Rose, S.H., Melton, L.J., III, Morrey, B.F., Ilstrup, D.M., and Riggs, B.L. (1982): Epidemiologic features of humerus fractures. *Clin. Orthop.*, 168:24–30.

220. Ruegsegger, P., Dambacher, M.A., Ruegsegger, E., Fischer, J.A., and Anliker, M. (1984): Bone loss in premenopausal and postmenopausal women. *J. Bone Joint Surg.*, 66-A:1015–1023.

221. Rundgren, A., and Mellstrom, D. (1984): The effect of tobacco smoking on the bone mineral content of the ageing skeleton. *Mech. Ageing Dev.*, 28:273–277.

222. Rydell, N.W. (1966): Forces acting on the femoral head-prosthesis. *Acta Orthop. Scand.*, 88:19, 1966.

223. Samaan, N.A., DeAsis, D.N., Buzdar, A.U., and Blumenschein, G.R. (1978): Pituitary-ovarian function in breast cancer patients on adjuvant chemoimmunotherapy. *Cancer*, 41:2084–2087.

224. Saville, P.D. (1965): Changes in bone mass with age and alcoholism. *J. Bone Joint Surg.*, 47-A:492–499.

225. Saville, P.D., and Nilsson, B.E.R. (1966): Height and weight in symptomatic postmenopausal osteoporosis. *Clin. Orthop.*, 45:49–54.

226. Saville, P.D., and Kharmosh, O. (1967): Osteoporosis of rheumatoid arthritis: Influence of age, sex and corticosteroids. *Arthritis Rheum.*, 10:423–430.

227. Schaadt, O., and Bohr, H. (1984): Bone mineral in lumbar spine, femoral neck and femoral shaft measured by dual photon absorptiometry with 153-gadolineum in prednisone treatment. In: *Glucocor-*

ticoid Effects and Their Biological Consequences. Advances in Experimental Medicine and Biology. Vol. 171, edited by L.V. Avioli, C. Gennari, and B. Imbim, pp. 201–208.

228. Scholz, D., Schwille, P.O., Schley, H.W., Hanisch, E., Bieger, D., Zeuner, E., and Engelhardt, W. (1983): Mineral metabolism and vitamin D status before and up to five years following highly selective vagotomy in duodenal ulcer patients. *Hepatogastroenterol.*, 30:102–106.

229. Schorn, D., and Mowat, A.G. (1977): Penicillamine in rheumatoid arthritis: Wound healing, skin thickness and osteoporosis. *Rheumatol. Rehabil.*, 16:223–230.

230. Schwartz, A.M., and Leonidas, J.C. (1984): Methotrexate osteopathy. *Skeletal Radiol.*, 11:13–16.

231. Seeman, E., Kumar, R., Hunder, G.G., Scott, M., Heath, H., III, and Riggs, B.L. (1980): Production, degradation, and circulating levels of 1,25-dihydroxyvitamin D in health and in chronic glucocorticoid excess. *J. Clin. Invest.*, 66:664–669.

232. Seeman, E., Wahner, H.W., Offord, K.P., Kumar, R., Johnson, W.J. and Riggs, B.L. (1982): Differential effects of endocrine dysfunction on the axial and the appendicular skeleton. *J. Clin. Invest.*, 69:1302–1309.

233. Seeman, E., Melton, L.J. III, O'Fallon, W.M., and Riggs, B.L. (1983): Risk factors for spinal osteoporosis in men. *Am. J. Med.*, 75:977–983.

234. Shapiro, J.R., and Rowe, D.W. (1984): Imperfect osteogenesis and osteoporosis. *N. Engl. J. Med.*, 310:1738–1740.

235. Shore, R.M., Chesney, R.W., Mazess, R.B., Rose, P.G., and Bargman, G.J. (1981): Osteopenia in juvenile diabetes. *Calcif. Tissue Int.*, 33:455–457.

236. Slovik, D.M. (1983): The vitamin D endocrine system, calcium metabolism, and osteoporosis. In: *Special Topics in Endocrinology and Metabolism*, Vol. 5, edited by M.P. Cohen, and P.P. Foà, pp. 83–148. Alan R. Liss, Inc., New York.

237. Smith, R. (1980): Idiopathic osteoporosis in the young. *J. Bone Joint Surg.*, 62-B:417–427.

238. Sotaniemi, E.A., Hakkarainen, H.K., Puranen, J.A., and Lahti, R.O. (1972): Radiologic bone changes and hypocalcemia with anticonvulsant therapy in epilepsy. *Ann. Intern. Med.*, 77:389–394.

239. Stellon, A.J., Webb, A., Compston J., and Williams, R. (1986): Lack of osteomalacia in chronic cholestatic liver disease. *Bone*, 7:181–185.

240. Stephenson, W.H., and Cohen, B. (1956): Post-irradiation fractures of the neck of the femur. *J. Bone Joint Surg.*, 38-B:830–845.

241. Storm, T.L., Sørensen, O.H., Lund, Bj., Lund, Bi., Christiansen, J.S., Andersen, A.R., Lumholtz, I.B., and Parving, H.-H. (1983): Vitamin D metabolism in insulin-dependent diabetes mellitus. *Metab. Bone Dis. Rel. Res.*, 5:107–110.

242. Suzuki, Y., Ichikawa, Y., Saito, E., and Homma, M. (1983): Importance of increased urinary calcium excretion in the development of secondary hyperparathyroidism of patients under glucocorticoid therapy. *Metabolism*, 32:151–156.

243. Sweet, M.B.E., Zwi, S., Mendelow, A., Kotler, M.N., and Graham, W.D. (1967): Fractured neck of femur: Associated morbidity and mortality. *S. Afr. J. Surg.*, 5:57–64.

244. Taylor, R.T. Huskisson, E.C., Whitehouse, G.H., and Hart, F.D. (1971): Spontaneous fractures of pelvis in rheumatoid arthritis. *Br. Med. J.*, 4:663–664.

245. Teitelbaum, S.L., Rosenberg, E.M., Richardson, C.A., and Avioli, L.V. (1976): Histological studies of bone from normocalcemic postmenopausal osteoporotic patients with increased circulating parathyroid hormone. *J. Clin. Endocrinol. Metab.*, 42:537–543.

246. Teotia, M., Teotia, S.P.S., and Singh, R.K. (1979): Idiopathic juvenile osteoporosis. *Am. J. Dis. Child.*, 133:894–900.

247. Tiegs, R.D., Body, J.J., Barta, M.M., and Heath, H., III (1986): Secretion and metabolism of monomeric human calcitonin: Effects of age, sex, and thyroid damage. *J. Bone Joint Surg.*, 1:339–349.

248. Tsai, K.-S., Heath, H., III, Kumar, R., and Riggs, B.L. (1984): Impaired vitamin D metabolism with aging in women: Possible role in pathogenesis of senile osteoporosis. *J. Clin. Invest.*, 73:1668–1672.

249. Uitto, J., Murray, L.W., Blumberg, B., and Shamban, A. (1986): Biochemistry of collagen in diseases. (UCLA Conference) *Ann. Intern. Med.*, 105:740–756.

250. Urovitz, E.P.M., Fornasier, V.L., Risen, M.I., and MacNab, I. (1977): Etiological factors in the pathogenesis of femoral trabecular fatigue fractures. *Clin. Orthop.*, 127:275–280.

251. Utz, J.P., Melton, L.J., O'Fallon, W.M., and Riggs, B.L. (1987): Risk of osteoporotic fractures in women with breast cancer: A population-based cohort study. *J. Chron. Dis.* (in press).

252. Vahvanen, V. (1971): Femoral neck fracture of the rheumatoid hip joint: A study of 20 operatively treated cases. *Acta Rheum. Scand.*, 17:125–136.

253. Vernejoul de, M.C., Bielakoff, J., Herve, M., Gueris, J., Hott, M., Modrowski, D., Kuntz, D., Miravet, L., and Ryckewaert, A. (1983): Evidence for defective osteoblast function: A role for alcohol and tobacco consumption in osteoporosis in middle-aged men. *Clin. Orthop.*, 179:107–115.

254. Wasnich, R.D., Benfante, R.J., Yano, K., Heilbrun, L., and Vogel, J.M. (1983): Thiazide effect on the mineral content of bone. *N. Engl. J. Med.*, 309:344–347.

255. Weinstock, R.S., Goland, R.S., Shane, E., Clemens, T.L., Tohme, J.F., Lindsay, R., and Bilezikian, J.P. (1986): Increased bone mineral density in women with non-insulin-dependent diabetes mellitus. *J. Bone Min. Res.*, 1(Suppl. 1):227 (abstract).

256. Weiss, N.S., Ure, C.L., Ballard, J.H., Williams, A.R., and Daling, J.R. (1980): Decreased risk of fractures of the hip and lower forearm with postmenopausal use of estrogen. *N. Engl. J. Med.*, 303:1195–1198.

257. Williams, A.R., Weiss, N.S., Ure, C.L., Ballard J., and Daling, J.R. (1982): Effect of weight, smoking, and estrogen use on the risk of hip and

forearm fractures in postmenopausal women. *Obstet. Gynecol.,* 60:695–699.

258. Williams, H.E., and Prien, E.L., Jr. (1977): Nephrolithiasis. In: *Metabolic Bone Disease,* edited by L.V. Avioli, and S.M. Krane, pp. 387–423. Vol. 1, Academic Press, New York.

259. Wiske, P.S., Wentworth, S.M., Norton, J.A., Jr., Epstein, S., and Johnston, C.C., Jr. (1982): Evaluation of bone mass and growth in young diabetics. *Metabolism,* 31:848–854.

260. Wyshak, G. (1981): Hip fracture in elderly women and reproductive history. *J. Gerontol.,* 36:424–427.

Osteoporosis: Etiology, Diagnosis, and Management, edited by B. Lawrence Riggs and L. Joseph Melton, III. Raven Press, New York © 1988.

7

Radiology of Osteoporosis

*,†Harry K. Genant, **James B. Vogler, and **Jon E. Block

*Department of Radiology and Medicine, University of California, School of Medicine, San Francisco, California 94143; **Department of Radiology, Duke University, Durham, North Carolina 27710; and †Department of Internal Medicine, Kaiser Permanente Medical Group, San Francisco, California 94143

The generalized osteoporoses represent the most common forms of metabolic bone diseases, and their radiologic features are the major focus of this chapter. The list of processes that are associated with or result in a generalized deficient quantity of bone (osteoporosis) is extensive (see Table 1). Histologically, the end result in each of these disorders is a deficient amount of osseous tissue, although different pathogenetic mechanisms may be involved. In essence, the generalized osteoporoses represent a heterogenous group of conditions encompassing many pathogenetic mechanisms variably associated with low, normal, or increased bone-remodeling states.

Because of the uncertainties of specific radiologic interpretation, the term osteopenia has been introduced as a generic designation for generalized radiographic signs of decreased bone density, such as "demineralization," "undermineralization," and "deossification." Each of these terms similarly has its disadvantages. Demineralization implies a specific loss of mineral without concomitant loss of organic component of bone, a phenomenon referred to as halisteresis, which does not occur on a large scale in bone. On the other hand, undermineralization implies inadequate accretion of mineral into an osteoid matrix; histologically, this represents osteomalacia. Finally, deossification

implies abnormal loss of bone, presumably by excessive resorption, and is an inappropriate descriptive term for conditions with normal rates of resorption. Thus, we are left with osteopenia (meaning "poverty of bone") as an acceptable, nonspecific, descriptive term for generalized rarefaction of the skeleton observed radiographically. This term may be broadly applied to describing diminished bone density when the histopathologic nature of the bone loss is uncertain. The term osteoporosis on the other hand is widely used clinically to mean generalized loss of bone density, or osteopenia, accompanied by relatively atraumatic fractures of the spine, wrist, hip or ribs.

INVOLUTIONAL OSTEOPOROSES (POSTMENOPAUSAL AND SENILE)

The term *involutional osteoporosis* has been used to describe the condition of gradual, progressive bone loss, often accompanied by fractures, seen in postmenopausal women and, with increasing age, in both men and women. It has been suggested that this broad category of involutional osteoporosis may represent two distinct syndromes—postmenopausal osteoporosis and senile osteoporosis. Although there is substantial overlap between these two subcate-

TABLE 1. *Disorders associated with generalized osteopenia or osteoporosis*

I. Disorders of multiple and/or uncertain etiology
  1. Involutional osteoporosis[a] (postmenopausal and senile)
  2. Idiopathic male osteoporosis
  3. Juvenile osteoporosis
II. Secondary bone disorders
  A. Endocrine
    1. Adrenal cortex[b]
      (a) Cushing's disease
      (b) Addison's disease
    2. Gonadal disorders
      (a) Postmenopausal osteoporosis[a]
      (b) Hypogonadism[b]
    3. Pituitary
      (a) Acromegaly
      (b) Hypopituitarism
    4. Pancreas
      (a) Diabetes mellitus[a]
    5. Thyroid
      (a) Hyperthyroidism
      (b) Hypothyroidism
    6. Parathyroid
      (a) Hyperparathyroidism[a]
  B. Marrow replacement and expansion
    1. Myeloma[a]
    2. Leukemia
    3. Lymphoma
    4. Metastatic disease[a]
    5. Gaucher's disease
    6. Anemias (sickle cell, thallasemia, hemophilia)[b]
  C. Drugs and substances
    1. Steroids[a,b]
    2. Heparin (osteoporosis)
    3. Anticonvulsants (osteomalacia)
    4. Immunosuppressants
    5. Alcohol[a]
  D. Chronic disease
    1. Chronic renal disease[a]
    2. Hepatic insufficiency[b]
    3. GI malabsorption syndromes
    4. Chronic inflammatory polyarthropathies
    5. Chronic debility/immobilization
  E. Deficiency states
    1. Vitamin D (rickets/osteomalacia)[a,b]
    2. Vitamin C (scurvy)
    3. Calcium
    4. Malnutrition
  F. Inborn errors of metabolism
    1. Osteogenesis imperfecta
    2. Homocystinuria

[a]Common causes of loss of bone density in adults
[b]Common causes of loss of bone density in children

gories, it is convenient to discuss them as separate entities because of differing clinical features and proposed pathoetiologies. The

separation is based primarily on the different patterns of bone loss and types of fractures that are observed in these two processes.

Postmenopausal osteoporosis (also termed type I osteoporosis) (31,33) is believed to represent that process occurring in a subset of postmenopausal women, typically between the ages of 50 and 65 years. This group is characterized by accelerated trabecular bone resorption related to estrogen deficiency and is identified by a fracture pattern that involves predominantly the vertebrae and distal forearm (Colles' fractures). Accelerated and disproportionate loss of trabecular bone in these areas structurally weakens the bone and predisposes them to fractures.

In senile osteoporosis (or type II osteoporosis) (31,33), there is a proportionate loss of cortical and trabecular bone, in contrast to the disproportionate loss of trabecular bone in postmenopausal osteoporosis. Senile osteoporosis is characterized by fractures of the hip, proximal end of the humerus, tibia, and pelvis in elderly men and women, usually 75 years of age or older. The etiology of senile osteoporosis is speculative. However, factors that play a role include age-related decrease in bone formation, diminished adrenal function, reduced intestinal calcium absorption, and secondary hyperparathyroidism.

Radiologic diagnosis:

Generalized osteopenia (most prominent in the spine)

Thinning and accentuation of the cortices

Accentuation of primary and loss of secondary trabeculae

Changes in vertebral body shape (wedge-shaped, biconcave, and compression)

Spontaneous or atraumatic fractures of the spine, wrist, hip, or ribs.

Radiographic-Pathologic Findings in Postmenopausal and Senile Osteoporosis

In the normal adult physiologic state, the rates of bone formation and bone resorption are roughly equal (i.e., coupled), allowing the total amount of osseous tissue to remain constant. In osteoporosis (14) this equilibrium is lost such that bone resorption prodominates. This is reflected radiographically as various patterns of trabecular and cortical bone resorption ultimately leading to osteopenia (Fig. 1).

Trabecular bone resorption in the axial skeleton, particularly in type I osteoporosis, results in marked thinning and dissolution of transverse trabeculae with relative preservation of the primary trabeculae or those aligned with the axis of stress. In areas in which trabecular bone predominates such as the spine and pelvis, the combination of osteopenia and reinforcement of primary trabeculae may produce a striated bony appearance (Fig. 2). The reinforced primary trabeculae have a sharp appearance in osteoporotic bones, which occasionally

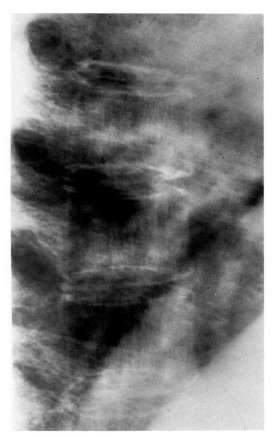

FIG. 2. Moderate postmenopausal osteoporosis of the thoracic spine. Overall there is loss of bone density. The cortices are thinned and the vertebral bodies have a "striated" appearance due to loss of secondary trabeculae and reinforcement of primary trabeculae.

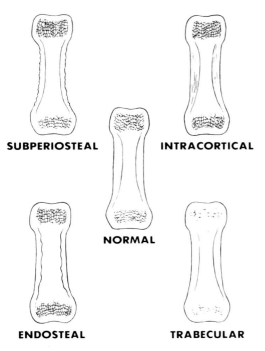

SUBPERIOSTEAL   **INTRACORTICAL**

NORMAL

ENDOSTEAL   **TRABECULAR**

FIG. 1. Four patterns of bone resorption. Subperiosteal bone resorption characterizes hyperparathyroidism, endosteal resorption is prominent in senile osteoporosis, while intracortical and trabecular resorption are features of postmenopausal osteoporosis and other high bone resorptive states.

aids in distinguishing osteoporosis from osteomalacia. In the latter, the trabeculae may appear indistinct or "fuzzy," a result of irregular resorption from accompanying secondary hyperparathyroidism and from trabeculae that become coated by a layer of partially unmineralized osteoid. The loss of trabecular bone mass also accentuates the cortical outline, producing the so-called "picture framing" or "empty box" seen in osteoporosis of the vertebral bodies (Fig. 3). The vertebral bodies become weakened and the intervertebral disc may

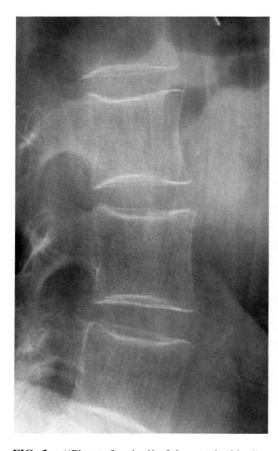

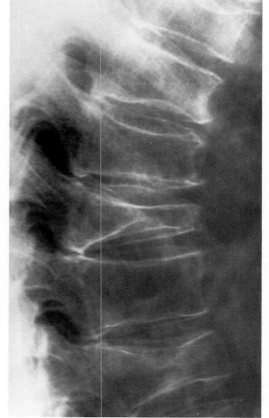

FIG. 3. "Picture framing" of the vertebral bodies in osteoporosis. Due to the loss of trabecular bone, there is osteopenia and accentuation of the cortices in this patient with involutional osteoporosis.

FIG. 4. Advanced osteoporosis of the thoracic spine. Changes in vertebral body shape have occurred as a result of involutional osteoporosis. Wedging of several of the vertebral bodies and complete compression fractures are noted.

protrude into the adjacent vertebral body. The degree of protrusion varies, ranging from bending and buckling of the endplates (biconcave appearance) to herniation of disc material into the vertebral body (Schmorl's node formation) (Fig. 4). In more advanced cases complete compression fractures of the vertebral bodies occur.

Bone loss in the appendicular skeleton is initially most apparent radiographically at the ends of long and tubular bones due to the predominance of cancellous bone in these regions. The epiphyseal-metaphyseal regions appear ra-

diolucent, and result in juxtaarticular osteopenia (Fig. 5). Endosteal resorption of bone has a prominent role, particularly in type II osteoporosis. The net result of this chronic process is widening of the medullary canal and thinning of the cortices, which is most pronounced in the appendicular skeleton. In late stages of senile osteoporosis, the cortices are "paper thin" and the endosteal surfaces are smooth (Fig. 6). In rapidly evolving postmenopausal osteoporosis, on the other hand, accelerated endosteal and intracortical bone resorption may be seen and can be directly assessed by high

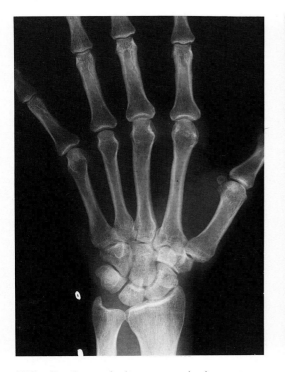

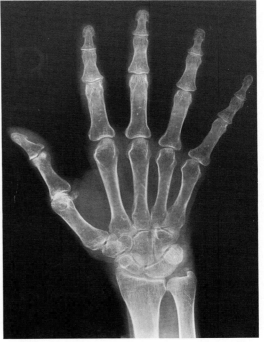

FIG. 5. Juxtaarticular osteopenia in postmenopausal osteoporosis. Due to the predominance of trabecular bone in the juxtaarticular regions, progressive loss of this spongy bone in patients with osteoporosis often results in a radiographic picture of juxtaarticular osteopenia.

FIG. 6. Cortical thinning in senile osteoporosis. The thinned appearance of the cortices is primarily the result of endosteal bone resorption.

resolution radiographic techniques (Figs. 7 and 8).

When there is an overall loss of bone mass, the skeletal system becomes weakened, and fractures occur. There appears to be a critical bone mass below which fractures become more frequent. Fractures are commonly seen in the vertebral bodies, femoral neck, distal radius, ribs, and pubis. These may be the result of minor trauma or even normal stress on the abnormal bone (insufficiency fracture). Vertebral body and wrist fractures (type I osteoporosis) are generally seen at an earlier age than fractures of the femur (type II osteoporosis). Occasionally, these osteoporotic fractures are not identified on initial radiographs but are identi-

fied by radionuclide bone scan, computed tomography, magnetic resonance imaging or by follow-up radiographic studies, as healing occurs (Fig. 9). The radiologic appearance in the setting of partial healing may suggest a metastatic neoplastic process, particularly with fractures of the vertebrae, sacrum, hip and pelvis (Fig. 10).

Semiquantitative Radiographic Assessment of the Spine and Hip in Osteoporosis

Spine

A number of radiologic criteria as discussed above, are associated with generalized verte-

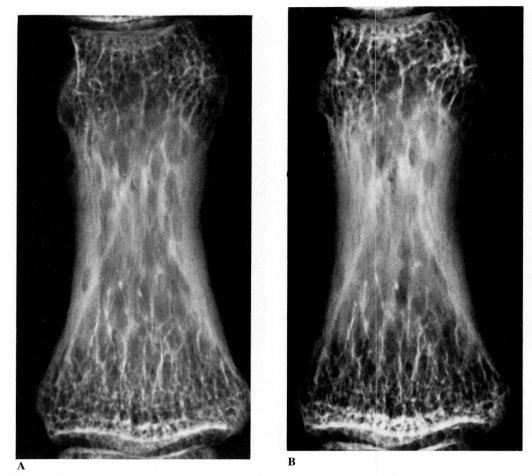

A   **B**

FIG. 7. Post-oophorectomy bone loss. Accelerated endosteal and intracortical bone resorption in the middle phalanx at baseline (**A**) and two years following (**B**) oophorectomy.

bral osteoporosis: increased lucency of the vertebral bodies, loss of horizontal trabeculae, reduction in cortex thickness of the vertebrae, endplate opaqueness, biconcavity of the vertebral body, and anterior wedging (5,12). However, factors such as breathing artifacts, variation in radiographic exposure and positioning errors make a qualitative assessment of vertebral body density, trabecular patterns, and cortical changes difficult and unreliable as an accurate indicator of osteoporosis (Fig. 11). Rather, emphasis might be placed on an overall assessment of the morphology of the vertebral bodies as an index of spinal osteoporosis.

Changes in vertebral body shape may be indicative of both the severity and degree of osteoporosis. A number of authors have attempted to define and quantify various morphological changes that constitute true vertebral fractures (12,32,33,36) (Fig. 12). These parameters have been used to determine the presence or absence of fractures (36), as well as the rate of change in fracture severity (17). Vertebral biconcavity may play a part in the diagnosis of osteoporosis, although this criterion has not been shown, in and of itself, to be associated with vertebral density or to be a reliable indicator of morphological change over time. Ante-

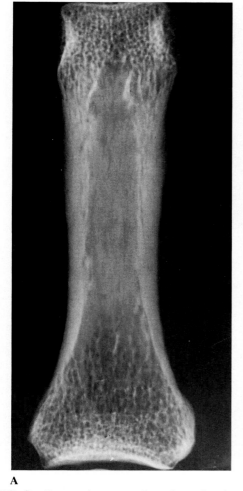 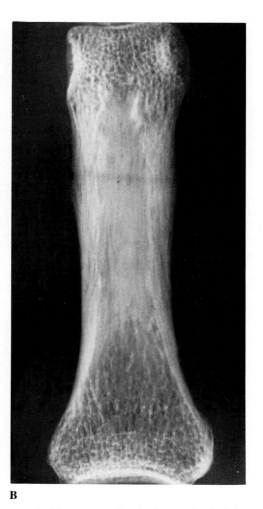

A **B**

FIG. 8. Post-oophorectomy bone loss. Accelerated intracortical bone resorption in the proximal phalanx at baseline (**A**) and two years following (**B**) oophorectomy.

rior wedging, on the other hand, has been shown to be associated with spinal density measurements, as well as being indicative of subsequent and more severe fractures (17,33). Although admittedly, such wedge deformity can infrequently represent residual change from remote trauma or Scheuermann's disease (juvenile epiphysitis) (Fig. 13).

There is widespread disagreement as to what degree of wedging constitutes a true fracture—estimates range from using a 15% to using a 25% reduction in anterior height relative to the posterior height of the same vertebra as the minimum criteria for designation as a fracture. Kleerekoper defines a vertebral fracture as a reduction in anterior height, with or without a concomitant reduction in posterior height, that is readily apparent on visual inspection (17). This definition probably restricts fracture identification to only those vertebrae where measured anterior height is reduced by at least 20%. Other morphological deformities would include advanced biconcavity, angling of the endplates, as well as complete compression

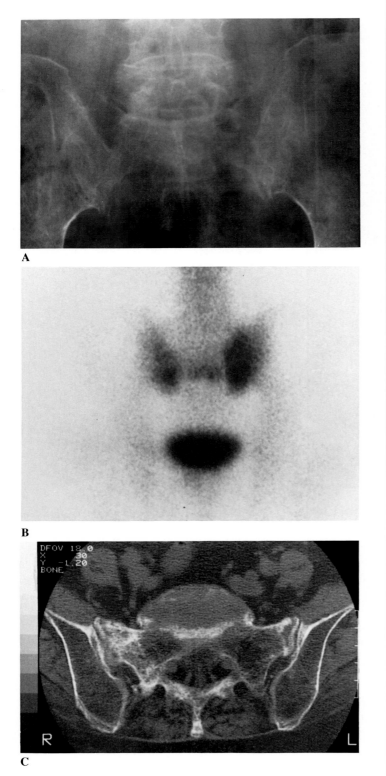

FIG. 9.   Occult insufficiency fractures of the sacrum. **A:** AP radiograph of the pelvis in an elderly osteoporotic woman presenting with low back pain. **B:** Posterior view bone scintigraphy showing bilateral increased uptake of Tc_{99m} MDP tracer most evident in the right sacrum and SI joint. **C:** Axial CT defining the region of sclerosis due to the right and left sacral insufficiency fractures in severely osteopenic bone.

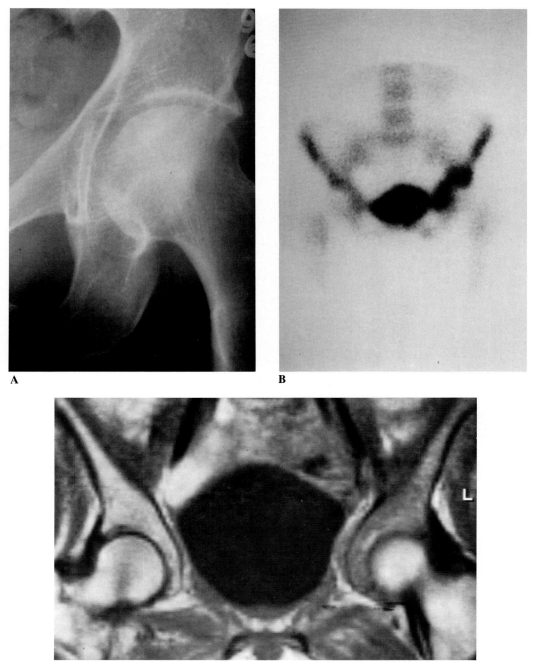

A

B

C

FIG. 10. Occult insufficiency fracture of the left acetabulum. **A:** Normal AP radiograph of left hip joint in an osteoporotic elderly woman presenting with acute onset of hip pain. **B:** Tc$_{99m}$ MDP bone scintigraphy, anterior view, showing increased uptake in the left supra-acetabular region. **C:** Coronal magnetic resonance imaging demonstrating nonspecific decreased marrow signal in left acetabulum and ilium on T1-weighted sequence.

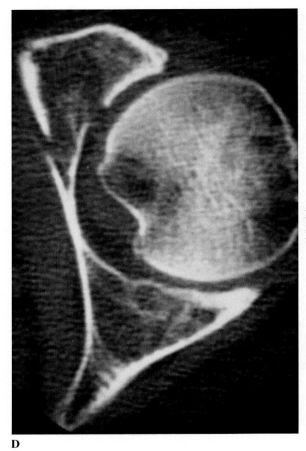

FIG. 10. *(continued)* **D:** Direct axial CT image demonstrating insufficiency fractures of quadrilateral plate.

D

fractures (i.e., reduction in both the anterior and posterior height by at least 25% relative to adjacent normal vertebrae, which is easily detectable upon inspection).

Vertebral fracture classification directly reflects the degree of vertebral body deformation either semiqualitatively or by direct measurement (7,17). Severity index scores commonly range from "absence of fractures" to "severe" osteoporosis (i.e., complete compression). In a grading scale we use, a 15 to 20% reduction (inclusive) of anterior height relative to posterior height indicates a "minimal" vertebral compression (grade one-half) but is not considered a true osteoporotic fracture; anterior wedging, greater than 20% and less than or equal to 25%, indicates a "mild" compression fracture (grade 1); further anterior wedging, or the aforementioned posterior or mid-height de-

formities represent a "moderate" fracture (grade 2); and lastly, marked deformity with loss of volume or projected area of greater than 40% relative to adjacent unfractured vertebrae represents a "severe" vertebral fracture (grade 3). An overall spinal fracture "index" is derived from the sum of the grades for T4 to L5. This graduated scale of vertebral morphological deformity may be useful in the classification of individual patients, in identifying rates of change in severity during follow-up studies, and in providing additional clinical information, along with other bone mineral measurements, for careful management decisions.

Hip

Conventional anteroposterior radiographs of the hips demonstrate a web-like configuration

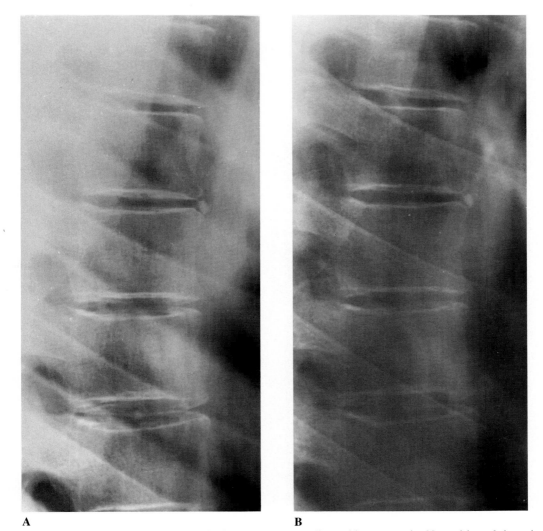

A   **B**

FIG. 11.   Effect of exposure and positioning on apparent radiographic osteopenia. Normal lateral thoracic spine (**A**) appears demineralized on over-penetrated (high kVp) radiograph (**B**)

of distinct segments of trabeculae that tend to resorb with increasing age and advanced osteoporosis. The cancellous bone of the proximal femur is composed of trabecular structural systems, which develop and form in response to compressive and tensile stresses placed upon this skeletal region during normal weight-bearing. A measurement technique, known as the Singh index, has been devised to evaluate the trabecular structure of the hip (10,18) (Fig. 14). With the progressive bone loss in osteoporosis, distinct areas of trabeculae are resorbed in an orderly and identifiable fashion. The order of disappearance of the trabeculae is presumably determined by the intensity of stresses normally carried by these trabeculae. The severity of osteoporosis is graded on a scale from six (normal) to one (severe osteoporosis). The Singh index has been shown to discriminate hip fracture cases from controls better than any other radiographic measurement of the hip (11), although its usefulness as a predictor of vertebral fracture has met with mixed success (3,38). Furthermore, use of the Singh index on

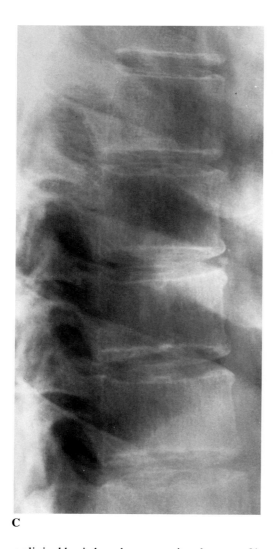

FIG. 11. *(continued)* and shows apparent biconcavity (**C**) when beam is obliqued to endplates.

C

a clinical basis has shown varying degrees of interobserver reliability (r = .41 − .97) and reproducibility; however, careful standardization of the technique can potentially alleviate this problem. The Singh index is not highly correlated with other measurements of bone mineral content or density. Bohr found a correlation of only r = 0.18 between mineral density of the hip by dual photon absorptiometry and Singh index (2). The Singh index is also poorly correlated with single photon measurements in the forearm (19). However, the Singh index provides information about the trabecular structure of the hip rather than mineral content or density; these different skeletal components may both make important contributions in the assessment of the integrity of the proximal femur (23).

IDIOPATHIC MALE OSTEOPOROSIS

Prior to the seventh decade, osteoporosis in men is unusual, unless such predisposing factors as alcoholism, corticosteroid therapy, chronic debilitating disease, or endocrine abnormalities exist. A small but distinct subset of men demonstrate symptomatic osteoporosis prior to the age of 60 years. Characteristically, these men have normal adrenal, parathyroid, thyroid, and gonadal function in addition to normal levels of vitamin D. Increased intesti-

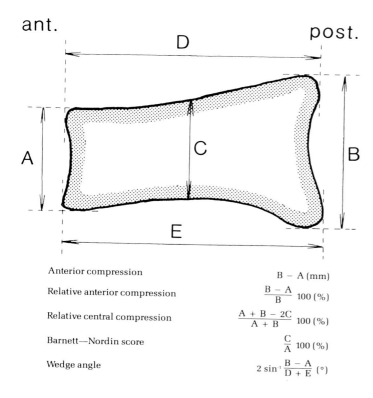

ant.   post.

Anterior compression $B - A$ (mm)

Relative anterior compression $\dfrac{B - A}{B}\ 100\ (\%)$

Relative central compression $\dfrac{A + B - 2C}{A + B}\ 100\ (\%)$

Barnett—Nordin score $\dfrac{C}{A}\ 100\ (\%)$

Wedge angle $2\ \sin^{-1}\dfrac{B - A}{D + E}\ (°)$

FIG. 12. Different methods of radiogrammetry have been proposed for semiquantitative assessment of vertebral compressions. From Hangartner, T.N. (1986): *J. Can. Assoc. Radiol.,* 37:143–152, with permission of the author and publisher.

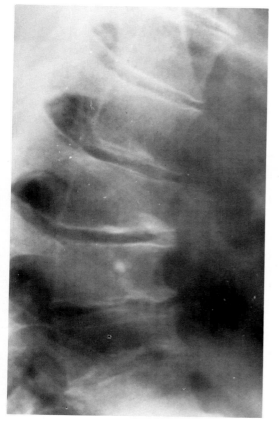

FIG. 13. Scheuermann's disease of spine simulating osteoporotic fractures. Vertebral wedge compression and Schmorl's nodes as residual deformity of "juvenile epiphysitis" or Scheuermann's disease.

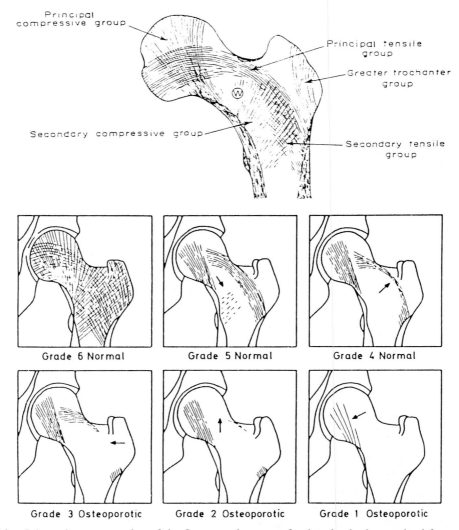

FIG. 14. Schematic representation of the five normal groups of trabeculae in the proximal femur. ''W'' indicates the location of Ward's triangle, from Singh (37).

nal absorption of calcium and hypercalciuria are inconstant findings. Initially accelerated bone turnover is present but in later stages bone turnover becomes diminished. The etiology is uncertain and the diagnosis is often one of exclusion.

Radiographically, men with idiopathic osteoporosis demonstrate generalized osteopenia, particularly of the axial skeleton with associated vertebral compression fractures (Fig. 15). There are no radiographic features that allow

differentiation of this entity from involutional osteoporosis.

Radiologic diagnosis:
Osteopenia predominantly of the axial skeleton
Fractures predominantly of the spine

IDIOPATHIC JUVENILE OSTEOPOROSIS

The etiology of this rare disorder (15,30) is not known. Children with idiopathic juvenile

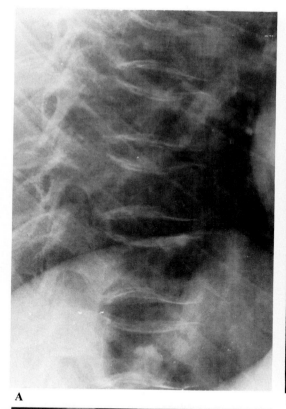

A

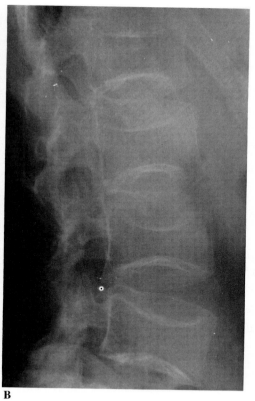

B

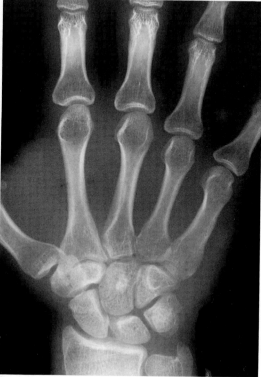

C

FIG. 15. Idiopathic male osteoporosis. Marked thoracic (**A**) and lumbar (**B**) osteoporosis with biconcave deformities. Appendicular cortical bone is normal in the hands (**C**).

osteoporosis typically present prior to puberty with rapidly progressive osteoporosis that later stabilizes. The findings occur predominantly in the axial skeleton but are otherwise similar to involutional osteoporosis. Fractures in the long bones generally involve the metaphyseal regions.

Radiologic diagnosis:
Osteopenia, particularly of the axial skeleton
Vertebral plana
Metaphyseal fractures

CUSHING'S DISEASE (ENDOGENOUS AND EXOGENOUS)

Cushing's disease (1,20,39) patients have chronic excess of endogenous or exogenous adrenocorticosteroids. Endogenous Cushing's disease is most frequently caused by adrenal hyperplasia and less frequently by tumors of the adrenal and pituitary glands. Exogenous Cushing's disease is far more common than endogenous and results from excessive corticosteroid administration.

Radiologic diagnosis:
Osteopenia, particularly of trabecular bone
Exuberant callus of compressed vertebral endplates (marginal condensation)
   and of fractured long bones and ribs
Osteonecrosis commonly of the hip, knee and shoulder
Skeletal growth retardation in children

Radiologic-Pathologic Considerations

As in osteoporosis, the equilibrium between bone formation and bone resorption is disrupted such that resorption predominates. Thus, the typical findings of osteoporosis are seen. These include generalized osteopenia from thinning of spongy and compact bone, accentuation of primary trabeculae giving the vertebral bodies a striated appearance, with ''picture framing'' and changes in vertebral body shape, particularly a biconcave appearance (fish vertebrae). Wedge and compression fractures are also seen. Histologically, exuberant endosteal callus formation is seen in compressed vertebrae and is manifested radiographically by increased density in the bony tissue adjacent to the vertebral endplate (Fig. 16). This excessive callus formation is also evident in fractures involving other bones including the ribs (which are commonly fractured in Cushing's disease).

Additional findings sometimes seen in Cushing's disease include a mottled appearance of the skull secondary to osteoporotic involvement. Osteonecrosis, particularly of the femoral heads, occurs commonly in cases of exogenous steroid administration but occurs infrequently in the endogenous cases for unknown reasons (20). Other less common findings seen principally in exogenous Cushing's disease are septic arthritis, neuropathic like joints, tendon rupture, and delayed skeletal maturation in children (28).

OSTEOMALACIA

Osteomalacia (26,27) is characterized by defective mineralization of osteoid in mature cancellous and cortical bone. Osteomalacia is a generic term describing similar histopathologic and radiologic changes that are seen in a large group of diverse disorders, generally resulting from a defect in vitamin D metabolism. The causes include: dietary deficiency, gastrointestinal malabsorption, liver disease, anticonvulsant drugs, renal insufficiency, vitamin D dependent rickets, renal tubular disorders, and hypophosphatasia.

Radiologic diagnosis:
Osteopenia
Looser's zones or pseudofractures
Intracortical bone resorption (cortical tunnelling)
Coarsened, unsharp trabecular pattern
Bowing of bones
True fractures (especially of the spine and femoral neck)

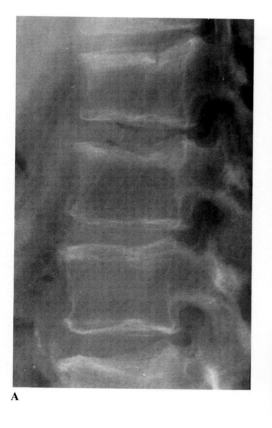

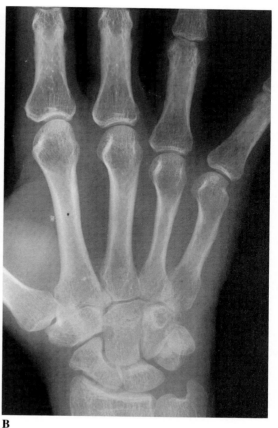

A

B

FIG. 16. Endogenous Cushing's disease in a 50-year-old man. Lateral view of the lumbar spine (**A**) demonstrates marked osteoporosis with vertebral collapse and characteristic marginal condensation. Hand radiograph (**B**) shows normal cortical bone and periarticular osteopenia.

Radiologic-Pathologic Considerations

Generalized osteopenia, frequent in osteomalacia, is sometimes distinguished radiographically from that of primary osteoporosis by the coarse and fuzzy appearance of trabecular and cortical surfaces particularly in the spine and pelvis (Fig. 17A). The unsharp and indistinct trabecular and cortical architecture results from the excessive partially-mineralized osteoid largely and from the bone resorption of secondary hyperparathyroidism.

Incomplete fractures with focal accumulations of osteoid occur in compact bone at right angles to the long axis of the bone (Fig. 18). Radiographically these are known as Looser's zones, Milkman's fractures or pseudofractures, and are distinguishing features of osteomalacia, although they may occur in Paget's and rarely in involutional osteoporosis (25). The exact etiology of Looser's zones is unclear, although they represent partial insufficiency fractures, which are often symmetrical in distribution and involve the pubic rami, femoral necks, scapulae, ribs, long bones, and metatarsals. While they may remain unchanged for months or even years, complete fractures may develop later in these weakened areas of bone.

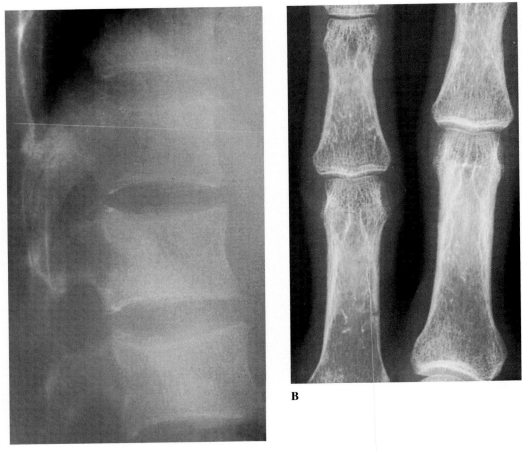

A

B

FIG. 17. Osteomalacia secondary to intestinal malabsorption in a 45-year-old man. **A:** Lateral view of the spine demonstrates osteopenia with indistinct cortical and trabecular outlines and biconcave deformities of the vertebral bodies. **B:** Magnification radiograph of the hand demonstrates osteopenia accompanied by increased intracortical tunneling due to associated secondary hyperparathyroidism.

Intracortical bone resorption or cortical tunnelling is observed in the tubular and long bones as a manifestation of the frequently associated secondary hyperparathyroidism (Fig. 17B) (28). High resolution magnification techniques are necessary to demonstrate these findings in the phalanges and metacarpals. Intracortical resorption or tunnelling is the most sensitive, although nonspecific, radiographic abnormality in osteomalacia, far more common radiographically than pseudofractures. This finding may help to differentiate osteomalacia from some low turnover osteoporoses such as senile osteoporosis.

Overall the bones in osteomalacia lose intrinsic strength with bowing and bending a result, unlike the brittle bones of osteoporosis. The vertebral bodies may assume a biconcave configuration uniformly involving the spine, which helps distinguish it from the focal collapse of involutional osteoporosis (Fig. 19). Bone "softening" in other areas of the body may result in basilar invagination, protrusio acetabuli and triradiate pelvis (27).

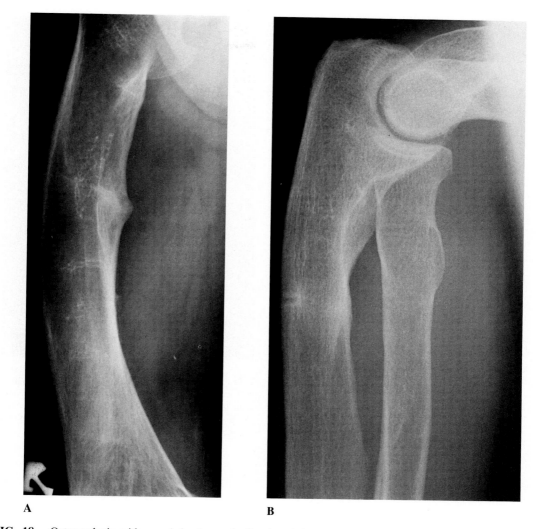

FIG. 18. Osteomalacia with pseudofractures. **A:** Bowing deformity of the femur with Looser's zones on the concave surface. **B:** Looser's zone of ulna.

RICKETS

Like the term osteomalacia, rickets (26) is a general term used to describe the histopathologic and radiologic changes resulting from a group of diverse disorders. The final common pathway of these disorders is a loss of orderly maturation and mineralization of cartilage cells at the growth plate resulting in similar pathologic and radiologic changes. Rickets represents osteomalacia in the growing and developing skeleton. Thus, inherent to all rachitic syndromes are osteomalacic radiographic changes in the portions of the skeleton that contain mature bone, and at sites containing immature, growing bone, characteristic radiographic changes of rickets.

Radiologic diagnosis:

Osteopenia and osteomalacia

Widening of the physis (growth plate)

Irregular metaphyseal margins (ill-defined zone of provisional calcification)

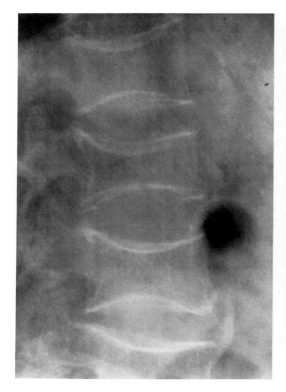

FIG. 19.   Osteomalacia. A lateral view of the lumbar spine in this patient with osteomalacia demonstrates moderate osteopenia involving the vertebral bodies with evidence of bone softening (bowing of the endplates).

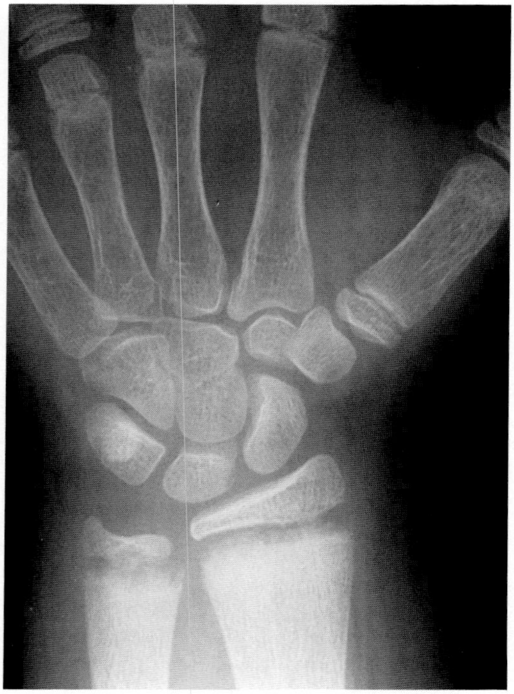

FIG. 20.   Wrist in a child with rickets. Widening and lengthening of the growth plates of the distal radius and ulna are evident. Also the zone of provisional calcification is indistinct and the metaphyseal margins appear irregular.

Splaying and cupping of the metaphyses
Growth retardation

Radiologic-Pathologic Considerations

The radiologic findings at the physeal plate are a reflection of the altered pathophysiology. The normal ordered maturation and mineralization of cartilage cells becomes disrupted. This occurs predominantly in the hypertrophic zone where the number of chondrocytes is seen to increase and the normal columnar formation of the cells is lost. There is a continued accumulation of cells resulting in the earliest radiographic finding of widening and irregularity of the physeal growth plate (Fig. 20). Defective

mineralization of the chondrocytes in the zone of provisional calcification yields the irregular frayed metaphyseal margins radiographically. As the cell mass in the hypertrophic zones continues to increase, it protrudes into the weakened metaphyseal region causing cupping and widening of the metaphyses (Fig. 21). While this process is occurring on the metaphyseal side of the growth plate, similar processes are occurring on the epiphyseal side. The defective maturation and mineralization seen here results in an epiphysis which is osteopenic and has irregular, unsharp borders. Overall, skeletal growth retardation occurs.

In the metaphysis and diaphysis, there is also defective mineralization of osteoid. In these areas, where mature bone is present, the

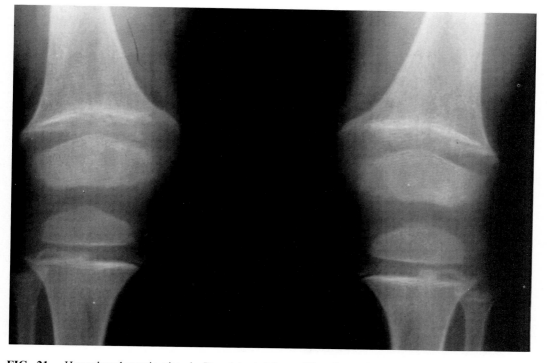

FIG. 21. Hypophosphatemic vitamin D-resistant rickets. AP radiograph of both knees demonstrates diffuse osteopenia. The growth plates of the distal femurs have widened and protrude into the weakened metaphyseal region causing cupping and widening of the metaphyses. Note also the irregular, unsharp borders of the femoral epiphyses.

radiographic findings of osteomalacia are produced.

Additional radiographic findings include prominence of the growth plates at the costochondral junctions producing the 'rachitic rosary'. The squared configuration of the skull, occasionally seen, results from abnormal remodeling. Because of the weakened and softened nature of the bones, there is often bowing resulting from normal weight-bearing and muscular stresses. Scoliosis, slipped capital femoral epiphyses, triradiate pelvis and basilar invagination may also be seen.

PRIMARY HYPERPARATHYROIDISM

This disorder results from a primary defect in the parathyroid gland with adenomatous or hyperplastic changes resulting in an increased secretion of parathyroid hormone (PTH). Increased bone turnover and remodeling with net increased bone resorption give the overall appearance of osteopenia, as well as characteristic radiographic features of localized bone resorption.

Radiologic diagnosis:
Osteopenia (rarely osteosclerosis)
Subperiosteal bone resorption of the phalangeal shafts and tufts
Bone resorption in intracortical, endosteal, subchondral, and subligamentous sites
Brown tumors
Chondrocalcinosis

Radiologic-Pathologic Considerations

A hallmark of hyperparathyroidism is accelerated bone resorption and fibrous proliferation of the bone marrow, known as osteitis fibrosa cystica. Bone resorption, a result of osteoclast stimulation, occurs at many different sites (intracortical, endosteal, trabecular, subchondral, and subligamentous). Subperiosteal bone resorption, which is most characteristic of hyperparathyroidism (40), is seen in approximately 10% of patients, most commonly on the radial aspects of the middle phalanges of the second and third digits (Fig. 22). Other sites commonly affected include the phalangeal tufts and the metaphyseal cut away zones of the medial aspects of the proximal humerus, femur and tibia. Intracortical bone resorption (cortical tunnelling or striation) (40) is seen in over half the patients with primary hyperparathyroidism

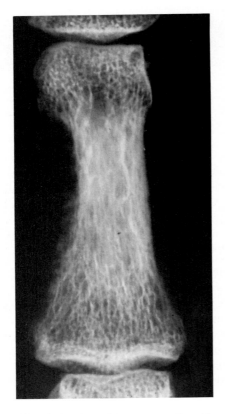

FIG. 22. Subperiosteal bone resorption of radial aspect of middle phalanx is characteristic of hyperparathyroidism.

and is detected with magnification techniques in the tubular bones of the hands. (Fig. 23) Erosions involving the sacroiliac joints, symphysis pubis, distal or medial ends of the clavicle and vertebral body endplates (aggressive Schmorl's nodes) are related to subchondral or subligamentous resorption at sites of mechanical stress and intrinsic high bone turnover. The skull occasionally shows a characteristic 'mottled' radiographic pattern that results from trabecular resorption and remodeling of the diploic space (30). Erosions of the calcaneus and inferior aspect of the distal clavicles are evidence of subligamentous resorption in these sites.

Osteopenia is an end result of these various patterns of bone resorption in many patients with primary hyperparathyroidism. Rarely, however, diffuse osteosclerosis may be demonstrated radiographically, perhaps related to stimulation of osteoblastic bone formation over osteoclastic bone resorption (Fig. 24) (28).

Brown tumors (osteoclastomas) represent focal, bone-replacing lesions most often occurring in the metaphyses and diaphyses of the long bones or the flat bones of the pelvis. Any skeletal site may be involved, however, and the lesions are often polyostolic. The radiographic appearance is diverse, ranging from lytic to sclerotic, benign to aggressive, and from purely destructive to principally expansile (Fig. 25). As a consequence, brown tumors are ''great mimickers'' since their radiographic appearance simulates that of a host of primary or metastatic neoplasms and infections. With restoration of normal parathyroid function, brown tumors may heal if underlying trabecular and cortical architecture has not been completely destroyed.

Chondrocalcinosis due to calcium pyrophosphate dihydrate crystal deposition (CPPD) occurs in 10 to 20% of patients with primary hyperparathyroidism (40). Characteristic chondrocalcinosis can be seen in the hyaline articular cartilage and fibrocartilage of the knee, symphysis pubis, and triangular cartilage of the wrist (Fig. 26).

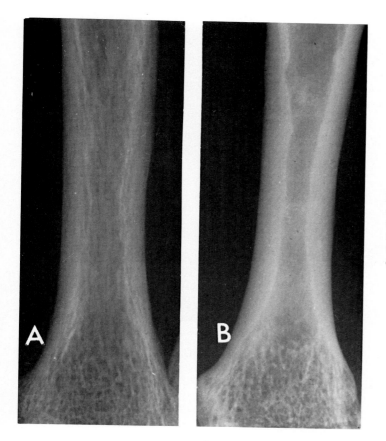

FIG. 23. Increased intracortical tunneling or resorption in the metacarpal of a hyperparathyroid patient (**A**) is contrasted with normal adult metacarpal cortex (**B**).

RENAL OSTEODYSTROPHY

The term renal osteodystrophy (13,22,34) represents the diverse spectrum of skeletal bony changes encountered in patients with chronic uremia due to a variety of renal parenchymal disorders.

Radiologic diagnosis:
Secondary hyperparathyroidism (subperiosteal resorption, intracortical tunnelling, brown tumors)
Osteomalacia/rickets (widened growth plate, splayed and frayed metaphyses, coarsened fuzzy trabeculae, Looser's zones)
Osteoporosis (osteopenia, thinned cortices)
Osteosclerosis (including 'Rugger-Jersey' spine)

Soft tissue calcifications (vascular and periarticular)

Radiologic-Pathologic Considerations

The mechanisms producing the pathologic and radiologic hyperparathyroid skeletal changes observed in renal osteodystrophy are the same as those operable in primary hyperparathyroidism, albeit the appearance is more severe in the former. Resorption of bone in the subperiosteal regions is a prominent feature (Figs. 27 and 28). Marked generalized bone resorption accounts for the frequently observed cortical thinning and overall loss of bone density or osteopenia.

Brown tumors may also be seen in patients

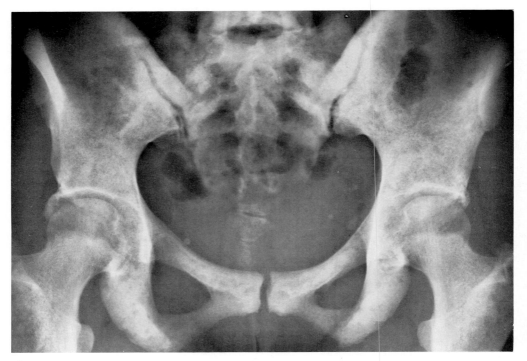

A

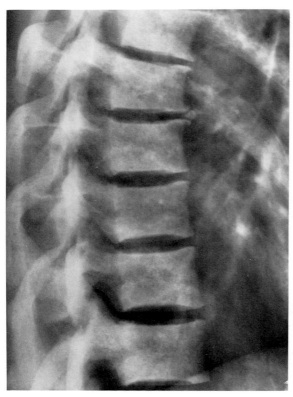

B

FIG. 24. Unusual diffuse osteosclerosis in primary hyperparathyroidism. **A:** The pelvis demonstrates advanced diffuse osteosclerosis of trabecular bone and (**B**) the spine shows diffuse trabecular osteosclerosis.

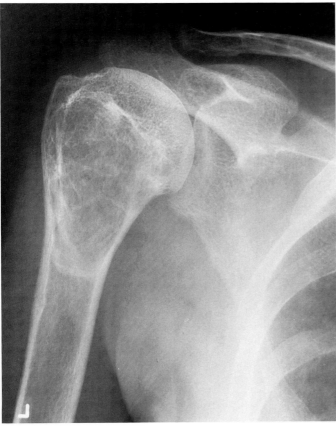

FIG. 25. The radiographic spectrum of brown tumors is shown with involvement of the proximal humerus (**A**).

A

with renal osteodystrophy as a manifestation of secondary hyperparathyroidism; they occur more commonly in uremic children than in adults. Brown tumors were at one time found mainly in patients with primary hyperparathyroidism, but today with earlier detection and treatment of patients with primary hyperparathyroidism and with increasing numbers of patients with chronic renal failure being maintained on dialysis, brown tumors are currently found more frequently in patients with secondary hyperparathyroidism (6).

Osteosclerosis is observed radiographically in approximately 15 to 20% of patients with renal osteodystrophy. The pathophysiology is conjectural, however, the presence of excessive osteoid on trabecular and endosteal surfaces may inhibit osteoclastic bone resorption, while simultaneously the elevated serum cal-

cium phosphate product may cause precipitation of mineral in areas of osteoid, notably, in the spongiosa (8). The typical signs of local osteosclerosis are the "Rugger-Jersey" spine, increased density of the pelvis or metaphyses of long bones, and sclerosis of the skull.

The prevalence of osteomalacic-rachitic alteration in patients with renal osteodystrophy is difficult to estimate due to the overlap of radiologic findings common to both secondary hyperparathyroidism and osteomalacia. However, typical Looser's zones (virtually diagnostic of osteomalacia) are seen in only about 1% of patients with chronic renal disease (34). On the other hand, bowing and bending of the thoracic cage (bell-shaped appearance) and of the pelvis (triradiate appearance) occur in advanced stages.

Insufficiency fractures are occasionally seen

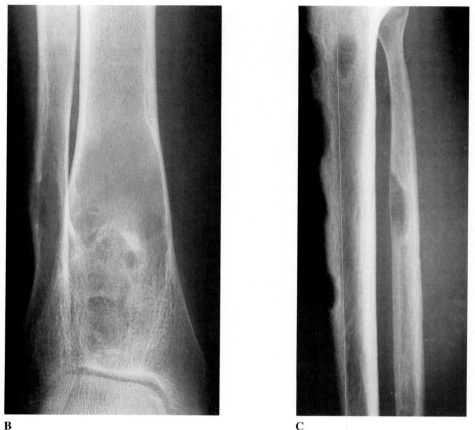

B   C

FIG. 25. *(continued)* Distal tibia (**B**), and tibial shafts (**C**).

in patients with renal osteodystrophy. These may occur as a result of a combination of osteomalacic, osteoporotic and hyperparathyroid changes in the bones. Of note in children is the well-recognized phenomenon of metaphyseal resorption with bowing and fracture leading to slipped epiphyses (Fig. 29), particularly of the capital femoral epiphyses, which occurs in approximately 10% of chronic uremic children with this disorder (32).

Soft tissue calcifications are another prominent feature of renal osteodystrophy. They may be present in vessels, subcutaneous tissue, and viscera (heart, lungs, stomach and kidneys). Large, globular, periarticular calcifications may also be seen especially in patients with severe secondary hyperparathyroidism and elevated calcium phosphate product.

SCURVY

Scurvy (14,29) is a disorder that results from long-term deficiency of vitamin C, the major source of which, is dietary. This disorder, rare in western societies, is more frequently encountered in children (particularly in infants) than in adults and, for the most part, results from a diet of pasteurized or boiled milk (29).

Radiologic diagnosis:

Osteopenia

Increased density and widening of the zone of provisional calcification (white line of Frankl)

Metaphyseal spurs of marginal fractures (Pelkan's sign)

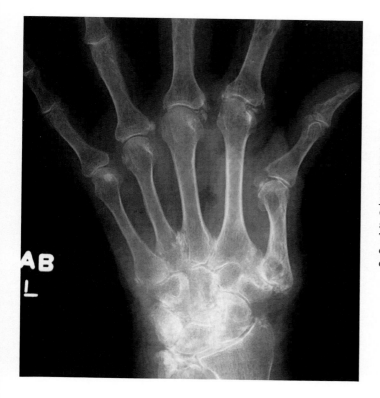

FIG. 26. Marked chondrocalcinosis in a patient with primary hyperparathyroidism. There is hyaline articular cartilage calcification evident at the MCP joints (*open arrows*) and fibrocartilage calcification of the triangular cartilage (*closed arrow*). These findings are characteristic of calcium pyrophosphate dihydrate deposition disease (CPPD).

Transverse zone of radiolucency in the metaphysis ('scurvy line' or Trummerfeld zone) subjacent to the zone of provisional calcification.

Ring of increased density surrounding the epiphysis (Wimberger's sign)

Periosteal elevation

Radiologic-Pathologic Considerations

The pathologic changes seen in scurvy are the results of depression of normal cellular activity such that the ability of supporting tissue to produce and maintain intracellular substance is markedly impaired (3). This suppression also occurs in the osteoblasts resulting in the cessation of normal bone formation. However, resorption continues with resulting osteoporosis.

At the growth plate, although cartilage proliferation is reduced, mineralization is unimpaired and, as a result, the zone of provisional calcification becomes wider and dense (white line of Frankl sign of scurvy) (Fig. 30). Similar changes occur around the epiphyseal ossification center resulting in a thin ring of increased density surrounding the epiphysis (Wimberger's sign of scurvy). Vascular invasion in the zone of provisional calcification ceases and with the suppression of osteoblastic activity, there is a decrease in the formation of bony matrix. This results in sparse trabeculae in the zone of primary and secondary spongiosa. Radiographically, this is seen as a transverse band of radiolucency (the Trummerfeld zone or 'scurvy line') subjacent to the zone of provisional calcification. This represents an area of weakened bone which shows a tendency to fracture with subsequent hemorrhage into the site. The zone of provisional calcification extends beyond the margins of the metaphyses resulting in periosteal elevation and

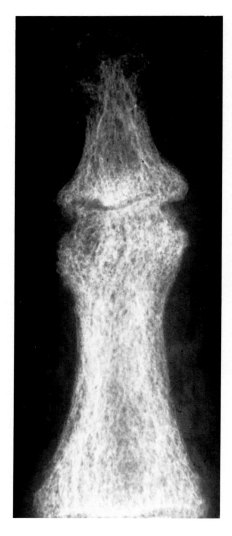

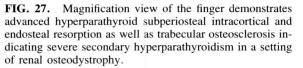

FIG. 27. Magnification view of the finger demonstrates advanced hyperparathyroid subperiosteal intracortical and endosteal resorption as well as trabecular osteosclerosis indicating severe secondary hyperparathyroidism in a setting of renal osteodystrophy.

marginal spur formation (Pelkan's sign). Subepiphyseal infractions ('corner sign') result in various degrees of separation of the epiphyseal plate from the metaphysis, and periosteal elevation from subperiosteal hemorrhage may be quite extensive (Fig. 31).

The above changes are most pronounced in regions of active endochondral bone growth and are best seen in the distal end of the femur (particularly the medial side), proximal and distal ends of the tibia and fibula, the distal end of the radius and ulna, the proximal end of the humerus and the sternal ends of the ribs. Despite the marked changes that occur in these active growth zones, permanent growth disturbances or other abnormalities after treatment are unusual.

HYPERTHYROIDISM

Hyperthyroidism usually occurs as a result of Graves' disease (toxic diffuse goiter), toxic

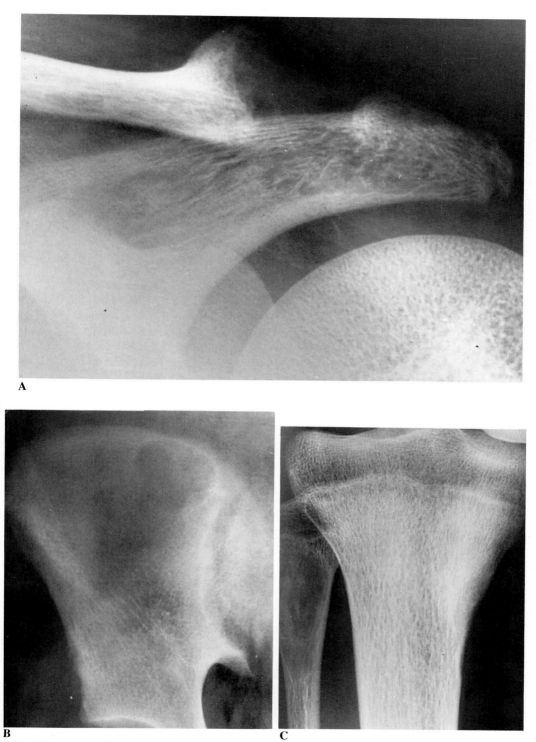

FIG. 28. Advanced renal osteodystrophy in an adolescent. **A:** The shoulder demonstrates classical erosion of the distal clavicle. **B:** The pelvis demonstrates diffuse trabecular sclerosis, erosion of the SI joint and a brown tumor of the iliac crest. **C:** The proximal tibia demonstrates sclerosis of metaphyseal trabecular bone, subperiosteal resorption of the metaphyseal cut away zone and a slightly expansile brown tumor of the proximal fibular metaphysis.

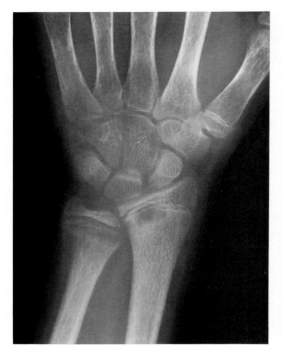

FIG. 29. Renal osteodystrophy. In this patient with secondary hyperparathyroidism a brown tumor is evident in the distal radial metaphysis and a fracture through the distal ulnar metaphysis results in slipping of the ulnar epiphysis.

multinodular goiter (35), or in response to excessive replacement therapy in patients with hypothyroidism. Resulting elevated levels of triiodothyronine (T3) and thyroxine (T4) cause a hypermetabolic state and accelerated bone resorption (14,24,35).

Radiologic findings:
Osteopenia
Osteoporotic fractures of spine, wrist and hips
Increased intracortical bone resorption in hands
Accelerated skeletal maturation (in children)

Radiologic-Pathologic Considerations

The hypermetabolic state present in hyperthyroidism results in catabolism of protein and subsequent loss of connective tissue. There is a net increase of bone resorption over bone formation ultimately contributing to generalized osteopenia. A prominent radiographic pattern is intracortical tunneling or striation most evident in the tubular bones of the hands and feet and occurring in approximately 50% of patients (Fig. 32) (21,24).

Bone resorption causes overall loss of bone density in the skull, spine, pelvis, and long

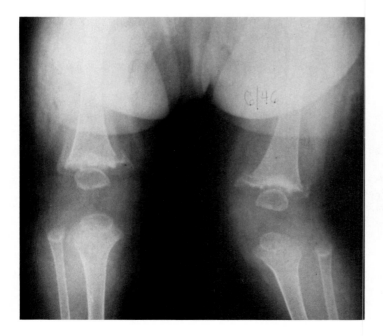

FIG. 30. Radiographic changes in scurvy. The zone of provisional calcification in both distal femora is becoming dense (white line of Frankl sign of scurvy). This zone is seen to extend beyond the margins of the metaphyses resulting in periosteal elevation and marginal spur formation (Pelkan's sign).

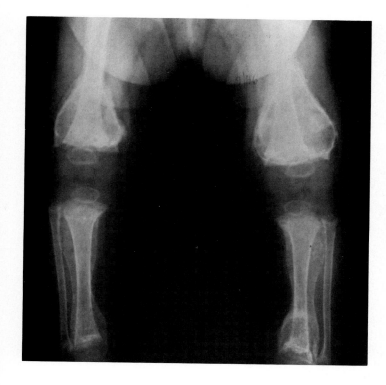

FIG. 31. Extensive periosteal elevation in scurvy. An AP radiograph of both lower extremities in a patient with scurvy demonstrates evidence of extensive subperiosteal hemorrhage with marked periosteal elevation.

bones. The spinal changes are similar to those found in involutional osteoporosis and include biconcave vertebral bodies ('codfish vertebrae') and wedge deformities with resultant kyphosis. Fractures may also be seen in other bones, especially the femoral neck. Soft tissue changes of pretibial myxoedema may be present.

OSTEOGENESIS IMPERFECTA

Osteogenesis imperfecta (OI) (9,16) is the most common heritable form of osteoporosis, although its occurrence is relatively uncommon. The term actually refers to a group of 4 diseases that are often congenital, always heritable, with either autosomal dominant or recessive inheritance. The classical clinical triad in this disease are: 1) fragility of the bones, 2) blue sclerae, and 3) deafness. Two forms are recognized: the congenita form in which life

expectancy is usually short, and the tarda form in which life expectancy is normal.

Radiologic diagnosis:
Generalized osteopenia
Multiple fractures with bowed bones
Wormian bones
Exuberant callus formation

Radiologic-Pathologic Considerations

The abnormal maturation of collagen in this disorder results in a primary defect in bone matrix and when accompanied by defective mineralization results in generalized osteopenia of the axial and appendicular skeleton (9). The long bones may either be thin and gracile, (usually in the tarda form) (Fig. 33), or they may be short and robust (exclusively in the congenita form) (Fig. 34). Multiple fractures (usually transverse) occur predominantly in the

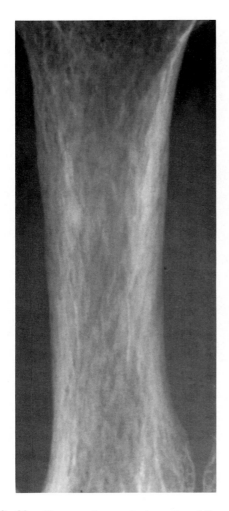

FIG. 32. Osseous changes in hyperthyroidism. A magnification radiograph of a metacarpal in this patient with thyrotoxicosis demonstrates prominent cortical tunneling or striations. This appearance is the result of increased intracortical bone resorption.

lower extremities, typically producing bowing deformities. This bowing may serve as an indication of the severity of the disease since it tends to correlate with the number of fractures (Fig. 35). Avulsion fractures are also common. Fracture healing is usually normal but demonstrates exuberant callus formation (Fig. 33) and sometimes pseudarthrosis. Inevitably, the ex-

tremities become shortened, which accounts for the short stature seen in most cases (16). Premature degenerative changes are often seen involving the joints, primarily from intra-articular fractures and ligamentous laxity.

The skull and axial skeleton also show typical changes. Wormian bones (or unfused accessory ossification centers in the occipital skull), enlargement of the paranasal sinuses, platybasia and basilar impression are frequent findings. Severe kyphoscoliosis, biconcave and wedged vertebral bodies, (Fig. 36), triradiate pelvis, and protrusio-acetabuli may be present.

Deafness, usually from otosclerosis, is present in about half of the patients. The patients often appear dwarfed with kyphoscoliosis. Translucent teeth (deciduous and permanent) result from defective dentine formation (dentinogenesis imperfecta). Hydrocephalus or spinal cord compression may occur and hypermobility of the joints is common.

OSTEOPENIA ASSOCIATED WITH MARROW REPLACEMENT AND EXPANSION

Disorders in which there is marrow replacement, infiltration, or expansion are sometimes associated with osteopenia or secondary osteoporosis. Although these processes do not meet the histologic criteria of osteoporosis because of abnormal marrow elements, their radiographic appearance may be similar to that of primary osteoporosis. Therefore, diffuse marrow disorders must be included in the differential considerations of generalized osteopenia. These conditions include multiple myeloma, leukemia, metastatic disease, Gaucher's disease, and chronic anemias (sickle cell and thalassemia). Multiple myeloma and metastatic disease follow the distribution of red marrow, thus, the axial skeleton demonstrates predominant involvement although the proximal appendicular skeleton may show prominent focal and diffuse endosteal scalloping (Fig. 37). In the

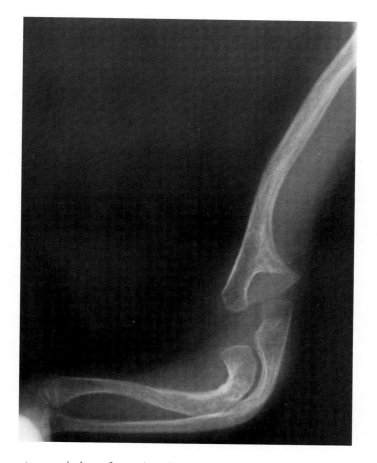

FIG. 33. Severe osteogenesis imperfecta. An AP radiograph of the right upper extremity in this child demonstrates severe bowing deformities of the long bones that are the result of numerous previous fractures and serve as an indication of the severity of the process.

case of myeloma, diffuse osteopenia is mediated by the osteoclast-activating factor (OAF), while in metastatic disease, osteopenia results from tumor destruction of bone tissue, and is more focal in appearance. Early, these disorders may be difficult to differentiate radiographically from the involutional osteoporoses. Clinical, laboratory, and computed tomographic studies are often necessary to distinguish these entities. Magnetic resonance imaging may play an important role here as well (Fig. 38).

The chronic anemias and Gaucher's disease produce osteoporosis, primarily by marrow expansion in the former and by combined marrow expansion and bone destruction in the latter (Fig. 39). Other helpful radiographic findings include bone modeling and remodeling errors ("Ehrlenmeyer flask" appearance) of the long bones in Gaucher's disease. Bone infarcts and avascular necrosis may be evident, particularly in sickle cell disease and Gaucher's disease. Other typical findings include "H-shaped" vertebrae (sickle cell) and a "hair-on-end" appearance of the skull in chronic anemias, especially thalassemia.

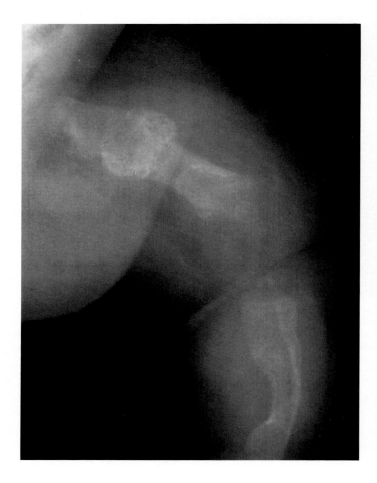

FIG. 34. Osteogenesis imperfecta (congenita form). Infant with OI demonstrates the long bones to be short and thick characteristic of the congenita form. A transverse fracture of the mid femur with exuberant callus formation is also evident.

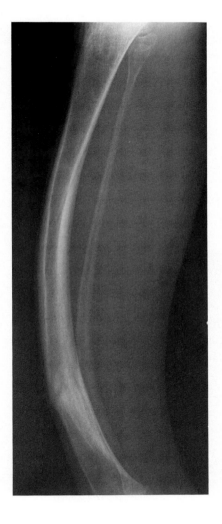

FIG. 35. Osteogenesis imperfecta (tarda form). In this adolescent patient with OI, a lateral radiograph demonstrates the tibia and fibula to be thin and gracile. In addition, note the bowing deformities and a healing fracture in the distal one-third of the tibia.

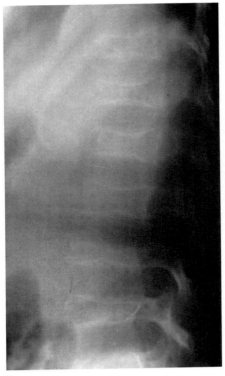

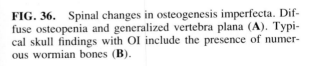

FIG. 36. Spinal changes in osteogenesis imperfecta. Diffuse osteopenia and generalized vertebra plana (**A**). Typical skull findings with OI include the presence of numerous wormian bones (**B**).

A

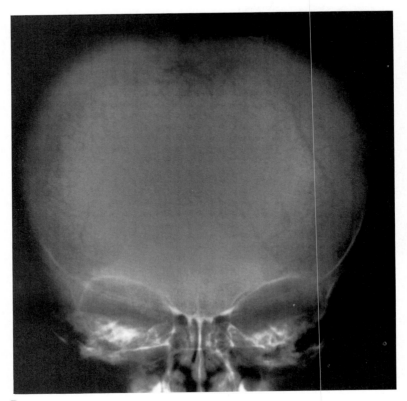

B

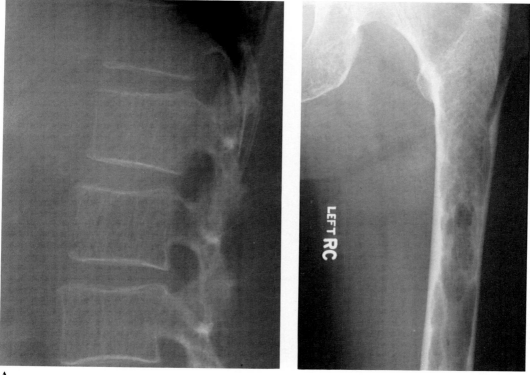

A   **B**

FIG. 37. Osteopenia in multiple myeloma. Lateral radiograph of the lumbar spine demonstrates severe mottled demineralization with compression deformities (**A**) and AP radiograph (**B**) of the femur demonstrates irregular endosteal scalloping in a patient with advanced multiple myeloma.

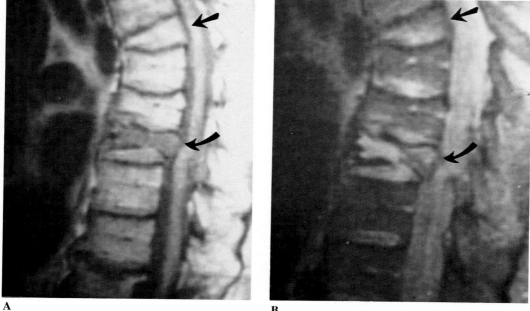

A   **B**

FIG. 38. Magnetic resonance study of an elderly woman with severe osteopenia and vertebral fractures due to simple osteoporosis (*straight arrow*) and to metastatic focus (*curved arrow*). On T1-weighted image (**A**), simple fracture has high signal from marrow fat comparable to adjacent levels, while metastatic fracture has low signal representing tumor. On T2-weighted image (**B**), metastatic tumor becomes bright (*curved arrow*) while simple fracture does not.

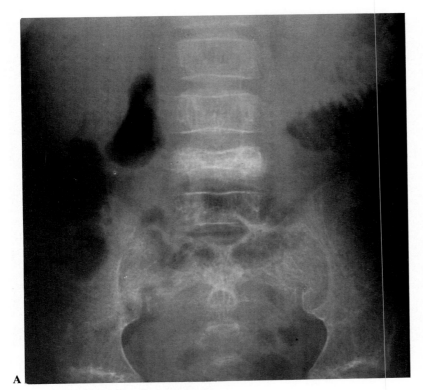

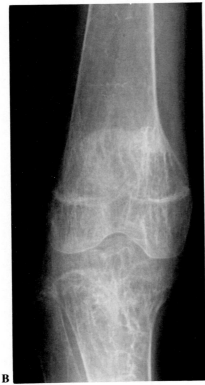

FIG. 39. Osteopenia in thalassemia. **A:** AP radiograph of the spine and pelvis demonstrates severe generalized osteopenia with marked accentuation of the trabecular pattern while AP radiograph of the knee (**B**) demonstrates expanded medullary canal, thinned cortices, and accentuated trabeculation in a child with advanced radiographic manifestations of thalassemia.

REFERENCES

1. Bondy, P.K. (1980): The adrenal cortex. In: *Metabolic Control and Disease*, 8th ed. edited by P.K. Bondy and L.E. Rosenberg, p. 1427. W. B. Saunders Co., Philadelphia.
2. Bohr, H., and Schadt, O. (1983): Bone mineral content of femoral bone and lumbar spine measured in women with fracture of the femoral neck by dual photon absorptiometry. *Clin. Ortho.*, 179:240–245.
3. Dequeker, J., Gautama, K., and Roh, Y.S. (1974): Femoral trabecular patterns in asymptomatic spinal osteoporosis and femoral neck fracture. *Clin. Radiol.*, 25:243–246.
4. Dodds, W.J., and Steinbach, H.K. (1968): Primary hyperparathyroidism and articular cartilage calcification. *A.J.R.*, 104:884–892.
5. Doyle, F.H., Gutteridge, D.H., Joplin, G.F., and Fraser, R. (1967): An assessment of radiologic criteria used in the study of spinal osteoporosis. *Brit. J. Radiol.*, 40:241–250.
6. Ehrlich, G.W., Genant, H.K., and Kolb, F.O. (1983): Secondary hyperparathyroidism and brown tumors in a patient with gluten enteropathy. *A.J.R.*, 141:381–383.
7. Genant, H.K. (1982): Radiography of acute and chronic osteopenia. *Med. Times*, May: 57s–70s.
8. Genant, H.K., Baron, J.M., Straus, F.H., et al. (1975): Osteosclerosis in primary hyperparathyroidism. *Am. J. Med.*, 59:104–113.
9. Goldman, A.B. (1981): Collagen diseases, epiphyseal dysplasias, and related conditions. In: *Diagnosis of Bone and Joint Disorders*, edited by D. Resnick and G. Niwayama, p. 2505. W. B. Saunders Co., Philadelphia.
10. Hall, M.C. (1961): The trabecular patterns of the neck of the femur with particular reference to changes in osteoporosis. *Can. Med. Ass. J.*, 85:1141–1144.
11. Horsman, A., Nordin, C., and Simpson, M. (1982): Cortical and trabecular bone status in elderly women with femoral neck fracture. *Clin. Ortho.* 166:143–151.
12. Hurxthal, L.M., Vose, G.P., and Dotter, W.E. (1969); Densitometric and visual observations of spinal radiographs. *Geriatrics*, 5:93–106.
13. Irby, R., Edwards, W.M., and Gatter, R. (1975): Articular complications of homotransplanation and chronic renal hemodialysis. *J. Rheumatol.*, 2:91–99.
14. Jaffe, H.L. (1972): *Metabolic, degenerative and inflammatory diseases of bones and joints*, p. 353. Lea & Febiger, Philadelphia.
15. Jowsey, J., and Johnson, K.A. (1972): Juvenile osteoporosis: Bone findings in seven patients. *J. Pediatr.*, 81:511–517.
16. King, J.D., and Bobechko, W.P. (1971): Osteogenesis imperfecta. An orthopaedic description and surgical review. *J. Bone Joint Surg.*, 53B:72–89.
17. Kleerekoper, M., Parfitt, A.M., and Ellis, B.I. (1984): Measurement of vertebral fracture rates in osteoporosis. *In: Osteoporosis*, edited by C. Christiansen, C.D. Arnaud, B.E.C. Nordin, A.M. Parfitt, W.A. Peck, and R.L. Riggs, pp. 103–109. Aalborg Stiftsborgtrykkeri, Glostrup, Denmark.
18. Koch, J.C. (1917): The laws of bone architecture. *Am. J. Anat.*, 21:177–298.
19. Kranendonk, D.H., Jurist, J.M., and Lee, H. (1972): Femoral trabecular patterns and bone mineral content. *J. Bone Joint Surg.*, 54A:1472–1478.
20. Madell, S.H., and Freeman, L.M. (1964): Avascular necrosis of bone in Cushing's syndrome. *Radiology*, 83:1068–1070.
21. Meema, H.E., and Schatz, D.L. (1970). Simple radiologic demonstration of cortical bone loss in thyrotoxicosis. *Radiology*, 97:9–15.
22. Mehls, O., Ritz, E., Krempien, B., Gilli, G., Link, K., Willich, E., and Scharer K. (1975): Slipped epiphyses in renal osteodystrophy. *Arch. Dis. Child*, 50:545–554.
23. Melton, L.J., Wahner, H.W., Richelson, L.S., O'Fallon, W.M., and Riggs, B.L. (1986): Osteoporosis and the Risk of Hip Fracture. *Am J Epidemial*. 124:254–261.
24. Meunier, P.J., S-Bianchi, G.G., Edouard, C.N., Bernard, J.C., Courpron, P., and Vignon, G.E. (1972): Bony manifestations of thyrotoxicosis. *Orthoped. Clin. North. Am.*, 3:745–752.
25. Perry, H.M., Weinstein, R.S., Teitelbaum, S.L., Avioli, L.V., and Fallon, M.D. (1982): Pseudofractures in the absence of osteomalacia. *Skel. Radiol.*, 8:17–19.
26. Pitt, M.J. (1981): Rachitic and osteomalacic syndromes. *Radiol. Clin. North Am.,*, 19:581–599.
27. Pitt, M.J. (1981): Rickets and osteomalacia. In: *Diagnosis of Bone and Joint Disorders*, edited by D. Resnick and G. Niwayama, p. 1682. W. B. Saunders Co., Philadelphia.
28. Resnick, D. (1981): Disorders of other endocrine glands and of pregnancy. In: *Diagnosis of Bone and Joint Disorders*, edited by D. Resnick and G. Niwayama, p. 1860. W. B. Saunders Co., Philadelphia.
29. Resnick, D. (1981): Hypervitaminosis and hypovitaminosis. In: *Diagnosis of Bone and Joint Disorders*, edited by D. Resnick and G. Niwayama, p. 1385. W. B. Saunders, Philadelphia.
30. Resnick, D., and Niwayawa, G. (eds.) (1981): *Diagnosis of Bone and Joint Disorders*. W. B. Saunders Co., Philadelphia, p. 1638.
31. Riggs, B.L., and Melton, J.L. (1983): Evidence of two distinct syndromes of involutional osteoporosis. *Am. J. Med.*, 75:899.
32. Riggs, B.L., and Melton, L.J. (1986): Involutional osteoporosis. *N. Eng. J. Med.*, 314(26):1676–1686.
33. Riggs, B.L., Seeman, E., Hodgson, S.F., Taves, D.R., and O'Fallon, W.M. (1982): Effect of the fluoride/calcium regimen on vertebral fracture occurrence in postmenopausal osteoporosis. *N. Eng. J. Med.*, 306(8):446–450.
34. Ritz, E., Krempien, B., Riedash, G., Kuhn, H., Hackeng, W., and Heuck, F. (1971): Dialysis bone disease. *Proc. Europ. Dial. Transpl. Assoc.*, 8:131–525.
35. Robbina, J., Rall, J.E., and Gorden, P. (1980): The thyroid and iodine metabolism. In: *Metabolic Control and Disease*, 8th ed. edited by P.K. Bondy and L.E. Rosenberg. W. B. Saunders, Co. Philadelphia.
36. Sartoris, D.J., Clopton, P., Nemcek, A., Dowd, C.,

and Resnick, D. (1986): Vertebral-body collapse in focal and diffuse disease. *Radiology,* 160:479–483.

37. Singh, M., Nagrath, A.R., and Maini, P.S. (1970): Changes in trabecular pattern of the upper end of the femur as an index of osteoporosis. *J. Bone Joint Surg.,* 52A(3):457–467.

38. Singh, M., Riggs, B.L., Beabout, J.W., and Jowsey, J. (1972): Femoral trabecular-pattern index for

evaluation of spinal osteoporosis. *Ann. Int. Med.,* 77:63–67.

39. Sissons, H.A. (1956): The osteoporosis of Cushing's syndrome. *J. Bone Joint Surg.,* 38B:418–433.

40. Steinbach, H.L., Gordon, G.S., Eisenberg, E., et al. (1961): Primary hyperparathyroidism: A correlation of roentgen, clinical and pathologic features. *A.J.R.,* 86:329–343.

Osteoporosis: Etiology, Diagnosis, and Management, edited by B. Lawrence Riggs and L. Joseph Melton, III. Raven Press, New York © 1988.

8

Quantitative Computed Tomography in Assessment of Osteoporosis

*,**Harry K. Genant, *,†Bruce Ettinger, **Steven T. Harris, *Jon E. Block, and *Peter Steiger

*Departments of Radiology, and **Medicine, University of California, San Francisco, California 94143; †Department of Internal Medicine, Kaiser Permanente Medical Group, San Francisco, California 94143

The recent attention given to osteoporosis by the media has been focused on informing women of the "silent epidemic" that results in an insidious loss of bone mass primarily evident through crush fractures of the vertebrae, and fractures of the wrist and hip. Public consciousness of this disorder has also been heightened by the toll in health care dollars measuring approximately four billion dollars annually. The growing importance of this public health issue has also been underscored by the recent U.S. Congressional Action designating one week in May as the Annual National Osteoporosis Week, by the convening of conferences at the National Institutes of Health on this subject in 1984 and 1987, and by the formation of a national foundation whose activities are specific to this condition. Among the conclusions reached by the NIH conference panel was a recommendation that studies be undertaken to develop accurate, safe and inexpensive methods for determining the level of risk for osteoporosis, early diagnosis of the condition, and assessment of the clinical course of the disease (50).

QUANTITATIVE BONE MINERAL ANALYSES

In recent years considerable effort has been expended in the development of methods for quantitatively assessing the skeleton so that osteoporosis can be detected early, its progression and response to therapy carefully monitored, and its risk effectively ascertained. There is not yet, however, a consensus on which method or methods are most efficacious for diagnosing and monitoring of the individual patient or for extensive screening of large populations. In this regard, the selection of anatomic sites and of methods for quantifying skeletal mass is of considerable current importance.

The skeleton as a whole is composed of about 80% cortical or compact bone and 20% trabecular or cancellous bone (2). The appendicular skeleton is composed of predominantly cortical bone, while the spine is composed of a combination of cancellous bone predominantly in the vertebral bodies and compact bone mostly in the dense endplates and posterior elements. Trabecular bone, because of its high surface-to-volume ratio, has a presumed turnover rate about eight times that of compact bone, and is highly responsive to metabolic stimuli (24,63). This high turnover rate in trabecular bone makes it a prime site for detection of early bone loss as well as the monitoring of response to various interventions. The clinical and epidemiological observation that osteoporotic fractures occur first in the vertebral bodies or distal radius, areas of predominantly trabecular bone, substantiates physiologic studies showing a differential early loss from this bone compartment (24).

Numerous methods have been used for quantitative assessment of the skeleton in osteoporosis with variable precision, accuracy and sensitivity. Precision here means longitudinal reproducibility in serial studies, accuracy means reliability that the measured value reflects true mineral content, and sensitivity means capacity to readily separate an abnormal from a normal population or to readily detect changes with time in a patient or in a population.

The first methods to be developed were radiogrammetry (26) and photon absorptiometry (8,44,64,67) which measure primarily cortical bone of the peripheral appendicular skeleton. Recently, techniques have become available that can quantify bone mineral content in the spine, the site of early osteoporosis. Quantitative computed tomography (QCT) (2,7,11–15,22,23,25,27–34,37,38,41,49,53–56,58,60–62,65) provides a measure of purely trabecular bone of the vertebral spongiosum, or other sites, while dual photon absorptiometry (DPA) (16,36,41,48,52,57,59,68) measures an integral of compact and calcellous bone of the spine, hip, or entire skeleton. The focus of this chapter is on the clinical application of QCT and its comparison with other methods commonly used to quantitatively assess the skeleton.

COMPUTED TOMOGRAPHY FOR BONE MINERAL ANALYSIS

Computed tomography (CT) has been widely investigated and applied in recent years as a means for noninvasive quantitative bone mineral determination (2,7,11–15,22,23,25,27–34,37,38,41,49,53–56,58,60–62,65). The usefulness of computed tomography for measurement of bone mineral lies in its ability to provide a quantitative image and, thereby, measure trabecular, cortical or integral bone, centrally or peripherally. For measuring the spine, the potential advantages of QCT (28,30,56) over other techniques are its capability for precise 3-dimensional anatomic localization providing a direct density measurement, and its capability for spatial separation of highly responsive cancellous bone from less responsive compact bone. The lumbar vertebrae contain substantial amounts of compact bone, with only part of the spinal mineral being high turnover trabecular bone. The sensitivity of a technique measuring an integral of compact and cancellous bone (such as area projection with DPA) may be low compared to QCT due to inclusion of low-turnover compact bone and extraosseous mineral such as osteophytes, sclerosis due to fractures and osteophytosis, or aortic calcification. The selective localization and the direct density measurement provided by QCT permit exclusion of these causes of low sensitivity or error and inclusion of purely trabecular bone.

QCT has been shown to measure changes in trabecular mineral content in the spine and in the radius and tibia with sensitivity and precision (2,7,11–15,22,23,25,27–34,37,38,41,49,53–56,58,60–62,65). The extraction of this quantitative information from the CT image, however, requires sophisticated calibration and positioning techniques and careful technical monitoring. Specifically designed, small-scale CT scanners using isotope or X-ray sources have also been developed and applied, principally on a research basis, for measurement of the appendicular trabecular and cortical skeleton (34,60).

TECHNICAL CONSIDERATIONS FOR VERTEBRAL QCT

Techniques developed at the University of California (15,27,28) allow quantitative measurements on commercially available CT scanners. The single energy measurement protocol requires that the patient be scanned with a reference standard (Fig. 1) containing solutions of varying K_2HPO_4 concentrations. Using a scout view for localization, one 8 to 10 mm thick slice is measured through the center of 2 to 4 noncompressed vertebral bodies (usually T12–L3) with the scanner gantry tilted such that the slice lies parallel to the endplates. Each vertebra is then evaluated as follows:

1. The mean Hounsfield units (HU) of the test solutions are plotted against their concentrations (BMD) and the linear regression with slope S and intercept I is calculated (Fig. 2)

$$HU = S \times BMD + I \qquad (1)$$

2. An elliptical region of interest (ROI) of approximately 3 to 4 cm^2 is placed in the purely trabecular anterior portion of the vertebral body avoiding the base venous complex and the cortical rim. The bone mineral density (BMD) in mg/cm^3 K_2HPO_4 equivalent can then be computed from the mean value of the ROI in Hounsfield units (HU) as (9):

$$BMD = \frac{HU - I}{S} \qquad (2)$$

For the dual energy technique each vertebrae is scanned twice at different energies. The bone mineral density can then be computed analogous to the single energy case as (37):

$$BMD = \frac{(HU_1 - I_1) - (HU_2 - I_2)}{S_1 - S_2}$$

Where:

HU_1: mean of ROI in Hounsfield units for energy 1

I_1: intercept of linear regression for energy 1 in HU

S_1: slope of linear regression for energy 1 in $HU/g\ cm^{-3}$

HU_2, I_2, S_2: as HU_1, I_1, S_1 for energy 2

A single energy study takes 10 min and the radiation exposure is approximately 100-300 mrem (1/10th of the dose of a routine CT study) (10). The radiation dose can be higher (up to 500 mrem) on some CT systems on which the manufacturers have restricted the capability for reducing kVp or mAs settings.

The precision (reproducibility) of vertebral QCT in humans is 1 to 3% for single-energy (80 kVp) and 3 to 5% for dual-energy (80 kVp/140 kVp) techniques (15,28,30). Recent improvements in CT scanner technology (with GE 9800 scanners) have further increased precision and reduced radiation exposure, i.e., a cadaver repositioned and scanned five times (at 100 mrem) resulted in a coefficient of variation of 0.32% for single-energy determination and 1.68% for dual-energy determination (30).

The accuracy of single-energy QCT is 1 to 2% for K_2HPO_4 solutions, and 5 to 15% for human vertebral specimens spanning a wide age-range (1,22,32,48) (Figs. 3 and 4, Table 1). The accuracy for QCT (and DPA), however, can be reduced in the elderly osteoporotic population (2,44,37,43). In the case of DPA, vertebral compression with callous formation, angular and scoliotic deformity, hypertrophy of articular facets, discogenic sclerosis or marginal osteophytosis, and extraosseous calcification, which are widespread in the elderly and are included in the integral measurement, may reduce accuracy as well as reproducibility of vertebral measurements (30). In the case of QCT, the sources of error are different but are partially correctable. The presence of fatty yellow marrow in the vertebral body reduces the spinal mineral equivalent by about 7 mg per 10% fat by volume (7,14,22,29); therefore, in the adult population, single energy QCT (SEQCT) with the GE9800 at 80 kVp is associated with an underestimation of bone mineral of about 20 to 30 mg/cm^3 (15,30). When scanning at higher energies, the relative fat error increases slightly (37,43), but does not preclude clinically meaningful single energy QCT measurements (7,14).

The underestimation of SEQCT can be partially corrected by applying an age-matched correction from the vertebral marrow fat data of Dunnill (17) and including the fat variation in the estimated error of the mean (Fig. 5). This leaves a residual uncertainty of 5 to 6 mg/cm^3 (1 SD), which is small when compared

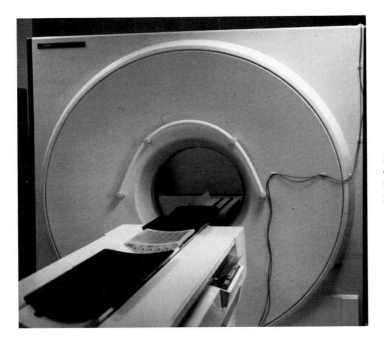

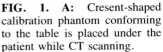

FIG. 1. A: Cresent-shaped calibration phantom conforming to the table is placed under the patient while CT scanning.

with the normal biologic variation of 15 to 20 mg/cm³ or with the large decrements observed from health to disease, typically on the order of 30 to 100 mg/cm³ (14,32,38). Since the fat-induced inaccuracy is only about 1/3 to 1/6 that of the biologic variation or pathologic range, age-based corrections for fat are generally not used. Alternatively, dual energy QCT (1,2,7,12,14,22,27,29,37) can be used to reduce the fat error to about 3 to 6%, but at a cost of lower longitudinal reproducibility, higher radiation exposure and some technical effort. Dual energy QCT is considered unnecessary, however, for most clinical applications. But, when highly accurate measurements are needed, as in special research applications, both single and dual-energy QCT can be performed initially at baseline, and then single-energy QCT alone can be applied for longitudinal follow-up, thus maintaining high precision.

CLINICAL AVAILABILITY OF QCT

Rapid technological advances in CT, including computed projection radiography, highly stable electronics and improved dose efficiency, mean that many of the advanced CT scanners worldwide may be adapted for QCT measurements relatively inexpensively. Recent reductions in patient scanning time and radiation exposure make this an attractive technique for noninvasive bone mass measurement. We have assessed (30,33) the scanner independence of vertebral QCT measurement by determining the interscanner variability on four separate CT scanners using these techniques (Fig. 6). A coefficient of variation between scanners of 3 to 4% was found, indicating that, with careful and appropriate calibration, normative data and clinical results obtained on a scanner at one site may be extrapolated to those obtained at different sites. Currently, QCT vertebral mineral determination by this approach has been implemented at over 800 sites encompassing a wide geographic distribution and a wide array of commercial scanners. With a worldwide distribution of approximately 8,000 advanced CT body scanners, the capability now exists for widespread application of vertebral bone mineral determination by quantitative computed tomography.

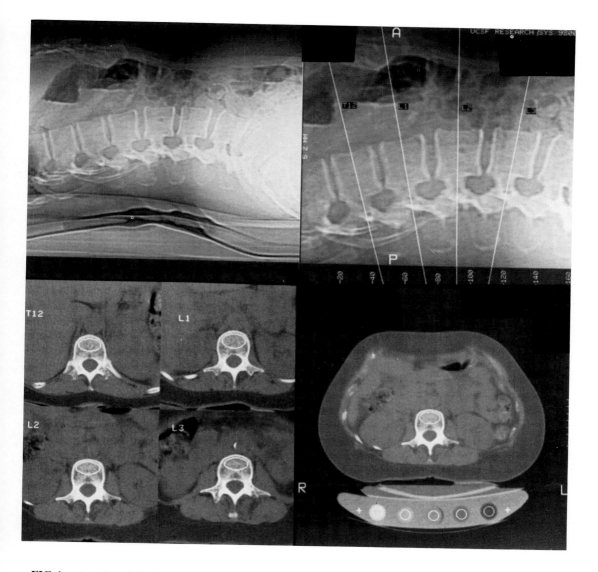

FIG 1. *(continued)* **B:** Quantitative CT using the GE 9800 CT scanner. Lateral scout view provides rapid and simple localization approach in which the midplane of 4 vertebral bodies are defined on the video monitor and a single 10-mm-thick section is obtained at each level. An oval region of interest, centered in the mid vertebral body, is used to determine cancellous bone mineral content (mg/cm^3), while circular regions of interest are used to quantify the K_2HPO_4 solutions in the calibration phantom.

CLINICAL APPLICATIONS OF QUANTITATIVE COMPUTED TOMOGRAPHY

The QCT techniques for vertebral mineral determination have been used to study skeletal changes in osteoporosis and other metabolic bone diseases. Longitudinal and cross-sectional bone mass measurements have been obtained at UCSF in over 2,500 patients seen clinically or on research protocols. The results presented here illustrate the use of QCT spinal mineral

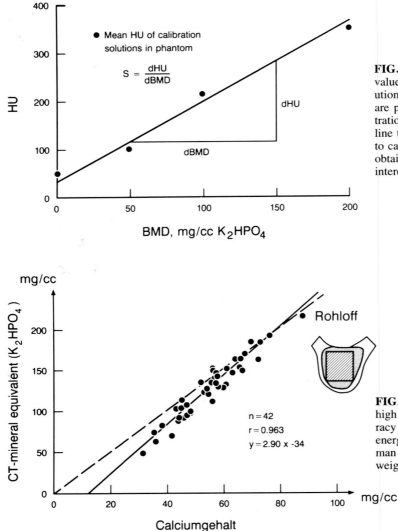

FIG. 2. The mean attenuation values (HU) of the K_2HPO_4 solutions in the calibration phantom are plotted against their concentrations (BMD). The regression line through these points is used to calibrate the mean attenuation obtained from the oval region of interest in the vertebral body.

FIG. 3. Rohloff (36) showed high correlation and high accuracy (8% dispersion) for single energy QCT measurement of human vertebrae versus ash weight.

measurement in the delineation of normal age-related bone loss, in the evaluation of estrogen effects on bone, in the assessment of fracture threshold and risk, and in the study of the effects of various exercise regimens on bone mineral.

Age-Related Bone Loss

The normal ranges of vertebral mineral and age-related bone losses were determined from cross-sectional studies (11,15,30,31,33) of 120 normal males and 203 normal females aged 20 to 80 years (Figs. 7A and B). The normal mean value for young males and females is approximately 175 mg/cm³. Males, by linear regression, lose an average 0.72%/year so that by age 75, the mineral content is reduced by 40% to approximately 110 mg/cm³. Females, by cubic regression, lose an average 1.2%/year, which is accelerated at menopause, and by age 75, mineral content is reduced by 50%

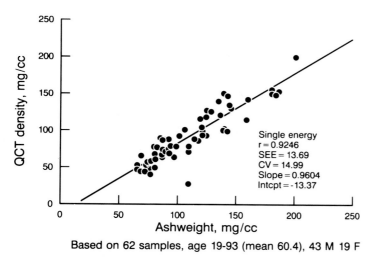

Based on 62 samples, age 19-93 (mean 60.4), 43 M 19 F

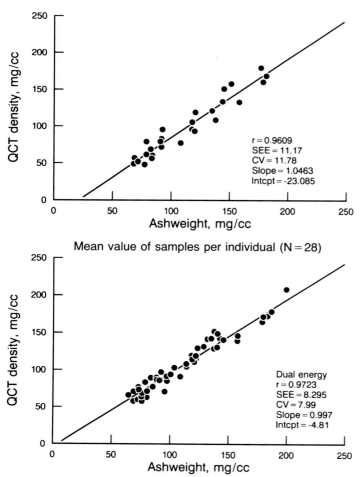

Mean value of samples per individual (N = 28)

Based on 62 samples, age 19-93 (mean 60.4), 43 M 19 F

FIG. 4. A. The accuracy of single energy QCT is shown for fresh vertebral specimen (derived from 62 samples) from 28 cadavers (20 males and 8 females with a mean age of 60). **B.** When the several vertebrae from each cadaver are averaged, as is done in clinical practice, the accuracy improves. The predictive error of 11 mg/cc is acceptable diagnostically because of the large decrements observed cross-sectionally from health to disease, typically 30 to 100 mg/cc. **C.** Dual energy QCT reduces accuracy errors (average underestimation and residual dispersion) approximately twofold over single energy QCT.

TABLE 1. *Comparison between spinal QCT and DPA*

	QCT	DPA
Measurement	Trabecular	Integral
Sensitivity	3X	1X
Precision	1.5– 5%	2–4%
Accuracy	5–15%	5%
Radiation	100–500mRem	10–20mRem
Time	10–15 min	30–45 min

to approximately 90 mg/cm³. Correcting for age-related marrow fat alters the observed rates of loss by only about 10%, e.g., in females, 1.08%/year versus 1.2%/year (Fig. 5) (15,30). These rates of loss are significantly greater than the cross-sectional results of approximately 0.7% per year found when integral spinal mineral was assessed by DPA in females from age 20 to 80 years (57) and by *in vitro* studies of integral lumbar spine density (6,66). However, other *in vitro* studies which have examined the purely trabecular portion of the spine have corroborated rates of loss by QCT with values of approximately 0.8% per year in men (3), and 1.2% per year in women (69).

Influence of Estrogen on Skeletal Integrity in Women

The importance of estrogen in maintaining skeletal mass in women has now been shown

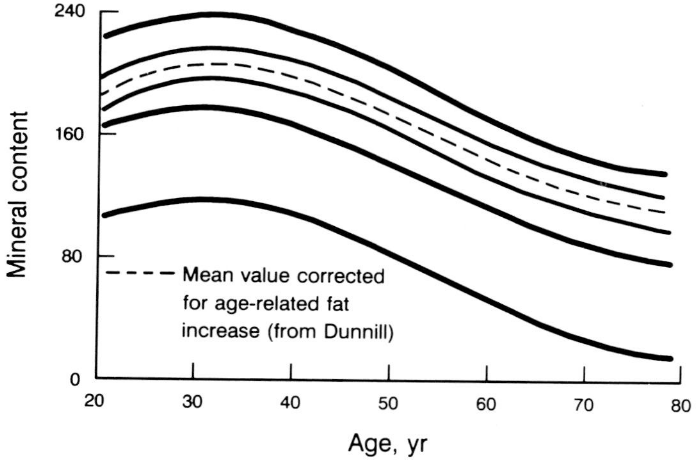

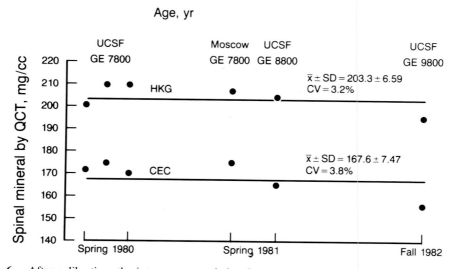

FIG. 5. Normal female vertebral cancellous mineral content (in mg/cm³ K_2HPO_4) versus age. (——) mean and 95% confidence interval; and (----) corrected mean value and 95% confidence interval of the corrected mean based upon age-related fat from Dunnill, ref. 51.

FIG. 6. After calibration, the interscanner variation for two individuals was 3 to 4% indicating that data from one scanner can be extrapolated from another.

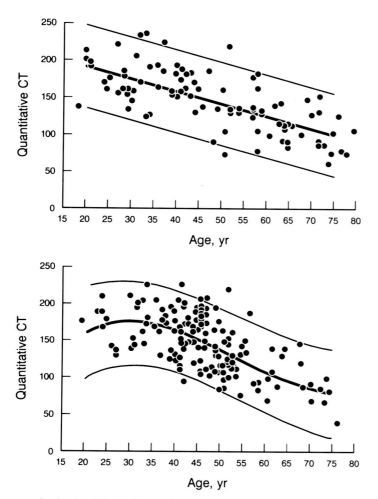

FIG. 7. A: Normal male values for vertebral cancellous mineral content by QCT, using a linear regression with 95% confidence intervals. B) Normal female values for vertebral cancellous mineral content by QCT, using a cubic regression with 95% confidence intervals; an accelerated loss is observed after menopause.

convincingly (18,19,39) and is supported by recent studies using spinal QCT. Furthermore, the natural rates of postmenopausal bone loss, and the dose response for estrogen replacement therapy are being established by noninvasive measurement techniques. Longitudinal studies (18) performed over 24 months in 75 climacteric women (within 3 years of menopause) show an alarming average cumulative vertebral mineral loss of 9% while a smaller loss of 1 to 2% is observed in the appendicular skeleton over two years (Figs. 8A and B). Furthermore, spinal QCT shows that treatment with 1500 mg calcium per day is ineffective (10% cumulative loss) while calcium plus 0.3 mg. conjugated estrogen daily is effective (+ 1.8%), and 0.625 mg conjugated estrogen alone is similarly effective (+ 1.6%) (20).

The rate of spinal trabecular loss is even more extreme with abrupt cessation of ovarian function following surgical menopause. Longitudinal studies (28) over 24 months in women following oophorectomy show an average 9% annual vertebral trabecular bone loss with peripheral cortical bone loss of about 2% (Fig. 9A–C). Of importance is the observation that appendicular cortical measurements do not reliably reflect spinal loss for the individual patient (Fig.10A) (28). In a subset of women losing bone rapidly, the rate of spinal trabecular loss is two to three times greater than spinal integral loss (Fig. 10B). This accelerated menopausal bone loss appears to differentially effect the trabecular bone envelope, as cross-sectional studies performed with DPA have not revealed distinct menopausal skeletal changes

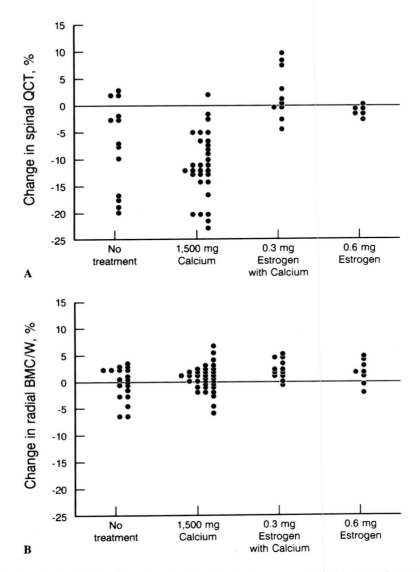

FIG.8. **A:** Vertebral trabecular bone loss in 83 climacteric women following natural menopause. The change in spinal QCT over 24 months (3-point data) is shown as a function of treatment. **B:** Only minimal changes are observed by the relatively insensitive radial BMC/W measurements.

(57). The large average annual losses of spinal trabecular bone are similar when measured by either single or dual energy QCT techniques (9.4 ± 2.2 vs 9.2 ± 5.2) indicating that marrow compositional changes with red to yellow conversion are not substantial (28). By quantitative computed tomography, the minimum protective dose of conjugated estrogen for preventing spinal bone loss following oophorectomy is 0.6 mg/daily (Fig. 9).

The effect of estrogen deprivation on younger premenopausal women has also been examined using QCT. We studied 38 women (17 to 49 years of age) with hypothalamic and hyperprolactinemic amenorrhea and premature ovarian failure (13). The hypothalamic amenorrhea group was made up primarily of athletes. Bone mass in the peripheral cortical bone was only slightly decreased from age-matched controls, but spinal trabecular bone was de-

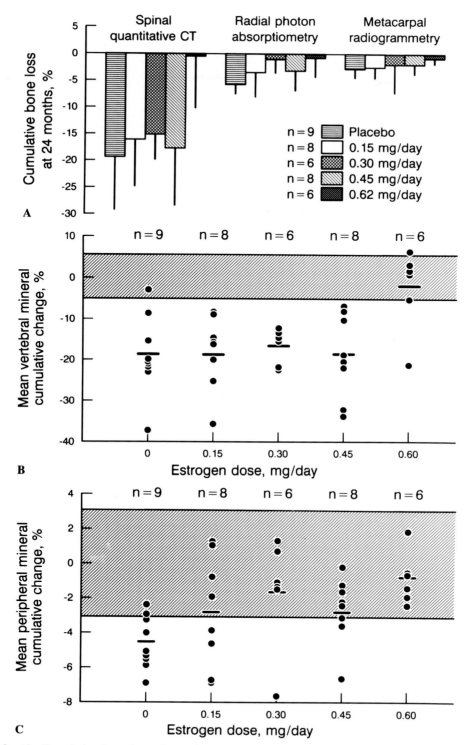

FIG. 9. **A:** Cumulative bone loss observed over a period of 24 months in 37 women as a function of quantitative technique and therapy with conjugated estrogen. The estrogen dose-response relationships determined by vertebral mineral (**B**) and mean peripheral cortical (**C**) measurements are shown for individual women at 24 months. The cross-hatched regions represent no significant change (that is, less than twice the coefficient of variation or precision of measurement).

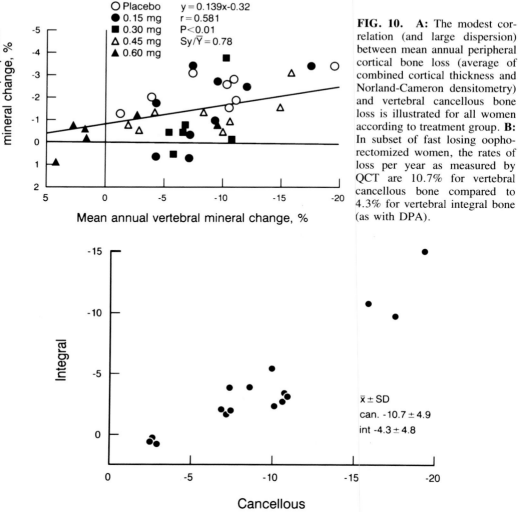

FIG. 10. A: The modest correlation (and large dispersion) between mean annual peripheral cortical bone loss (average of combined cortical thickness and Norland-Cameron densitometry) and vertebral cancellous bone loss is illustrated for all women according to treatment group. **B:** In subset of fast losing oophorectomized women, the rates of loss per year as measured by QCT are 10.7% for vertebral cancellous bone compared to 4.3% for vertebral integral bone (as with DPA).

creased 20 to 25% (Fig. 11). A subpopulation of this study included both amenorrheic and exercise-matched eumenorrheic athletes (42). In this study, eumenorrheic elite athletes (VO₂ max = 50 ml-kg/min) had more spinal mineral than sedentary controls, followed in order by amenorrheic elite athletes, amenorrheic causal (30 miles/week) athletes, and amenorrheic non-athletes. Thus, the exercise effect is apparent in women, but can be overridden by the strong effect of estrogen deprivation.

There is ample evidence that estrogen replacement therapy begun soon after spontaneous menopause or oophorectomy prevents bone loss. The *long-term* benefits of estrogen use on skeletal mass and integrity, however, are not well established. To quantify the degree to which estrogen replacement therapy prevents postmenopausal osteoporosis, we performed a retrospective study (19) comparing the occurrence of fractures in 245 long-term estrogen users and 245 case-matched controls, followed for an average of 17.6 years. Quantitative bone mineral assessments were obtained from 18 of these women using estrogen replacement therapy and their controls (average age, 73 years)

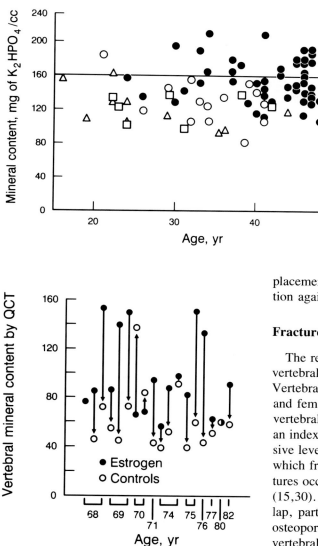

FIG. 11. Mineral content in lumbar vertebrae for normal controls *(black dots)* and women with amenorrhea due to hyperprolactinemia *(squares)*, hypothalamic causes *(triangles)*, and premature ovarian failure *(circles)*. Solid line is regression with age for controls showing negligible loss premenopausally. K_2HPO_4 indicates potassium phosphate mineral equivalents.

FIG. 12. Vertebral mineral content in the subset of 18 long-term estrogen treated women and their respective 17 controls.

(Fig. 12). Osteoporotic fracture incidence in estrogen users was 50% as great as in the controls (p = 0.01) (Fig. 13). Estrogen users showed significantly greater bone mineral: 54.2% greater spinal mineral (p = 0.0002), 19.4% greater forearm mineral (p = 0.0005), and 15.6% greater metacarpal cortical thickness (p = 0.0005). The results of this study strongly suggest that long-term estrogen re-

placement therapy confers significant protection against bone loss and fracture.

Fracture Threshold and QCT

The relationship between spinal fracture and vertebral mineral density has been examined. Vertebral QCT measurements in both males and females correlate well with the severity of vertebral fracture (25,32,40,56), and provide an index of fracture risk by revealing a permissive level at approximately 110 mg/cm³, above which fractures are rare and below which fractures occur more commonly (Figs. 14A and B) (15,30). There is, however, substantial overlap, particularly in older women, between the osteoporotic group, as defined by atraumatic vertebral fracture, and the normal population. This overlap reduces the predictive value of spinal QCT, as with all other measurements of bone mass, for the individual patient, and also underscores the potential importance of other factors such as quality of bone tissue or propensity for injury. Nevertheless, all studies (25,40,53–55,62) to date that have compared QCT and DPA in the same patients have found a better separation of spinal osteoporotics from normals or a better correlation with vertebral fracture for spinal trabecular measurement by QCT than for spinal integral measurement by DPA.

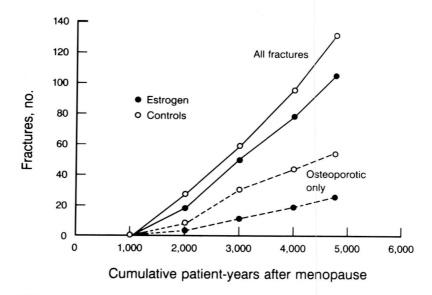

FIG. 13. A 50% reduction in osteoporotic fractures is observed in estrogen-treated women.

Exercise and Spinal Bone Mineral

Types of exercise programs, as well as intensity and duration of exercise, have not been well studied or described in research dealing with skeletal health. As a step toward elucidating the independent effects of exercise upon the skeleton, we have studied spinal bone mineral in 46 young men, 28 of whom engaged in regular and vigorous exercise programs (4). Measurements of spinal trabecular bone mineral density (mg/cc) and vertebral integral bone mass (g) were obtained for all subjects by QCT. Spinal trabecular bone density was greater by 14% in the exercise group (p = .0001) and integral bone mass was greater by 10% (p = .04). Subjects in the exercise group were further categorized to reflect their particular fitness regimen. Individuals engaged in a program that utilized both weight-training and aerobic forms of exercise had a mean value of trabecular bone density of 197.3 mg/cc while those engaged in a purely weight-training regimen had a mean value of 183.1 mg/cc, and an aerobic group had a mean value of 172.9 mg/cc, respectively. Control males were lowest with a mean value for tra-

becular bone density of 161.3 mg/cc (Fig. 15). An analysis of variance across all four activity levels indicated a significant difference between groups for trabecular bone density (p = .0001), although differences in total integral bone mass (g) did not reach statistical significance.

COMPARISON OF SPINAL QCT WITH APPENDICULAR SPA AND CCT IN METABOLIC BONE DISEASES

In order to investigate the effects of specific metabolic bone disorders on skeletal mass at different anatomic sites and to determine the associations among various methods for noninvasive measurement of bone mineral, we studied 269 subjects (56). The study group consisted of 34 patients with hyperparathyroidism, 24 patients with steroid-induced osteoporosis, and 38 men with idiopathic osteoporosis. These subjects were compared with a group of 173 normal women, of whom 51 were premenopausal, 94 were perimenopausal, and 28 were postmenopausal. The measurements taken on these 269 subjects included QCT of

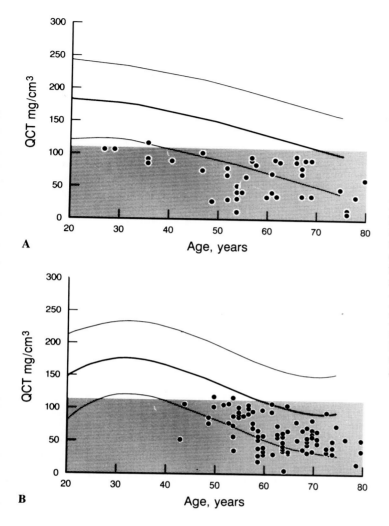

A

B

FIG. 14. **A:** Males with idiopathic osteoporosis and vertebral fractures are plotted as closed circles against the normal curve drawn with 95% confidence intervals. **B:** Females with postmenopausal osteoporosis and crushed or wedged vertebrae are plotted against the normal curve. For both males and females a fracture threshold or permissive level is observed below approximately 110 mg/cm³ *(crosshatched area).*

the lumbar spine (mg/cm³), combined cortical thickness (CCT) of the second metacarpal shaft (mm), and Norland-Cameron single photon absorptiometry of the radial diaphysis (NCD) and metaphysis (NCM) (g/cm). The latter two measurements were divided by bone width to yield two size-corrected measurements, NCDW and NCMW (g/cm²), whose ratio was then calculated (NCDW/NCMW). Mean values for each test were then expressed in terms of the mean percent increment/decrement from age- and sex-matched normals. The normative data used for calculating percent increment/decrement were extracted from published normal values

for QCT (15,31), CCT (26), NCDW, and NCDW (44). Lateral thoracolumbar radiographs were evaluated semi-quantitatively, and a spinal fracture index (FXI) was calculated (32).

A Spearman correlation matrix for the different skeletal mineral measurements performed in this study is shown in Table 2. The measurements of appendicular bone correlated moderately well (r = 0.54 − 0.66) with each other. The appendicular measurements correlated less well with the spinal QCT measurements (r = 0.33 − 0.41) (Fig. 16). The spinal FXI correlated best with QCT (r = −0.74)

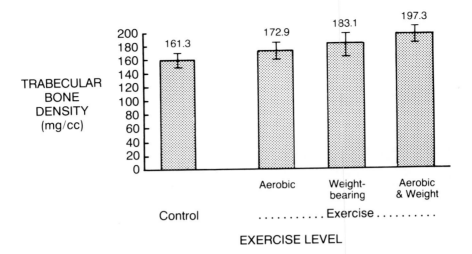

FIG. 15. This bar graph, showing mean trabecular bone density by exercise level, shows progressively greater vertebral trabecular bone mineral through each exercise type.

(Fig. 17) and less well with the appendicular measurements $(r = -0.20 - -0.33)$ (Fig. 18). The appendicular ratio NCDW/NCMW correlated poorly with the appendicular and axial measurements as well as with the FXI. A fracture threshold of about 110 mg/cm^3 by QCT was noted for the group as a whole. Furthermore, below a level of approximately 60 mg/cm^3, fractures were common and absence of fractures was uncommon.

The idiopathic osteoporotic men, the hyperparathyroid patients, and the corticosteroid

TABLE 2. *Spearman correlation matrix*

	CT	CCT	NCD	NCDW	NCM	NCMW	NCDW NCMW	FXI
AGE	−0.60972 0.0001 259	−0.43969 0.0001 266	−0.15230 0.0127 267	−0.39689 0.0001 266	−0.17956 0.0051 242	−0.36982 0.0001 242	0.03348 0.6050 241	0.50067 0.0001 255
CT		0.38778 0.0001 259	−0.00333 0.9574 260	0.32837 0.0001 259	0.10223 0.1181 235	0.40685 0.0001 235	−0.17430 0.0075 234	−0.73982 0.0001 248
CCT			0.43558 0.0001 268	0.63361 0.0001 268	0.44808 0.0001 242	0.54489 0.0001 242	−0.07034 0.2757 242	−0.32923 0.0001 256
NCD				0.75405 0.0001 268	0.81586 0.0001 243	0.42884 0.0001 243	0.18566 0.0037 242	0.04527 0.4699 257
NCDW					0.71001 0.0001 242	0.65716 0.0001 242	0.12875 0.0454 242	−0.20359 0.0011 256
NCM						0.60836 0.3745 243	−0.05734 0.6299 242	−0.03167 234
NCMW							−0.59443 0.0001 242	−0.24691 0.0001 234
NCDW NCMW								0.10042 0.1264 233

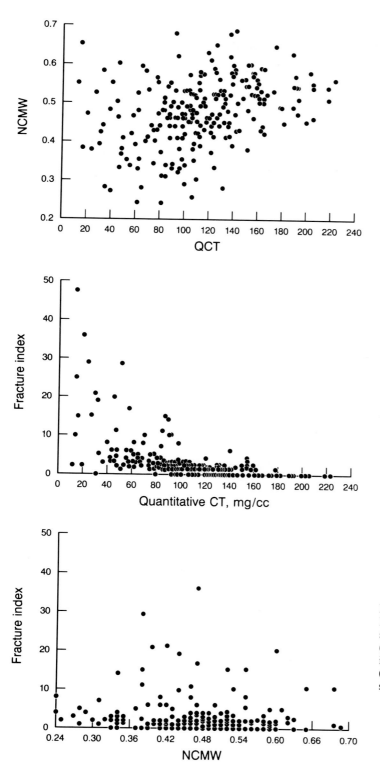

FIG. 16. Scatter plot of Norland-Cameron metaphyseal measurement vs. quantitative CT. Poor correlation (r = .40) is observed between these two measures.

FIG. 17. Scatter plot of quantitative CT versus spinal fracture index. Moderate correlation (r = .74) is observed between these two measurements.

FIG. 18. Scatter plot of Norland-Cameron metaphyseal measurement divided by width (NCMW) versus spinal fracture index. There is weak correlation (r = .25) between these two measurements.

treated patients differed significantly from their age- and sex-matched controls in virtually all of the tests (p = .0001 – .01) (Table 3). Plots of the percent decrement/increment for each patient in these three subgroups are shown in Figs. 19–21. The largest percent decrements in the spine were seen in the idiopathic osteoporotic men and corticosteroid groups, reflecting the severity of the disease process on axial trabecular bone. The largest decrements in the appendicular indices were seen in the idiopathic osteoporotic men and hyperparathyroid groups. NCDW was the strongest discriminator of the appendicular indices, while NCDW/NCMW was the weakest.

From this study, we concluded that knowledge of appendicular cortical mineral status is important in its own right, but is not a valid predictor of axial trabecular mineral status, which may be disproportionately decreased in certain diseases. Furthermore, quantitative CT provides a reliable means of assessing the latter region of the skeleton and correlates well with the spinal fracture index, a semiquantitative measurement of end-organ failure.

COMPARISON BETWEEN QCT AND DPA IN NORMAL AND OSTEOPOROTIC WOMEN

To investigate the associations among the principal methods for the noninvasive measurement of spinal and appendicular bone mass, we studied 40 normal early postmenopausal

TABLE 3. *Percent decrement/increments for bone mineral measurements (56)*

	Idiopathic osteoporotic males	Primary hyper- parathyroidism	Steroid-induced osteoporosis
Mean age	59.1 ± 11.3	59.1 ± 11.1	45.9 ± 16.8
Number	38	34	24
CT			
Mean ± SD	59.9 ± 27.0	94.9 ± 27.1	88.3 ± 45.2
% change	−52.8 ± 21.8	−17.1 ± 19.4	−37.9 ± 30.6
p	.0001	.0001	.0001
n	38	34	23
CCT			
Mean ± SD	4.67 ± .852	3.92 ± .842	4.33 ± 1.20
% change	−12.5 ± 15.5	−17.1 ± 13.4	−14.1 ± 17.8
p	.0001	.0001	.0025
n	38	34	22
NCDW			
Mean ± SD	.711 ± .085	.544 ± .128	.673 ± .127
% change	−15.9 ± 9.57	−22.3 ± 14.4	−10.2 ± 11.2
p	.0001	.0001	.0003
n	38	34	22
NCMW			
Mean ± SD	.482 ± .095	.370 ± .077	.489 ± .123
% change	−21.8 ± 14.6	−27.3 ± 12.1	−9.88 ± 15.4
p	.0001	.0001	.1433
n	37	32	7
NCDW/ NCMW			
Mean ± SD	1.519 ± .326	1.481 ± .242	1.381 ± .136
% change	10.9 ± 23.8	8.17 ± 17.7	−1.87 ± 7.57
p	.0085	.0139	.5713
n	37	32	6

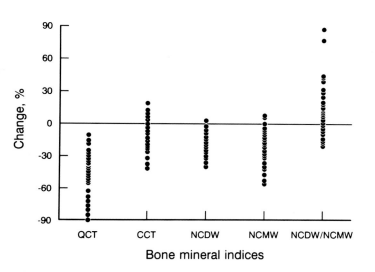

FIG. 19. Percent increment/ decrement for idiopathic osteoporotic males.

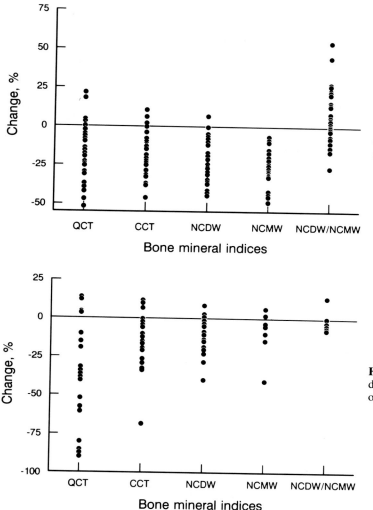

FIG. 20. Percent increment/decrement for patients with primary hyperparathyroidism.

FIG. 21. Percent increment/decrement for patients with steroid-induced osteoporosis.

women and 68 older postmenopausal women with mild to moderate osteoporosis (55). Specifically, the purposes of the study were: (1) to examine the associations among the major methods for noninvasive bone mineral measurement in both normal postmenopausal women and osteoporotic women; (2) to assess the discrimination capability of these techniques for detecting bone loss and spinal fracture; and (3) to provide a basis for understanding disparate results, when comparing bone mineral measurements of different bone compartments such as cortical and trabecular bone, different anatomic sites in the axial and appendicular skeleton, and different measuring techniques such as linear scanning with area projection and direct volume-density measurements. The methods for determining bone mineral content included single and dual energy QCT and DPA of the lumbar spine, single photon absorptiometry of the distal one third of the radius (SPA) and CCT of the second metacarpal shaft. Lateral thoracolumbar radiography was evaluated and a spinal fracture index was calculated. The normal early postmenopausal women ranged in age from 44 to 58 years with a mean age of 52.6 years. The postmenopausal osteoporotic women (with mild-to-moderate vertebral compression fractures) ranged in age from 54 years to 75 years with a mean age of

64.1 years. The means, standard deviations, coefficients of variation (percent standard deviation) and ranges of values for early postmenopausal and postmenopausal osteoporotic women are given in Tables 4 and 5, respectively.

The greatest decrements in mean bone mineral content between the two populations were found by QCT. There was a difference of 42.3 mg/cm³ (or 35.6%) by SEQCT (t = 9.369, p = 0.0001) and of 38.7 mg/cm³ (or 28.2%) by DEQCT (t = 9.244, p = 0.0001). The difference measured by DPA was 13.7% (t = 4.604, p = 0.001), while those measured by SPA, SPA/W and CCT were 13.8% (t = 4.955, p = 0.0001), 10.5% (t = 2.869, p = 0.01) and 15.0% (t = 5.752, p = 0.0001), respectively.

The correlation coefficients and levels of significance for both patient groups are shown in Table 6 and 7. There were high correlations (r = 0.97 and r = 0.95) between SEQCT and DEQCT in both populations (Figs 22A and B). SEQCT showed a good correlation (r = 0.87) with DPA for early postmenopausal and a

TABLE 4. *Early postmenopausal women (n = 40)*

Variable	Mean	STD dev	Coefficient variable	Minimum	Maximum
AGE	52.650	3.371	6.402	44.000	58.000
SEQCT	118.749	24.244	20.416	71.710	168.740
DEQCT	137.257	21.502	15.665	100.760	177.500
DPA	1.067	0.173	16.241	0.802	1.433
SPA	0.846	0.119	14.143	0.663	1.142
SPA/W	0.697	0.068	9.803	0.525	0.845
CCT	4.783	0.640	13.386	3.600	5.950

TABLE 5. *Postmenopausal osteoporotic women (n = 68)*

Variable	Mean	STD dev	Coefficient variable	Minimum	Maximum
AGE	64.103	5.456	8.511	54.000	75.000
SEQCT	76.400	19.739	25.837	33.950	114.720
DEQCT	98.553	20.086	20.381	57.640	138.300
DPA	0.921	0.132	14.388	0.595	1.288
SPA	0.731	0.112	15.281	0.486	0.968
SPA/W	0.624	0.152	24.305	0.467	1.365
CCT	4.064	0.605	14.898	2.650	5.500
FXI	4.735	2.717	57.385	1.000	12.000

TABLE 6. *Pearson correlation coefficients early postmenopausal women (n = 40)*

	SEQCT	DEQCT	DPA	SPA	SPA/W	CCT
SEQCT		0.9734	0.8661	0.3824	0.4874	0.5363
		0.0001	0.0001	0.0149	0.0014	0.0004
SEQCT	0.9734		0.8156	0.3716	0.4345	0.5345
	0.0001		0.0001	0.0182	0.0051	0.0004
DPA	0.8661	0.8156		0.4673	0.5396	0.5029
	0.0001	0.0001		0.0024	0.0003	0.0009
SPA	0.3824	0.3716	0.4673		0.7307	0.3650
	0.0149	0.0182	0.0024		0.0001	0.0206
SPA/W	0.4874	0.4345	0.5396	0.7307		0.5466
	0.0014	0.0051	0.0003	0.0001		0.0003
CCT	0.5363	0.5345	0.5029	0.3650	0.5466	
	0.0004	0.0004	0.0009	0.0206	0.0003	

moderate correlation (r = 0.53) for postmenopausal osteoporotic women (Figs 23A and B). DEQCT did not improve these correlations with DPA. The appendicular cortical measurements correlated only moderately (r = 0.37 – 0.54) with the axial measurements for early postmenopausal women and even less well (r = 0.16 – 0.36) for postmenopausal osteoporotic women. The appendicular cortical measurements correlated moderately (r = 0.37 – 0.73) among themselves for early postmenopausal women and also moderately (r = 0.25 – 0.58) for postmenopausal osteoporotic women. The spinal fracture index correlated best (r = −0.91) with SEQCT (Fig. 24A), and DEQCT did not improve this correlation with fracture severity. Spinal fracture correlated only moderately (r = −0.44) with DPA (Fig. 24B) and poorly with SPA, SPA/W and CCT.

Comparison Between SEQCT and DEQCT

Our results show a small but significant decrease in the correlation between SEQCT and DEQCT from the younger to the older population, likely due to the increased vertebral fat in the older osteoporotic females. Nevertheless, generally excellent correlations were observed between DEQCT and SEQCT in both populations. Furthermore, the failure of DEQCT to improve the correlation with DPA or with fracture, to substantially reduce the normal biolog-

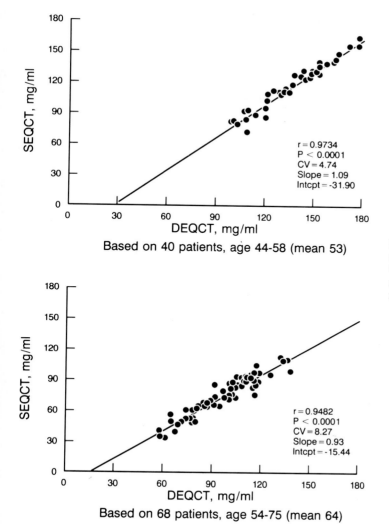

Based on 40 patients, age 44-58 (mean 53)

FIG. 22. High correlation is shown for SEQCT versus DE-QCT for (**A**) normal early post-menopausal women and (**B**) post-menopausal osteoporotic women.

Based on 68 patients, age 54-75 (mean 64)

TABLE 7. *Pearson correlation coefficients postmenopausal osteoporotic women (n = 68)*

	SEQCT	DEQCT	DPA	SPA	SPA/W	CCT	FXI
SEQCT		0.9482	0.5310	0.2005	0.2390	0.2285	−0.9102
		0.0001	0.0001	0.1012	0.0497	0.0609	0.0001
DEQCT	0.9482		0.4245	0.2005	0.2133	0.2366	−0.8817
	0.0001		0.0003	0.1012	0.0809	0.0521	0.0001
DPA	0.5310	0.4245		0.3633	0.1622	0.2522	−0.4399
	0.0001	0.0003		0.0023	0.1864	0.0380	0.0002
SPA	0.2005	0.2005	0.3633		0.4021	0.5788	−0.0775
	0.1012	0.1012	0.0023		0.0007	0.0001	0.5316
SPA/W	0.2390	0.2133	0.1622	0.4021		0.2522	−0.2195
	0.0497	0.0809	0.1864	0.0007		0.0381	0.0720
CCT	0.2285	0.2366	0.2522	0.5788	0.2522		−0.1720
	0.0609	0.0521	0.0380	0.0001	0.0381		0.1610
FXI	−0.9102	−0.8817	−0.4399	−0.0775	−0.2195	−0.1720	
	0.0001	0.0001	0.0002	0.5316	0.0720	0.1610	

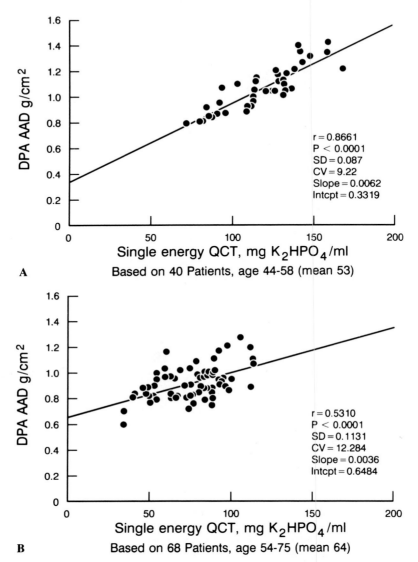

FIG. 23. A: Moderately good correlation is shown for DPA versus SEQCT for normal early postmenopausal women. **B:** Modest correlation is shown for DPA versus SEQCT for postmenopausal osteoporotic women.

ical variation, or to enhance the discrimination between normal and osteoporotic women, all strongly suggest that DEQCT is generally unnecessary in the assessment of postmenopausal women, and that SEQCT is adequate.

Comparison Between QCT and DPA

Widely differing correlations between QCT and DPA have been reported in apparently similar groups of patients (Table 8). Some reported correlations observed may be poor because of the small number of patients measured by DPA and QCT (35,51,53). Our results show good correlation ($r = 0.82$, and $r = 0.87$) between SEQCT or DEQCT and DPA in early postmenopausal osteoporotic women, and moderate correlations ($r = 0.42$, and $r = 0.53$) in postmenopausal women, even though we averaged the values of T12 to

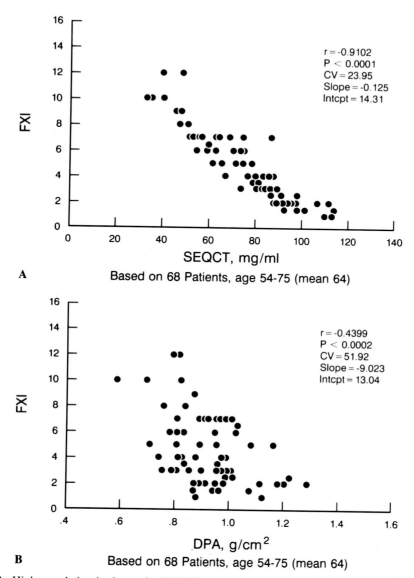

FIG. 24. **A:** High correlation is shown for SEQCT versus spinal fracture index. **B:** Modest correlation is shown for DPA versus spinal fracture index.

L3 by QCT in mg/cm^3 and of L2 to L4 by DPA in g/cm^2. Using DEQCT instead of SEQCT does not improve the correlation with DPA, suggesting that the variable vertebral fat content—and its effect on SEQCT accuracy—is not a major factor in degrading the correlation between QCT and DPA. Furthermore, the modest correlation observed in osteoporotic women, while statistically significant, shows sufficient dispersion that a reliable prediction

of QCT value from DPA value or vice versa is precluded for the individual patient.

Some authors (32,45) have tried to improve the correlation between QCT and DPA by measuring the same bone envelopes with both methods and expressing the quantities measured in dimensionally similar units (32,62). Genant (32) showed, in a mixed group of 52 patients, that the modest correlation (r = 0.67) between the anatomically and di-

TABLE 8. *Correlations between QCT, DPA and SPA*

Authors	SEQCT/DPA	SEQCT/SPA	DPA/SPA
Cann et al. (15)	–	0.48	–
Genant et al. (32)	0.67–0.88	0.40–0.47	0.47–0.55
Kilcoyne et al. (35)	0.32	–	–
Ott et al. (51)	0.26–0.46	0.44–0.51	0.54–0.60
Powell et al. (53)	0.40	0.48	0.56
Richardson et al. (56)	–	0.33–0.41	–
Sambrook et al. (62)	0.65–0.80	0.30	0.38
Reinbold et al. (55)	0.53–0.87	0.20–0.49	0.16–0.54

mensionally dissimilar integral DPA in g/cm^2 and trabecular QCT in mg/cm^3 was significantly improved when both techniques measured the same parameters. For example, integral mass in gm by DPA correlated well (r = 0.88) with integral mass by QCT; likewise, integral density in mg/cm^3 by DPA correlated well (r = 0.84) with integral density by QCT. Nevertheless, the strongest correlation (r = 0.91) was observed between trabecular and integral density when both were measured by QCT. Thus, the differences observed between QCT and DPA were not explained entirely by anatomic considerations, which suggests that residual fundamental differences exist between these techniques, perhaps related to their respective abilities to define bone edges, regions of interest, baseline measurements, and volumes, and to their respective other sources of error.

Mazess and Vetter (45) examined comparable bone envelopes in 10 excised vertebrae using QCT and DPA. They found that the mineral mass obtained by integrating all bone voxels by DEQCT correlated highly (r = 0.97) with the mass determined by DPA. The mineral density by DPA correlated highly (r = 0.87) with the density by DEQCT of the total vertebra including all processes, whereas the correlation with the density of the body was lower (r = 0.82), and even lower (r = 0.79) with the density of a section from the spongiosum of the anterior vertebral body, i.e., correlations between DPA and QCT weakened when integral density was compared with the more labile trabecular bone density.

Comparison Between Normal and Osteoporotic Women

The current study showed that older postmenopausal osteoporotic women have less bone mineral than early postmenopausal women and the magnitude of the difference depends upon the method used for measurement. The mean differences observed were 35.6% by SEQCT, 28.2% by DEQCT, 13.7% by DPA, 13.7% by SPA, and 15.1% by CCT. The larger difference measured by SEQCT than by DEQCT is explained by the fact that DEQCT reduces the fat error of SEQCT, which is increased in the older osteoporotic population and results in a slight overestimation of about 10% in the age-related rate of loss of mineral density (14,30).

The substantial decrement observed by QCT suggests that measurement of spinal trabecular bone density by QCT discriminates those women with spinal osteoporosis from younger postmenopausal normals better than measurements of spinal integral bone mineral content by DPA or appendicular cortical bone mass by SPA or CCT. This observation is supported by the work of Laval-Jeantet et al. (38) showing disproportionate loss of trabecular relative to compact bone in the spine, both in aging and in osteoporosis (Table 9). We also have previously shown, in a prospective study (28) of bone mineral changes following oophorectomy, that the loss of spinal trabecular bone is three-fold greater than spinal integral bone and five-fold greater than appendicular cortical bone. Furthermore, two recent studies (Table 10) have compared the differences between young normals and osteoporotics measured by QCT and by DPA. Sambrook (62) found a 54% (p = 0.0001) decrement by QCT and a 23% (p = 0.002) decrement by DPA, while Gallagher (25) found a 65% (p = 0.001) decrement by QCT and 16% (p = 0.06) decrement by DPA (Table 10). Finally, Raymakers (54), tested the ability of these two tests to dis-

TABLE 9. Relative density and attenuation by QCT of trabecular[a], compact, and integral[b] bone of the vertebrae in normal and osteoporotic females

| | Density (mg/cm³) | | | Attenuation |
	Trabecular	Compact	Integral	Trabecular integral
Normals Age 50 to 60	120 ± 27	225 ± 50	186 ± 40	.220 ± .04
Osteoporotics Age 50 to 60	74 ± 21	223 ± 56	161 ± 39	.167 ± .03
Normals Age 60 to 70	95 ± 27	192 ± 25	155 ± 23	.208 ± .03
Osteoporotics Age 60 to 70	35 ± 30	170 ± 27	102 ± 21	.144 ± .10

[a]Trabecular analysis.
[b]Integral analysis.

criminate between women with crush fractures and age-matched normals. QCT was slightly better, showing a sensitivity and specificity of 83% and 83% respectively, compared to 73% and 76% for DPA.

The range of values and coefficients of variation of trabecular bone density measured by QCT are greater than those of integral bone content determined by DPA, both across the two populations and within each population. This indicates a substantially greater pathologic range or physiologic sensitivity of spinal trabecular bone compared to that of spinal compact bone (32,56). The wide range of values

TABLE 10. *Comparison between QCT and DPA in young normals and osteoporotics with vertebral fractures*

	QCT	DPA
Gallagher et al. (25)	(mg/cm³)	(g/cm²)
Normals	119	1.029
Osteoporotics	42	0.859
Decrement	65%	16%
Significance	(p < 0.001)	(p < 0.06)
Sambrook et al. (62)	(mg/cm³)	(g/cm)
Normals	98.1 ± 11.8	3.39 ± 0.26
Osteoporotics	45.2 ± 25.5	2.62 ± 0.62
Decrement	54%	23%
Significance	(p < 0.0001)	(p < 0.002)
Reinbold et al. (55)	(mg/cm³)	(g/cm²)
Normals	118.7 ± 24.2	1.067 ± 0.17
Osteoporotics	76.4 ± 19.7	0.921 ± 0.13
Decrement	35.6%	13.7%
Significance	(p < 0.0001)	(p < 0.001)

found for QCT bone mineral density in early postmenopausal women may be explained, in part, by the fact that some of these women have already experienced substantial bone loss. This observation is supported by comparing current data with that from a previous study (28) of 47 normally menstruating women with an average age of 42 years who showed a mean baseline bone mineral density of 165.8 mg/cm³ ± 25.5 mg/cm³ by SEQCT. By contrast, our early postmenopausal women with an average age of 53 years (and on the average two years postmenopausal) had a mean bone density by SEQCT of 118.75 mg/cm³ ± 24.24 mg/cm³ representing a decrement of 47.05 mg/cm³ or 28%. It remains to be determined what portions of this perimenopausal bone loss occur before, during or after alteration in ovarian function, although we have previously shown (18,21) in a longitudinal study that spinal trabecular bone loss averages about 5% annually for the first several years after natural menopause.

Correlations with Spinal Fracture Index

In our postmenopausal osteoporotic women, the index of spinal fracture severity correlated highly (r = −0.91) with SEQCT and moderately (r = −0.44) with DPA. These results are supported by the *in vitro* studies of Brassow (5), who demonstrated a good correlation between absorption values by QCT and breaking load of vertebral bodies and of McBroom

(46), who showed a high correlation between trabecular bone density measured by QCT and fracture load of vertebral bodies. All vertebral bodies, in the latter study failed by compression of the endplate, suggesting that the cortical shell of the vertebra has only a modest structural role. Mack (40) showed that spinal fracture prevalence correlates better with spinal QCT ($r = -0.45$) than with spinal DPA ($r = -0.023$). Powell (53) demonstrated a significant correlation ($r = -0.66$) between QCT and FXI and no significant correlation ($r = -0.07$) between DPA and FXI. However, by eliminating the few extreme fracture cases and re-analysis of the data, he found stronger correlations for both techniques (QCT versus FXI, $r = -0.83$; DPA versus FXI, $r = -0.50$). Gallagher (25) showed the high sensitivity of QCT for fracture discrimination by demonstrating a close relationship between QCT spinal density and the number of vertebral fractures, as an index of fracture severity. Richardson (56) showed a good correlation ($r = -0.74$) between spinal fracture index and spinal QCT. Genant (32) showed a better correlation for QCT versus spinal fracture index ($r = -0.83$) than for DPA versus spinal fracture index ($r = -0.47$) (31). Table 11 summarizes the correlations between spinal fracture index and bone mineral measurements given by different authors.

Comparison of Appendicular and Axial Skeleton

Various authors (15,32,35,51,53,56,62) have reported different correlations among

TABLE 11. *Correlations between FXI, SEQCT and DPA*

Authors	FXI/QCT		FXI/DPA	
	r	p	r	p
Genant et al. (32)	−0.83	0.0001	−0.47	0.0006
Mack et al. (40)	−0.45	0.001	−0.023	NS
McBroom et al. (46)	−0.91	0.061	−	−
Powell et al. (53)	−0.83	0.01	−0.50	0.02
Richardson et al. (56)	−0.74	0.0001	−	−
Reinbold et al. (55)	−0.91	0.0001	−0.44	0.0002

QCT, DPA and SPA (Table 8). In the current study we found moderate correlations ($r = 0.37 - 0.54$) between axial and appendicular bone mineral measurements in normal postmenopausal women and weaker correlations ($r = 0.16 - 0.36$) in osteoporotic women. The best appendicular to axial correlation ($r = 0.54$) was observed between the dimensionally similar DPA and SPA/W, both measurements in g/cm^2, for early postmenopausal women. Correlations between measurement of purely trabecular bone by spinal QCT and measurements of peripheral cortical bone by SPA, SPA/W, and CCT were lower ($r = 0.20 - 0.54$), particularly for the older women.

Although it may be important to measure skeletal mineral content at both axial and appendicular sites to differentiate the effects of certain endocrine disorders (28,47,56,57), the relatively poor ability of all peripheral cortical measurements to predict axial bone mineral content is apparent, and reflects differences in the dynamic nature of cortical and trabecular bone change at the two sites. Besides anatomic and physiologic differences between the appendicular and axial skeleton, the quantities of mineral measured are generally expressed and compared in terms that have different units.

Several studies of postmenopausal women have shown that radial cortical bone mineral content decreases gradually, while vertebral trabecular bone mineral content declines more rapidly (28,47). Our current study of early postmenopausal women and postmenopausal osteoporotic women also shows greater losses of the vertebral spongiosum than of the peripheral cortex with aging and from health to disease.

Since there is poor predictive value of spinal bone mineral content from appendicular cortical measurement, it is not surprising that there is also relatively poor prediction of spinal fracture from a peripheral cortical bone measurement. All correlations between appendicular cortical measurements and spinal fracture index or bone mineral content are poor, or moderate at best; therefore, these measurements probably have limited value as screening tests to identify women with early bone loss or women with the greatest risk of vertebral fractures.

Conclusions

The correlations between spinal measurements by QCT and DPA are good in normal early postmenopausal women and are only modest in postmenopausal osteoporotic women. The correlations between spinal measurements by either QCT or DPA and appendicular cortical measurements by SPA or CCT are modest in normal women and are poor in osteoporotic women. Although measurements of bone mineral content by QCT, DPA, SPA and CCT are positively correlated, their relationships are not strong enough and their dispersions are too large to predict one measure by another for the individual patient. The strongest correlation with vertebral fracture severity is provided by QCT measurement and the weakest by SPA. The correlation is high between single energy QCT and dual energy QCT, suggesting that errors due to fat uncertainties are not substantial in these postmenopausal women. The failure of dual energy QCT compared to single energy QCT to improve correlations with DPA or with the fracture index suggests that single energy QCT may be adequate and perhaps preferable for assessing postmenopausal women. Finally, measurement of spinal trabecular bone density by QCT discriminates osteoporotic women from younger normal women more sensitively than measurements of spinal integral bone by DPA or appendicular cortical bone by SPA or CCT.

SUMMARY

Osteoporosis is a common disorder with considerable health risk and medical care cost. Recent advances in technology have provided new opportunities for evaluating bone mass noninvasively that may impact substantially on the detection and course of osteoporotic conditions.

The laboratory and clinical results presented herein indicate that quantitative computed tomography provides a reliable means to evaluate and monitor the many forms of osteoporosis and the various interventions aimed at ameliorating this condition. The greatest advantages of spinal QCT for noninvasive bone mineral measurement lie in the high precision of the technique, the high sensitivity of the vertebral spongiosa measurement site, and the potential for widespread application.

REFERENCES

1. Adams, J.E., Chen, S.Z., Adams, P.H., and Isherwood, I. (1982): Measurement of trabecular bone mineral by dual energy computed tomography. *J. Comput. Assist. Tomogr.*, 6:601–607.
2. Adams, J.E., Pullan, B.R., and Adams, P.H., et al. (1982): Dual energy computed tomography (CT) and the estimation of bone mass. *J. Comput. Assist. Tomogr.*, (Abstr.) 6:204.
3. Arnold, J.S. (1970): External and trabecular morphologic changes in lumbar vertebrae in aging. In: *Progress in Methods of Bone Mineral Measurement*, edited by G.D. Whedon, and J.R. Cameron. U.S. Department of Health, Education and Welfare, Washington, DC.
4. Block, J.E., Genant, H.K., and Black, D. (1986): Greater vertebral bone mineral mass in exercising young men. *West J. Med.*, 145:39–42.
5. Brassow, F., Cone-Muenzebrock, W., Weh, L., Kranz, R., Eggers-Stroeder, G. (1982): Correlations between breaking load and CT absorption values of vertebral bodies. *Europ. J. Radiol.*, 2:99–101.
6. Broman, G.E., Trotter, M., and Peterson, R.R. (1958): The density of selected bones of the human skeleton. *Am. J. Phys. Anthro.*, 16:197–211.
7. Burgess, A.E., Colborne, B., and Zoffman, E. (1985): Vertebral bone mineral content. *Proceedings of the 5th International Workshop on Bone and Soft Tissue Densitometry*. Bretton Woods, New Hampshire, Oct. 14–18.
8. Cameron, J.R., Mazess, R.B., and Sorenson, J.A. (1968): Precision and accuracy of bone mineral determination by the direct photon absorptiometric method. *Invest Radiol.*, 3:141–150.
9. Cann, C.E., and Genant, H.K. (1980): Precise measurement of vertebral mineral content using computed tomography. *J. Comput. Assist. Tomogr.*, 4:493–500.
10. Cann, C.E. (1981): Low-dose CT scanning for quantitative spinal mineral analysis. *Radiology*, 140:813–815.
11. Cann, C.E., and Genant, H.K. (1982): Cross-sectional studies of vertebral mineral using quantitative computed tomography. *J. Comput. Assist. Tomogr.*, 6:216.
12. Cann, C.E., and Genant, H.K. (1983): Single versus dual-energy CT for vertebral mineral quantification. *J. Comput. Assist. Tomogr.* 7(3):551.
13. Cann, C.E., Martin, M.C., and Genant, H.K. (1984): Decreased spinal mineral content in amenorrheic women. *J.A.M.A.* 251:626–629.
14. Cann, C.E., Ettinger, B., and Genant, H.K. (1985): Normal subjects versus osteoporotics: No evidence

using dual energy computed tomography for disproportionate increase in vertebral marrow fat. *J. Comput. Assist. Tomogr.* 9:617–618.

15. Cann, C.E., Genant, H.K., Kolb, F.O., Ettinger, B. (1985): Quantitative computed tomography for prediction of vertebral fracture risk. *Metab. Bone Dis. Rel. Res.*, 6:1–7.

16. Dalen, N., and Jacobsen, B. (1976): Bone mineral assay: Choice of measuring sites. *Invest. Radiol.*, 9:174.

17. Dunnill, M.S., Anderson, J.A., and Whitehead, R. (1967): Quantitative histological studies on age changes in bone. *J. Pathol. Bacteriol.*, 94:274–291.

18. Ettinger, B., Genant, H.K., and Cann, C.E. (1985): Menopausal bone loss can be prevented by low dose estrogen with calcium supplements. *J. Comput. Assist. Tomogr.*, 9:633–634.

19. Ettinger, B., Genant, H.K., and Cann, C.E. (1985): Long-term estrogen replacement therapy prevents bone loss and fracture. *Ann. Intern. Med.*, 102:319–324.

20. Ettinger, B., Genant, H.K., and Cann, C.E. (1987): Postmenopausal bone loss is prevented by low-dosage estrogen with calcium. *Ann. Intern. Med.* (in press).

21. Ettinger, B., Ettinger, V., Genant, H.K., and Cann, C.E. (1985): Menopausal bone loss: Low dose conjugated estrogen used with calcium prevents spinal mineral loss. In: *Proceedings of the 5th International Workshop on Bone and Soft Tissue Densitometry Using Computed Tomography*, p. 162. Bretton Woods, New Hampshire, Oct. 14–18.

22. Faul, D.D., Couch, J.L., Cann, C.E., Boyd, D.P., and Genant, H.K. (1982): Composition-selective reconstruction for mineral content in the axial and appendicular skeleton. *J. Comput. Assist. Tomogr.*, 6:202–203.

23. Firoonzia, H., Golimbu, C., Rafii, M., Schwartz, M.S., Alterman, A. (1984): Quantitative computed tomography assessment of spinal trabecular bone. I. Age-related regression in normal men and women. *CT*, 91–97. 97.

24. Frost, H.M. (1964): Dynamics of bone remodeling. In: *Bone Biodynamics*, edited by H.M. Frost, Little-Brown, Boston, Massachusetts.

25. Gallagher, C., Golgar, D., Mahoney, P., and McGill, J. (1985): Measurement of spine density in normal and osteoporotic subjects using computed tomography: Relationship of spine density to fracture threshold and fracture index. *J. Comput. Assist. Tomogr.*, 9:634–635.

26. Garn, S.M. (1970): The earlier gain and later loss of cortical bone. In: *Nutritional Perspective*, edited by S.M. Garn, p. 146. CC Thomas, Springfield, Illinois.

27. Genant, H.K., and Boyd, D.P. (1977): Quantitative bone mineral analysis using dual-energy computed tomography. *Invest. Radiol.*, 12:545–551.

28. Genant, H.K., Cann, C.E., Ettinger, B., and Gordan, G.S. (1982): Quantitative computed tomography of vertebral spongiosa: A sensitive method for detecting early bone loss after oophorectomy. *Ann. Int. Med.*, 97:699–705.

29. Genant, H.K., Boyd, D.P., Rosenfeld, D., Abols, Y., and Cann, C.E. (1981): Computed tomography. In: *Non-invasive Measurements of Bone Mass and*

Their Clinical Application, edited by S.H. Cohn, pp. 121–149. CRC Press, Boca Raton.

30. Genant, H.K., Cann, C.E., Boyd, D.P., Kolb, F.O., Ettinger, B., and Gordan, G.S. (1983): Quantitative computed tomography for vertebral mineral determination. In: *Clinical Disorders of Bone and Mineral Metabolism*, edited by B. Frame and J.T. Potts, pp. 40–47. Excerpta Medica, Amsterdam-Oxford-Princeton.

31. Genant, H.K., Cann, C.E., Pozzi-Mucelli, R.S., and Kanter, A.S. (1983): Vertebral mineral determination by quantitative CT: Clinical feasibility and normative data. *J. Comput. Assist. Tomogr.*, 7:554.

32. Genant, H.K., Powell, M.R., Cann, C.E., Stebler, B., Rutt, B.K., Richardson, M.L., and Kolb, F.O. (1984): Comparison of methods for in vivo spinal mineral measurement. In: *Osteoporosis*, edited by C. Christiansen, C.D. Arnaud, B.E.C. Nordin, A.M. Parfitt, W.A. Peck, and B.L. Riggs, pp. 97–102. Aalborg Stiftsbogtrykkeri, Glostrup, Denmark.

33. Genant, H.K., Cann, C.E., Ettinger, B., Gordan, G.S., Kolb, F.O., Reiser, U., and Arnaud, C.D. (1985): Quantitative computed tomography for spinal mineral assessment: Current status. *J. Comput. Assist. Tomogr.*, 9(3):602–604.

34. Hangartner, T.N., and Overton, T.R. (1983): The Alberta gamma CT system. *J. Comput. Assist. Tomogr.*, 6:1156.

35. Kilcoyne, R.F., Hanson, J.A., Ott, S.M., Mack, L., and Chesnut, C.H. (1984): Vertebral bone mineral content measured by two techniques of computed tomography and compared with dual photon absorptiometry. *J. Comput. Assist. Tomogr.*, 8:1164–1167.

36. Krolner, B., and Pors Nielsen, S. (1980): Measurement of bone mineral content (BMC) of the lumbar spine. I. Theory and application of a new two-dimensional dual-photon attenuation method. *Scand. J. Clin. Lab. Invest.*, 40:485–487.

37. Laval-Jeantet, A.M., Cann, C.E., Roger, B.M., Dallant, P. (1984): A post-processing dual energy technique for vertebral CT densitometry. *J. Comput. Assist. Tomogr.*, 9:1164–1167.

38. Laval-Jeantet, A.M., Jones, C.D., Bergot, C., Laval-Jeantet, M.H., and Genant, H.K. (1985): Comparison of bone loss from spongiosa and from compact vertebral bone in the aging process and in osteoporotics. *Proceedings of the 5th International Workshop on Bone and Soft Tissue Using Computed Tomography*. Bretton Woods, New Hampshire, Oct. 15–18.

39. Lindsay, R., Hart, D.M., Forrest, C., and Baird, C. (1976): Prevention of spinal osteoporosis in oophorectomized women. *Lancet*, 1:1038–1040.

40. Mack, L.A., Hanson, J.A., Kilcoyne, R.F., Ott, S.M., Gallagher, J.C., and Chesnut, C.H. (1985): Correlation between fracture index and bone densitometry by CT and dual photon absorptiometry. *J. Comput. Assist. Tomogr.*, 9:635–636.

41. Madsen, M., Peppler, W., and Mazess, R.B. (1975): Vertebral and total body bone mineral content by dual photon absorptiometry. Proceedings of the Eleventh European Symposium on Calcified Tissues.

42. Marcus, R., Cann, C.E., Madvig, P., Minkoff, J., Goodard, M., Bayer, M., Martin, M., Gaudiani, L.,

Haskell, W., and Genant, H.K. (1985): Menstrual function and bone mass in elite women distance runners. *Ann. Intern. Med.*, 102:158–163.

43. Mazess, R.B. (1983): Errors in measuring trabecular bone by computed tomography due to marrow and bone composition. *Calcif. Tissue Int.*, 35:148–152.

44. Mazess, R.B. and Cameron, J.R. (1973): Bone mineral content in normal US whites. In: *International Conference on Bone Mineral Measurements*, edited by R.B. Mazess, pp. 228–237. US Department of Health, Education and Welfare. Publication # IHO 75-683, Chicago, Illinois.

45. Mazess, R.B., and Vetter, J. (1985): Comparison of dual-photon absorptiometry and dual-energy computed tomography for vertebral mineral. *J. Comput. Assist. Tomogr.*, 9:624–625.

46. McBroom, R.J., Hayes, W.C., Edwards, W.T., Goldberg, R.P., and White, A.A. (1985): Prediction of vertebral body compressive fracture using quantitative computed tomography. *J. Bone Joint Surg.*, 67:1206–1214.

47. Meier, D.E., Orwoll, E.S., and Jones, J.M. (1984): Marked disparity between trabecular and cortical bone loss with age in men. Measurement by vertebral computed tomography and radial photon absorptiometry. *Ann. Int. Med.*, 101:605–612.

48. Nilas, L., Bord, J., Gordfredsen, A., Christiansen, C. (1985): Comparison of single- and dual-photon absorptiometry in postmenopausal bone mineral loss. *J. Nucl. Med.*, 26:1257–1261.

49. Orphanoudakis, S.C., Jensen, P.S., Rauschkolb, E.N., Lang, R., and Rasmussen, H. (1979): Bone mineral analysis using single energy computed tomography. *Invest. Radiol.*, 14:122–130.

50. Osteoporosis: Consensus Conference (1984): *J.A.M.A.*, 252:799–802.

51. Ott, S.M., Chesnut, S.H., Hanson, J.A., Kilcoyne, R.F., Murano, R., and Lewellen, T.K. (1984): Comparison of bone mass measurements using different diagnostic techniques in patients with postmenopausal osteoporosis. In: *Osteoporosis*, edited by C. Christiansen, C.D. Arnaud, B.E.C. Nordin, A.M. Parfitt, W.A. Peck, and B.L. Riggs, pp. 97–102. Aalborg Stiftsbogtrykkeri, Glostrup, Denmark.

52. Peppler, W.W., and Mazess, R.B. (1981): Total body bone mineral and lean body mass by dual photon absorptiometry., *Calcif. Tissue Int.*, 33:

53. Powell, M.R., Kolb, F.O., Genant, H.K., Cann, C.E., and Stebler, B.G. (1983): Comparison of dual photon absorptiometry and quantitative computed tomography of the lumbar spine in the same subjects. In: *Clinical Disorders of Bone and Mineral Metabolism*, edited by B. Frame and J.T. Potts, pp. 58–61., Excerpta Medica, Amsterdam.

54. Raymakers, J.A., Hoekstra, O., Van Putten, J., Kerkhoff, H., and Duursma, S.A. (1987): Osteoporotic fracture prevalence and bone mineral mass measured with CT and DPA. *Skel. Radiol.*, (in press).

55. Reinbold, W.D., Reiser, U.J., Harris, S.T., Ettinger, B., and Genant, H.K. (1986): Measurement of bone mineral content in early postmenopausal and postmenopausal osteoporotic women. A comparison of methods. *Radiology*, 160:469–478.

56. Richardson, M.L., Genant, H.K., Cann, C.E., Ettinger, B., Gordan, G.S., Kolb, F.O., and Reiser, U.J. (1985): Assessment of metabolic bone disease by quantitative computed tomography. *Clin. Orth. Rel. Res.*, 195:224–238.

57. Riggs, B.L., Wahner, H.W., Dunn, W.L., Mazess, R.B., Offord, K.P., and Melton, L.J. (1981): Differential changes in bone mineral density of the appendicular and axial skeleton with aging. *J. Clin. Invest.* 67:328–335.

58. Rohloff, R., Hitzler, H., Arndt, W., and Frey, W. (1983): Vergleichende Messungen des Kalksalzgehaltes spongioser knochen mittels Computertomographie und J-125-Photonen-Absorptiomethode. In: *CT '82*, edited by J. Lissner, and J.L. Doppman, pp. 126–30. Schnetztor-Verlag, Konstanz.

59. Roos, B., Rosengren, B., and Skoldborn, H. (1970): Determination of bone mineral content in lumbar vertebrae by a double gamma-ray technique. In: *Proceedings of the Bone Measurement Conference*, USAEC Conf-700515, edited by J.R. Cameron, pp. 243–254. Clearinghouse for Federal scientific and technical information, National Bureau of Standards, U.S. Dept. of Commerce, Springfield, Virginia.

60. Ruegsegger, P., Elsasser, U., and Anliker, M., et al. (1976): Quantification of bone mineralization using computed tomography. *Radiology*, 121:93–97.

61. Ruegsegger, P., Dambacher, M.A., and Ruegsegger, M.S., et al. (1984): Bone loss in premenopausal and postmenopausal women. *J. Bone Joint Surg.*, 66A:1015–1023.

62. Sambrook, P.N., Bartlett, C., Evans, R., Hesp, R., Katz, D., and Reeve J. (1985): Measurement of lumbar spine bone mineral: A comparison of dual photon absorptiometry and computed tomography. *Br. J. Radiol.*, 58:621–624.

63. Snyder, W. (1975): Report of the task group on reference man, pp. 62–98. Pergamon Press, Oxford.

64. Sorenson, J.A., and Mazess, R.B. (1970): Effects of fat on bone mineral measurements. In: *Proceedings of the Bone Measurement Conference*, edited by J.R. Cameron, pp 255–262. USAEC Conference 700515, Chicago, Illinois.

65. Stebler, B., and Ruegsegger, P. (1983): Special-purpose CT-system for quantitative bone evaluation in the appendicular skeleton. *Biomed. Tech. (Berlin)*, 28:196–205.

66. Trotter, M., and Hixon, B.B. (1974): Sequential changes in weight, density, and percentage ash weight of human skeletons from an early fetal period through old age. *Anat. Rec.*, 179(1):1–18.

67. Wahner, H.W., Eastell, R., and Riggs, B.L. (1985): Bone mineral density of the radius: Where do we stand? *J. Nucl. Med.*, 26:1339–1341.

68. Wahner, H.W., Dunn, W.L., Mazess, R.B., Towsley, M., Lindsay, R., Markhard, L., and Dempster, A. (1985): Dual-photon Gd-153 absorptiometry of bone. *Radiology*, 156:203–206.

69. Weaver, J.K., and Chalmers, J. (1966): Cancellous bone: Its strength and changes with aging and an evaluation of some methods for measuring its mineral content. *J. Bone Joint Surg.*, 48(2):289–298.

70. Weissberger, M.A., Zamenhoff, R.G., Aronow, S., and Neer, R.M. (1978): Computed tomography for the measurement of bone mineral in the human spine. *J. Comput. Assist. Tomogr.*, 2:253–262.

Osteoporosis: Etiology, Diagnosis, and Management, edited by B. Lawrence Riggs and L. Joseph Melton, III. Raven Press, New York © 1988.

9

Nuclear Medicine and Densitometry

Richard B. Mazess, and *Heinz M. Wahner

*Department of Medical Physics, University of Wisconsin, Madison, Wisconsin 53706; and *Division of Nuclear Medicine, Mayo Clinic, Rochester, Minnesota 55905*

Several reports and books over the past decade have summarized bone measurement methods (48,49,52,62,67,209,212–215). This chapter serves as an update on those with particular reference to nuclear medicine approaches to bone density and skeletal uptake. Bone densitometry approaches include single-photon absorptiometry (SPA) and dual-photon absorptiometry (DPA), neutron activation of calcium, Compton scattering, ultrasound measurements and uptake of diphosphonates. Of these only SPA and DPA are used clinically; the other methods are largely experimental or investigational. Radiographic morphometry, radiographic indices, and X-ray QCT are dealt with in Chapters 7 and 8.

In earlier reports (212,213) the suggestion was made that the location of bone measurement could prove more significant than the methodologic approach, or its implementation, in obtaining valuable clinical results. The last several years of research have confirmed that suggestion. It is now apparent that there are dramatic differences between peripheral and axial measurement sites and even among local areas on the peripheral skeleton or on the axial skeleton. Bone turnover differences among the sites are reflected by differences in bone density and in skeletal uptakes. Local measurements on the peripheral skeleton are variably associated with total skeletal measures and even less reliably associated with measurements of the axial skeleton. Our previous notion of a monolithic skeleton, or even a relatively unitary axial skeleton, has now given way to the concept that there are regional differences within both axial and peripheral sites (99,210,291,292).

All these skeletal sites differ with respect to (a) sensitivity to disease processes, (b) responsivity to therapy, and (c) intrapopulation variation. These functional differences in turn seem to relate to (a) the relative amount of trabecular bone, (b) the amount of red marrow, (c) bone cellular activity, and perhaps (d) weight-bearing or other muscular stress.

BONE MEASUREMENT AND BONE STRENGTH AT FRACTURE SITES

Many factors are implicated in increasing the relative risk of osteoporotic fracturing (121,325) but all seem to act by affecting the amount of bone at fracture sites.

Research studies over the past 20 years have shown definitively that bone strength is directly dependent on bone mineral content (33,60). About 80 to 90% of the variance in strength is accounted for by mass or density. The small remaining variance may be due to structural factors such as anisotropy or microfractures. In addition factors such as muscle strength (10) probably influence fracture *in vivo*. In the spine the critical measure of skeletal integrity to load resistance (245) is directly related to the integral bone mass in the entire vertebral cross-section, including the outer shell of "compacted" trabecular bone (129,244,297). Values of density determined in small areas of the vertebral body relate to load resistance of the entire body only to the extent that such densities correlate with integral mass (244) or are corrected for vertebral size (23). Since there are large interindividual differences in vertebral size, and since the size of the body may change with aging (244,268), it becomes critical in the evaluation of risk for compression fracture to have a noninvasive measurement that reflects the total vertebral body, and not just a small portion of it. Measurement of the anterior body, as is done with one popular approach to computed tomography (104,301), does give an indication of fracturing (280) but use of larger areas could provide an improvement (13).

There seems to be greater confusion about the role of bone density in hip fracture than in spine fracture (57). It has been demonstrated, however, that strength of the femoral neck in compression is accounted for almost entirely by the bone mineral content across the neck (60,185,358) though ash content has some influence (357). The critical region for integrity of the neck appears to be the Ward's triangle zone (358). This is the trabecular area in which bone loss first appears (163), based on three-dimensional computed tomography, and the area in which there is a 50% difference between hip fracture patients and age-matched controls (359). The import of this zone has been noted in qualitative scoring with the Singh Index (331). Measurements at adjacent sites are not as markedly abnormal (376) so it is not surprising that Cummings (57), in his survey of densitometry at "remote" sites, found little evidence of osteopenia in hip fracture patients.

Epidemiologic studies (242,243,291) using dual-photon absorptiometry for direct measurement of density at fracture sites, have shown that there is a gradient of fracture risk. Each 10% decrease of density increases the relative risk of fracture two- to three-fold. Since skeletal osteopenia is usually systemic and not local, one also can expect that decreases of density at remote sites will reflect increased risk at fracture sites. However measurements at remote sites will be less sensitive and specific than direct measurement. This appears to be true even for spinal measurements, or iliac crest biopsies (1), in relation to hip fracture. About 95% of the attributable risk of fracture is associated with subnormal density.

It has been commonly assumed that axial osteoporosis can be considered as one disease, which it may well be, but recent evidence suggests that its manifestation differs in spinal fractures and femoral fractures (153,290). Epidemiologic studies show that there is a remarkable increase of spinal compression fractures beginning at the menopause. The average age of females presenting with compression fractures is about 65 to 70 years. At this age there is normally only about 20% less bone in the spine than at peak bone mass, while in osteoporotic patients the difference is 30% (289). In contrast, fractures of the proximal femur do not increase substantially until age 70 years and the average age of a "hip" fracture group is about 75 years. Normal subjects at this age have about a 30% bone diminution in the femoral neck. This bone loss reflects a 20% loss of compact bone and a 40% loss of the trabecular component at this site (15.21). In osteoporotic patients there is a 45% loss from the femoral neck (15,233) reflecting an approximate 20% loss of compact bone and a 60% loss of trabecular bone. Figure 1 shows a comparison of the bone profile across the femoral neck in a younger woman and in an osteoporotic patient with a femoral fracture. There is clearly preferential loss from the trabecular zone. The profile is similar in appearance to the profile of a bone from this area in which all the trabecular bone has been experimentally removed. Identification of a comparable region of vertebral loss critical for spinal fracture has not been made.

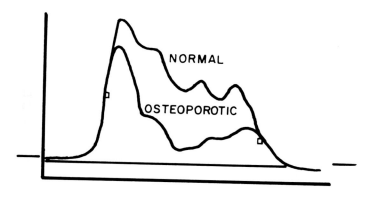

PERIPHERAL VERSUS AXIAL DENSITOMETRY

Osteoporotic fractures occur mainly in the axial skeleton in areas such as the spine, proximal femur, proximal humerus, and pelvis. These areas are highly trabecular and are particularly affected by the menopause (30,57). It has, therefore, been assumed that accelerated trabecular bone loss led to decreased strength in these zones and that trabecular bone anywhere in the skeleton, including that of the limbs, would reflect this process (59). At the same time it is fairly well-accepted that measurements of compact bone on the peripheral skeleton do not indicate axial densities with exactitude (227,280,291,292).

There is evidence of some preferential aging loss in the more trabecular regions of the peripheral skeleton, such as the distal radius (251,273); however, this may not reflect preferential loss of trabecular bone (210). Investigators using high-resolution ^{125}I computed tomography (136,137,305,306) showed that there was little aging loss in the purely trabecular bone of the distal radius or the proximal tibia (Table 1). Chalmers (35) arrived at similar conclusions in examination of the os calcis. The losses that occur in these regions may be from surrounding compact bone. In fact it has been demonstrated that the aging loss in women at the distal radius is due mostly to cortical thinning and not to trabecular osteopenia (150). However, trabecular bone at these sites is lost in osteoporosis. Consequently, measurements in these more trabecu-

lar areas of the peripheral skeleton do not reflect normal aging changes of trabecular bone in the axial skeleton. Changes of compact bone might indicate axial osteopenia equally well because these changes can be measured with better precision and accuracy (363,364).

There is, in general, good correlation between bone density in the peripheral skeleton and total skeletal state and between total skeletal state and the axial skeleton, but the relationship between peripheral sites and axial sites is more tenuous (see Fig. 2) and is affected to an even greater degree by the age, sex and clinical state of the subjects (58,227,324,378). This is discussed in greater detail in the section on SPA. This lack of a strong appendicular-axial association becomes critical in monitoring therapy, for not only may the degree of response be underestimated at peripheral sites (24,265) but the response may be dramatically opposite in axial bone (279). On the other hand estrogen

TABLE 1. *Changes in trabecular bone density (expressed as linear attenuation coefficient, cm^{-1}) using low-energy QCT on the tibia and the distal radius (137,305,306).*

	Tibia		Radius	
	n	*Mean*	*n*	*Mean*
20–29	26	.69	18	.64
30–39	21	.69	11	.64
40–49	25	.74	21	.64
50–59	23	.68	24	.62
60–69	28	.69	24	.61
70–70	18	.59	10	.58

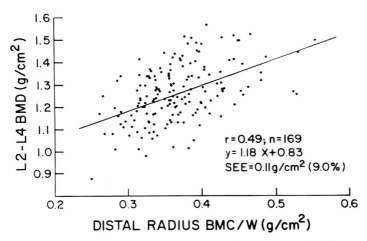

FIG. 2. Relation of SPA of the radius to DPA of the spine in young normal women. Despite the obvious correlation, the prediction error of 0.13g/cm^2 precludes accurate extrapolation from the radius.

therapy for the menopause seems to produce a fairly uniform, positive effect on all skeletal areas (114,115). In some centers, however, where the unusual precision errors of the methods were larger than the biological changes, no conclusions could be reached regarding the associations among sites (260).

Measurements using various methods can be made on the appendicular and axial skeleton (Table 2). Most methods are used for research only and have not found their way into clinical practice. SPA, however, has been used in clinical practice for over a decade. There have been at least ten manufacturers of commercial SPA instruments. The major differences in SPA approaches involve: (1) the location of measurement; (2) the radiation source; and (3) rectilinear or linear scanning. Dual-photon absorptiometry is the most common method used for measurement of the axial skeleton and there are at least six commercial devices. Quantitative computed tomography (QCT) is an alternative method that is used for spine densitometry but not as yet for femoral measurements. Several commercial QCT packages are available for implementation on scanners in addition to software available from the scanner manufacturers.

SINGLE-PHOTON ABSORPTIOMETRY (SPA)

SPA involves use of a narrow beam (usually < 6mm) of monoenergetic radiation for bone

quantitation *in vivo* (27,253). The beam flux is detected with a collimated radiation detector, usually a scintillation detector, that gives linear results over a wide dynamic range. The narrow radiation beam and detector collimation are used to minimize detection of scattered radiation from the area of interest on the appendicular skeleton. The radiation energy is nearly always under 70 KeV to ensure good contrast between bone and soft-tissue (367). ^{125}I at 27 KeV is ideal for forearm bones, where there is slight (< 8 cm) covering of soft-tissue, while ^{241}Am at 60 KeV is used on thicker areas, such as the upper arms. ^{241}Am also has been used on the forearm (3,4,205,206) but the poor contrast

TABLE 2. *Methods of appendicular and axial measurement and estimated values of precision and accuracy errors*

Appendicular	Precision	Accuracy
Compton scattering	5%	15%
Radiographic photodensitometry	3–5%	15%
Radiographic morphometry	3–5%	15%
Ultrasound–speed of sound	2%	—
Ultrasound–attenuation	5%	—
Neutron activation analysis	3%	3%
Single-photon–linear	3%	< 3%
Single photon–rectilinear	1%	< 3%
Low-energy computed tomography	1%	< 3%
Axial		
Neutron activation	5%	10%
Quantitative computed tomography	< 5%	15–30%
Dual–photon absorptiometry	1–3%	< 3%

due to the smaller bones requires a great reduction in scan speed.

SPA measurements must be made with the bone embedded in a constant thickness of soft-tissue. In some areas, this can be achieved by compression of the soft-tissue but in areas such as the distal forearm a water-bag, waterbath or tissue-equivalent gel, is used to equalize thickness. The latter is most convenient and less error-prone.

The integrated attenuation of the beam as it passes across bone is compared to the beam intensity in adjacent soft-tissue as an indication of mineral mass (27). This is described by: $(I = I_o \exp(-\mu_{BM} BM - \mu_s ST)$ where I is the resultant beam intensity, Io is the initial beam intensity in soft-tissue, $\mu_B M$ and μ_{ST} are the attenuation coefficients of bone and soft-tissue respectively and M_B and M_s are the mass of bone mineral and of soft-tissue.

SPA has been demonstrated to be inherently accurate (1 to 3%) on phantoms and actual bone specimens, and SPA results are not affected by location of the bone in the beam or by overlying tissue thickness (28,216,338). Bone mineral content determined in this way is directly proportional to bone strength (22). The effects of scan geometry on accuracy are usually small and are compensated for by scanning standards (366). Of greater concern has been apparent interunit variation among scanners and apparent miscalibrations (226,311). Other sources of variation are the effects of subcutaneous fat and intraosseous fat. Older scanners determined the soft-tissue baseline (Io) immediately lateral to the radius. In some subjects this was an area of subcutaneous fat that did not extend across the bone (190,384). Conversely some scanners determined the soft-tissue baseline in a waterbath adjacent to the forearm and this baseline also did not adequately represent the actual, somewhat fatter, soft-tissue in the forearm (251). Finally, measurements in areas containing large amounts of marrow relative to mineral, such as the distal radius or os calcis, are subject to substantial errors due to variable marrow composition. This is particularly the case when a higher energy source (such as ^{241}Am) is used. (173,339,381).

Older commercial instruments for SPA used an analog computer initially-designed at the University of Wisconsin (218). All newer systems use microcomputers for control of the mechanical scanners, analysis of data, normalization of data, and maintenance of the database (215). Use of computers not only facilitates analysis but allows novel changes of procedure. For example, the tin filter that once was used with ^{125}I sources can be removed, thereby doubling count rate and extending source life. This can be done provided a beam-hardening algorithm (compensation for selective absorption of lower-energy beam components) is implemented in the data analysis program (313).

One of the major advances in SPA over the past decade has been the advent of rectilinear scanners. These allow measurements over a small area a few centimeters in length rather than a single traverse (effectively having only a 3-mm width). Area scanning halves the precision error of older linear scans from about 3% to 1 to 2% on the radius shaft, and permits measurements on anatomically variable areas (44,219,249,353). The precision error on the latter areas is usually double that on the radius shaft. Unless routine calibration on a standard is done, however, the precision error can be double or triple this low level (251). Careful orientation of the arm or heel also is necessary to ensure reliable results (319). Alternate methods of area determinations, such as proportional counters (18,126,127,140,386) or gamma-cameras (64,65,182,343), are less satisfactory because of: (1) poor detection efficiency, (2) poor spatial resolution, (3) high cost, and (4) contributions of scattered radiation.

When SPA first became available 15 years ago, it was demonstrated on skeletal series that measurements on long-bones correlated highly (r about 0.94) with total skeletal mineral (138,208). Subsequently, it was shown that SPA measurement in vivo correlated highly with total body calcium (TBCa) from neutron activation analysis (51,141); there was a common regression line for normals and abnormals, and both males and females, with a prediction error less than 10%. In recent years, more detailed studies using DPA for total body bone mineral (TBBM) have shown that at a given BMC the TBBM is usually lower in patients than normals (113,114,228,250). Osteoporotic patients have lower TBBM values than normals at a given radius BMC (228). The Danish investigators also have demonstrated that at any radius BMC: (1) women have a TBBM about 5% lower than men (113,114), and (2) gastrectomy patients have TBBM values 10% lower than normal (250). The general relationship of TBBM with radius BMC, however, is adequate for roughly outlining group differences and/or changes with diseases or therapy. Still the large variance ($\pm$ 10%) among the regression slopes for different populations precludes exact prediction of TBBM in an individual case although a common regression slope can be chosen to minimize systematic offsets.

Gotfredsen et al. (113,114) showed that changes in forearm BMC correlated fairly well with changes of TBBM in postmenopausal women (both with and without estrogen supplementation). However, Aloia et al. (7) failed to find an association between changes of TBCa by neutron activation and radius BMC by SPA. Hesp et al. (137) showed that such local changes were a good indication of changes in total calcium balance. This could be expected since 80% of skeletal mass is compact bone with a responsivity similar to that encountered at sites on the peripheral skeleton. Thus, local measurements of BMC, particularly on the shafts of long bones, are of value because they reflect total skeletal state. On the other hand, changes in the radius do not always reflect changes in the spine either with aging or with therapy (104,292).

SPA measurements on the peripheral skeleton do not reflect axial bone density very well at a given time (138,227,251), so it is understandable that they do not reflect the dynamic state of the axial skeleton. Several studies have now confirmed that the correlation between appendicular and axial BMC is only about 0.5 and that the prediction error (standard error of estimate) in estimating spine or femoral density

is about 12 to 15% (120,170,198,227,251). The prediction error can be smaller in a narrowly defined group such as young women but the regression over a narrow age range may not apply to older groups of patients. This is true not only for sites on purely compact bone, but for the distal radius and even for the purely trabecular os calcis (83,195). In contrast, two studies have indicated that there is a strong correlation of radius density to trabecular bone volume (TBV) on iliac crest biopsy (200,249).

The clinical deficiencies of SPA on the appendicular skeleton have led several investigators to reinvestigate measurements on more trabecular areas (Figs. 3 and 4), such as the distal radius or os calcis (12,120,363–365). These areas were first investigated twenty years ago and were found to be not clinically useful because of high variability. The usual distal radius site (5 to 10% of the forearm length or a radius-ulna spacing of 4 to 8 mm) contains about 20 to 40% trabecular bone (78,241,318). Large changes in trabecular content are associated with only small (1 mm) shifts in location (Table 3).

It is possible to measure at an "ultradistal" site where the radius and ulna conjoin, and where trabecular content is 60 to 75%, but this area is no more highly correlated with axial densities than conventional sites on the shaft (214). The ultradistal site appears to be more sensitive than usual distal sites, or shaft sites, in relation to Colles' fracture (132,137), lactation (362), and arthritis, (77) but not osteoporosis (78). The os calcis, which is over 80% trabecular, is no more highly correlated with the spine and femur than other peripheral sites (365) and is no better at discrimination of abnormality than the radius shaft or distal radius (382). The spine has at least twice the diagnostic sensitivity.

Clinical Applications

SPA has been used to define normal age-increases in infants and children, and bone loss in adults (118,220,310,333,345,346). Most normal bone loss with aging is associated with

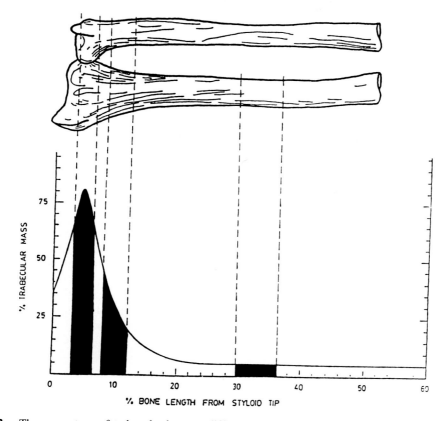

FIG. 3. The percentage of trabecular bone at different radius sites. Adapted from Schlenker et al. ref. 318, with permission.

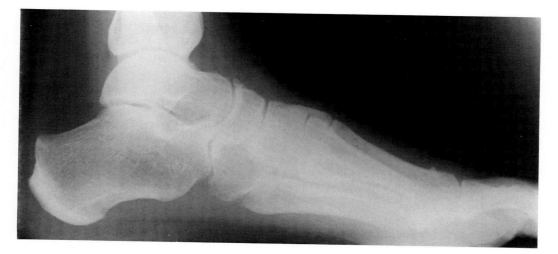

FIG. 4. Os calcis X-ray showing **(A)** variability of density distribution in the os calcis, and **(B)** the unusual soft-tissue cover.

TABLE 3. *The percentage trabecular bone at typical scan sites on the forearm.[a] The first site is now referred to as "ultradistal." The latter three sites are typical "distal" sites.*

Site description	% Trabecular			
	Radius		Ulna	
	Mean	Range	Mean	Range
A band 7 mm wide, 1 cm from ulnar styloid tip	53	42–61	52	45–48
2 cm from the ulnar styloid tip	24	17–30	21	11–30
0.1 of the ulna length from the ulnar styloid tip	13	6–24	13	4–26
3 cm from the radial styloid tip	13	10–18	12	4–20

[a]From Schlenker, ref. 318, with permission.

endosteal resorption from the medullary canal (102,210,239) but a few percent of the loss in normal subjects, and about twice that amount in osteoporotic patients, is associated with intracortical porosity (177,284). There is a strong genetic component in BMC of the appendicular skeleton within any ethnic group (196,334), and there are major differences among ethnic groups. Blacks are about 5 to 10% higher in BMC than whites, (50,207). Orientals in the U.S. are comparable to whites (110), but first generation Japanese in Hawaii are 5 to 10% lower (382,383).

A variety of clinical applications have been investigated (119,209,244). These include: hyperthyroidism, (189); intestinal bypass (288); hyperparathyroidism (286); gastrointestinal disorders (294); rheumatoid arthritis (8,77,372); dental pathology (354,355); anticonvulsant osteomalacia (43) and osteomalacia (265). Perhaps the most common use of SPA has been in monitoring skeletal complications of renal disease (25,249). While positive responses to therapy can be seen readily and rapidly in the appendicular bone of children (36,37), therapeutic intervention often is undetectable in the radius and ulna in adults (265). SPA on the radius and metacarpals has been the standard tool to examine the consequences of estrogen therapy in early postmenopausal women (114, 192,193). Positive results have been seen on the peripheral skeleton after treatment for hyperprolactinemia (165).

SPA at peripheral skeletal sites has been less successful for clinical diagnosis and monitoring of osteoporosis than was believed possible when the method was first developed. Several studies have shown that a substantial proportion (30% or more of osteoporotic patients with well-defined crush fractures or Colles' fractures, have radius BMC values within the normal range (78,131,132,149,172,254,255,326,333). This is also the case for hip fracture patients (4,131,151). This overlap of normal and abnormal is especially the case for the more "trabecular" sites, such as the distal radius and os calcis (14,78,109,120,131,269,364) because in such areas there is a wider intrapopulation variation than at shaft sites. For example, Wasnich (364) showed that the intrapopulation variation of the os calcis in both osteoporotic patients and age-matched controls was about 0.08g/cm^2 which at a mean density of about 0.32g/cm^2 amounted to a 25% variation! Spinal and femoral variability from DPA are about half this (i.e., 10 to 14%). The percentage reduction of bone at such "trabecular" appendicular sites may be greater than for purely compact bone, and may even approach that of axial bone, but the Z-score (difference divided by the standard deviation) that measures the statistical difference is invariably lower (Fig. 5). Even in young adults the wide normal range partially overlaps the range within which fractures occur. Still, these trabecular sites, like those on diaphysial bone, do reflect risk of fracture in prospective studies (169,364) and hence, they have some diagnostic validity, at least in older subjects.

The os calcis also has been measured using dual-photon absorptiometry using ^{153}Gd, and using a pair of low-energy nuclides, ^{125}I and ^{57}Co (307). The effects of smoking and exercise have been examined (307–309). Use of a

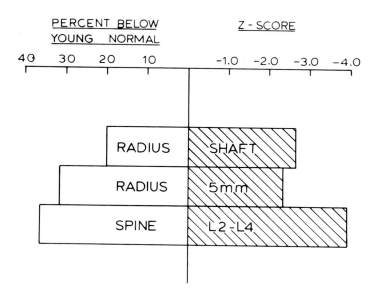

PERCENT BELOW YOUNG NORMAL — Z-SCORE

RADIUS SHAFT

RADIUS 5mm

SPINE L2-L4

FIG. 5. The percent reduction of bone in the distal radius (5 mm site), the radius shaft (33%) and lumbar spine in osteoporotic patients and in young normal women. The Z-score is lower for the distal radius than for the shaft, and both sites are less sensitive than the spine itself (121).

dual-photon source on this fat-containing bone (about 600 mg/cm^3 of fat versus 200 mg/cm^3 in vertebrae) can eliminate some of the inaccuracies caused by variation in marrow fat (40,381).

DUAL-PHOTON ABSORPTIOMETRY

Dual-photon absorptiometry (DPA) like SPA, involves the relative attenuation of monoenergetic radiation but two discrete energies rather than a single energy is used. This allows determination of the masses of the two-component mixture of bone mineral (BM) and soft-tissue (ST), without the necessity of a constant thickness of soft-tissue as is the case with SPA. The dual-energy radiation source can be a combination of radionuclides such as 241-AM/137-Cs (60 KeV and 662 KeV), I-125/241-Am (27 and 60 KeV) or, as is more usual, a dual energy emitter such as 153-Gd (44 and 100 KeV). When two sources are used it may be appropriate to use the term "dual-beam" absorptiometry, but for ^{153}Gd it is a misnomer.

The simultaneous equations describing attenuation at the two energies of a two component system consisting of BM and ST are readily solved (156,379).

$$ST = \mu_{BM}{}' \ln(I/I_0) + \mu_{BM} \ln(I'/I_0')/\mu_{st} \mu'_{BM} - \mu_{st}{}' \mu_{BM}$$

$$BM = - \mu_{st} \ln(I'/I_0' + \mu_{st}{}' \ln(I/I_0)/\mu_{st} \mu_{BM}{}' - \mu_{st}{}' \mu_{BM}$$

where I and I_0 are the attenuated and unattenuated photon intensities, μ_{st} and μ_{BM} are the mass attenuation coefficients (cm^2/g) for components ST and BM and the prime superscript indicates the same quantities at the second energy. The attenuation coefficients are known, or readily determined, and photon intensities can be measured directly. Hence the two masses (BM and ST in g/cm^2) are the only unknown quantities; and these can be obtained by solving the equations.

DPA was first developed at the University of Wisconsin over 20 years ago using a combination of ^{125}I and ^{241}Am sources for measurements of both bone mineral content and soft-tissue composition on the limbs (27,217). Later, European researchers used the ^{241}Am/^{137}Cs combination on the limbs and on the spine (278,301,375). During this same period, the Wisconsin Bone Mineral Laboratory developed procedures for spine, femur and total body measurement using the dual-energy emitter ^{153}Gd (44 and 100 KeV) (156,157,221, 379), while investigators at Vanderbilt examined the spine (274). These procedures were later refined in several laboratories (76,111, 112,168,169,267).

Rectilinear scanners are usually used for DPA; scans require about 20 min for local areas (spine, proximal femur or humerus, knee) or 40 to 70 min for the total skeleton. Gamma-cameras could be used for DPA (187) but for several limitations: (a) the requisite spatial resolution of 1 to 2 mm is several-fold greater than that of the best cameras; (b) scattered radiation must be minimized; (c) source nonuniformities can cause nonlinearity; (d) energy resolution at 44 KeV is inadequate with most cameras; (e) high count rates cause instabilities in camera systems, and (f) the difference of spatial resolution at the upper and lower energies causes a partial volume artifact. Other types of area detectors such as multiwire proportional collimators have been tried with DPA but have not been adopted (139).

The initial studies, and all subsequent studies on DPA, have shown that it is a precise and accurate method for bone measurement (156,300,316,361). Typically, precision of repeat spinal measurements *in vivo* is about .02 to .03 g/cm^2 or about 2 to 3% (183,225, 360,316). The results are not affected by the fat content of marrow or by the thickness or composition of surrounding soft-tissue (361). Appropriate correction factors have been documented (267,336). When suitable corrections are made for scattered radiation, larger collimation can be used on the detector to allow more rapid scanning and/or extended source life (350). One of the major sources of uncertainty in obtaining adequate results is the difficulty in establishment of suitable soft-tissue baselines. A 1% uncertainty in the baseline leads to a 5% uncertainty in bone mineral content (302). This critical determination, as well as determination of bone edges, is now done under computer control in commercial instruments (Fig. 6).

Spinal Density

Most studies using DPA have concentrated on the spine, particularly the lumbar vertebrae,

(168,171,289) because of the import of this zone in crush fracture osteoporosis. The initial reports on changes of density with age in this zone appeared controversial (198,289) because these cross-sectional data suggested that bone density decreased continuously from young adulthood onward with little apparent influence of the menopause. An early onset of spinal bone loss has been confirmed in some later studies using DPA (107,130,232) though others disagree (171,345). An early onset of axial bone loss has been demonstrated in anatomic series (11,35,201,212,213,232). Clearly estrogen changes at the menopause do influence this loss (191,287). When data are analyzed in regard to years-since-menopause rather than chronologic age, this menopause effect becomes clearer (68,107). The DPA changes in the first postmenopausal years are about 3 to 4% annually or only slightly less than the 4%/year change seen with better QCT methods (85).

Variation in DPA results at the menopause cannot simply be due to technical considerations, as suggested by Smith and Tothill (336), but probably reflects sample selection in relation to the menopause. There is a preferential spinal loss by DPA in amenorrheic younger women (74,188). This loss is regained when such women become eumenorrheic (75,188); spinal density is positively correlated to estradiol in both normal and amenorrheic women (88,247). Johnston et al. (152) showed that spinal bone loss occurred in perimenopausal women with irregular menses whereas radius bone loss did not begin until after complete cessation of menses. Estrogen contraceptives seem to protect against vertebral bone loss (193).

Lumbar scans are usually done in an anterior-posterior projection. The legs are elevated to minimize lordosis and to achieve better intervertebral spacing. Lateral scans of the spine are also possible, but scans in this projection require narrow collimation (to achieve adequate resolution) which reduces the flux two-to ten-fold. Attenuation of the beam in the lateral projection is ten to twenty-fold greater than in

Left: 51   **Right: 83**

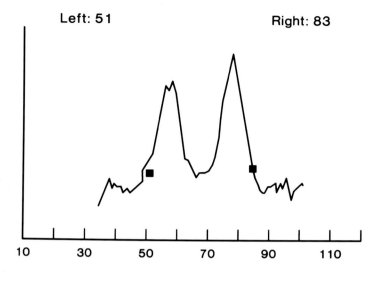

FIG. 6. Soft-tissue baselines and edges on the spine must be selected with care to achieve good precision and a low intra-population variance.

the AP projection. As a consequence, lateral scans require source activities many times greater and scan times several-fold longer than conventional AP scans. In addition lateral scans have a much greater precision error than AP scans. Since the results between the two projections correlate fairly highly, only the AP view is used clinically. Lateral spine scans of normal young women demonstrate another problem, high intrapopulation variance (374). The mean BMD in one series was 0.78 ± 0.25 g/cm². This intrapopulation variance in normals was 33% compared to the variance of 10% in the AP projection where mean BMD was 1.25 ± 0.12 g/cm². The normal-abnormal difference has to be 2.5 × greater in the lateral projection to give the *same* diagnostic sensitivity as the more reliable AP projection.

Bone mineral content of lumbar vertebrae measured by DPA has been shown to be directly related ($r = 0.9$) to bone strength (129). As a consequence, spinal density measured by either DPA (242,291) or QCT (31,101) is related to the risk of spinal fracture. Similarly, bone density of the proximal femur is directly related to its strength (60,185,358,359). Consequently, variations of femur density are directly related to the incidence of femoral fracture (243).

Studies have now demonstrated that spinal bone density is preferentially diminished relative to bone density of the appendicular skeleton in postmenopausal osteoporosis characterized by crush fractures and in corticosteroid-induced osteoporosis (55,78,120,168,228, 233,289,290). Low-level use of corticosteroids does not result in a substantial (> 5 to 10%) osteopenia (312,352). This preferential axial loss is most apparent in patients below age 60 to 70 years (360), but at 70 to 80 years of age, the age group used in many retrospective studies, axial and appendicular losses are similar (82,120). Even at this age, however, the relative low variance of spinal BMD measurements (< 15%) compared to the large variance in some appendicular measurements (< 25%) gives the former twice the diagnostic discrimination power as the latter (78). Not all DPA scanners produce this low intrapopulation variance for spinal density and consequently normal-abnormal differences will be obscured when deficient instruments or procedures are used (260,280). In fact the DPA instruments at these two leading institutions gave diagnostic sensitivity *poorer* than SPA! In patients with hip fracture, spinal density, either by DPA or by QCT, is not substantially reduced below age-matched controls (though it is much lower than in young normal subjects) (20,87,289, 290). Spinal density is not very highly correlated (*r* about 0.5 to 0.7) with femoral density (Fig. 9) and cannot be used to predict risk of femoral fracture.

Femoral Density

There are essentially two distinct approaches to measurement of the proximal femur using DPA. The traditional approach, developed at Mayo Clinic and the University of Wisconsin, involves rectilinear scanning of the entire proximal femur (76). This procedure takes about 15–20 min. Regions-of-interest (ROI) can be isolated by the operator using the graphical display of the data or they can be automatically selected, under computer control, based upon pattern recognition programs. The algorithms place one ROI across the femoral neck perpendicular to the neutral axis, and also delineate the low-density "Ward's triangle" region as well as a trochanteric region. The Ward's triangle region is the site of earliest bone loss (163). This approach gives readily reproducible results (Table 4) which are anatomically "correct", that is they adjust for differences in the angle of the femoral neck.

A simpler alternative has been attempted by European investigators. Scans are made diagonally in the proximal femur region at a fixed angle (53°) in an attempt to transverse the femoral neck perpendicular to the neutral axis (20). A series of parallel passes are made in the general area based on external landmarks. Though this requires a scan of only 10 min duration, the setup procedure may require another

10 min and repeat determinations may be necessary if the scan does not properly traverse the neck region. Reproducible results can be attained with considerable practice but the accuracy of even acceptable scans could be questioned simply because the angle of the scan may not be exactly perpendicular to the neutral axis. There is a standard deviation of 5° in the angle so values can vary from 45 to 60°. Small changes of angulation and of position can alter results (Fig 7). In addition, this diagonal scanning approach does not provide desirable data on the Ward's triangle and trochanteric regions.

When less optimal scan procedures are used and regions are not defined under computer control, the precision error in measurements is even larger than the usual 2 to 3% value, and the intrapopulation variance is increased to 0.2 g/cm² or more (20,290). With a good procedure the intrapopulation SD at the femoral neck is about 0.1 g/cm² (232). The use of pro-

TABLE 4. *Reproducibility of femur scans by DPA on isolated bones, a femur phantom, a torso phantom, and in vivo*

	In vitro bones	In vitro phantom	In vitro torso	In vivo
Cases	7	1	1	15
Observations	35	263	56	43
OBS/Case	5	263	56	3
Neck	2.2%	2.6%	2.1%	1.9%
Ward's	1.8%	2.0%	2.6%	3.2%
Trochanter	2.9%	2.1%	2.6%	3.1%

From Mazess et al., ref. 233, with permission.

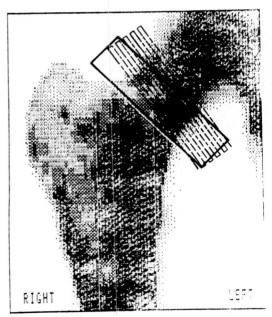

FIG. 7. The ROI can be taken at different angles on femoral neck but it is best to use an ROI perpendicular to the neutral axis rather than an arbitrarily fixed axis.

cedures or instrumentation giving a greater intrapopulation variance will decrease the discrimination of femoral abnormality.

All radiographic methods for analysis of density in the proximal femur must take into account the femoral anteversion (20 to 30%) that usually is evident. This is usually achieved by inward rotation of the leg. In older patients it may be desirable to use a foam wedge beneath the thigh to avoid femoral stress. This procedure helps ensure that views in the anterior-posterior projection will not be overly oblique, and it also provides better separation between the lesser trochanter and the pelvis.

The typical reproducibility of femoral densities in these regions is about 0.02 to 0.04 g/cm^2 (about 2 to 4%), while the total variance, assessed from right-left femoral differences is about 0.04 to 0.05 g/cm^2. The correlation between the left and right femur is usually about 0.97 to 0.98 (270) so only one femur needs to be measured. Thus, the uncertainty in femoral measurements is at least 50% if not 100% greater than that for the spine. Monitoring therapeutic effects on the femur is almost as feasible as on the spine, but both areas give less sensitive results than total skeletal scanning (for those agents having general skeletal affects). Obviously, those agents such as fluoride or exercise, that seem to have preferential positive effects on the spine (24,330) or corticosteroids, which cause preferential spinal osteopenia (106,317), require spinal assessment.

Bohr and Schaadt (21) demonstrated that bone was lost from the femoral neck with aging at a far faster rate than from the shaft. The latter area was, in fact, rather stable. Moreover, within the neck region itself there was preferential loss from the trabecular middle portion while the compact bone of the medial zone was retained much as the bone of the femur shaft was retained.

Several reports (1,57) have suggested that bone density in femoral fracture patients does not differ significantly from that in so-called age-matched controls. However, several factors preclude the mistaken conclusion that density is not a factor in fracture. First, in nearly all cases density was not measured across the femoral neck nor was density measured in the critical Ward's triangle area. Since bone loss is not uniform throughout the skeleton it is quite conceivable that measurements of the spine, pelvis or even femoral head (84,376) do not indicate the state of trabecular bone at the fracture site itself and certainly measurements at remote nonaxial sites such as the radius, metacarpals or os calcis would be even less likely to indicate density of the proximal femur.

Second, the control group against which the fracture group is usually compared often contains frankly osteoporotic patients, thereby biasing results. Certainly, subjects with existing osteoporotic fractures at sites other than the femur must be excluded from a control group. There is even some question of the validity of using age-matched controls since after age 70, when femoral fractures occur, many individuals are already substantially osteopenic.

Third, there has been a large intrapopulation variance (20%) in femoral neck measurements due to the difficulties of determining baselines, edges and ROI in this anatomically complex zone (20,21,290). New methods allow a lower variance (10 to 12%) with better discrimination of abnormality (15,232). Sensitivity of 85% can be achieved with an 85% specificity by using both BMC and BMD in the femoral neck determination (Fig. 8). Femoral measurement by DPA compares favorably to the poor discrimination achieved by spinal QCT (Fig. 9).

The lack of ability of the spine to specifically indicate femoral osteopenia and fracture risk (87,290) probably results from the only moderate association between these two zones (Fig. 10). The prediction of femoral density from the spine is only slightly better than that achieved using peripheral skeletal sites (i.e., SEE of about 0.15 g/cm^2).

Total Body Bone Mineral

Total body bone mineral (TBBM) is a direct indication of total bone calcium (TBCa) since calcium is a virtually constant component (37%) of mineral. TBBM can be measured us-

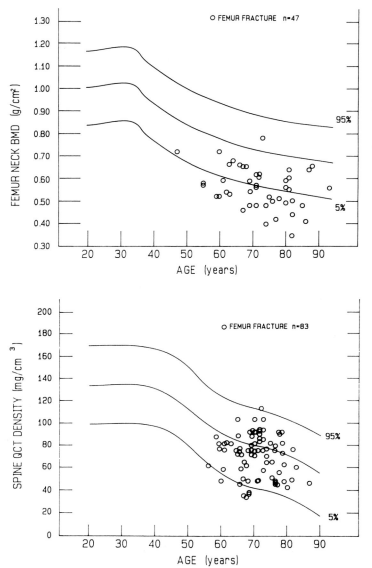

FIG. 8. The femoral neck density by DPA was an excellent discriminator of hip fracture risk. Adapted from Mazess et al., ref. 233, courtesy of Lunar Radiation Corp.

FIG. 9. The spinal density from QCT_{SE} was entirely normal in 83 hip fracture cases without concomitant spine fracture. From Firooznia et al., ref. 87, courtesy of Lunar Radiation Corp.

ing DPA by rectilinear scanning of the entire body (222,267). Total body measurement involves a low radiation exposure (< 1 mrem) and requires about 60 to 70 min because of the large area (170 cm × 60 cm) that is covered. Newer scanning procedures almost halve the time required by increasing scan speed in nonskeletal areas. TBBM determinations have been shown to be accurate on skeletons (with various tissue thicknesses and composition) and the results also correlate well ($r > 0.9$) with TBCa determined by neutron activation analysis *in vivo* (112,224). TBBM measurements also correlate highly with trunk calcium from neutron activation (223).

Over the past decade, the precision of TBBM measurements have been determined to be about 3% (112,228,293) but newer procedures have allowed total skeletal density (TBBD) to be measured with a precision of

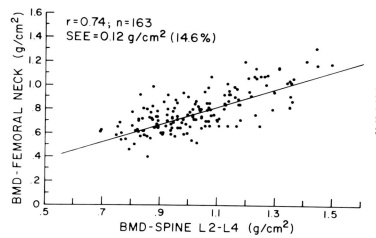

FIG. 10. Relationship of spine BMD to femoral neck BMD in a mixed sample of women (20 to 80 years).

about 0.5 to 1% in normal females and 0.75 to 1.25% in osteoporotic patients. The excellent precision of TBBD makes it particularly useful for monitoring skeletal changes with disease or with therapy (113,293). Also total body determinations, because of a generally high correlation with axial densities, provide discrimination between normals and osteoporotic patients that is comparable to that achieved with axial densitometry (228).

Total body scans also provide information on regional bone mineral densities though not with the excellent precision of TBBD (Fig. 11). Commercial instruments utilize computer algorithms to automatically divide the skeleton into four major regions (head, arms, trunk and legs); the trunk is further divided into four regions (thoracic spine, lumbar spine, pelvis, ribs).

X-RAY ABSORPTIOMETRY

Single and Dual

The low output of radionuclide sources and the inability to adjust energies to be optimal for given tissue thicknesses led to the use of single-energy X-ray sources (146,337). Usually the X-ray beam is filtered heavily to gain effective monochromaticity. Alternatively, stimulated fluorescent X-rays can be used (18,72). Typically, a narrow radiation beam is used,

coupled with a scintillation detector. There is little problem with scattered radiation in such a "narrow-beam" configuration. More rapid determinations can be done if a broad beam of radiation is used with a linear or area detector (such as an array of diodes or an image analyzer). Scattered radiation in such a configuration can be greatly reduced by using moving slits over the tube (to narrow the beam), perhaps coupled with a grid at the detector. A system for quantitative bone measurement (roentgen video absorptiometry) at the University of Wisconsin utilized the latter configuration (71). Precision of measurements on the proximal femur, distal radius and lumbar spine was about 2%. The method also has been implemented experimentally in dual-energy configurations for measurement of both the spine and the femur (166,282,283,314). A radiation detector with good energy resolution can be used to reject the contribution from scattered radiation or to measure attenuation at a series of narrow energy bands (155,303).

The initial work on radionuclide absorptiometry actually developed out of research on X-ray-based methods conducted over a 50-year period (197,356). These first approaches used broadbeam X-ray exposures of radiographs. The bone image on the film was quantified using scanning photodensitometers, hence the name "photodensitometry." Compensation for variations in beam energy, exposure, and film

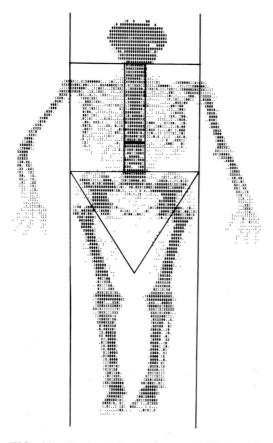

FIG. 11. Regional densities from TBBM can be selected automatically.

development was partially achieved by use of calibration standards (step or continuous wedges) exposed on the patient's film. While reasonable results could be achieved with care (17,54), the uncertainties in the process have led to a disenchantment with the method. The large contribution of scattered radiation to the film image have limited the approach to areas of the body with minimal soft-tissue cover such as the hands or forearms (239), areas which are of less clinical nature.

PERIPHERAL CT

Computed tomography of peripheral skeletal sites (Fig. 12) is an extension of the basic transmission scanning approach at those same

locations (81,305). In the original approach, a low-energy radionuclide source (^{125}I) is used together with a single scintillation detector and scans are made at a series of angles around the bone of interest (rotate-translate). Later manifestations of this approach have used (a) alternative movement approaches (123,142,321), (b) multiple sources and detectors (148), (c) X-ray sources, and (d) solid state detectors.

The reproducibility of ^{125}I-QCT of the distal radius or proximal tibia, typical sites of application, is about 1%, (305) but better precision is available with low-energy X-ray sources, particularly when multiple slices are performed along the longitudinal axis of the bone. By taking a series of successive 1 mm slices, and by careful use of pattern analysis to recognize the same region in independent determinations, it is possible to get precision better than 0.5% (261).

Measurements of peripheral trabecular bone by ^{125}I-QCT and X-ray QCT have shown that the normal rate of bone loss from these areas with aging is slower than in trabecular bone of the axial skeleton or even in adjacent compact bone (150,306). Peripheral trabecular bone is poorly to moderately correlated with axial trabecular bone (195,299). Measurements of the distal radius using ^{125}I-QCT showed a correlation of only 0.3 with spinal bone density by X-ray QCT (342). Moreover, the regression relationship in osteoporotic patients differs from that in normals (26). At any given radius density the spinal density in osteoporosis is about one standard deviation below that of age-matched controls. Our results from the University of Wisconsin (320) show that ^{125}I-QCT measurements in normal women correlated only moderately (about 0.6) with femoral and spinal densities using DPA. The prediction error was no better than for SPA measurement on the distal radius or radius shaft. As Hangartner et al. (124) pointed out, the error in predicting axial density from peripheral QCT is 15 to 20%, a figure too high to allow it to be clinically useful for exact diagnosis. However, since trabecular bone density in the peripheral skeleton does *not* show age decreases until age

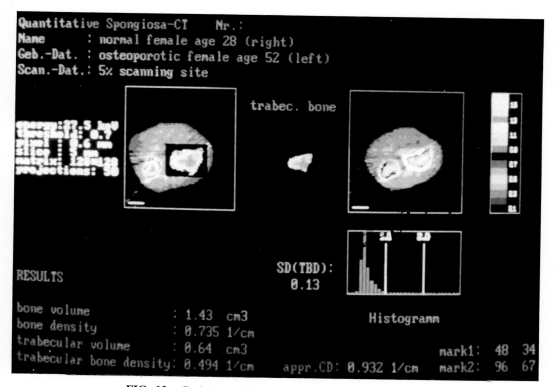

FIG. 12. Peripheral QCT image showing the distal radius.

70 (137,306) but does show pathologic changes (Colles' fracture cases are 10 to 15% low and crush fracture cases are 20 to 25% low) such measurements can be used for screening.

Peripheral QCT also could be useful for monitoring the response to therapy because the low precision errors that are achievable make it easier to reliably detect small changes. However, studies using sodium fluoride show only small changes, a few percent annually at most, despite larger spinal changes that occur with the same agent (61,63). Changes with 1,25-vitamin D have been larger (125). These changes could be due to or at least influenced by increases of osteoid and/or red marrow associated with these therapeutic agents rather than to bone mineral increases. Consequently, peripheral QCT would best be applied to monitoring the effects of stabilizing agents, such as estrogen, which seemingly have less effect on osteoid and hematopoietic tissue.

THE RELATIONSHIP OF DPA TO QCT

Both DPA and QCT are used to measure vertebral mass and density. While it is expected that there would be a fairly high correlation between them, there are several reasons why the correlation *in vivo* is imperfect. First, typical QCT measurements are usually limited to a small volume (2 to 5 cm³) of the anterior body. This volume constitutes only a few percent of vertebral mass and under 5% of the mass of the vertebral body (230,231). Measurement of a larger area of the body (13) undoubtedly helps both precision and accuracy. In contrast, DPA measures the entire vertebra minus the transverse processes (or about 85% of the total mass). Second, QCT results are usually expressed as a volumetric density of mineral (ash or K_2HPO_4 equivalent in mg/cm^3). DPA results are expressed as an area density, or mass per unit projected area (g/cm^2). When the integral bone mass is measured by QCT and DPA, or when the DPA mass is converted to a density by dividing it by the bone volume determined from QCT, then there is a good correlation ($r > 0.9$) between the methods (230,312). Third, a variety of technical factors (scattered radiation, beam hardening, position in the beam, slice orientation) contribute to errors in QCT (30,380). These errors were shown by Cann to be about 14 mg/cm^3 in mineral-equivalent density. Finally, both QCT and DPA may be subject to artifacts which inhibit accurate measurement of the different quantities they purport to measure. DPA provides an accurate (1% error) indication of bone mass on phantoms simulating bone, or on bone specimens. Area density (BMD) is also measured accurately (1% error) on phantoms, but on actual vertebral specimens the accuracy is somewhat reduced (3 to 5%). Artifacts such as osteophytes, etc. can lead to greater inaccuracies. As preferential loss of the anterior body occurs with aging and disease the relationship of the anterior region as measured by spinal QCT to total vertebral body density will decrease. QCT also becomes increasingly inaccurate with aging and with bone disease because of the variable composition of marrow (Fig. 13) and the variable content of osteoid matrix (105,211,262,231,373). QCT density predicts bone strength with an error at least five times greater [30% error (237, Fig. 14)] than DPA measurement [$r = 0.90$ (129)]. Moreover, DPA can measure integral BMC, the variable that best reflects the load resistance that is the critical factor in compression (244), whereas QCT measures strength in only a small region. DPA theoretically provides a better index of resistance to crush fracture.

In normal elderly individuals the SEE in predicting actual mineral density from single energy QCT was 16 mg/cm^3 at 85 kVp and 19 mg/cm^3 at 130 kVp (176,178,179). These errors amount to only 10 to 15% of the average value in a young normal person, 15 to 20% of the average value in healthy older women or female patients with hip fracture, and 30 to 50% of the values seen in women with spinal fractures. This large variance was due mostly to the uncertainties in single-energy QCT introduced by the variability of marrow fat (276,298). There is also a systematic error due to fat in addition to the random error (about 16 mg/cm^3) associated with variable fat (179, 231,262,276). Most studies, including the original work (105) but not the later work of the UCSF group (280), have shown that single-energy QCT gives results that are 10 to 30 mg/cm^3 lower than dual-energy QCT due to the inaccuracy resulting from influence of fat using the single-energy approach. The results from single-energy QCT overestimate aging loss by about 100% due to fat increases (178,234). Dual-energy QCT using post-reconstruction methods does not fully correct for this (262,276). The effect of fat on QCT values is very evident since actual mineral density in elderly subjects rarely is lower than 70 mg/cm^3 even in osteoporosis (11,244). In contrast QCT densities below 70 mg/cm^3 are common and even negative values are seen in clinical studies.

The fat-induced error (15 to 20 mg/cm^3) and the technical uncertainties (15 mg/cm^3) produce a total error of 20 to 25 mg/cm^3 in QCT densities. Despite this problem, QCT in competent hands has proven useful in discriminating patients with spinal osteoporosis from normal subjects (31,85,86,101,262). DPA measurements, even when less sophisticated, show statistically greater differences than QCT (277) though where DPA variance is excessive the opposite has been observed (280). The sensitivity of both DPA and QCT for spinal fracture is comparable (about 40 to 70% at the usual 95% specificity, i.e., at the 5th percentile (see Table 5). The increased vertebral fat content in patients with spinal osteoporosis (300 to 400 mg/cm^3 vs 250 mg/cm^3) decreases the apparent QCT density by at least 10 to 20

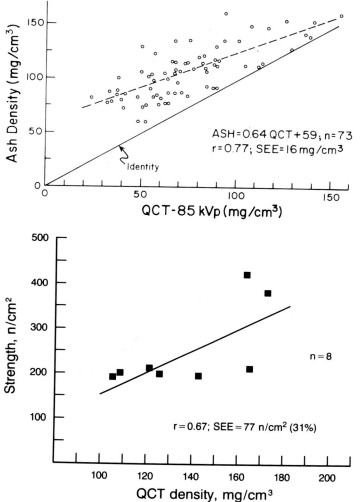

FIG. 13. Error in predicting physical density from QCT at 85 kVp; the error was 19 mg/cm³ at 130 kVp. Adapted from Laval-Jeantet et al., ref. 179, with permission.

ASH = 0.64 QCT + 59; n = 73
r = 0.77; SEE = 16 mg/cm³

FIG. 14. QCT density vs strength. Adapted from Mc-Broom et al., ref. 237.

n = 8

r = 0.67; SEE = 77 n/cm² (31%)

TABLE 5. *Sensitivity of DPA and QCT in spinal osteoporosis*

Method	Source	Within 2 SD of young normal	<2 SD below age-matched (%)
DPA	Mazess (228)	2%	72
DPA	Wahner (360)	2%	70
DPA	Mazess (233)	5%	40
DPA	Eastell et al. (78)	–	38
QCT	Firooznia (87)	15%	68
QCT	Cann (31)		21
QCT	Gallagher (101)	0	70
QCT	Pacifici (262)		50
QCT	Reinbold (281)		10

mg/cm³ to values 40 mg/cm³ (or 1.51 SD) below that of age-matched controls (and 30 to 50 mg/cm³ below the actual mineral density).

Part of the controversy concerning DPA and QCT derives from the unique achievements of researchers at UCSF using a dedicated CT scanner, achievements that have not been approximated in clinical practice (see Table 6). It is most obvious that at UCSF the radiation dose is low and the precision and accuracy are substantially better than in most institutions (32). Also the DPA instrument used at UCSF produced uniquely poor results (280).

TABLE 6. *Comparison of dual-photon absorptiometry and QCT.*

	DPA	QCT (most)	QCT (UCSF)
Precision (%)	1–3	3–9	1–3
Accuracy (%)	1–5	15–30	5–15
Marrow dose (mrem)	2	>1000	100–300
Time (min)	25	30	10–15
Sensitivity (spine)[a] (%)	40	50	20
Sensitivity (hip)[a] (%)	70	10	?
Cost	$125	>$300	$100
Sites	Various	Spine	Spine

[a]At 90% specificity.

QCT of the spine gives slightly better discrimination of spinal osteoporosis in older patients but comparable or lower discrimination than DPA in younger subjects. DPA of the femur is necessary for discrimination of hip fractures.

Density of the spine, even when determined with minimal error, has little relation to the risk of hip fracture (87,290). DPA measurements of the femur, in contrast, provide a good indication of hip fracture risk (compare Figs., 7 and 8). The development of QCT methods for scanning the proximal femur (315) offers some hope for use of the QCT method in relation to this critical problem.

ULTRASONIC MEASUREMENTS

Several investigators have examined ultrasound properties of bone and defined the properties of this tissue (2,9,16,56,174,202,285). Greenfield et al. (116,117) used speed-of-sound in compact bones. The results suggested that, at best, this method gives an inexact measure of cortical thickness. There was no incremental value of such measurement compared to single-photon absorptiometry alone (100). This is probably also true for ultrasound measurements of bone thickness (332).

Speed-of-sound has been measured *in vitro* and shown to correlate with trabecular bone volume (285). The method has been used as an indicator of "bone status" in race horses (147,349). However, speed-of-sound is greatly influenced by surrounding tissue and by marrow. Since measurements are largely confined to appendicular sites (os calcis, distal radius) there will be limited direct relevance to axial bone disease.

Attenuation of ultrasound (16) has been applied to assessment of bone density by Langton et al. (175). These studies showed that attenuation in cancellous bone reflected trabecular bone volume and that measurements *in vivo* separated femoral fracture patients from controls. Measurement on the os calcis correlated well ($r = 0.9$) with bone density of the radius (272).

NEUTRON ACTIVATION ANALYSIS

Neutron activation analysis (NAA) for calcium determination *in vivo* usually involves activation of the trace inert isotope ^{48}Ca to ^{49}Ca. This approach was developed 15 years ago (49,246,264,377). The ^{49}Ca is a high-energy γ-emitter with a short half-life (8.8 min). This short half-life requires that counting measurements be done immediately after activation and that high-efficiency scintillation detectors be used in order to achieve the best precision and accuracy at the lowest patient dose. A second activation approach, in which gaseous ^{37}Ar is produced from the common ^{40}Ca isotope (263), has not proven reliable despite its feasibility.

NAA can be done on the total body to measure total body calcium (TBCa) or on limited regions such as the hand (79,235,236), spine (5,181), or entire trunk (238). NAA of the hand measures mostly compact bone and correlates poorly (r about 0.3) with TBV of iliac crest biopsies in hemodialized and osteoporotic patients (236). Localized spine measurements can be done with a precision of 2 to 3% (335), but there are problems with (a) uniformity and specificity of irradiation, and (b) with the efficiency of counting (leading to high radiation doses of about 5000 mrem). NAA of the entire trunk provides somewhat poorer precision (5% error *in vivo*) albeit at a lower dose, 300 mrem (133). However, this trunk area is diagnostically less sensitive than the spine itself and it does not correlate much better with spinal density than does peripheral densitometry (224).

Still, because this measurement includes the spine, significant changes have been observed with agents like sodium fluoride that increase spinal density (134).

Total body NAA for TBCa has been deemed more desirable than regional measurement despite the greater difficulty (41,49,280), but the number of facilities in the world doing this determination is still less than a dozen. The high cost of NAA, both irradiation and counting, limits its implementation. The usual radiation dose is 2000 to 5000 mrem and the typical precision is 4 to 5% with conventional shadow-shield detectors (159,340,377). The accuracy error may be 5 to 10% (280,340) particularly in those facilities where limited detectors and less sophisticated counting instrumentation prevents precise correction. Only in the advanced facility at Brookhaven National Laboratory (7,148) can TBCa by NAA be considered a "gold standard." The large area detectors and sophisticated electronics at this facility reduce dose to 300 mrem and allow good precision and accuracy (2% error). TBCa could prove to be the "fools gold standard" in centers at the low end of the precision and accuracy spectrum (41).

Recent clinical results on TBCa from Brookhaven have been encouraging with regard to the diagnostic utility of TBCa at that facility (53). These improved results derive in part from the normalization procedure utilized at that facility. Normalization reduces the intra-population variation from 15 to 8% and thereby increases diagnostic sensitivity (53). Longitudinal studies at the same center have shown that calcium and exercise had minimal effects on TBCa and that aging changes in the radius did not correlate highly with those in skeletal mass (7). TBCa studies using less-advanced instrumentation have produced results which are questionable physiologically at least in control groups (38–40,160).

COMPTON SCATTERING

There are now numerous approaches to measuring bone density *in vivo* using detection of the radiation scattered from a small area of interest, typically 2 to 10 cm^3 (368). The intensity of Compton-scattering depends on the electron density.

The initial scattering method was developed approximately 15 years ago at about the same time by the two Canadian research groups (47,103,160) and by German investigators (282). Simpler approaches were taken by Israeli workers (135,184). The dose with these methods was high, about 2000 mrem, and there were substantial errors due to (a) multiple scattering, and (b) geometrical uncertainties.

The method was improved by using lower energy radionuclide and x-ray sources with detection of scattered radiation at smaller angles (143,258,369). The geometric uncertainties were better controlled (144,161) and the dose greatly reduced. This approach has given reasonably accurate and precise data *in vivo* (295,327).

An alternative approach uses the ratio of coherent to Compton-scattering with ^{241}Am, ^{153}Gd, or ^{153}Sm (35,108,158,162,186,259,275). The coherent-Compton method gives information on both electron density and atomic number of the irradiated area. A high purity Ge(Li) detector is needed to separately count the coherent and Compston scatter because their close energy proximity makes conventional scintillation detectors unusable. A 3% precision error has been achieved with a dose of about 500 mrem (328). The recent use of X-ray sources for this application (128,370,371) allows rapid measurements with even better precision.

All of these methods currently focus on peripheral sites, such as the distal radius and os calcis (295,296). Thus, even when performed successfully, they are subject to the inherent deficiency associated with these areas of marginal clinical interest. In particular, it has been demonstrated that (a) Compton density of the os calcis is highly influenced by body weight and physical activity (295), and (b) the observed longitudinal changes in Compton density are too large to correspond to relevant physiological changes (296). Because of problems with inherent errors, high radiation dose, disagreements on optimal approach and lack of commercial instrumentation, there have not been significant technical or clinical advances in this area for the past several years.

NORMALIZATION

Normalization refers to the procedures used to compare observed values for a subject or a group of subjects to those for a normal population. The observed values can be compared to the mean of the referent population and the difference expressed as a percentage, a Z-score, a percentile, or some other index. This type of comparison has been used since the inception of the first quantitative approaches to radiologic densitometry and has been the standard clinical practice for photon absorptiometry over the past twenty years.

Comparison to Normals and Abnormals

The most common comparison is made by expressing the observed value of a subject as a percentage of the mean value in a referent population. Usually that population consists of a definite ethnic group, such as U.S. whites, who are free of chronic diseases, are not using medications affecting skeletal metabolism, and are free of nontraumatic fractures. The defect of this approach is that it does not take into account the intrapopulation variance. A 10% deviation is almost 2 SD different from the mean in young normals for a radius shaft SPA measurement while it is only 0.4 SD different for QCT of the spine. Difference can be expressed relative to the standard deviation as a Z-score (difference divided by the standard deviation). Such Z-scores are proportional to the centiles derived from a normal curve (Table 7) and to sensitivity and specificity. Alternatively, centiles can be expressed directly (66).

The implicit assumption in such normalization is that deviancy below normal is indicative of "abnormality". However, this is not uniformly the case for different measurement sites or methods. For example, the mean spine and femur values in young normal women (using

TABLE 7. *Discrimination of spinal and hip fracture osteoporosis relative to age-matched controls using Z-scores*

	Z-scores		Extrapolated centiles	
	Spine	Hip	Spine	Hip
Age (years)	65	75		
SPA-distal radius[c]	−1.0	−0.8	16	21
QCT-distal radius[c]	−0.7	−0.6	24	27
QCT-spine[c]	−1.6	−0.8	5	21
QCT-spine[b]	−1.6	−0.5	5	30
TBV-biopsy[c]	−0.6	−0.5	27	31
DPA-spine[a]	−1.4	−0.8	8	20
DPA-hip[a]	−1.0	−1.5	15	6

The Z-scores were transformed into extrapolated centiles at which the osteoporotic mean value occurs.
[a]From Mazess et al., ref. 233, with permission.
[b]From Firooznia et al., refs. 86, 87.
[c]From Harma et al., refs. 131, 132.

DPA) are 1.27 and 1.01 g/cm², respectively, while the values in osteoporotic patients, with fractures at these sites, average 0.86 and 0.56 g/cm². In the first case, the difference is 0.41 g/cm² while in the latter it is 0.45 g/cm². The former site shows a 32% reduction (3.2 SD) in osteoporosis, while the latter exhibits a 45% reduction (4.5 SD) despite the fact that the absolute magnitude of bone diminution is similar. Normal women 70 years of age average about 1.02 g/cm² (− 20% or 2.0 SD) for the spine and 0.75 g/cm² (− 26% or 2.6 SD) for the femur. Considering these site differences it could be advantageous to express clinical results relative to the normal-abnormal difference. For the normal women noted above, the spine score would be ([1.27 − 1.02]/0.41)*100 or 61 while the femur score would be ([1.01 − 0.75]/0.45)*100 or 58. Scoring in this way ignores purely statistical deviancy (Z-scores and percentiles) in favor of a rating scale that is proportional to fracture risk. The fracture "threshold," the deviancy level where fractures first become evident, occurs at a score of about 70 for both spine and femur. Such a scoring approach could prove more understandable clinically, than the commonly used measures of deviancy (centiles below normal, Z-scores, percentages). Alternatively results can be expressed directly in terms of the centile distribution in a population with fractures. The "normal" 70-year-old woman noted above lies at the 61st centile for spinal osteoporosis and at the 97th centile of femoral fracture.

Adjustment for Ethnic Group

Bone mass and density seem to be remarkably uniform in the white population of the U.S. and Europe (220,310) but do vary among other ethnic groups at least according to data on the peripheral skeleton. Blacks have bone density values that average 5 to 10% above those for comparable whites (50,110,220,351) while orientals have values that are 5 to 10% lower (383). The difference is consistent with blacks having a fracture rate about 30 to 50% that of whites. The lower density in orientals in part reflects the smaller body size of oriental populations and may not directly translate into higher fracture risk.

Adjustment for Bone and Body Size

It is obvious that larger individuals have bigger skeletons and will, therefore, show higher values for noninvasive measurements of bone mass. Males, for example, have a bone mineral content that is about 30% greater than that of females (220). Males also tend to have "denser" bones, at least in the peripheral skeleton, than females (214,248). Part of this sex difference is due simply to the larger body size of males. Even within each sex, however, larger individuals have bigger bones and a higher bone density. It has been considered useful, therefore, to adjust for bone and body size.

Nilas et al. (252) have reviewed adjustments of radius, spinal and total body bone mineral in 161 women during the early post-menopausal years. They found that TBBM was closely correlated ($r = 0.92$) with projected skeletal area; normalization for skeletal size reduced the SD in TBBM from 15 to 6%. On the distal radius, adjustment for bone size decreased the SD from about 14 to about 12%. Adjustment of lumbar spine BMC for bone size also reduced the SD only slightly (from 16 to 13%). Further corrections of these adjusted values for body size were not explored. The same research group previously showed that adjustments of the BMC on the very distal radius for height, weight, and lean body mass had little influence on variances (45).

Densities could also be influenced by strength and muscle size as well as bone and body weight. Chow et al. (42) demonstrated a moderate correlation between trunk calcium and oxygen intake. Sinaki and McPhee (330) showed that spinal BMD was influenced to a small degree by height, weight, and strength of the back extensor muscles. Psoas width is apparently reduced some time before osteoporosis is evident (271). Doyle et al. (73) also showed psoas size was related to ash density of the third lumber vertebra. Pocock et al. (270) showed that spine density by DPA was moderately correlated to maximal oxygen uptake ($r = 0.5$) and femoral density even more highly associated ($r = 0.6$). It is not clear as yet if adjustments should be made for muscle strength or size.

Adjustments may have value in reducing extraneous variance but will not enhance diagnostic sensitivity if the normal-abnormal difference is reduced as well. Krolner (167) examined various approaches to ajdust spinal BMD (DPA) for bone width and area. He found these reduced the SD from about 27 to 15% but that such adjustment did not greatly increase the significance of the difference between normal and osteoporotic women.

DIAGNOSTIC VALUE

The relative diagnostic value of different measurement approaches or sites is extremely difficult to evaluate because different procedures and population samples are used in the various reports in the literature. Most comparisons of older osteoporotic patients with "age-matched controls" are flawed because at the time the study is performed, axial loss probably has stabilized while ongoing appendicular loss has caught up with axial loss (53,82,120). Thus the situation differs from that in younger subjects who would actually be the target for early diagnosis. Second, the values in the age-matched group depend critically on its age composition and the exclusion criteria for disease and/or drug use. When fractures, chronic diseases and chronic drug use (including aluminum antacids) are excluded the variance even in an elderly population is similar to that in a younger population. Third, differing and arbitrary thresholds of fracture risk are used in comparisons (385). These problems can be avoided in part by using a fixed, functional criteria as a threshold in separating normal and abnormal groups and by comparing young normal subjects to osteoporotic patients. This was done in Table 4 where specificity (= true negatives) was examined at an 84% sensitivity (i.e., the threshold was taken as the mean density level in osteoporotic patients plus one standard deviation). Conversely, sensitivity (true positives) was examined at an 84% specificity (i.e., the threshold was taken as the mean density in normal subjects minus one SD). ROC analyses of this sort depend critically on the intrapopulation variances as well as on the intergroup difference. This has led to failures in discrimination of abnormality in studies where the procedures, instrumentation and sample selection led to much larger intrapopulation variances than usual (52,260,277,280).

The os calcis appears to be the least favorable of the peripheral sites for diagnostic use, while the radius shaft is the most sensitive. The distal radius provides specificity comparable to the shaft site but not the sensitivity (269). The three peripheral sites were markedly inferior to the axial sites; both false positives and false negatives were at least 10 to 20 times more common at peripheral sites. Of the two axial sites, the femur provided better discrimination of abnormality than the spine. These figures are, of course, only approximate given the lack of detailed studies, but do show the diagnostic value of axial and total body

TABLE 8. *Bone density values at local sites and for the total skeleton in young normal and osteoporotic patients, together with sensitivity (at 84% specificity) and specificity (at 84% sensitivity)*

	Young normal		Osteo-porotic		Speci-ficity	Sensi-tivity
	X	SD	X	SD	%	%
Femoral neck	1.01	.11	.56	.10	99.9	99.9
Lumbar spine	1.26	.12	.86	.13	98.5	98.3
Radius-shaft	.71	.06	.54	.10	89.4	87.3
Radius-distal	.42	.06	.28	.07	87.9	88.8
Os calcis	.44	.07	.31	.08	77.9	78.8
Total skeleton	1.07	.15	.80	.15	78.8	78.8

measurements compared to measurements at any peripheral site.

SKELETAL UPTAKE

Efforts to develop techniques for nontraumatic measurements of bone metabolism and turnover have in general been less successful than those directed towards the development of noninvasive bone mineral measurements. Initial radiochemical studies with alkaline earths and fluorine have been largely replaced by technetium labeled diphosphonates.

A sizeable literature has accumulated over the last two decades that describes qualitative and quantitative approaches to skeletal uptake measurements of diphosphonates in different metabolic bone diseases. Techniques with acceptable accuracy and precision are now available. Virtually diagnostic scintigraphic images have been described in advanced metabolic bone disease. Groups of patients with metabolic bone disease have been distinguished from normal control groups by quantitative studies. Yet the routine clinical usefulness of diphosphonate uptake procedures is still controversial. This is mainly because of the complex uptake mechanism of these diphosphonates that does not closely reflect a single diagnostically important bone parameter, such as bone resorption or bone formation, and the uptake variations are not as well-documented as more common histomorphometric analyses of bone biopsy. The uptake mechanism and the importance of this technique in diagnosis and management of osteoporosis is reviewed.

Mechanism of Diphosphonate Uptake

The radiopharmaceuticals of interest for assessment of metabolic bone disease are diphosphonates, specifically disodium methylene diphosphonate (MDP), disodium hydroxymethelene diphosphonate (HMDP), and hydroxyethylene diphosphonates (NEDP). The compounds bind reduced technetium and apatite in a complex bond (69). The preparation injected for clinical use is probably a mixture of very similar but not identical complexes.

The three compounds differ in blood clearance, soft tissue retention, skeletal uptake and kidney excretion (194) (Fig. 15). Compounds with greater lipophilic activity have higher tissue retention which is unwarranted for imaging and quantitation (97,98). Of the three compounds HMDP shows the highest and HEDP the lowest body retention. Several comparisons of different agents are available in the literature (96,97,266). Changes in uptake affect the entire skeleton but vary in extent in different portions of the skeleton (95). This is of importance for selection of skeletal sites when regional measurements are made.

The radioisotope of Technetium (^{99m}Tc) is eluted as sodium pertechnetate (Na^{99m}TcO$_4$) from commercially available Molybdenum (^{99}Mo) generators. For effective complexing with a bone seeking chemical it is reduced to ^{99m}Tc cation (III, IV, or V) with stannous ion. This step should be performed just prior to intravenous injection, since the type of complexes formed and with it the skeletal uptake vary with time. In general ^{99m}Tc diphosphonates are stable up to 4 to 6 hr after preparation. Some vendors add sterilizing agents to reduce degradation.

Almost 70% of an intravenously administered dose of MDP is excreted by the normally functioning kidneys within 6 hr, and 24 hr retention is almost entirely in the skeleton (2).

Uptake and retention in any tissue appears to be a function of the calcium content (329). In bone tissue however blood flow, metabolic activity and surface area exert an additional influence on uptake. Maximal bone uptake occurs between 2 and 4 hr but may take longer in bone tumors. (46,199). Lesion to bone and bone to soft tissue ratios continue to rise up to 4 to 6 hr depending on the compound used. (91,92,199).

The uptake of ^{99m}Tc-labeled diphosphonates in bone is a complex mechanism that can be conceptualized as depending on several steps which are, however, difficult to evaluate independently. These are: (1) blood flow, (2) diffusion out of the vascular compartment into the interstitial space, (3) chemadsorption onto the surface of bone, and (4) fate of the complexes at the bone surface. Of these steps the last is least well-understood.

Although vascular supply is *sine qua non* for diphosphonate uptake other factors are significantly involved even at early measurements. Therefore diphosphonate bone uptake cannot be used to accurately measure skeletal blood flow. The unusual early high uptake of diphosphonate agents at sites of rapid bone formation such as healing fractures, epiphyseal growth plates, and bone tumors cannot be explained on the basis of blood flow alone. (180).

Autoradiographic studies show a striking selectivity of diphosphonates or ^{99m}Tc diphosphonate complexes for the mineral component (Ca-P surface) of bone. This is after exclusion of deposition in the organic matrix. (122,348). Francis found that the adsorption on the immature calcium phosphate (low Ca/P ratio) was higher than on the mature crystalline hydroxyapatite (97). The intense bone uptake seen in osteomalacia is not readily explained by this mechanism, however, and additional factors not well known at present, may play a role. (98).

It is not known whether the complexes, once adsorbed onto the hydroxyapatite surface, remain intact or break down on the surface. In the latter case the ^{99m}Tc (IV) ion might hydrolyse, migrate and adsorb separately on the

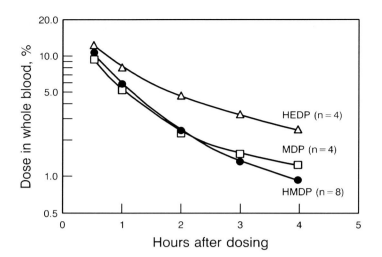

FIG. 15. Blood clearance of three diphosphonate compounds in dogs as a function of time. Adapted from Bevan et al., ref. 19, with permission.

bone surface as highly insoluble[99m]Tc_2 (98). The tin behaves similar to calcium and also is found in the mineral phase (70).

Clinical Use of Diphosphonate Uptake

In contrast to bone mineral measurements, that reflect the amount of bone present at the time of examination, the information from bone scintigraphy performed under standardized conditions is related to the rate of bone formation (osteoblastic activity) and blood flow and is thought to reflect bone metabolism in a broad sense. The retention of different radiopharmaceuticals is not the same, but the interrelationship between different bones is remarkably constant for each radiopharmaceutical (Fig. 15). Data obtained with different compounds have to be compared with this in mind. Bones with primarily trabecular bone with very thin cortices have a higher retention with all three agents, while bones that are largely cortical with relatively low metabolic activity show lower retention with MDP. The femurs constitute only slightly more than 10% of total body retention while the ribs contribute over 40%. (95). Superimposed on this normal pattern, in active metabolic bone disease, bone loss usually occurs in the entire skeleton, but trabecular bone sites show earliest and most pronounced involvement. On normal scintigrams,

therefore, moderately to markedly increased uptake is seen in the skull, mandible, ends of femurs, and proximal ends of tibias (listed in approximate order of frequency of occurrence). The highest uptake is generally in the sacroiliac joints, followed in descending order by thoracic spine, lumbar spine, sternum and ilia, kidneys, ischia, mandible, skull, and ends of femurs and tibias. (240). In patients with high rates of bone loss, scintigraphy may reveal characteristically abnormal patterns of uptake that can be useful in the differential diagnosis.

There is variation in skeletal uptake in normal subjects with age, kidney function, hydration and other factors affecting soft tissue retention. These factors have to be considered in the interpretation of the standard total body scintigram, taken 2 to 4 hr post-injection, generally used for the diagnosis of focal bone disease. Because of this, slightly increased tracer uptake throughout the entire skeleton is difficult to detect by visual inspection alone. In more severe cases, however, the standard bone scintigram can show striking abnormalities.

Fogelman et al. (92) have described bone scintigraphic patterns of metabolic bone disease. If three or more of the seven generalized features they described are present, metabolic bone disease should be suspected (Table 9). These findings on bone scintigraphy, however, are not specific for any particular condition or

TABLE 9. *Bone scintigraphic patterns in patients with metabolic bone disease*

Generalized features
Increased tracer uptake in axial skeleton
Increased tracer uptake in long bones
Increased tracer uptake in periarticular areas
Prominent calvaria and mandible
Beading of the costochondral junctions
Increased tracer uptake in sternum (tie sternum, striped tie sign) Faint or absent kidney images (only in absence of kidney disease)

Occasionally associated findings
Focal tracer uptake involving one or more entire vertebrae (spinal compression fracture)
Focal tracer uptake in ribs or other skeletal areas (fractures, pseudofractures, stress microfractures)
Abnormal tracer uptake in kidneys (renal disease)
Soft tissue tracer uptake (soft tissue calcification)

Modified from Fogelman et al., ref. 92.

group of metabolic bone disorders and only suggest a generalized increase in skeletal remodeling. This can occasionally be seen in normal adolescents which suggest that caution should be used in interpretation when this pattern is seen in young subjects. In patients with metabolic bone disease this generalized increase is often accompanied by focal uptake suggestive of superimposed focal pathologic processes (Table 9) not seen in the normal young adult.

Reports about diphosphonate uptake are available in a number of metabolic bone diseases (Table 10). However bone scintigrams and quantitation are rarely useful in the diagno-

TABLE 10. *Scintigraphy in metabolic bone disease. Diffuse skeletal uptake pattern*

Renal osteodystrophy
Primary hyperparathyroidism
Osteomalacia
Al-induced osteomalacia
Osteoporosis
NaF-treated osteoporosis
Reflux sympathetic dystrophy
Hyperthyroidism
Acromegaly
Hyperparathyroidism
Systemic mastocytosis
Hyperphosphatasia
Osteopetrosis
Cushing's syndrome

---

sis or management of idiopathic osteoporosis and the information provided is less reliable than this from standard radiographs (93). A washed-out pattern has been described and been related to "end stage" disease with a low bone mass and markedly low bone turnover. Sy observed these features in 72% of his patients with osteoporosis (344). Fogelman reports this number to be smaller in his series. (93). A few patients, however, demonstrate increased uptake. These patients have been thought to have high ratios of bone turnover, extensive bone involvement, or other etiologic factors that have contributed to the bone loss (89). This observation needs further clarification. Recent spinal compression fractures appear as foci of increased uptake on the scintigram. (Fig. 16) Occasionally, the bone scintigram may be used to determine the age of an asymptomatic radiographically detected vertebral fracture. In a study by Matin, (204) the minimal time for tracer uptake to return to normal levels after a vertebral fracture was 7 months. Of all vertebral fractures in that study, 59% showed normal tracer uptake within 1 year and 31% within 2 years; after 3 years, 10% still showed abnormal tracer uptake.

In women with osteoporosis and on NaF and Ca treatment, Schultz et al. (322) have described new focal areas of increased tracer uptake particularly in the peripheral skeleton at sites of trabecular bone such as the metaphysis 6 months after the treatment was initiated. These areas were interpreted as focal areas of intense bone remodeling in response to NaF therapy and were considered evidence for an effect of the NaF and Ca regimen on the peripheral skeleton.

O'Duffy et al. (257) found similar results in patients with osteoporosis who had developed the lower extremity pain syndrome while on a similar NaF treatment regimen. Patients on the treatment regimen had higher numbers of foci of abnormal bone remodeling than controls on calcium alone. Abnormal uptake was always found at sites of bone pain but many additional asymptomatic focal areas of uptake were noted. In about half of the patients with the

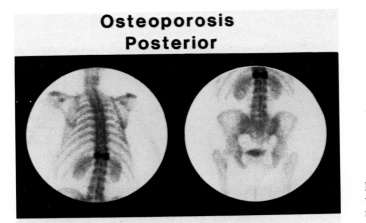

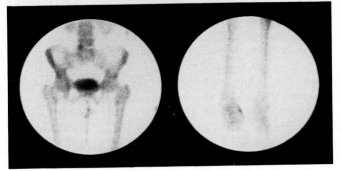

FIG. 16. Skeletal scintigram of woman with documented osteoporosis. A radiographically confirmed recent compression fracture is noted in T12. Focal degenerative changes are present at the right side of L5–S1. The remainder of the scintigram is normal.

pain syndrome a stress fracture was identified radiographically. It was concluded that the pain resulted from acute focal bone remodeling which may be complicated by stress microfracture. (Fig. 17)

Attempts have been made to quantitate the maximal skeletal uptake and to study dynamic aspects of this uptake to better detect abnormal bone metabolism at early stages when the scintigraphic findings are still inconclusive. Several approaches have been proposed, all of which necessitate rigid adherence to a standardized protocol. (Table 11).

The ratio of bone to soft tissue uptake provides a rough estimate of the uptake in bone but may lead to a falsely low estimation because of the high level of background activity in soft tissue that has been affected by hypercalcemia, dehydration, or poor renal function (92,323) (Fig. 18). Increase in skeletal uptake

TABLE 11. *Standardized protocol for quantitative evaluation of methylene diphosphonate uptake in bone*

Visual inspection of bone scintigrams[92,344]
Ratio measurements with use of bone scintigrams
   Comparison with presumably normal bone
   Comparison of bone and soft tissue
   Comparison with a simultaneously imaged phantom[240]

Regional blood flow and clearance measurements[256,323]
   Early vascular phase
   Early uptake phase
   Above with correction for glomerular filtration rate

Whole body retention at 24 hr[28,90,94]
   Whole body counter
   Gamma camera
   Thyroid-uptake probe[34]
   24-hr urine collection

in patients with non-osseous malignances has been noted. The 24-hr whole body retention method has received the most attention but is technically demanding and tends to overesti-

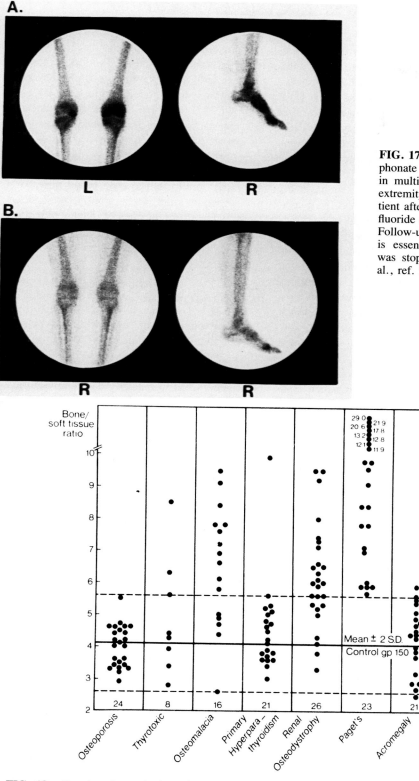

FIG. 17. **A:** Increased diphosphonate uptake on scintigraphy in multiple bones of the lower extremity in a symptomatic patient after six months of sodium fluoride and calcium therapy. **B:** Follow-up scan 15 months later is essentially normal. Therapy was stopped. From O'Duffy et al., ref. 257, with permission.

FIG. 18. Results of quantitation of bone-to-soft tissue ratio of scintigraphic skeletal uptake for early detection of metabolic bone disorders. The values of eight patients with Paget's disease that exceeded the upper limits of this graph are specified at the top of the chart. From Fogelman et al., ref. 92, by permission of the European Nuclear Medicine Society and Springer-Verlag.

mate skeletal uptake in patients with abnormal uptake of tracer in soft tissues and those with associated focal bone disease. (29,90,94,203). Approaches using a simple thyroid probe (34) or gamma camera make the procedure more accessible than the whole body counters used in experimental laboratories. Whole body retention shows age and sex related changes. (Fig. 19)

Measurements of tracer uptake in the skull with use of single-photon emission CT or conventional scintigraphy of the head in conjunction with a reference standard and film densitometry for quantitation have been described as sensitive methods for the assessment of bone remodeling activity (80) (Fig. 20). Corrections for glomerular filtration rate have been proposed to measure more specifically the removal of diphosphonate from the blood (256).

The results from such quantitations obtained mostly from studies of small groups of patients, show that patients with certain metabolic bone diseases can be distinguished from normal persons, but results with patients with osteoporosis have been disappointing. How-ever for other metabolic bone diseases such as renal osteodystrophy, Paget's disease, osteomalacia and hyperparathyroidism, interesting observations have been made. (90,94,145, 203,304,347) (see Figs. 18,20). Acceptance of this approach for the management of patients by estimation of bone loss has been slow. The major criticism is that uptake of the radiopharmaceutical agents is dependent not only on osteoblastic activity but also on blood flow, kidney function, and other poorly understood factors. The different rates of uptake shown by various phosphate compounds further obscure the issue, and make a review of the available literature confusing.

CONCLUSIONS

Several methods are now widely available for noninvasive bone measurement in metabolic bone disease (SPA, DPA, QCT), but others are still experimental in that the equipment is confined to major research laboratories and likely will be for the foreseeable future (neutron activation, peripheral QCT, Compton

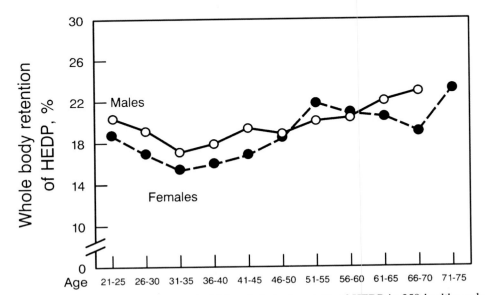

FIG. 19. Age and sex related changes in 24 hr whole-body uptake of HEDP in 250 healthy volunteers. From Fogelman et al. (1980): *J. Nucl. Med.*, 23:296–300, with permission.

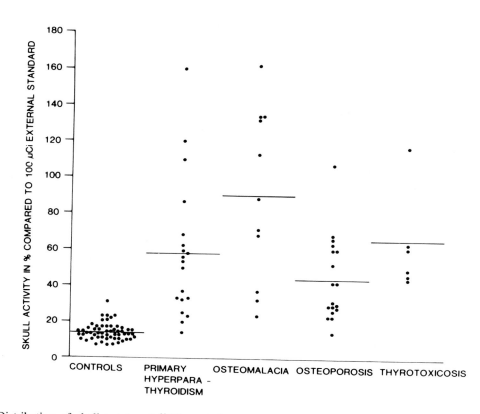

FIG. 20. Distribution of skull uptake of ^{99m}Tc-methylene diphosphonate and mean values *(horizontal lines)* of control group and four groups of patients with metabolic bone disease. From Meindock et al., ref. 240, with permission of Chapman and Hall, London.

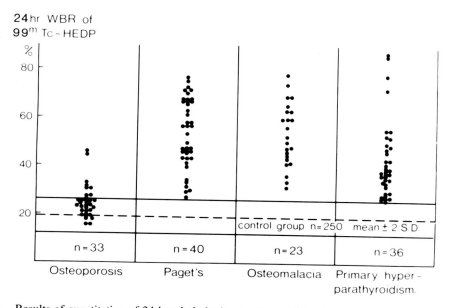

FIG. 21. Results of quantitation of 24-hr whole-body retention of ^{99m}Tc-hydroxyethylidene diphosphonate for early scintigraphic detection of metabolic bone disorders. From Fogelman, ref. 89, with permission of Futura Publishing Company.

scattering). Other methods, like the potentially more accessible ultrasound approach have not yet been demonstrated to have clinical value. Significant questions still remain on the incremental value of diphosphonate uptake studies but the wide availability of gamma-cameras may make them useful in the future.

Bone measurement by single and dual-photon absorptiometry using radionuclide sources offers the clinician the possibility of direct skeletal evaluation at minimal cost, effort, and with very low radiation dose. SPA measurements on the limbs have been most useful in pediatric applications and for renal osteodystrophy, but have been less successful in the early diagnosis of osteoporosis and monitoring of its therapy. SPA on the radius shaft, where precision error is low, could be useful for monitoring estrogen therapy but many gynecologists and internists still give estrogen without monitoring in hopes that the dose will be appropriate. Newer instrumentation utilizing rectilinear scanning has allowed extension of the original SPA approach, that was largely confined to the shafts of long bones, to more irregularly shaped regions such as the ultradistal radius and the os calcis. The preliminary studies at these sites, however, have indicated that compared to the older shaft sites: (a) they are no more diagnostically sensitive, at least in osteoporosis; (b) they are not better correlated with bone density at axial fracture locations and (c) they are equally unresponsive to therapies.

DPA allows low-cost, low-dose measurements at key fracture sites, the spine and proximal femur, as well as total skeletal density. The diagnostic sensitivity of the DPA method is far superior to alternatives on the peripheral skeleton, and DPA offers monitoring capabilities hitherto unavailable. Certainly the major advantages of low-cost, low radiation exposure, accessibility, and patient acceptance as well as a freedom from technical and compositional uncertainties make DPA preferable for spinal assessment. DPA is the only method practiced for femoral and total skeletal assessment.

The new developments in bone densitometry and diphosphonate uptakes provide not only an avenue for clinical research but major advances in clinical management of patients with bone disease.

REFERENCES

1. Aaron, J.E., Gallagher, J.C., Anderson, J. Stasiak, L., Longton, E.B., Nordin,B.E.C., and Nicholson, M. (1974): Frequency of osteomalacia and osteoporosis in fractures of the proximal femur. *Lancet, L:229–233.*
2. Abendeschein, W., and Hyatt, G.W. (1970): Ultrasound and selected physical properties of bone. *Clin. Orthop.* 69:294–301.
3. Alhava, E.M., and Karjalainen, P. (1973): The mineral content and mineral density of bone of the forearms in healthy persons measured by Am-241 gamma ray attenuation method. *Ann. Clin. Res.,* 5:238–243.
4. Alhava, E.M., and Karjalainen, P. (1973): Mineral content and density of the forearm bones measured by Am-241 gamma ray attenuation method in 80 patients with osteoporosis hip fractures. *Ann. Clin. Res.,* 5:244–247.
5. Al-Hiti, K., Thomas, B.J., Al-Tikrity, S.A., Ettinger, K.V., Fremlin, J.H., and Dabek, J.T. (1976): Spinal calcium: its *in vivo* measurement in man. *Inter. J. Appl. Rad. Isot.* 27:97–102.
6. Aloia, J.F. (1982): Estrogen and exercise in prevention and treatment of osteoporosis. *Geriatrics,* 37:81–85.
7. Aloia, J.F., Ross, P., Vaswani, A., Zanzi, I., and Cohn, S.H. (1982): Rate of bone loss in postmenopausal and osteoporotic women. *J. Am. Physiol.* 242 (Endoc. Metab. 5): E82–E86.
8. Als, O.S., Gotfredsen, A., Riss, B.J., and Christiansen C. (1985): Are disease duration and degree of functional impairment determinants of bone loss in rheumatoid arthritis. *Ann. Rheum. Dis.,* 44:406–411.
9. Andre, M.P., Craven, J.D., and Greenfield M.A. (1980): Measurement of the velocity of ultrasound in the human femur *in vivo. Med. Phys.,* 7:324–330.
10. Aniansson, A., and Zetterberg, C. (1984): Impaired muscle function with aging. A background factor in the incidence of fractures of the proximal end of the femur. *Clin. Ortho.,* 191:193–201.
11. Arnold, J. (1973): Amount and quality of trabecular bone in osteoporotic vertebral fractures. *Clin. Endocr. Metab.,,* 2:221–238.
12. Awbrey, B.J., Jacobson, P.C., Grubb, S.A., McCartney, W.H., Vincent, L.M., and Talmage, R.V. (1984): Bone density in women: a modified procedure for measurement of distal radial density. *J. Orthrop. Res.,* 2:314–321.
13. Banks, L.M., and Stevenson, J.C. (1986): Modified method of spinal computed tomography for trabecular bone mineral measurements. *J. Comp. Assist. Tomog.,* 10(3):463–467.
14. Banzer, D.H., Schneider, U., Risch, W.D., and

Botsch, H. (1976): Roentgen signs of vertebral de-mineralization and mineral content of peripheral cancellous bone. *Am. J. Roentgen.*, 126:1306–1308.

15. Barden, H., Mazess, R.B. and Ettinger, M. (1986): Bone mineral density in femoral fractures. *J. Bone Min. Res.*, 1:284.

16. Barger, J.E. (1979): Attenuation and dispersion of ultrasound in cancellous bone. In: *Ultrasonic Tissue Characterization II,* edited by M. Linzer. NBS Publication 525, U.S. Government Printing Office, Washington, D.C.

17. Baylink, D.J., Vose, G.P., Dotter, W.E., and Hurxthala, L.M. (1964): Two methods for the study of osteoporosis and other metabolic bone diseases. II. Radiographic densitometry. *Lahey Clin. Bull.*, 13:217–277.

18. Bellazzini, R., Brez, A., Del Guerra, A., Massai, M.M., and Torquati, M.R. (1984): Digital imaging with a pressurized xenon filled MWPC working at a high data rate. *Nucl., Inst. Meth.*, 228:193–200.

19. Bevan, J., et al. (1979): *Proceedings Second International Symposium on Radiopharmaceuticals,* March 19–22, 1979 Seattle, Washington pp., 645–654. Society of Nuclear Medicine, New York.

20. Bohr, H., and Schaadt, O. (1983): Bone mineral content of femoral bone and the lumbar spine measured in women with fracture of the femoral neck by dual photon absorptiometry. *Clin. Orthol.*, 179:240–245.

21. Bohr, H., and Schaadt, O. (1985): Bone mineral content of the femoral neck and shaft: relation between cortical and trabecular bone. *Calcif. Tissue Int.*, 37:340–344.

22. Borders, S., Peterson, K.R., and Orne, D. (1977): Prediction of bending strength of long bones from measurements of bending stiffness and bone mineral content. *J. Biomechan. Eng.*, 99:40–44.

23. Brassow, F., Crone-Munzebrock, W., Weh, L., Kranz, R., and Eggers-Stroeder, G. (1982): Correlations between breaking load and CT absorption values of vertebral bodies. *Europ. J. Radiol.*, 2:99–101.

24. Briancon, D., and Meunier, P.J. (1981): Treatment of osteoporosis with fluoride, calcium and vitamin D. *Orthop. Clin. North Am.*, 12:629–648.

25. Buccianti, G., Bianchi, M.L., Valenti, G., and Ortolani, S. (1983): Direct photon absorptiometry for long term monitoring of uremic osteodystrophy. *Nephron,* 34:135–137.

26. Bydder, G.M., Elsasser, U., Hesp, R., Reeve, J., and Spinks, T.J. (1982): The relationship between CT measurements on the radius and results obtained by other techniques. *J. Comput. Assist., Tomogr.*, 6:212–213.

27. Cameron, J.R., and Sorenson, J. (1963): Measurement of bone mineral *in vivo:* an improved method. *Science,* 142:230–232.

28. Cameron, J.R., Mazess, R.B., and Sorenson, J.A. (1968): Precision and accuracy of bone mineral determination by the direct photon absorptiometric method. *Invest. Radiol.*, 3:141–150.

29. Caniggia, A., and Vattimo, A. (1980): Kinetics of ^{99m}technetium-tin-methylenediphosphonate in normal subjects and pathological conditions: a simple index of bone metabolism. *Calcif. Tissue Int.*, 30:5–13.

30. Cann, C.E., Genant, H.K., Ettinger, B., and Gordon, G.S. (1980): Spinal mineral loss in oophorectomized women. *JAMA* 244:2056–2059.

31. Cann, C.E., Genant, H.K., Kolb, F.O., and Ettinger, B. (1985): Quantitative computed tomography for prediction of vertebral fracture risk. *Bone,* 6:1–7.

32. Cann, C.E. (1987): Quantitative CT applications: comparison of current scanners. *Radiology,* 162:257–261.

33. Carter, D.R., and Hayes, W.C. (1976): Bone compressive strength: the influence of density and strain rate. *Science,* 194:1174–1175.

34. Castronovo, F.P., Jr., McKusick, K.A., Dann, J., Proout, G.R., and Strauss, H.W. (1985): A simplified technique for quantifying 24-hr whole body retention of ^{99m}Tc-labeled methylene diphosphonate (MDP). *Int. J. Nucl. Biol.*, 12(3):209–214.

35. Chalmers, J. (1973): Distribution of osteoporotic changes in the aging skeleton. *Clin. Endoc. Metab.*, 2:203–220.

36. Chesney, R.W., Mazess, R.B., Rose, P., Hamstra, A.J., DeLuca, H.F., and Breed, A.L. (1983): Long-term influence of calcitriol (1,25-dihydroxyvitamin D) and supplemental phosphate in x-linked hypophosphatemic rickets. *Pediatrics,* 71(4:559–567.

37. Chesney, R.W., Mazess, R.B., Rose, P.G., and Jax, D.K. (1977): Bone mineral status measured by direct photon absorptiometry in childhood renal disease. *Pediatrics,* 60:864–872.

38. Chesnut, C.H., Ivey, J.L., Nelp, W.B., and Baylink, D.J. (1979): Assessment of anabolic steroids and calcitonin in the treatment of osteoporosis. In: *Osteoporosis II,* edited by U.S. Barzell, pp. 135–150. Grune & Stratton, New York.

39. Chesnut, C.H., III, Gruber, H.E., Baylink, D.J., Ivey, J.L., Matthews, M., Sisom, K., and Nelp, W.B. (1981): Treatment of postmenopausal osteoporosis with synthetic salmon calcitonin—an update. *Osteoporosis,* edited by J. Menczel, G.C. Robin, M. Makin. and R. Steinberg, pp. 389–393. *The Proceedings of an International Symposium,* Jerusalem Osteoporosis Center, Jerusalem.

40. Chesnut, C.H. III, Gruber, H.E., Ivey, J.L., Matthews, M., Sisom, K., Nelp. W.B., and Baylink, D.J. (1981): Stanozolol, an anabolic steroid, in the treatment of postmenopsusal osteoporosis—an update. *Osteoporosis,* edited by J. Menczel, G.C. Robin, M. Makin, and R. Steinberg, pp. 385–388. *The Proceedings of an International Symposium,* Jerusalem Osteoporosis Center, Jerusalem.

41. Chesnut, C.H., Nelp, W.B., and Lewellen, T.K. (1981): Neutron activation analysis for whole body calcium measurements. In: *Osteoporosis—Recent Advances in Pathogenesis and Treatment,* edited by H.F. DeLuca, H.M. Frost, W.S.S. Jee, C.C. Johnston Jr., and A.M. Parfitt. University Park Press, Baltimore.

42. Chow, R.K., Harrison, J.E., Brown, C.F., and Hajek, V. (1986): Physical fitness effect on bone mass in postmenopausal women. *Arch. Phys. Med. Rehabil.*, 67:231–234.

43. Christiansen, C., Rodbro, P., Munck, O., Munck,

O. (1975): Actions of vitamin D_2 and D_3 and 25-OHD$_3$ in anticonvulsant osteomalacia. *Br. Med. J.,* 2:363–365.

44. Christiansen, C., and Robdro, P. (1977): Long-term reproducibility of bone mineral content measurements. *Scand. J. Clin. Lab. Invest.,* 37:321–323.

45. Christiansen, M.S., Christiansen, C., Naestoft, J., McNair, P., and Transbol, I. (1981): Normalization of bone mineral content to height, weight, and lean body mass: implication for clinical use. *Calcif. Tissue Int.,* 33:5–8.

46. Citrin, D.L., Bessent, R.B., McGinlay, E., and Gordon, D. (1975): Dynamic studies with ^{99m}Tc-HEDP in normal subjects and in patients with bone turnovers. J. Nucl. Med., 16:886–890.

47. Clarke, R.L., and Van Dyk, G. (1973): A new method for measurement of bone mineral content using both transmitted and scattered beams of gamma-rays. *Phys. Med. Biol.,* 18:532–539.

48. Cohn, S.H. (ed.) (1980): *Non-invasive measurements of bone mass and their clinical application.* CRC Press, West Palm Beach, Florida.

49. Cohn, S.H. (1981): *In vivo* neutron activation analysis: State of the art and future prospects. *Med. Phys.* 8(2):145–154.

50. Cohn, S.H., Abesamis, C., Yasumura, S., Aloia, J.F., Zanzi, I., and Ellis, K.J. (1977): Comparative skeletal mass and radial bone mineral content in black and white women. *Metabolism,* (26)2:171–177.

51. Cohn, S.H., Ellis, K.J., Caselnova, R.C., and Letteri, J.M. (1975): Correlation of radial bone mineral content with total body calcium in chronic renal failure. *J. Lab. Clin. Med.,* 86:910–919.

52. Cohn, S.H., and Parr, R.M. (1985): Nuclear-based techniques for the *in vivo* study of human body composition. *Clin. Phys. Physiol. Meas.,* 6(4)275–301.

53. Cohn, S.H., Aloia, J.F., Vaswani, A.N. Yeun, K., Yasumura, S., and Ellis, K.J. (1986): Women at risk for developing osteoporosis: determination by total body neutron activation analysis and photon absorptiometry. *Calcif Tissue Int.,* 38:9–15.

54. Colbert, C., and Bachtell, R.S. (1981): Radiographic absorptiometry (photodensitometry). In: *Non-invasive Measurements of Bone Mass and Their Clinical Application,* edited by S.H. Cohn, pp. 51–84. CRC Press, West Palm Beach, Florida.

55. Coutris, G., Talbot, J.N., Kiffel, T., Paus, L., and Milhaud, G. (1985): Risque fracturaire vertebral apres la menopause: detection des sujets a haut risque par absorptiometrie biphotonique. *Biomed. Pharmacother.,* 39:35–39.

56. Craven, J.D., Constantini, M.A., and Greenfield, M.A. (1973): Measurement of the velocity of ultrasound in human cortical bone and its potential clinical importance. *Invest. Radiol.,* 8:72–77.

57. Cummings, S.R. (1985): Are patients with hip fractures more osteoporotic? *Am. J. Med.,* 78:487–494.

58. Dalen, N., and Jacobson, B. (1974): Bone mineral assay: choice of measuring sites. *Invest. Radiol.,* 9:174–185.

59. Dalen, N., Lamke, B., and Wallgren, A. (1974): Bone mineral losses in oophorectomized women. *J. Bone Joint Surg.,* 56–A:1235–1238.

60. Dalen, N., Hellstrom, L.G., and Jacobson, B. (1976): Bone mineral content and mechanical strength of the femoral neck. *Acta Ortho. Scand.* 47:503–508.

61. Dambacher, M.A., Ittner, J., and Ruegsegger, P. (1985): Fluoride therapy of postmenopausal osteoporosis and its complications. In: *Osteoporosis,* edited by C. Christiansen, C.D. Arnaud, B.E.C. Nordin, A.M. Parfitt, W.A. Peck, and B.L. Riggs, Vol 2. Aalborg Stiftsbogtrykken, Glostrup, Denmark.

62. Dambacher, M.A., and Ruegsegger, P. (1985): Nichtinvasive Untersuchungsmethoden bei osteoporosen. *Therapeutische Umschau/Revue therapeutique,* Va42:339–350.

63. Dambacher, M.A., Ittner, J., and Ruegsegger, P. (1986): Long-term fluoride therapy of postmenopausal osteoporosis. *Bone,* 7:199–205.

64. DePuey, E.G., and Burdine, J.A. (1972): Determination of bone mineral content using the scintillation camera. *Radiology,* 105:607–610.

65. DePuey, E.G., Thompson, W.L., Alagarsamy, V., and Burdine, J.A.(1975): Bone mineral content determined by functional imaging. *J. Nucl. Med.,* 16:891–895.

66. Dequeker, J., Wielandts, L., and Nijs, S. (1980): Evaluation of bone mineral content data using isowidths and percentile curves. In: *Fourth International Conference on Bone Measurement,* edited by R.B. Mazess, pp. 69–80. NIH Publication 80-1938 U.S. Department HEW, Bethesda, Maryland.

67. Dequeker, J., and Johnson, C.C. (ed.) (1981): *Non-invasive bone measurements,* pp. 59–72, IRL Press, Oxford.

68. Dequeker, J., and Geusens, P. (1985): Contributions of aging and estrogen deficiency to postmenopausal bone loss. *New Engl. J. Med.,* 313(7):453.

69. Duetsch, E., and Barnett, B.L. (1983): Synthetic and structural aspects of technetium chemistry as related to nuclear medicine. In: *Inorganic Chemistry in Biology and Medicine,* edited by A.E. Martell, pp. 103–119. ACS symposium series No. 140.

70. Dewanjee, M.K., and Wahner, H.W. (1979): Pharmacodynamics of Stannous Chelates Administered with ^{99m}Tc-labelled Chelates. *Radiology,* 132:711–716.

71. Dobbins, J.T. III, Pedersen, P.L., Mazess, R.B., Cameron, J.R., Hansen, J.L., and Hefner, L.V. (1984): A scanning slit x-ray videoabsorptiometric technique for bone mineral measurement. *Med. Phys.,* 11(5):582–588.

72. Doi, K., Vyborny, C.J., and Holje G. (1982): Development of a rigid fluorescent x-ray source for monoenergetic radiation studies in radiographic imaging. *Radiology,* 142:233–236.

73. Doyle, F., Brown, J., and Lachance, C. (1970): Relation between bone mass and muscle weight. *Lancet,* 391:393.

74. Drinkwater, B.L., Nilson, K., Chestnut, C.H. III, Bremmer, W.J., Shainholtz, S., and Southworth, M.B. (1984): Bone mineral content of amenorrheic and eumenorrheic athletes. *N. Engl. J. Med.,*

(311)5:277–281.

75. Drinkwater, B.L., Nilson, K., Ott, S., and Chestnut, C.H. III. (1986): Bone mineral density after resumption of menses in amenorrheic athletes. *JAMA*, 256:380–382.

76. Dunn, W.L., Wahner, H., and Riggs, B.L. (1980): Measurement of bone mineral content in human vertebrae and hip by dual-photon absorptiometry. *Radiology*, 136:485–487.

77. Dykman, T.R., Gluck, O.S., Murphy, W.A., Hahn, T.J., and Hahn, B.H. (1985): Evaluation of factors associated with glucocorticoid-induced osteopenia in patients with rheumatic diseases. *Arth. Rheum.*, (28)4:361–368.

78. Eastell, R., Wahner, H.W., Melton, L.J., O'Fallon, W.M., and Riggs, B.L. (1986): Comparison of bone mineral density of the lumbar spine and ultradistal radius in women with vertebral fractures. *Bone Min. Res.*, 1:271.

79. Ebifegha, M.E., Harrison, J.E., McNeill, K.G., Krishnan, S.S., and Ssengabi, J. (1986): A system for *in vivo* measurement of bone calcium by local neutron activation of the hand. *Appl. Rad. Isot.* (*Int. J. Rad. Appl. Inst.*, Part A), (37)2:159–164.

80. Ell, P.J., Jarrit, P.H., Cullum, I., and Lui, D. (1984): The MDP skull uptake test: a new diagnostic tool. *J. Nucl. Med.*, 25:24. (abstr.)

81. Elsasser, U. (1977): Quantifizierung der Spongiosadichte an Rohreknochen mittels computer-tomographie. Ph.D. Thesis University of Zurich, Zurich, Switzerland.

82. Ettinger, M. (1985): The relation of radius and spinal bone mineral in a mixed patient population. Program American Society for Bone and Mineral Research, Washington, D.C. abstr. 236.

83. Evans, H., LeBlanc, A., Schneider, V., Marsh, C., Johnson, P., and Jhingran, S. (1984): Lumbar spine vs. calcaneus bone mineral density. *Med. Phys.*, 11:744.

84. Fazzalari, N.L., Darracott, J., and Bernon-Roberts, B. (1985): Histomorphometric changes in the trabecular structure of a selected stress region in the femur in patients with osteoarthritis and fracture of the femoral neck. *Bone*, 6:125–133.

85. Firooznia, H., Golimbu, C., Rafii, M., Schwartz, M.S., and Alterman, E.R. (1984): Quantitative computed tomography assessment of spinal trabecular bone. I. Age-related regression in normal men and women. *J. Comp. Assist. Tomogr.*, 8:91–97.

86. Firooznia, H., Golimbu, C., Rafii, M., Schwartz, M.S., and Alterman, E.R. (1984): Quantitative computed tomography assessment of spinal trabecular bone. II. In osteoporosis women with and without vertebral fractures. *J. Comp. Assist. Tomogr.* 8:99–103.

87. Firooznia, H., Rafii, M., Golimbu, C., Schwartz, M., and Ort, P. (1986): Trabecular mineral content of the spine in women with hip fracture: CT measurement. *Radiology*, 159:737–740.

88. Fisher, E.C., Nelson, M.E., Frontera, W.R., Turksoy, R.N., and Evans, W.J. (1986): Bone mineral content and levels of gonadotropins and estrogens in amenorrheic running women. *J. Clin. Endocrin. Metab.*, 62(6):1232–1236.

89. Fogelman, I. (1984): Bone scanning in metabolic bone disease. In: *Bone Scintigraphy, edited by* E.B. Silberstein. Futura Publishing Company, Mount Kisco, New York.

90. Fogelman, I., Bessent, R.G., Turner, J.G., Citrin, D.L., Boyle, I.T., and Greig, W.R. (1978): The use of whole-body retention of Tc-99m diphosphonate in the diagnosis of metabolic bone disease. *J. Nucl. Med.*, 19:270–275.

91. Fogelman, I., Citrin, D.L., McKillop, J.H., Turner, J.G., Bessent, R.G., and Greig, W.R. (1979): A clinical comparison of Tc[99m] HEDP and Tc[99m] MDP in the detection of bone metastases: Concise Communication. *J. Nucl. Med.*, 20:98–101.

92. Fogelman, I., Citrin, D.L., Tuner, J.G., Hay, I.D., Bessent, R.G., and Boyle, I.T. (1979): Semi-quanitative interpretation of the bone scan in metabolic bone disease: definition and validation of the metabolic index. *Eur. J. Nucl. Med.*, 4:287–289.

93. Fogelman, I., and Carr, D. (1980): A comparison of bone scanning and radiology in the evaluation of patients with metabolic bone disease. *Clin. Radiol.*, 31:321–326.

94. Fogelman, I., Bessent, R.G., Cohen, H.N., Hart, D.M., and Lindsay R. (1980): Skeletal uptake of diphosphonate: method for prediction of postmenopausal osteoporosis. *Lancet*, 2:667–670.

95. Fogelman, I., Pearson, D.W., Bessent, R.G., Toft, A.J., and Francis, M.D. (1981): A comparison of skeletal uptakes of three diphosphonates by whole body retention: Concise Communication. *J. Nucl. Med.* 22:880–883.

96. Fogelman, I. (1982): Diphosphonate bone scanning agents—current concepts. *Eur. J. Nucl. Med.*, 7:506–509.

97. Francis, M.D., Ferguson, D.L., Tofe, A.J., Bevan, J.A., and Michels, S.E. (1980): Comparison evaluation of three diphosphonates: in vivo adsorption (C[14] labelled) and in vivo osteogenic uptake (Tc99M complexed) *J. Nucl. Med.* 21:1185–1189.

98. Francis, M.D., and Fogelman, I. (1984): [99m]Tc Diphosphonate uptake mechanism in bone. In: *Bone Scanning in Clinical Practice*, edited by I. Fogelman, pp. 7–11. Springer Verlag, Berlin-Heidelberg.

99. Frisch, B., and Eventov, I. (1986): Hematopoiesis in osteoporosis-preliminary report comparing biopsies of the femoral neck and iliac crest. *Israel J. Med. Sci.*, 22:380–384.

100. Fujita, T., Fukase, M., Yoshimoto, Y., Tsutsumi, M., Fukami, T., Imai, Y., Sakahuchi, K., Abe, T., Sawai, M., Seo, I., Yaguchi, T., Enomoto, S., Droke, D.M., and Avioli, L.V. (1983): Basic and clinical evaluation of the measurement of bone resonant frequency. *Calcif. Tissue Int.*, 35:153–158.

101. Gallagher, C., Goldgar, D., Mahoney, P., and McGill, M. (1985): Measurement of spine density in normal osteoporotic subjects using computed tomography: relationship of spine density to fracture threshold and fracture index. *J. Comput. Assist. Tomogr.*, 9:634–635.

102. Garn, S.M. (1970): *The Earlier Gain and the Later Loss of Cortical Bone.* Charles C Thomas, Springfield.

103. Garnett, E.E., Kennett, T.J., Kenyon, D.B., Webber, C.E., and Phil, M. (1973): A photon scattering technique for the measurement of absolute bone density in man. *Radiology,* 106:209–212.

104. Genant, H., Boyd, D., Rosenfeld, D., Abols, Y., and Cann, C.E. (1981): Non-invasive measurements of bone mass and their clinical application. *Comp. Tomogr.,* 121–150.

105. Genant, K.K., and Boyd, D. (1977): Quantitative bone mineral analysis using dual energy computed tomography. *Invest. Radiol.,* 12:545–551.

106. Gennari, C., and Imbimbo, B. (1985): Effects of prednisone and deflazacort on vertebral bone mass. *Calif. Tissue Int.,* 37:592–593.

107. Geusens, P., Dequeker, J., Verstraeten, A. and Nijs, J. (1986): Age-, sex-, and menopause-related changes of vertebral and peripheral bone: population study using dual and single photon absorptiometry and radiogrammetry. *J. Nucl. Med.,* 27:1540–1549.

108. Gigante, G.E., and Sciuti, S. (1985): A large angle coherent Compton scattering method for measurement *in vitro* of trabecular bone mineral concentration. *Med. Phys.,* 12(3):321–326.

109. Goldsmith, N.F., Johnston, J.O., Ury, H., Vose, G., and Colbert, C. (1971): Bone mineral estimation in normal and osteoporotic women. *J. Bone Joint Surg.,* 53A:83–100.

110. Goldsmith, N.F., Johnston, J.O., Picetti, G., et al. (1973): Bone mineral in the radius and vertebral osteoporosis in an insured population. *J. Bone Joint Surg.,* 55A:1276–1293.

111. Gotfredsen, A., Borg J., Christiansen, C., and Mazess, R. (1984): Total body bone mineral *in vivo* by dual-photon absorptiometry. I. Measurement procedures. *J. Clin. Physiol.,* 4(4):343–355.

112. Gotfredsen, A., Borg J., Christiansen, C., and Mazess, R.B. (1984): Total body bone mineral *in vivo* by dual photon absorptiometry. II. Accuracy. *J. Clin. Physiol.,* 4:357–362.

113. Gotfredsen A., Borg, J., Nilas, L., Tjellesen, L., and Christiansen, C. (1986): Representativity of regional to total bone mineral in healthy subjects and anticonvulsive treated epileptic patients. Measurements by single and dual photon absorptiometry. *Eur. J. Clin. Invest.,* 16:198–203.

114. Gotfredsen, A., Nilas, L., Riis, B.J., Thomsen, K., and Chirstiansen, C. (1986): Bone changes occurring spontaneously and caused by oestrogen in early postmenopausal women: a local or generalized phenomenon? *Br. Med. J.,* 292:1098–1100.

115. Gotfredsen, A., Riis, B.J., and Christiansen, C. (1986): Total and local bone mineral during estrogen treatment: a placebo controlled trial. *Bone Mineral,* 1:167–173.

116. Greenfield, M.A., Craven, J.D., and Wishko, D.S. (1975): The modulus of elasticity of human cortical bone: an *in vivo* measurement and its clinical implications. *Radiology,* 115:163–166.

117. Greenfield, M.A., Craven, J.D., Huddleston, A., Kehrer, M.L., Wishko, D., and Steen, R. (1981): Measurement of the velocity of ultrasound in human cortical bone *in vivo. Radiology,* 138:701–710.

118. Greer, F.R., Lane, J., Wiener, S., and Mazess, R.B. (1983): An accurate and reproducible absorptiometric technique for determining bone mineral content in newborn infants. *Pediat. Res.,* 17:259–262.

119. Griffiths, H.J., and Zimmerman, R.E. (1978): The clinical application of bone mineral analysis. *Skeletal Radiol.,* 3:1–9.

120. Grubb, S.A., Jacobson, P.C., Awbrey, B.J., McCartney, W.H., Vincent, L.M., and Talmage, R.V. (1984): Bone density in osteopenic women: a modified distal radius density measurement procedure to develop an "at risk" value for use in screening women. *J. Orthop. Res.,* 2:322–327.

121. Gruber, H.E., and Baylink, D.J. (1981): The diagnosis of osteoporosis. *J. Am. Geriat. Soc.,* 29(11):490–497.

122. Guillemart, A., LePape, A., Gaby, G., and Besnard, J.C. (1980): Bone kinetics of Calcium. 45 and pyrophosphate labelled with technetium-96. An autoradiographic evaluation. *J. Nucl. Med.,* 21:466–470.

123. Hangartner, T.N., and Overton, T.R. (1982): Quantitative measurement of bone density using gamma-ray computed tomography. *J. Comp. Assist. Tomogr.,* 6(6):1156–1162.

124. Hangartner, T.N., Overton, T.R., and Regal, W.M. (1983): Comparison of trabecular bone density at axial and peripheral sites using computed tomography. In: *Clinical Disorders of Bone and Mineral Metabolism,* edited by B. Frame and J.T. Potts, Jr., pp. 54–57. Excerpta Medica, Amsterdam.

125. Hangartner, T.N., Overton, T.R., Harley, C.H., van den Berg, L., and Crockford, P.M. (1985): Skeletal challenge: An experimental study of pharmacologically induced changes in bone density in the distal radius, using gamma-ray computed tomography. *Calcif Tissue Int.,* 37:19–24.

126. Hanson, J.A. (1979): Absorptiometry with a linear position-sensitive proportional counter. Ph.D. Thesis, University of Wisconsin-Madison, Wisconsin.

127. Hanson, J.A. (1979): Design and properties of a multianode, cylindrical proportional counter for position sensing at high count rates. *Rev. Sci. Instrum.,* 50(10):1318–1319.

128. Hanson, J.A., Moore, W.E., Figley, M.M., and Duke, P.R. (1984): Compton scatter with polychromatic sources for lung densitometry. *Med. Phys.,* (11)5:633–637.

129. Hansson, T., Roos, B., and Nachemson, A. (1980): The bone mineral content and ultimate compressive strength of lumbar vertebrae. *Spine,* 5:46–55.

130. Hansson, T., and Roos, B. (1986): Age changes in the bone mineral of the lumbar spine in normal women. *Calcif. Tissue Int.,* 38:249–251.

131. Harma, M., Karjalainen, P., Hoikka, V., and Alhava, E. (1985): Bone density in women with spinal and hip fractures. *Acta Orthop. Scand.,* 56:380–385.

132. Harma, M., and Karjalainen, P. (1986): Trabecular osteopenia in Colles' fractures. *Acta. Orthop. Scand.*, 57:38–40.

133. Harrison, J.E., McNeill, K.G., Hitchman, A.J., and Britt, B.A. (1979): Bone mineral measurements of the central skeleton by *in vivo* neutron activation analysis for routine investigation of osteopenia. *Invest. Radiol.*, 14:27–34.

134. Harrison, J.E., Bayley, T.A., Josse, R.G., Murray, T.M., Sturtridge, W., Williams, C., Goodwin, S., Tam, C., and Fornasier, V. (1986): The relationship between fluoride effects on bone histology and on bone mass in patients with postmenopausal osteoporosis. *Bone Mineral*, 1:321–333.

135. Hazan, G., Leichter, I., Loewinger, E., and Weinreb, A. (1977): The early detection of osteoporosis by Compton gamma ray spectroscopy. *Phys. Med. Biol.*, 22:1073–1084.

136. Hesp, R., Deacon, A.C., Hulme, P., and Reeve, J. (1983): Trends in trabecular and cortical bone in the radius compared with whole body calcium balance in osteoporosis. *Clin. Sci.*, 66:109–112.

137. Hesp, R., Dore, C., Page, L., and Summers, R. (1985): Normal values for trabecular and cortical bone in the radius measured by computed tomography. *Clin. Phys. Physiol. Meas.*, 4:303–310.

138. Horsman, A., Bulusu, L., Bentley, H.B., and Nordin, B.E.C. (1970): Internal relationships between skeletal parameters in twenty-three male skeletons: In: *Proceeding Bone Measurement Conference*, edited by J.R. Cameron, pp. 365–382. U.S. Atomic Energy Commission Conference 700515; U.S. Department of Commerce, Springfield, Virginia.

139. Horsman, A., Reading, D.H., Connolly, J., Glasgow, W., and McLachlan, M.S.F. (1976): Bone imaging using a gadolinium 153 source and a xenon-filled multiwire proportional counter as detector. *Am. J. Roentgenol.* 126:1273. (abstr.)

140. Horsman, A., Reading, D.H., Connolly, J., Bateman, E., Glasgow, W., and McLachlan, M.S.F. (1977): Bone mass measurement using a xenon filled multiwire proportional counter as a detector. *Phys. Med. Biol.*, 22(6):1059–1072.

141. Horsman, A., Burkinshaw, L., Pearson, D., Oxby, B., and Milner, R.M. (1983): Estimating total body calcium from peripheral bone measurements. *Calcif. Tissue Int.*, 35:135–144.

142. Hosie, C.J., Richardson, W., and Gregory, N.L. (1985): A gamma-ray computed tomography scanner for the quantitative measurement of bone density. *J. Biomed. Eng.*, 7(1):30–34.

143. Huddleston, A.L., and Bhaduri, D. (1979): Compton scatter densitometry in cancellous bones. *Phys. Med. Biol.*, 24(2):310–318.

144. Huddleston, A.L., Bhaduri, D., and Weaver, J. (1979): Geometrical considerations for Compton scatter densitometry. *Med. Phys.*, 6(6):519–522.

145. Hyldstrup, L., Morgensen, J., Jensen, G.F., McNair, P., and Transbol, I. (1984): Urinary 99m-Tc-diphosphonate excretion as simple method to quantify bone metabolism. *Scand. J. Clin. Lab. Invest.*, 44:105–109.

146. Jacobson, B. (1964): X-ray spectrophotometry *in vivo*. *Am. J. Roentgenol.*, 91:202–210.

147. Jeffcott, L.B., and McCartney, R.N. (1985): Ultrasound as a tool for assessment of bone quality in the horse. *Vet. Rec.*, 116:337–342.

148. Jelinek, J., and Overton, T.R. (1985): Reordering schemes for multiple-rotation fan-beam CT scanner. *IEEE Trans Med. Imag.*, (MI-4)4:215–221.

149. Jensen, G.F., Christiansen, C., Boesen, J., Hegedus, V., and Transbol, I. (1982): Epidemiology of postmenopausal spinal and long bone fractures. *Clin. Orthop.*, 166:75–81.

150. Jensen, P.S., and Orphanoudakis, S.C. (1985): Clinical results from longitudinal determinations of bone mass using quantitative computed tomography. *J. Comput. Assist. Tomogr.*, 9:627.

151. Johnell, O., and Nilsson, B.E. (1984): Bone mineral content in men with fractures of the upper end of the femur. *Int. Orthol.*, 7:229–231.

152. Johnston, C.C., Hui, S., Witt, R.M., Appledorn, R., Baker, R.S., and Longcope, C. (1985): Early menopausal changes in bone mass and sex steroids. *J. Clin. Endocrinol. Metab.*, 61(5):905–911.

153. Johnston, C.C., Norton, J., Khairi, M.R.A., Kernek, C., Edouard, C., Arlot, M., and Meunier, P.J. (1985): Heterogeneity of fracture syndromes in postmenopausal women. *J. Clin. Endocrinol. Metabl.*, 61:551–556.

154. Jones, K.P., Ravnikar, V.A., Tulchinsky, D., and Schiff, I. (1985): Comparison of bone density in amenorrheic women due to athletics, weight loss, and premature menopause. *Obstet. Gynecol.*, 66(1):5–8.

155. Jonson, R., Roos, B., and Hansson, T. (1986): Bone mineral measurement with a continuous roentgen ray spectrum and a germanium detector. *Acta Radiol. Diagn.*, 27:105–109.

156. Judy, P.F. (1971): A dichromatic attenuation technique for the *in vivo* determination of bone mineral content. Ph.D. Thesis for Radiological Sciences, University of Wisconsin-Madison, Wisconsin.

157. Kan, W.C., Wilson, C.R., and Witt, W., et al. (1974): Direct readout of bone mineral content with dichromatic absorptiometry, In: *Proceeding International Symposium Bone Mineral Measurement*, edited by R.B. Mazess, pp. 66–72. U.S. Government Printing Office, Washington, D.C.

158. Karellas, A., Leichter, I., Craven, J.D., and Greenfield, M.A. (1983): Characterization of tissue via coherent-to-Compton scattering ratio: sensitivity considerations. *Med. Phys.*, (10)5:605–609.

159. Kennedy, N.S.J., Eastell, R., Ferrington, C.M., Simpson, J.D., Smith, M.A., Strong, J.A., and Tothill, P. (1982): Total body neutron activation analysis of calcium: calibration and normalization. *Phys. Med. Biol.*, 27:697–707.

160. Kennett, T.J., Garnett, E.S., Webber, C.E., and Phil, M. (1972): An *in vivo* measurement of absolute bone density. *J. Assoc. Canad. Radiol.*, 23:168–170.

161. Kennett, T.J., and Webber, C.E. (1976): Bone density measured by photon scattering. II. Inherent sources of error. *Phys. Med. Biol.*, 215:770–780.

162. Kerr, S.A., Kouris, K., Webber, C.E., and Kennett, T.J. (1980): Coherent scattering and the assessment of mineral concentration in trabecular bone. *Phys. Med. Biol.*, 25(6):1037–1047.

163. Kerr, R., Resnick, D., Sartoris, D.J., Kursunoglu, S., Pineda, C., Haghighi, P., Greenway, G., and Guerra, J. Jr. (1986): Computerized tomography of proximal femoral trabecular patterns. *J. Orthop. Res.*, 4:45–56.

164. Khairi, R.A., Cronin, J.H., Robb, J.A., Smith, D.M., and Johnston, C.C. (1976): Femoral trabecular pattern index and bone mineral content measurement by photon absorption in senile osteoporosis. *J. Bone Joint Surg.*, 58-A,2:221–226.

165. Klibanski, A., and Greenspan, S.L. (1986): Increase in bone mass after treatment of hyperprolactinemic amenorrhea. *New Engl. J. Med.*, 315:542–546.

166. Krokowski, E. (1970): Calcium determination in the skeleton by means of x-ray beams of different energies. In: *Symposium Ossium*, edited by A.M. Jelliffe and B. Strickland. E.S. Livingstone, Edinburgh.

167. Krolner, B. (1982): Osteoporosis and normality: how to express the bone mineral content of lumbar vertebrae. *Clin. Physiol.*, 2:139–146.

168. Krolner, B. (1985): Lumbar spine bone mineral content by photon beam absorptiometry. *Dan. Med. Bull.*, 32(3):152–170.

169. Krolner, B., and Pors Nielsen, S. (1980): Measurement of bone mineral content (BMC) of the lumbar spine. I. Theory and application of a new two-dimensional dual-photon attenuation method. *Scand. J. Clin. Lab. Invest.*, 40:653–663.

170. Krolner, B., Pors Nielsen, S., Lund, B., Lund, B.J., Sorensen, O.H., and Uhrenholdt, A. (1980): Measurement of bone mineral content (BMC) of the lumbar spine. II. Correlation between forearm BMC and lumbar spine BMC. *Scand. J. Clin. Lab. Invest.*, 40:665–670.

171. Krolner, B., and Pors Nielsen S (1982): Bone mineral content of the lumbar spine in normal and osteoporotic women: cross sectional and longitudinal studies. *Clin. Sci.*, 62:329–336.

172. Kruse, H.P., Kuhlencordt, F., and Ringe, J.D. (1976): Correlation of clinical, densitometric and histomorphometric data in osteoporosis. In: *Calcified Tissues 1975*, edited by S. Pors Nielsen and E. Hjorting-Hansen, pp. 457–461. FADL Publishing, Copenhagen, Denmark.

173. Lahtinen, T., Vaananen, A., and Karjalainen, P. (1980): Effect of intraosseous fat on the measurement of bone mineral of distal radius. *Calcif. Tissue Intern.*, 32:7–8.

174. Lakes, R., Sub Yoon, H., and Katz, L. (1986): Ultrasonic wave propagation and attenuation in wet bone. *J. Biomed. Eng.*, (8):143–148.

175. Langton, C.M., Palmer, S.B., and Porter, R.W. (1984): The measurement of broadband ultrasonic attenuation in cancellous bone. *Eng. Med.*, 13:89–91.

176. Laval-Jeantet, A-M., Lamarque, J.L., and Demoulin, B. (1979): Evaluation de la mineralization osseuse vertebrale par tomographie computerisee. *J. Radiol.*, 60:87–93.

177. Laval-Jeantet, A-M., Bergot, C., Carroll, R., and Garcia-Schaefer, F. (1983): Cortical bone senescence and mineral bone density of the humerus. *Calcif. Tissue Intern.*, 35:268–272.

178. Laval-Jeantet, A-M., Roger, B., de Vernejoul, M.C., and Laval-Jeantet, J. (1985): Testing of dual-energy postprocessing method of QCT densitometry. *J. Comp. Assist. Tomogr.*, 9:616–617.

179. Laval-Jeantet, A-M., Roger, B., Bouysse, S., Bergot, C., and Mazess, R.B. (1986): Influence of vertebral fat content on quantitative CT density. *Radiology*, 159:463–466.

180. Lavender, J.P., Khan, R.A.A., and Hughes, S.P.F. (1979): Blood flow and tracer uptake in normal and abnormal canine bone: comparisons with Sr-85 microspheres, Kr-81 m and Tc 99m MDP. *J. Nucl. Med.*, 20:413–418.

181. LeBlanc, A.D., Evans, H.J., Johnson, P.C., and Loeffler, S.H. (1980): Partial body activation analysis using a Californium-252 source. In: *Fourth International Conference on Bone Measurement*, edited by R.M. Mazess. U.S. Department HEW, NIH Publication 80-1938, Washington, D.C.

182. LeBlanc, A.D., Evans, H., Jhingran, S., and Johnson, P. (1984): High resolution bone mineral densitometry with a gamma camera. *Phys. Med. Biol.*, 29:25–30.

183. LeBlanc, A.D., Evans, H.J., Marsh, C., Schneider, V., Johnson, P.C., and Jhingran, S.G. (1986): Precision of dual photon absorptiometry measurements. *J. Nucl. Med.*, 27:1362–1365.

184. Leichter, I., Weinreb, A., Hazan, G., Loewinger, E., Robin, G.C., Steinberg, R., Menczel, J., and Makin, M. (1981): The effect of age and sex on bone density, bone mineral content and cortical index. *Clin. Orthop.*, 156:232–239.

185. Leichter, I., Margulies, J.Y., Weinreb, A., Mizrahi, J., Robin, G.C., Conforty, B., Makin, M., and Bloch, B. (1982): The relationship between bone density, mineral content, and mechanical strength in the femoral neck. *Clin. Orthop.*, 163:272–281.

186. Leichter, I., Karellas, A., Craven, J.D., and Greenfield, M.A. (1984): The effect of the momentum transfer on the sensitivity of a photon scattering method for the characterization of tissues. *Med. Phys.*, 11(1):31–36.

187. Levy, L.M., Hoory, S., and Bandyopadhyay, D. (1985): Estimation of bone mineral content using gamma camera: A real possibility? *J. Nucl. Med.*, 26(5):24.

188. Lindberg, J.S., Fears, W.B., Hunt, J.M., Powell, M.R., Boll, D., and Wade, C.E. (1984): Exercise-induced amenorrhea and bone density. *Annal Intern. Med.*, (1)5:647–648.

189. Linde, J., and Friis, T. (1979): Osteoporosis in hyperthyroidism estimated by photon absorptiometry. *Acta Endocrinol.*, 91:437–448.

190. Lindergard, B., and Naverstein, Y. (1980): Bone mineral content by photon absorptiometry: the influences of fat and of different absorption profiles. In: *Proceedings Fourth International Conference Bone Mineral Measurements*, edited by R.B. Mazess, 80-1938:29–40. NIH Publishing, Bethesda, Maryland.

191. Lindquist, O., Bengtsson, C., Hansson, T., and Jonsson, R. (1983): Changes in bone mineral content of the axial skeleton in relation to aging and the menopause. *Scand. J. Clin. Lab. Invest.*, 43:333–338.

192. Lindsay, R. (1983): Can estrogen prevent bone loss? In: *Clinical Disease and Bone Mineral Measurement*, edited by B. Frame, and J.T. Potts, Jr. pp. 346–348. Excerpta Medica, Amsterdam.

193. Lindsay, R., Thome, J., and Kanders, B. (1986): The effect of oral contraceptive use on vertebral bone mass in pre-and post-menopausal women. *Contraception*, 34(4):333–340.

194. Littlefield, J.L., and Rudd, T.G. (1980): Tc-99m hydroxymethylene diphosphonate and Tc-99 methylene diphosphonate: biological and clinical comparison: Concise Communication. *J. Nucl. Med.*, 24:463–466.

195. Luther, R. (1974): Correlation of os calcis and spinal bone by Compton scattering. In: *International Conference on Bone Mineral Measurement*, edited by R.B. Mazess, pp. 161–168. DHEW Publ. 75 683. NIH, Bethesda, Maryland.

196. Lutz, J. (1986): Bone mineral, serum calcium and dietary intakes of mother/daughter pairs. *Am. J. Clin. Nutr.*, 44:99–106.

197. Mack, P.B., Brown, W.N., Jr., and Trapp, H.D. (1949): The quantitative evaluation of bone density. *Am. J. Roentgen Radiol. Ther.*, 61:808–825.

198. Madsen, M. (1977): Vertebral and peripheral bone mineral content by photon absorptiometry. *Invest. Radiol.*, 12:185–188.

199. Makler, P.T., and Charkes, N.D. (1980): Studies of skeletal tracer kinetics IV. Optimum time delay for Tc99m (Sn) methylene diphosphonate bone imaging. *J. Nucl. Med.*, 21:641–645.

200. Manicourt, D.H., Orloff, S., Brauman, J., and Schoutens, A. (1981): Bone mineral content of the radius: Good correlations with physicochemical determinations in iliac crest trabecular bone of normal and osteoporotic subjects. *Metabolism*, 30(1):57–62.

201. Marcus, R., Kosek, J. Pfefferbaum, A., and Horning, S. (1983): Age-related loss of trabecular bone in premenopausal women: a biopsy study. *Calcif. Tissue Int.* 35:406–409.

202. Martin, B., and Haynes, R.R. (1970): The relationship between the speed of sound and stiffness of bone. In: *Proceedings of the Bone Measurement Conference*, edited by J.R. Cameron. U.S. Atomic Energy Commission Conference 700515. CFSTI, Springfield, Virginia.

203. Martin, W., Fogelman, I., and Bessent, R.G. (1981): Measurement of 24-hour whole-body retention of Tc-99m HEDP by a gamma camera. *J. Nucl. Med.*, 22:542–545.

204. Matin, P. (1979): The appearance of bone scans following fractures including immediate and long-term studies. *J. Nucl. Med.*, 20:1227–1231.

205. Mautalen, C., Tau C., Casco, C., and Fromm, G. (1984): Contenido mineral oseo en la problacion normal de buenos aires. *Medicina* (Buenos Aires), 44:356–360.

206. Mautalen, C., Reyes, H.R., Chiringhelli, G. and Fromm, G. (1986): Cortical bone mineral content in primary hyperparathyroidism. Changes after parathyroidectomy. *Acta Endocrinol.*, 111:494–497.

207. Mayor, G.H., Sanchez, T.V., and Garn, S.M. (1980): Adjusting photon absorptiometry norms for whites to the black subject. In: *Proceedings Fourth International Conference Bone Mineral Measurements*, edited by R.B. Mazess, 80-1938, pp. 99–106, NIH Publishing, Bethesda, Maryland.

208. Mazess, R.B. (1971): Estimation of bone and skeletal weight by direct photon absorptiometry. *Invest. Radiol.*, 6:52–60.

209. Mazess, R.B. (ed) (1980): *Fourth International Conference on Bone Measurement*. U.S. Department, HEW, NIH Publication 80-1983. Bethesda, Maryland.

210. Mazess, R.B. (1982): On aging bone loss. *Clin. Orthop.*, 162:239–252.

211. Mazess, R.B. (1983): Errors in measuring trabecular bone by computed tomography due to marrow and bone composition. *Calcif. Tissue Int.*, 35:148–152.

212. Mazess, R.B. (1983): Noninvasive bone measurements. In: *Skeletal Research II*, edited by A. Kunin, pp. 277–343. Academic Press, New York.

213. Mazess, R.B. (1983): The noninvasive measurements of the skeletal mass. In: *Bone and Mineral Research Annual I*, edited by W.A. Peck, pp.223–279. Excerpta Medica, Amsterdam.

214. Mazess, R.B. (1984): Advances in single-and dual-photon absorptiometry. In: C. Christiansen, C.D. Arnaud, B.E.C. Nordin, A.M. Parfitt, W.A. Peck, B.L. Riggs, eds. *Osteoporosis, Proceedings of the Copenhagen International Symposium on Osteoporosis*. Aalborg Stiftsbogtrykkeri, Glostrup, Denmark.

215. Mazess, R.B. (1987): Computers used for single and dual photon absorptiometry. In: *Computers in Nuclear Medicine*, edited by M. Gelfand. (in press)

216. Mazess, R.B., Cameron, J.R., O'Connor, R., and Knutzen, D. (1964): Accuracy of bone mineral measurement. *Science*, 145:388–389.

217. Mazess, R.B., Cameron, J.R., and Sorenson, J.A. (1970): Determining body composition by radiation absorption spectrometry. *Nature*, 228:771–772.

218. Mazess, R.B., Cameron, J.R., and Miller, H. (1972): Direct readout of bone mineral content using radionuclide absorptiometry. *Intern. J. Appl. Radiol.*, 23:471–479.

219. Mazess, R.B., Judy, P.F., Wilson, C.R., and Cameron, J.R. (1973): Progress in clinical use of photon absorptiometry. In: *Clinical Aspects of Metabolic Bone Disease*, 270, edited by B. Frame, et al., pp. 37–43. Excerpta Medica Found International Congress, Amsterdam.

220. Mazess, R.B., and Cameron, J.R. (1974): Bone mineral content in normal U.S. whites, In: *International Conference on Bone Mineral Measurements*, edited by R.B. Mazess, pp. 228–238. Department Health Education & Welfare Publ., Washington, D.C.

221. Mazess, R.B., Wilson, C.R., Hanson, J., Kan,

W., Madsen, M., Pelc, N., and Witt, R. (1974): Progress in dual photon absorptiometry of bone. In: *Proceedings Symposium on Bone Mineral Determinations,* vol. 2, edited by P. Schmeling, pp. 40–52. Aktiebolaget Atomenergi Publ. AE-489, Studsvik, Nykoping, Sweden.

222. Mazess, R.B., and Peppler, W. (1977): Total body bone mineral by photon absorptiometry. *Calcif. Tissue Res.,* 22(Suppl):452–453.

223. Mazess, R.B., Peppler, W.W., Chestnut, C.H., Nelp, W.B., Cohn, S.H., and Zanzi, I. (1981): Total body bone mineral and lean body mass by dual-photon absorptiometry. II. Comparison with total body calcium by neutron activation analysis. *Calcif. Tissue Int.,* 33:361–363.

224. Mazess, R.B., Peppler, W.W., Harrison, J.E., and McNeill, K.G. (1981): Total body bone mineral and lean body mass by dual-photon absorptiometry. III. Comparison with trunk calcium by neutron activation analysis. *Calcif. Tissue Int.,* 33:365–368.

225. Mazess, R.B., and Young, D. (1982): Measurement of spine and total body mineral by dual-photon absorptiometry. In: *International Symposium Space Physiology.* Toulouse, France.

226. Mazess, R.B., and Witt, R. (1983): Interlaboratory variation in a commercial bone mineral analyzer. *Am. J. Radiol.,* 141:789–791.

227. Mazess, R.B., Peppler, W.W., Chesney, R.W., Lange, T.A., Lindgren, U., and Smith, E., Jr. (1984): Does bone measurement on the radius indicate skeletal status? *J. Nucl. Med.,* 25:281–288.

228. Mazess, R.B., Peppler, W.W., Chesney, R.W., Lange, T.A., Lindgren, U., and Smith, E., Jr. (1984): Total body and regional bone mineral by dual-photon absorptiometry in metabolic bone disease. *Calcif. Tissue Int.,* 36:8–13.

229. Mazess, R.B., Barden, H., and Towsley, M., et al. (1985): Bone mineral density of the spine and radius in normal young women. Presented at the American Society of Bone Mineral Research, Washington, D.C.

230. Mazess, R.B., and Vetter, J. (1985): Comparison of dual-photon absorptiometry and dual-energy computed tomography for vertebral mineral. *J. Comput. Assist. Tomogr.,* 9:624–625.

231. Mazess, R.B., and Vetter, J. (1985): The influence of marrow on measurement of trabecular bone using computed tomography. *Bone,* 6:349–351.

232. Mazess, R.B., Barden, H.S., Ettinger, M., Johnston, C., Dawson-Hughes, B., Baran, D., Powell, M., and Notelovitz, M. (1987): Spine and femur density using dual-photon absorptiometry in normal US white women. *Bone and Mineral,* 2:211–219.

233. Mazess, R.B., Barden, H., Ettinger, M., and Schulz, E. (1987): Bone density of the radius, spine and proximal femur in osteoporosis. J. Bone Min. Res. (in press).

234. Mazess, R.B., Vetter, J., and Weaver, D.S. (1987): CT bone changes in oophorectomized monkeys. *J. Comp. Assist. Tomogr.* (in press).

235. Maziere, B. (1981): Partial body neutron activation-hand. In: *Non-invasive measurements of bone mass and their clinical application,* edited by S.H.

Cohn, pp. 151–164. CRC Press, West Palm Beach, Florida.

236. Maziere, B., Kunz, D., Comar, D., and Ryckewaert, A. (1979): *In vivo* analysis of bone calcium by local neutron activation of the hand: results in normal and osteoporotic subjects. *J. Nucl. Med.,* 20:85–91.

237. McBroom, R.J., Hayes, W.C., Edwards, W.T., Goldberg, R.P., and White, A.A., III (1985): Prediction of vertebral body compressive fracture using quantitative computed tomography. *J. Bone Joint Surg.,* 67A(8):1206–1214.

238. McNeill, K.G., Thomas, B.J., Sturtridge, W.C., and Harrison, J.E. (1973): *In vivo* neutron activation analysis for calcium in man. *J. Nucl. Med.,* 14:502–506.

239. Meema, H.E., and Meema, S. (1981): Radiogrammetry. In: *Non-invasive measurements of bone mass and their clinical application,* edited by: S.H. Cohn, pp. 5–50. CRC Press, West Palm Beach, Florida.

240. Meindock, J., Rapport, A., Oreopoulos, O.G., Rabinovich, S., Meema, H.E., and Meema, S. (1985): Quantitative radionuclide scanning in metabolic bone disease. *Nucl. Med. Commun.,* 6:141–148.

241. Melsen, F., Nielsen, H.E., Christensen, P., Mosekilde, Li, and Mosekilde, Le. (1980): Some relations between photon-absorptiometric and histomorphometric measurements of bone mass in the forearm. In: *Fourth International Conference on Bone Measurement,* edited by R.B. Mazess, No. 80-1938, pp. 45–50. NIH Publ., Bethesda, Maryland.

242. Melton, L.J., Wahner, H.W., Richelson, L.S., O'Fallon, W.M., Dunn, W.L., and Riggs, B.L. (1985): Bone-density specific fracture risk: a population-based study of the relationship between osteoporosis and vertebral fractures. *J. Nucl. Med.,* 26:24.

243. Melton, L.J., Wahner, H.W., Richelson, L.S., O'Fallon, W.M., and Riggs, B.L. (1986): Osteoporosis and the risk of hip fracture. *Am. J. Epidemiol.,* (124)254–261.

244. Mosekilde, L., and Mosekilde, L. (1986): Normal vertebral body size and compressive strength: Relations to age and to vertebral and iliac trabecular bone compressive strength. *Bone,* 7:207–212.

245. Nachemson, A. (1966): The load on lumbar disks in different positions of the body. *Clin. Orthop.,* 45:107–122.

246. Nelp. W.B., Palmer, H.E., Murano, R., Pailthorp, K., Hinn, G.M., Rich, C., Williams, J.L., Rudd, T.G., and Denney, J.D. (1972): Absolute measurements of total body calcium (bone mass) *in vivo. J. Lab. Clin. Med.,* 79:430–438.

247. Nelson, M.E., Fisher, E.C., Catsos, P.D., Meredith, C.N., Turksoy, R.N., and Evans, W.J. (1986): Diet and bone status in amenorrheic runners. *Am. J. Clin. Nutr.,* 43:910–916.

248. Newton-John, H.F., and Morgan, D.B. (1970): The loss of bone with age, osteoporosis and fractures. *Clin. Orthop.,* 71:229–252.

249. Nielsen, H.E. (1981): Uremic bone disease before

and after renal transplantation. Clinical and biochemical aspects, bone mineral content and bone morphometry. M.D. Thesis, Aarhus University, Laegeforeningens forlag, Aarhus, Denmark.

250. Nilas, L., Gotfredsen, A., and Christiansen, C. (1984): Relationship between local and total bone mineral content after gastric surgery. *Scand. J. Gastroenterol.,* 19(5):591–595.

251. Nilas, L., Borg, J., Gotfredsen, A., and Christiansen, C. (1985): Comparison of single and dual-photon absorptiometry in postmenopausal bone mineral loss. *J. Nucl. Med.,* 26:1257–1262.,

252. Nilas, L., Gotfredsen, A., and Christiansen, C. (1986): Total and local bone mass before and after normalization for indices of bone and body size. *Scand. J. Clin. Invest.,* 46:53–57.

253. Nilsson, B. (1970): radiometry of bone *in vivo.* In: *Symposium Ossium,* edited by A.M. Jelliffe and B. Strickland. E.S. Livingston, Edinburgh.

254. Nilsson, B.E., and Westlin, N.E. (1974): The bone mineral content in the forearm of women with Colles' fracture. *Acta Orthop. Scand.,* 45:836.

255. Nilsson, B.E., and Westlin, N.E. (1977): Bone mineral content and fragility fractures. *Clin Orthop.,* 125:196.

256. Nisbet, A.P., Edwards, S., Lazarus, C.R., et al (1984): Chromium 51 EDTA/technetium 99m MDP plasma ratio to measure total skeletal function. *Br. J. Radiol.,* 57:677–680.

257. O'Duffy, J.D., Wahner, H.W., O'Fallon, W.M., Johnson, K.A., Muhs, J., and Riggs, B.L. (1986): Mechanism of acute lower extremity pain syndrome in fluoride-treated osteoporotic patients. *Am. J. Med.,* 80:561–566.

258. Olkkonen, H. and Karjalainen, P. (1975): A [170]Tm gamma scattering technique for the determination of absolute bone density. *Br. J. Radiol.,* 48:594–597.

259. Olkkonen, H., Puumalainen, P., Karjalainen, P., and Alhava, E.M. (1981): A coherent/Compton scattering method for measurement of trabecular bone mineral density in the distal radius. *Invest. Radiol.,* 16:491–495.

260. Ott, S.M., Kilcoyne, R.F., and Chesnut, C.H. (III). (1986): Longitudinal changes in bone mass after one year as measured by different techniques in patients with osteoporosis. *Calcif. Tissue Int.,* 39:133–138.

261. Overton, T.R., Macey, D.J., Hangartner, T.N., and Battista, J.J. (1985): Accuracy and precision in x-ray CT and γ-ray CT measurement of bone density: identification and evaluation of some sources of error in quantitative studies. *J. Comput. Assist. Tomogr.,* (9):3:606–607.

262. Pacifici, R., Susman, N., Carr, P.L., Birge, S.J., and Avioli, L.V. (1987): Single and dual energy tomographic analysis of spinal trabecular bone: a comparative study in normal and osteoporotic women. *J. Clin. Endocrinol. Metab.,* 64(2):209–214.

263. Palmer, H.E. (1973): Feasibility of determining total-body calcium in animals and humans by measuring 37-Ar in expired air after neutron irradiation. *J. Nucl. Med.,* 14:522–527.

264. Palmer, H.E., Nelp. W.B., Murano, R., and Rich, C. (1968): The feasibility of *in vivo* neutron activation analysis of total body calcium and other elements of body composition. *Phys. Med. Biol.,* 13:269–279.

265. Parfitt, A.M., Sudhaker Rao, D., Stanciu, J., Villanueva, A.R., Kleerekoper, M., and Frame, B. (1985): Irreversible bone loss in osteomalacia. *J. Clin. Invest.,* 76:2403–2412.

266. Pauwels, E.K.J., Blom, J., Camps, J.A.J., and Herman, J.R. (1983): Comparison between the diagnostic efficiency of ^{99m}Tc-MDP, [99m]TC-DPD and ^{99m}Tc-HDP for the detection of bone metastasis. *Eur. J. Nucl. Med.,* 8:118–122.

267. Peppler, W.W., and Mazess, R.B. (1981): Total body bone mineral and lean body mass by dual-photon absorptiometry. I. Theory and measurement procedure. *Calcif. Tissue Int.,* 33,353–359.

268. Pesch, H.J., Scharf, H.P., Lauer, G., and Seibold, H. (1980): Der altersabhangige Verbundbau der Lendenwirbelkorper, Eine Struktur and Formanalyse. *Virchows Arch. A Path. Anat.,* 368:21–41.

269. Pocock, N.A., Eisman, J.A., Yeates, M.G., Sambrook, P.N., Eberl, S., and Wren, B.G. (1986): Limitations of forearm bone densitometry as an index of vertebral or femoral neck osteopenia. *J. Bone Min. Res.,* 1:369–375.

270. Pocock, N.A., Eisman, J.A., Yeates, M.G., Sambrook, P.N., and Eberl, S. (1966): Physical fitness is a major determinant of femoral neck and lumbar spine bone mineral density. *J. Clin. Invest.,* 78:618–621.

271. Pogrund, H., Bloom, R.A., and Weinberg, H. (1986): Relationship of psoas width to osteoporosis. *Acta Orthop. Scand.,* 57:208–210.

272. Poll, V., Cooper, C., and Cawley, M.I.D. (1986): Broadband ultrasonic attenuation in the os calcis and single photon absorptiometry in the distal forearm: a comparative study. *Clin. Phys. Physiol. Meas.,* 7(4):375–379.

273. Price, R.I., Rettallack, R.W., and Gutteridge, D.H. (1984): Choice of measurement sites in forearm bone mineral measurements using photon absorptiometry and roentgenography. In: *Osteoporosis, Proceedings of the Copenhagen International Symposium on Osteoporosis,* edited by C. Christiansen, C.D. Arnaud, B.E.C. Nordin, A.M. Parfitt, W.A. Peck, B.L. Riggs. Aalborg Stiftsbogtrykkeri, Glostrup, Denmark.

274. Price, R.R., Wagner, J., Larsen, K., Patton, J., and Brill, A.B. (1976): Regional and whole-body bone mineral content measurement with a rectilinear scanner. *Am. J. Roentgen,* 126:1277–1278.

275. Pummalainen, P., Uimarihuhta, A., Olkkonen, H., and Alhava, E.M. (1982): A coherent/Compton scattering method employing an x-ray tube for measurement of trabecular bone mineral content. *Phys. Med. Biol.,* 27:425–429.

276. Rao, G.U., I. Yaghmai, A.O. Wist, and G. Arora. (1987): Systematic errors in bone-mineral measurements by quantitative computed tomography. *Med. Physics,* 14(1):62–69.

277. Raymakers, J.A., Hoekstra, O., van Putten, J., Kerkhoff, H., and Duursma, S.A. (1986): Fracture

prevalence and bone mineral mass in osteoporosis measured with computed tomography and dual energy photon absorptiometry. *Skeletal Radiol.,* 15:191–197.

278. Reed, G.W., West, R.R., and Atkinson, P.J. (1970): The measurement of bone mineralization *in vivo* using monoenergetic radiation. In: *Symposium Ossium,* edited by A.M. Jelliffe and B. Strickland, pp. 267–269. E.S. Livingstone, Edinburgh.

279. Reeve, J., Meunier, P.J., Parsons, J.A., Bernat, M., Bijvoet, Olav, L.M., Courpron, P., Edouard, C., Klenerman, L., Neer, R.M., Renier, J.C., Slovik, D., Vismans, F., Jon, F.E., and Potts, J.T. Jr. (1980): Anabolic effect of human parathyroid hormone fragment on trabecular bone in involutional osteoporosis: a multicentre trial. *Br. Med. J.* 1340–1344.

280. Reid, D.M. (1986): Measurement of bone mass by total body calcium: a review. *J. Roy. Soc. Med.,* 79:33–37.

281. Reinbold, W.D., Genant, H.K., Reiser, U.J., Harris, S.T., and Ettinger, B. (1986): Bone mineral content in early-postmenopausal and postmenopausal osteoporotic women; comparison of measurement methods. *Radiology,* 160:469–478.

282. Reiss, K.H., and Steinle, B. (1973): Medical application of the Compton effect. *Siemens Forsch-u. Enfwickl.,* 2:16–25.

283. Reiss, K.H., Killig, K., and Schuster, W. (1974): Dual photon x-ray beam applications. In: *International Conference on Bone Mineral Measurement,* edited by R.B. Mazess, pp. 80–87. Department of Health, Education & Welfare Publications, Washington, D.C.

284. Revak, C.S. (1980): Mineral content of cortical bone measured by computed tomography. *J. Comp. Asst. Tomogr.,* 4:342–350.

285. Rich, C., Klink, E., Smith, R., Graham, B., and Ivanovich, P. (1966): Sonic measurement of bone mass. In: *Progress in the Development of Methods in Bone Densitometry,* edited by Whedon, et al. National Aeronautics and Space Administration Publications, NASA SP-64, Washington D.C.

286. Richardson, M.L., Pozzi-Mucelli, R.S., Kanter, A.S., Kolb, F.O., Ettinger, B., and Genant, H.K. (1986): Bone mineral changes in primary hyperparathyroidism. *Skeletal Radiol.,* 15:85–95.

287. Richelson, L.S., Wahner, H.W., Melton, L.J., and Riggs, B.L. (1984): Relative contributions of aging and estrogen deficiency to post-menopausal bone loss. *New Engl. J. Med.,* 311(20):1273–1275.

288. Rickers, H., Balsley, I., Foltved, H., and Rodbro, P. (1981): Bone mineral content before and after intestinal bypass operation in obese patients. *Acta Med. Scand.,* 209:203–207.

289. Riggs, B.L., Wahner, H.W., Dunn, W.L., Mazess, R.B., Offord, K.P., and Melton, L.J. III. (1981): Differential changes in bone mineral density of the appendicular and axial skeleton with aging. *J. Clin. Invest.,* 67:328–335.

290. Riggs, B.L., Wahner, H.W., Seeman, E., Offord, K.P., Dunn, W.L., Mazess, R.B., Johnson, K.A., and Melton, L.J. III. (1982): Changes in bone mineral density of the proximal femur and spine with aging: differences between the postmenopausal and senile osteoporosis syndromes. *J. Clin. Invest.,* 70:716–723.

291. Riggs, B.L., and Melton, L.J. III. (1986): Involutional osteoporosis. *New Engl. J. Med.,* 314:1676–1686.

292. Riggs, B.L., Wahner, H.W., Melton, L.J. Richelson, L.S., Judd, H.L., and Offord, K.P. (1986): Rates of bone loss in the appendicular and axial skeletons of women. *J. Clin. Invest.,* 77:1487–1491.

293. Riis, B.J., Thomsen, K., and Christiansen, C. (1986): Does $24R,25(OH)_2$-Vitamin D_3 prevent postmenopausal bone loss? *Calcif. Tissue Int.,* 39:128–132.

294. Ringe, J.D. (1985): Value of single photon absorptiometry as a screening method for osteopenia in different gastrointestinal disorders. *J. Comput. Assist. Tomogr.,* 9:627.

295. Roberts, J.G., DiTomasso, E., and Webber, C.E. (1982): Photon scattering measurements of calcaneal bone density: results of *in vivo* cross-sectional studies. *Invest. Radiol.,* 17:20–28.

296. Roberts, J.G., Lien, J.W.K., Woolever, C.A., and Webber, C.E. (1984): Photon scattering measurements of calcaneal bone density: results of *in vivo* longitudinal studies. *Clin. Phys. Physiol. Meas.,* 5(3):193–200.

297. Rockoff, S.D., Sweet, E., and Bleustein, J. (1969): The relative contribution of trabecular and cortical bone to the strength of human lumbar vertebrae. *Calcif. Tissue Res.,* 3:163–175.

298. Rohloff, R., Hitzler, H.,, Arndt, W., Frey, K.W., and Lissner, J. (1982): Influence of fat content of bone marrow on bone mineral measurements by CT and photon absorptiometry in trabecular bone. *J. Comput. Assist. Tomogr.,* (6)1:212–213.

299. Rohloff, R., Mayr, R., Radlmeier, A., Schattenkirchner, W., and Frey, K.W. (1984): Evaluation of mineral content by photon absorptiometry (ulna, os calcis) and CT (lumbar spine) in patients with rheumatoid arthritis. *Fourth International Workshop on Bone and Soft Tissue Densitometry Using Computed Tomography,* p. 61. Fontevraud, France.

300. Roos, B.O. (1975): Dual photon absorptiometry in lumbar vertebrae. II. Precision and reproducibility. *Acta Radiol.,* 14:291–303.

301. Roos, B., and Skoldborn, H. (1974): Dual photon absorptiometry in lumbar vertebrae. I. Theory and method. *Acta Radiol.,* 13:1–15.

302. Roos, B.O., Hansson, T.H., and Skoldborn, H. (1980): Dual photon absorptiometry in lumbar vertebrae. *Acta Radiol. [Oncol.],* 19:111–114.

303. Roos, R.J., and Hansson, T. (1986): Bone mineral measurement with a continuous roentgen ray spectrum and germanium detector. *Acta Radiol. Diagr.,* (27)1:105–109.

304. Rosenthall, L., and Azoumanian, A. (1983): Total body retention measurements of Tc-99m MDP using a simple detector. *Clin. Nucl. Med.,* 8:210–213.

305. Ruegsegger, P., Anliker, M., and Dambacher, M. (1981): Quantification of trabecular bone with low dose computed tomography. *J. Comput. Assist. Tomogr.,* 5(3):384–390.

306. Ruegsegger, P., Dambacher, M.A., Ruegsegger,

E., Fischer, J.A., and Anliker, M. (1984): Bone loss in premenopausal women. *J. Bone Joint Surg.,* 66A:1015–1023.

307. Rundgren, A., Aniansson, A., Ljungberg, P., and Wetterqvist, H. (1984): Effects of a training programme for elderly people on mineral content of the heel bone. *Arch. Gerontol. Geriatr.,* 3:243–248.

308. Rundgren, A., Eklund, S., and Jonsson, R. (1984): Bone mineral content in 70- and 75-year old men and women. An analysis of some anthropometric background factors. *Age Ageing,* 13:6–13.

309. Rundgren, A., and Mellstrom, D. (1984): The effect of tobacco smoking on the bone mineral content of the ageing skeleton. *Mechan. Aging Develop.,* 28:273–277.

310. Runge, P.H., Fengler, F., Franke, J., and Koall, W. (1980): Ermittlung des peripheren knochenmineral-gehaltes bei normalpersonen und patienten mit verschiedenen knochenerkrankungen, bestrinmt mit hilfe der photonabsorptions-technik am radius. *Radiologe,* 20:505–514.

311. Rustgi, S.N., Siegel, J.A., Braunstein, M., Craven, J.D., and Greenfield, M.A. (1980): Accuracy of bone mineral. *Am. J. Roentgenol.,* 135:275–277.

312. Sambrook, P.N., Bartlett, C., Evans, R., Hesp, R., Katz, D., and Reeve, J. (1985): Measurement of lumbar spine bone mineral: a comparison of dual-photon absorptiometry and computed tomography. *Br. J. Radiol.,* 58(691):621–624.

313. Sandrik, J.N., and Judy, P.F. (1973): Effects of the polyenergetic character of the specturm of 125-I on the measurement of bone mineral content. *Invest. Radiol.,* 8:143–149.

314. Sartoris, D.J., Sommer, F.G., Kosek, J., Gies, A., and Carter, D. (1985): Dual-energy projection radiography in the evaluation of femoral neck strength, density, and mineralization. *Invest. Radiol.,* 20:476–485.

315. Sartoris, D.J., Andre, M., Resnick, C., and Resnick, D. (1986): Trabecular bone density in the proximal femur: quantitative CT assessment. *Radiology,* 160:707–712.

316. Schaadt, O., and Bohr, H. (1981): Bone mineral by dual photon absorptiometry. Accuracy-precision-sites of measurements. In: *Non-Invasive Bone Measurements,* edited by J. Dequeker and C.C. Johnston, pp. 59–72. IRL Press, Oxford.

317. Schaadt, O., and Bohr, H. (1981): Loss of bone mineral in axial and peripheral skeleton in aging, prednisone treatment and osteoporosis. *Non-Invasive Bone Measurements: Methodological Problems* edited by J. Dequeker, and C.C. Johnston, pp. 207–214.

318. Schlenker, R.A., and VonSeggen, W.W. (1976): The distribution of cortical and trabecular bone mass along the lengths of the radius and ulna and the implications for *in vivo* bone mass measurements. *Calcif. Tissue Res.,* 20:41–52.

319. Schlenker, R.A., and Kotek, T.J. (1979): Effect of arm orientation on bone mineral mass and bone width measured using the Cameron-Sorenson technique. *Med. Phys.,* 6:105–109.

320. Schneider, P., Borner, W., Mazess, R.B., and Barden, H. (1987): The relationship of peripheral to axial bone density. (submitted).

321. Schneider, V.P., Berger, P., Moll, E., Reiners, C., and Borner, W. (1985): Getrennte messung von kompakta und spongiosadichte mit einem transversal rotations scanner. *Fortschr. Rontgenstr.,* 143(2):178–182.

322. Schultz, E.E., Libanate, C.R., Farlay, S.M., Kirk, G.A., and Baylink, D.J. (1984): Skeletal scintigraphic changes in osteoporosis treated with sodium fluoride: Concise Communication. *J. Nucl. Med.,* 25:651–655.

323. Schumichem, C., Fegert, J., Gaeda, J., and Straub, E. (1982): Improved diagnosis of renal osteodystrophy (i.a) by use of Tc99m MDP bone clearance. *J. Nucl Med.,* 23:50 (abstr.).

324. Seeman, E., Wahner, H.W., Offord, K.P., Kumar, R., Johnson, W.J., and Riggs, B.L. (1982): Differential effects of endocrine dysfunction on the axial and the appendicular skeleton. *J. Clin. Invest.,* 69:1302–1309.

325. Seeman, E., Melton, L.J., O'Fallon, W.M., and Riggs, B.L. (1982): Risk factors for spinal osteoporosis in men. *Am. J. Med.,* 75:977–983.

326. Shapiro, J.R., Moore, W.T., Jorgensen, H., Reid, J., Epps, C.H., and Whedon, D. (1975): Osteoporosis: evaluation of diagnosis and therapy. *Arch. Int. Med.,* 135:563–567.

327. Shukla, S.S., Karellas, A., Leichter, I., Craven, J.D., and Greenfield, M.A. (1985): Quantitative assessment of bone mineral by photon scattering: accuracy and precision considerations. *Med. Phys.,* 12(4):447–448.

328. Shukla, S.S., Leichter, I., Karellas, A., Craven, J.D., and Greenfield, M.A. (1986): Trabecular bone mineral density measurement in vivo: use of the ratio of coherent to Compton-scattered photons in the calcaneus. *Radiology,* 158:695–697.

329. Silberstein, E.D., Francis, M.D., Tofe, A.J., and Slough, C.L. (1975): Distribution of ^{99m}TcSn-diphosphonate and free ^{99m}Tc pertechnetate in selected soft and hard tissues. *J. Nucl. Med.,* 16:58–61.

330. Sinaki, M., and McPhee, M.C. (1986): Relationship between bone mineral density of spine and strength of back extensors in healthy postmenopausal women. *Mayo Clin. Proc.,* 61:116–122.

331. Singh, M., Riggs, B.L., Beabout, J.W., and Jowsey, J. (1973): Femoral trabecular pattern index for evaluation of spinal osteoporosis. *Mayo Clin. Proc.,* 48:184–189.

332. Singh, S., Saha, S., Giyanani, V.L., Thompson, H.E., and Albright, J.A. (1984): Measurements of cortical bone thickness by ultrasound, cat-scan and micrometer. In: *Biomedical Engineering III: Recent Developments,* edited by L. Sheppard, pp. 82–85. Pergamon Press, New York.

333. Smith, D.M., Khairi, M.R.A., and Johnston, C.C. Jr. (1975): The loss of bone mineral with aging and its relationship to risk of fracture. *J. Clin. Invest.,* 56:311–318.

334. Smith, D.M., Nance, W.E., Kang, K.W., Christian, J.C., and Johnston, C.C. Jr. (1973): Genetic factors in determining bone mass. *J. Clin. Invest.,* 52:2800–2808.

335. Smith, M.A., Eastell, R., Kennedy, N.S.J., McIntosh, L.G., Simpson, J.D., Strong, J.A., and Tothill, P. (1981): Measurement of spinal calcium by *in vivo* neutron activation analysis in osteoporosis. *Clin. Phys. Physiol. Meas.*, 2:45–48.

336. Smith, M.A., and Tothill, P. (1982): The crossover correction in dual photon absorptiometry with ^{153}Gd. *Phys. Med. Biol.*, 27:1515–1521.

337. Smith, N.J.D. (1970): The measurement of bone mineral *in vivo* using two parallel scintillation counting circuits. In: *Symposium Ossium,* edited by A.M. Jelliffe and B. Stickland. E.S. Livingstone, Edinburgh.

338. Sorenson, J.A., and Cameron, J.R. (1967): A reliable *in vivo* measurement of bone mineral content. *J. Bone Joint Surg.*, 49A:481–497.

339. Sorenson, J.A., and Mazess, R.B. (1970: Effects of fat on bone mineral measurements. In: *Proceedings of Bone Measurement Conference,* edited by J.R. Cameron, U.S. Atomic Energy Commission Conference 700515.

340. Spinks, T.J. (1979): Effects of size and ocmposition of the body on absolute measurement of calcium *in vivo*. *Phys. Med. Biol.*, 24(5):976–987.

341. Stalp, J.T., and Mazess, R.B. (1980): Determination of bone density by coherent-Compton scattering. *Med. Phys.*, 7:723–726.

342. Stevenson, J.C., Banks, L.M., MacIntyre, I., Hesp, R., Padwick, M., Endacott, J.A., and Whitehead, M.I. (1986): Axial and peripheral CT scanning: findings in the early post-menopause. *J. Bone Min. Res.*, 1:277.

343. Strash, A.M., and Bright, R.W. (1976): Recent advances in skeletal transimaging. *Am. J. Roentgenol.*, 126:1278.

344. Sy, W.M. (1981): *Gamma Immagery in Benign and Metabolic Bone Diseases,* pp. 223–239. CRC Press, Boca Raton, Florida.

345. Talmage, R.V., Stinnett, S.S., Landwehr, J.T., Vincent, L.M., and McCartney, W.H. (1986): Age-related loss of bone mineral density in non-athletic and athletic women. *Bone Mineral*, 1:115–125.

346. Thomsen, K., Gotfredsen, A., and Christiansen, C. (1986): Is postmenopausal bone loss an age-related phenomenon? *Calcif. Tissue Int.*, 39:123–127.

347. Thomsen, K., Nilas, L., Mogensen, T., and Christiansen, C. (1986): Determination of bone turnover by urinary excretion of ^{99m}Tc-MDP. *Eur. J. Nucl. Med.*, 12:342–345.

348. Tilden, R.L., Jackson, J., and Enneking, W.F. (1973): ^{99m}Tc polyphosphate histological localization in human femurs by autoradiography. *J. Nucl. Med.*, 14:576–578.

349. Tomioka, Y., Hasegawa, T., Kaneko, M., and Oikawa, M. (1985): Morphological and chemical examination of relationship between ultrasonic pulse velocity and bone properties of the third metacarpal and metatarsal bone in thoroughbreds. Bull. Equine Res. Insti., 22:8–15.

350. Tothill, P., Smith, M.A., and Sutton, D. (1983): Dual photon absorptiometry of the spine with a low activity source of gadolinium 153. *Br. J. Radiol.*, 56:829–835.

351. Trotter, M., Broman, G.E., and Peterson, R.R. (1960): Densities of bones of white and negro skeletons. *J. Bone Joint Surg.*, 42A:50–58.

352. Verstraeten, A., and DeQueker, J. (1986): Vertebral and peripheral bone mineral content and fracture incidence in postmenopausal patients with rheumatoid arthritis: effect of low dose corticosteroids. *Ann. Rheum. Dis.* 45:852–857.

353. Vogel, J.M., and Anderson, J.T. (1972): Rectilinear transmission scanning of irregular bones for quantification of mineral content. *J. Nucl. Med.*, 13:13–18.

354. Von Wowern, N. (1974): A new method of gamma-ray osteodensitometry of the mandible. *Int. J. Oral Surg.* 3:353–357.

355. Von Wowern, N. (1986): Bone mass of mandibles. In vitro and in vivo analyses. *Danish Med. Bull.* (33)1:23–44.

356. Vose, G.P. (1966): Factors affecting the precision of radiographic densitometry of the lumbar spine and femoral neck. In: *Progress in Development of Methods in Bone Densitometry* edited by G.D. Whedon, W.F. Neuman, and D.W. Jenkins, NASA, Washington, D.C.

357. Vose, G.P., and Kubala, A.L., Jr. (1959): Bone strength—its relationship to x-ray determined ash content. *Human Biol.*, 31:261–270.

358. Vose, G.P., and Mack, P.B. (1963): Roentgenologic assessment of femoral neck density as related to fracturing. *Am. J. Roentgenol.*, 89:1296–1301.

359. Vose, G.P., and Lockwood, R.M. (1965): Femoral neck fracturing—its relationship to radiographic bone density. *J. Gerontol.* 20(3):300–305.

360. Wahner, H.W., Dunn, W.L., and Riggs, B.L. (1983): Noninvasive bone mineral measurements. *Sem. Nuc. Med.*, 13:282–289.

361. Wahner, H., Dunn, W., Mazess, R.B., Towsley, M., Lindsay, R., Markhardt, L., and Dempster, D. (1985): Dual-photon (153-Gd) absorptiometry of bone. *Radiology,* 156:203–206.

362. Wardlaw, G., and Pike, A.M. (1986): The effect of lactation on peak adult shaft and ultra-distal forearm bone mass in women[1-3]. *Am. J. Clin. Nutr.,* 283–286.

363. Wasnich, R., Yano, K., and Vogel, J. (1983): Postmenopausal bone loss at multiple skeletal sites: relationship to estrogen use. *J. Chron. Dis.,* 36(II):781–790.

364. Wasnich, R.D., Ross, P.D., Heilbrun, L.K., and Vogel, J.M. (1985): Prediction of postmenopausal fracture risk with bone mineral measurements. *Am. J. Obstet. Gyn.,* 153:745–751.

365. Wasnich, R.D., Ross, P.D., and Vogel, J.M. (1985): Evaluation of a screening test for fracture risk prediction: a prospective study of bone mineral content and fracture incidence. *West Regional SNM,* Oct. 1985.

366. Watt, D.E. (1973): Beam diameter and scan velocity effects on linear bone mass measurement by photon attenuation. *Phys. Med. Biol.*, 18:673–685.

367. Watt, D.E. (1975): Optimum photon energies for the measurement of bone mineral and fat fractions. *Br. J. Radiol.*, 48:265–274.

368. Webber, C.E. (1981): Compton scattering meth-

ods. In: *Non-Invasive Measurements of Bone Mass and Their Clinical Application,* edited by S.H. Cohn, pp. 101–120. CRC Press, West Palm Beach, Florida.

369. Webber, C.E., Phil, M., and Kennett, T.J. (1976): Bone density measured by photon scattering. I. A system for clinical use. *Phys. Med. Biol.,* 21:760–769.

370. Webster, D.J., and Lillicrap, S.C. (1985): Coherent Compton scattering for the assessment of bone mineral content using heavily filtered x-ray beams. *Phys. Med. Biol.,* 30(6):531–539.

371. Webster, D.J., Manser, S.A., and Lillicrap, S.C. (1986): Enhancement of tungsten kα characteristic x-rays for measurement of coherent and Compton scattering. *Phys. Med. Biol.,* 31(6):651–656.

372. Weisman, M.H., Orth, R.W., Catherwood, B.D., Manolagas, S.C., and Deftos, L.J. (1986): Measures of bone loss in rheumatoid arthritis. *Arch. Intern. Med.,* 146:701–704.

373. Weissberger, M.A., Zamenhof, R.G., Aronow, S., and Neer, R.M. (1978): Computed tomography scanning for measurement of bone mineral in the human spine. *J. Comp. Assist. Tomogr.,* 2:253–262.

374. Wellman, H.N., Appledorn, C.R., Klatte, E.C., Kosegi, J.E., Witt, R.M., and Swingle, B. (1986): Lateral vertebral imaging of trabecular bone mineral content using dual photon absorptiometry. *Proceedings European Nuclear Medicine Congress.* (129).

375. West, R.R., and Reed, G.W. (1970): The measurement of bone mineral *in vivo* by photon beam scanning. *Br. J. Radiol.,* 43:886–893.

376. Wicks, M., Garrett, R., Vernon-Roberts, B., and Fazzalari, N. (1982): Absence of metabolic bone disease in the proximal femur in patients with fracture of the femoral neck. *J. Bone Joint Surg.,* 64B:319–322.

377. Williams, E.D., Boddy, K., Harvey, I., and Haywood, J.K. (1978): Calibration and evaluation of a system for total body *in vivo* activation analysis using 14 MeV neutrons. *Phys. Med. Biol.,* 23:405–415.

378. Wilson, C.R. (1977): Bone-mineral content of the femoral neck and spine versus the radius and ulna. *J. Bone Joint Surg.,* 59A:665–669.

379. Wilson, C.R., and Madsen, M. (1977): Dichromatic absorptiometry of vertebral bone mineral content. *Invest. Radiol.,* 12:180–184.

380. Wilson, C.R., and James, C.D. (1980): Quantitative computed tomographic bone mineral measurement. In: *Porceedings Fourth International Conference Bone Mineral Measurements,* edited by R.B. Mazess, pp. 274–283. NIH Publ. 80-1938, Bethesda, Maryland.

381. Wooten, W.W., Judy, P.F., and Greenfield, M.A. (1973): Analysis of the effects of adipose tissue on the absorptiometric measurement of bone mineral mass. *Invest. Radiol.,* 8:84–87.

382. Yano, K., Wasnich, R.D., Vogel, J.M., and Heilbrun, L.K. (1984): Bone mineral measurements among middle-aged and elderly Japanese residents in Hawaii. *Am. J. Epidemiol.* 119:751–761.

383. Yano, K., Heilbrun, L.K., Wasnich, R.D., Hankin, J.H., and Vogel, J.M. (1985): The relationship between diet and bone mineral content of multiple skeletal sites in elderly Japanese-American men and women living in Hawaii. *Am. J. Clin. Nutrit.,* 42:877–888.

384. Zeitz, L. (1972): Effect of subcutaneous fat on bone mineral content measurements with the "single-energy" photon absorptiometry technique. *Acta Radiol.,* 11:401–410.

385. Zemcov, A., Barclay, L.L., Sansone, J., and Metz, C.E. (1985): Receiver operating characteristic analysis of regional cerebral blood flow in Alzheimer's disease. *J. Nuc. Med.,* 26:1002–1010.

386. Zimmerman, R.E., Lanza, R.C., Tanaka, T., Bolon, G.G., Griffiths, H.J., and Judy, P.F. (1976): A new detector for absorptiometric measurement. *Am. J. Roentgenol,* 126:1272.

Osteoporosis: Etiology, Diagnosis, and Management, edited by B. Lawrence Riggs and L. Joseph Melton, III. Raven Press, New York © 1988.

10

Biochemical Markers of Bone Turnover in Osteoporosis

Pierre D. Delmas

INSERM Unit 234 and Department of Rheumatology and Metabolic Bone Diseases, Hôpital Edouard Herriot, 69437 Lyon, France

Bone is constantly renewed by two opposite activities, the resorption of old bone by osteoclasts and the formation of new bone by osteoblasts. Bone mass results from the equilibrium from these two activities and it is crucial to be able to quantitate them precisely in osteoporosis. Measuring bone formation and resorption by noninvasive methods is rather easy in diseases characterized by dramatic changes of bone turnover such as Paget's disease of bone and renal osteodystrophy. It is much more difficult in osteoporosis, a condition where subtle modifications of the bone remodeling activity can lead to a substantial loss of bone mass after a long period of time. Actually, most conventional markers of bone turnover are usually normal in an osteoporotic patient and incredibly, after 40 years of investigation, it is not clear whether bone loss in osteoporosis results from increased bone resorption, decreased bone formation or both. Invasive techniques such as bone histomorphometry and radiocalcium kinetics have provided new insights but both have limitations and there is obviously a need for sensitive biochemical markers of bone turnover.

Bone is a two-phase tissue comprised of an inorganic mineral phase (hydroxyapatite crystals) and of an organic matrix which represents about 35% of the total weight. The organic matrix is composed mainly (90%) of type I collagen. The noncollagenous compartment of the bone matrix has been extensively studied in the last 10 years, because it contains several proteins, such as osteocalcin (also called bone gla-protein), matrix gla-protein, osteonectin, bone sialoprotein, and proteoglycans (83,112), some of them being specific for bone tissue. The rate of formation or degradation of the bone matrix can be assessed either by measuring an enzymatic activity specific of the bone forming or resorbing cells, such as alkaline and acid phosphatase activity, or by measuring bone matrix components released into the circulation during formation or resorption (Table 1). As discussed below, these markers are of unequal specificity and sensitivity.

BIOCHEMICAL MARKERS OF BONE FORMATION

Serum Alkaline Phosphatase

Structure and Function

Alkaline phosphatase [EC 3.1.3.1. ; ortho phosphoric-mono-ester phospho-hydrolase (al-

TABLE 1. *Biochemical markers of bone turnover*

Formation	Resorption
Serum	**Plasma**
Total alkaline phosphatase	Total hydroxyproline
Bone specific alkaline	Tartrate-resistant acid
phosphatase	phosphatase
osteocalcium (BGP)	
Procollagen I carboxy-ter-	
minal extension peptide	
Urine	**Urine**
Nondialyzable hydroxypro-	Total and dialyzable hy-
line.	droxyproline
	Hydroxylysine glycosides

kaline optimum)] activity in serum has been extensively studied in the past 50 years. Its determination was first applied to the investigation of metabolic bone diseases after Robinson had shown the association between an increased alkaline phosphatase activity in serum and an increased osteoblastic activity in bone (94). Robinson showed that growing bone is very rich in phosphatase activity and that the optimum pH of the enzyme is alkaline. It was suggested that alkaline phosphatase allows bone mineralization by releasing inorganic phosphate that contributes to the deposition of calcium-phosphate complexes into the osteoid matrix. Alkaline phosphatase might also promote mineralization by hydrolyzing the inorganic pyrophosphate, a potent inhibitor of hydroxyapatite crystal formation and dissolution (1,28), within the extracellular calcifying matrix vesicles. Finally, a role for alkaline phosphatase in bone mineralization is strongly suggested by a rare and severe form of rickets, hypophosphatasia. Indeed, these patients are characterized by a very low alkaline phosphatase activity in serum and bone, which could explain the mineralization defect (91). Despite these evidences, the precise role of alkaline phosphatase in mineralization and its mechanism of action remain unclear.

Alkaline phosphatase is not part of the extracellular matrix of bone, but it circulates in blood. Since the observation of Roberts that increased serum alkaline phosphatase activity often accompanied hepatobiliary disease, particu-larly in cases of biliary stasis (93), the existence of different tissue specific forms of alkaline phosphatase has been established. It has been recently shown that three different genes code for a placental, an intestinal and a "bone-liver-kidney" alkaline phosphatase isoenzyme (97). Hypophosphatasia is characterized by a specific inherited autosomal recessive defect of the latter isoenzyme (5). Liver, bone and kidney alkaline phosphatase differ in electrophoretic mobility and resistance to inactivation by heat (71,72). These differences are thought to reflect posttranslational modification of the carbohydrate side-chains of these glycoprotein enzymes, but it is generally believed that these three tissue "secondary" isoenzymes are encoded by a single locus, with tissue-specific variations introduced during its expression in different types of cells (70).

Circulating Total Alkaline Phosphatase

The total alkaline phosphatase activity of plasma or serum is commonly estimated by an automated procedure based upon the enzymatic hydrolysis of P-nitrophenyl phosphate during incubation at 37°5 C (53,68). Total alkaline phosphatase activity of serum is contributed by at least two isoenzymes, one presumably derived from bone, the other from liver. Isoenzyme analysis has shown that a small amount of intestinal alkaline phosphatase is present in about 25% of sera from normal subjects and is probably responsible for the increase in total alkaline phosphatase activity that can occur after eating (57). The renal alkaline phosphatase does not contribute to the serum activity of normal subjects. The placental alkaline phosphatase isoenzyme is detectable in the blood from the 16th to 20th week of pregnancy. In addition to these physiologic conditions, the total alkaline phosphatase activity can be increased by a considerable number of perturbations unrelated to bone metabolism. An increase of the liver alkaline phosphatase activity is responsible for the increased levels of total serum alkaline phosphatase that are found in a variety of hepatobiliary diseases and with a large number of medications (66). Also, total serum alkaline phosphatase may be increased in hepatoma and a variety of other malignancies because of the secretion by the tumor of a carcinoplacental isoenzyme of alkaline phosphatase (27,66). The possible influence of these extraskeletal sources of alkaline phosphatase should be kept in mind when assessing bone turnover by measuring serum alkaline phosphatase. Finally, the turnover rate of alkaline phosphatase in serum is markedly different from one isoenzyme to the other. Thus, the half-life is less than an hour for the intestinal isoenzyme (51), approximately 1 to 2 days for the skeletal isoenzyme (81,113) and 7 days for the human placental one (8).

Serum alkaline phosphatase is thought to reflect skeletal growth and maturation in healthy children. The enzyme levels are about three times higher than the upper limit of normal adult levels throughout childhood and early adolescence and decline to adult levels during the late teens. These changes are parallel to bone growth assessed by the height increase (7) and they appear to reflect the simultaneous changes in bone mineral content (54). Isoenzyme studies indicate that bone alkaline phosphatase is the major fraction of the total activity in sera of children. In the blood of healthy adults, the total alkaline phosphatase activity represents approximately equal contributions by the bone and the liver isoenzyme. Between 30 and 80 years of age, there is a slight but significant increase of serum alkaline phosphatase that is accounted for by an increase of both the liver and the bone isoenzymes determined by a quantitative heat-inactivation technique (70). When data obtained from men and women are analyzed separately, the increase in serum alkaline phosphatase with aging is of greater magnitude in women than in men (48). The modification of serum alkaline phosphatase with aging and the specific influence of menopause have deserved special attention. Comparing two groups of pre- and postmenopausal women that were matched for age to exclude the effect of age *per se*, Crilly et al. (9) found that the serum alkaline phosphatase level was approxi-

mately 40% higher in postmenopausal women. We have measured total serum alkaline phosphatase in 174 women aged 30 to 94 years and values were correlated with other biochemical markers and with bone density (20). Serum alkaline phosphatase increased slightly but significantly ($r = 0.31$, $p < 0.001$) with a predicted mean at age 90 years that was 30% more than the predicted mean at age 30 years.

Serum alkaline phosphatase was positively correlated with other biochemical markers and negatively correlated with the bone mineral density measured at the lumbar spine ($r = -0.34$, $p < 0.001$). These data suggest that the increase in serum alkaline phosphatase activity with age in women, more pronounced at menopause, reflects an increase of bone turnover which accounts for postmenopausal bone loss (20).

Serum alkaline phosphatase is increased in metabolic bone diseases characterized by an increased bone turnover such as primary hyperparathyroidism, hyperthyroidism, and Paget's disease of bone, the latter condition being associated with the highest recorded levels of the enzyme (47). However, increased levels of serum alkaline phosphatase activity can also reflect a mineralization defect such as in most types of rickets and osteomalacia (47). The difficulty of interpreting increased levels of serum alkaline phosphatase activity is illustrated by renal osteodystrophy where it can be associated with a markedly increased bone turnover (secondary hyperparathyroidism) or with osteomalacia. This ambiguity should be kept in mind when analyzing serum alkaline phosphatase activity in patients with osteoporosis.

Total Serum Alkaline Phosphatase in Postmenopausal Osteoporosis

The majority of patients with osteoporosis have normal serum alkaline phosphatase activity. In the absence of hepatic disorder, a substantial increase of serum alkaline phosphatase in a patient with crushed vertebrae should be analyzed carefully. Because the alkaline phosphatase activity of fracture callus is usually greater than that of normal bone, increased serum levels are sometimes attributed to a recent vertebral fracture (44). Actually, fractures, even when multiple, do not result in marked increases in serum alkaline phosphatase activity (80). High turnover osteoporosis is rarely associated with a marked increase of serum alkaline phosphatase activity (see below) and the possibility of occult osteomalacia should always be suspected (78). Some information can be derived from measurement of serum alkaline phosphatase in a large group of patients with osteoporosis. In a group of 100 postmenopausal women with ill defined spinal osteoporosis (apparently some of the patients did not show radiologic evidence of vertebral collapse), Hulth et al. (43) found a mean serum alkaline phosphatase of 6.7 ± 2.0 units for a normal range of 2 to 8 units. Twelve patients had high values ranging from 10 to 14 units without histologic evidence of osteomalacia. There was a weak but significant negative correlation between serum alkaline phosphatase and the bone mineral content of the forearm measured by photon absorptiometry (43). We (23) have measured total serum alkaline phosphatase activity in a well-defined population of 62 postmenopausal women with spinal osteoporosis defined by one or more nontraumatic vertebral fractures. All of them had normal routine biochemical tests including serum level of 25-hydroxyvitamin D and none had received specific treatment during the last 6 months. Serum alkaline phosphatase levels of the patients were compared with values of 142 normal women. In order to exclude a possible influence of age, individual values of patients were expressed as standard deviation from the predicted mean for normal subjects obtained from the regression equation which predicts serum alkaline phosphatase as a function of age. In patients with postmenopausal osteoporosis, serum alkaline phosphatase was significantly increased with a mean increase of 27% and a Z score of + 0.97 ($p < 0.001$). The distribution of values was normal but 22.5% of patients had values > 2.S.D. There was no significant

correlation between serum alkaline phosphatase activity and the bone mineral density of the lumbar spine measured by dual photon absorptiometry suggesting that serum alkaline phosphatase cannot be used as a marker of bone loss in osteoporosis (23). Conversely, the observation of a mild but significant increase of the mean value of the serum enzyme suggests an increased bone turnover that needs to be analyzed further.

There are many clinical observations showing that serum alkaline phosphatase is a valid index of bone turnover, but most of them have been applied to diseases characterized by a dramatic increase of bone turnover, such as Paget's disease. Furthermore, because bone formation and bone resorption are usually tightly coupled, these studies cannot determine if serum alkaline phosphatase is a specific marker of bone formation. The crucial question is to know if serum alkaline phosphatase is a sensitive and reliable marker of bone formation in a disease—osteoporosis—where the range of variations of bone turnover and alkaline phosphatase are quite narrow. Serum alkaline phosphatase can be compared to the rate of bone formation and bone resorption measured by two techniques: calcium kinetic studies have significant limitations for assessing bone remodeling in osteoporotic states because of technical problems (short- and long-term exchanges of isotope between blood and bone compartments, role of decreased bone mass on isotope retention, etc.). However, a significant correlation ($r = 0.69$, $p < 0.01$) was found by Laufferburger et al. (58) between the Ca^{47} accretion rate, which reflects bone formation rate, and serum alkaline phosphatase activity in 15 untreated postmenopausal women with spinal osteoporosis. After treatment with sodium fluoride (100 mg/day for 6 months) both serum alkaline phosphatase and Ca^{47} accretion rate rose, but the increase of the latter was of lesser magnitude, probably because of the mineralization defect induced by the high doses of fluoride. Although it was significantly correlated with calcium accretion rate, serum alkaline phosphatase was not related to the osteoid and osteoblastic surfaces (r = 0.17 and r = 0.13, respectively) measured in the same patients on iliac crest biopsy (58). Shifrin (100) did not find a significant correlation between serum alkaline phosphatase and bone formation measured on bone biopsy in a heterogenous group of patients including 25 postmenopausal osteoporotics. Similarly, White et al. did not find significant correlation between serum alkaline phosphatase and the osteoid parameters in 26 females with osteopenia, some of them having been previously treated (114). We have evaluated the value of serum alkaline phosphatase to predict bone turnover in 31 postmenopausal women with untreated spinal osteoporosis, all of them having nontraumatic vertebral fractures. There was a weak and nonsignificant correlation between serum alkaline phosphatase and histologic parameters reflecting bone formation, with the best correlation (r = 0.32) obtained with the bone formation rate evaluated at the tissue level (Table 2). As expected, serum alkaline phosphatase was not correlated with bone resorption. When patients were classified according to the bone remodeling activity measured in trabecular bone (4), serum alkaline phosphatase activity was not significantly different among the groups with low formation (3.2 ± 0.5 BU/1), high formation (3.4 ± 0.3 BU/1) and normal formation (4.0 ± 0.4 BU/1). Thus, total serum alkaline phosphatase activity is a valid marker of the level of bone formation in conditions with dramatic increases of bone turnover like Paget's disease of bone, but its measurement does not appear to be a sensitive marker in primary osteoporosis, a condition where the bone remodeling activity fluctuates within a rather narrow range. Serum alkaline phosphatase measurement is unable to detect the decrease of bone formation that occurs in some of the osteoporotic patients. This lack of sensitivity is probably related to the lack of specificity, as serum activity arises from both bone and liver alkaline phosphatase. In an attempt to improve the specificity and the sensitivity of serum alkaline measurement, techniques have been developed to differentiate alkaline phosphatase isoenzymes.

Circulating Bone Alkaline Phosphatase

Several techniques have been used to quantitate the different forms of alkaline phosphatase in serum. These techniques rely on three general methods: the use of differentially effective activators and inhibitors (heat, phenylalanine and urea), separation by electrophoresis (starch and polyacrylamide gel, cellulose acetate, disc electrophoresis and gel filtration chromatography), and separation by specific antisera (70). The possible contribution of intestinal and placental alkaline phosphatases can be easily detected and measured because these two isoenzymes are specifically inhibited after treatment of serum by L-phenylalanine. Actually, the major problem is to differentiate between bone and liver alkaline phosphatase which contribute approximately equally and represent 60 to 95% of serum alkaline phosphatase activity. These two enzymes cannot be completely separated by electrophoretic techniques and there are no marked catalytic or immunologic differences between them. It has been found that the bone alkaline phosphatase is more sensitive to urea inhibition than is the liver alkaline phosphatase, and that the bone enzyme is more heat labile at 56° C than other tissue isoenzymes (3,72). A combination of heat and urea inhibition is usually applied to the quantitative deter-

TABLE 2. *Correlations between serum alkaline phosphatase and bone turnover measured in trabecular bone in 31 untreated patients with postmenopausal osteoporosis*

Histomorphometric parameter	Linear correlation		
	N	r	P
Osteoid surfaces	31	0.19	NS
Osteoid volume	31	− 0.02	NS
Mineralization rate	29	− 0.07	NS
Tetracycline double-labelled surfaces	26	0.30	NS
Tetracycline total-labelled surfaces	26	0.11	NS
Bone formation rate (tissue level)	25	0.32	NS
Bone formation rate (BMU level)	25	0.13	NS
Resorption surfaces	31	− 0.11	NS
Osteoclast count	31	− 0.08	NS

mination of bone and liver phosphatases, but they are tedious and time-consuming techniques that require skill and careful attention during the procedure. Furthermore, quantitative data can be markedly affected by slight variations in temperature, pH, protein and substrate concentrations (70). These limitations explain why few data are available on serum levels of bone alkaline phosphatase in osteoporosis. On a large population of healthy subjects, it has been shown that the bone isoenzyme is mainly responsible for the variation associated with age, sex, puberty and to some extent with menopause. Bone alkaline phosphatase increases after 30 years of age in females but not in males with a 30% rise after the menopause (96). In a group of 50 patients with ill-defined osteoporosis, Stepan et al. (106) found that serum bone alkaline phosphatase was significantly higher (mean 16.4 μ/1, range 11.1–24.4) than in controls (mean 9.2 μ/1, range 7.1–12.0, $p < 0.001$). Bone phosphatase was increased in 60% of the patients, in contrast to the total activity of serum alkaline phosphatase that was increased in 22% of patients. Interestingly there was no overlap of bone alkaline phosphatase between patients with osteoporosis and 35 patients with osteomalacia who had much higher values (mean 70.2, range 33.1–148.7). Finally, a good correlation was found between serum bone alkaline phosphatase and urinary hydroxyproline in osteoporotic patients ($r = 0.80$, $p < 0.001$). Farley et al. (26) have developed a technique for measuring bone alkaline phosphatase using the heat inactivation method optimized by including organ-derived internal standards of skeletal, intestinal and biliary alkaline phosphatase to minimize between-assay variations. Serum bone alkaline phosphatase was found to be slightly higher in 43 untreated patients with postmenopausal osteoporosis than in age-matched controls (10.4 ± 7.24 U/1 vs 7.05 ± 3.63) and did not correlate with total serum alkaline phosphatase. Seven patients who responded to sodium fluoride therapy (88 mg/day for 3 to 8 years) by increased bone density and bone formation assessed histologi-

cally, had a mean value of serum bone alkaline phosphatase after treatment that was 100% higher than in age-matched controls. Finally, after a short term treatment with Stanozolol, 10 osteoporotic patients had a significant increase of bone, but not of total, alkaline phosphatase in serum (26).

Osteocalcin

Structure, Function, and Metabolism

Osteocalcin, also called bone gla-protein or BGP, is one of the most abundant proteins of bone making up 15 to 20% of the non collagenous matrix (41,86). Osteocalcin is a single chain protein of low molecular weight (5800 daltons) with four isomeric forms of identical molecular weight having a pI ranging from 3.95 to 4.5 (21). The aminoacid sequence of osteocalcin established for several species includes the presence of three residues of gamma carboxyglutamic acid (82), a calcium-binding aminoacid that results from the posttranslational carboxylation of glutamic acid in the presence of vitamin K. In contrast to gla that is present in a variety of mineralized tissues (33), osteocalcin has been found only in bone and in minute amounts in tooth dentin, experimental calcifications and atherosclerotic plaques.

Because of the presence of gla, osteocalcin binds to calcium and more strongly to hydroxyapatite and the protein undergoes calcium dependent conformational changes (19,39). The secretion of osteocalcin by rat osteogenic sarcoma cells and by human bone cells in vitro is dependent on 1,25 dihydroxyvitamin D (2,84). Despite these fascinating properties, the potential role of osteocalcin in the mineralization process is unknown. A possible role of osteocalcin in the local regulation of bone metabolism is suggested by its chemotactic activity (64) and by the fact that implanted osteocalcin-deficient bone particles are resistant to resorption (61). It should be stressed, however, that the physiological role of osteocalcin is unknown.

The metabolism of osteocalcin is only partially known. Several experiments demonstrate that osteocalcin is synthesized by bone and osteoblasts are the most likely candidates for this synthesis (2,60,73,74). Whether osteocalcin derives or not from a larger precursor protein is debated (21,40). After its synthesis, osteocalcin is incorporated into bone matrix but its precise cell and tissue distribution, using techniques such as immunohistochemistry, have not been investigated. Osteocalcin circulates in blood, where it can be measured by radioimmunoassay (85) and is probably eliminated by the kidney like most of small proteins. It has been shown in rat that osteocalcin is almost entirely cleared from the plasma by kidney filtration (88), but few data are available in humans. Osteocalcin is not found in urine, where it is probably degraded, and we have shown that plasma levels of osteocalcin show an hyperbolic increase when the glomerular filtration rate is lower than 30 ml/min/1.73 m^2 (22). Conversely, circulating levels are not affected by kidney filtration when the renal failure is mild to moderate (22). Price et al. (88) have shown in rat that bone resorption does not contribute significantly to serum osteocalcin, and we will see that it is also the case in humans. Actually, osteocalcin released during resorption has probably been broken down by the osteoclast into short oligopeptides that are not recognized by most antisera (13,14), a situation similar to what happens with collagen. Assuming that the half-life of serum osteocalcin is 12 hr and that the protein has the same volume of distribution as insulin (MW = 5000), and assuming that the theories of Frost (30) on bone-remodeling rates are correct, Parfitt (76) has estimated that approximately 15% of the osteocalcin synthesized is released into the circulation, and 85% incorporated into bone where it binds to the mineral. Actually, these data were calculated with a concentration of osteocalcin in bone of 1 mg/g, a number which applies to bovine but not to human bone. Assuming a likely 0.1 mg of osteocalcin per g of bone, the fraction of osteocalcin incorporated into bone should be lower than the one of os-

teocalcin released into the circulation, approximately 30 and 70% respectively. These theoretical numbers are important to interpret pathological variation of serum osteocalcin.

Measurement of Serum Osteocalcin

Because bovine and human osteocalcin differ only by 5 aminoacids, most radioimmunoassays of osteocalcin are developed with antisera raised against bovine osteocalcin and cross react with purified human osteocalcin (20,25,35,37,77,85). When tested, these assays have shown that all the immunoreactivity in human sera from normal individuals coelutes with purified intact osteocalcin on gel filtration chromatography and all of them exhibit parallel dilutions of bovine standard and human serum. All these assays provide a normal mean value of serum osteocalcin in adults ranging from 4.2 to 7 ng/ml according to the assay, with individual values ranging from 2 to 13 ng/ml (20,25,35,37,85). In contrast, Catherwood et al. (6) have recently reported a radioimmunoassay based on an antiserum raised against a small fragment (12 aminoacids) of human osteocalcin which provides much higher values, with a calculated mean of 15 ng of intact osteocalcin/ml in normal adults. Furthermore, individual values show a wide normal range from 0 to an extraordinary high 40 ng/ml, suggesting that this antiserum might also recognize fragments of osteocalcin and/or other proteins. Because the specificity of this assay has not yet been documented, the serum values in normal and pathologic conditions should be interpreted cautiously.

Using conventional assays, increased values of serum osteocalcin have been reported in diseases characterized by an increased bone turnover such as primary hyperparathyroidism, renal osteodystrophy, Paget's disease of bone and hyperparathyroidism (23,36,63,87,104). In contrast, serum osteocalcin is decreased in hypoparathyroidism, a condition associated with a low bone turnover (23,87). Several lines of evidence suggest that serum osteocalcin reflects more bone formation than bone resorption in various metabolic bone diseases (18). For example, serum osteocalcin values are dissociated from indices of bone resorption after treatment of primary hyperparathyroidism (16). In patients on chronic maintenance dialysis, serum osteocalcin correlates better with bone formation than with bone resorption assessed histologically (63). In a group of 23 patients with endocrine disorders characterized by a low bone turnover (corticosteroid treated patients), or a high bone turnover (primary hyperparathyroidism and hyperthyroidism), serum osteocalcin was found to be significantly correlated with bone formation, but not with bone resorption, measured on iliac crest biopsies. These data suggest that measurement of circulating osteocalcin might be useful in the investigation of metabolic bone diseases and to monitor the effects of specific treatments. However, in cases where the texture of bone is not normal, such as Paget's disease of bone, serum osteocalcin does not seem to be a reliable marker of bone turnover (17).

Osteocalcin and Osteoporosis

In a group of 174 women, aged 30 to 94 years that were randomly selected from the population of Rochester, Minnesota, we found that serum osteocalcin increased linearly with aging from a mean value of 4.4 ng/ml in the fourth decade to 8.9 ng/ml in the tenth decade (20). This increase correlated inversely with concomitant decreases in bone mineral density measured at the lumbar spine and at the radius. This increase of serum osteocalcin, that is accompanied by a less marked but significant increase of serum alkaline phosphatase and urinary hydroxyproline, reflects an increase in overall bone turnover with aging. It is noteworthy that changes of osteocalcin are more pronounced after a surgical menopause, with a mean value that doubles 6 months after the menopause, an increase which is sustained up to 24 months after oophorectomy (29). When postmenopausal women are treated with estrogen for 2 to 8 weeks, there is a significant and marked decrease (50 to 70%) of serum osteo-

calcin but a moderate fall of serum alkaline phosphatase (108). In contrast to women, the age-related increase of serum osteocalcin is mild in men, who also have an age-related bone loss of lesser magnitude than women (25).

In patients with postmenopausal osteoporosis and vertebral fractures, the mean level of serum osteocalcin has been reported to be either normal (4,36) or slightly elevated (23,87) but with a wide scatter of individual values that can explain the differences according to the population studied. When the data obtained from 62 untreated osteoporotic females and 83 normal postmenopausal normals were pooled, there was a negative correlation (r = 0.36, p < 0.001) between serum osteocalcin and the lumbar density (23). Because osteoporosis is a heterogenous disorder with a wide spectrum of histologic bone turnover, we chose to assess the significance of circulating osteocalcin by comparing its value with the bone remodeling activity measured on iliac crest biopsy. Twenty-six patients with untreated postmenopausal osteoporosis were studied and 22 of them had previously received two courses of tetracycline (4). Serum osteocalcin was significantly correlated with all parameters reflecting trabecular bone formation such as the osteoid parameters, the tetracycline labelled surfaces and the bone formation rate (Table 3 and Fig. 1), but not with parameters reflecting bone resorption. When patients were classified according to the histologic level of bone turnover, serum osteocalcin was significantly lower in the subgroup of patients with a low osteoblastic activity (2.9 ± 0.9 ng/ml) and higher in the group of patients with high turnover (9.7 ± 0.8 ng/ml) than in the group of patients with normal turnover (4). In this study, histologic measurements were applied to the trabecular envelope only. Because the subcortical endosteal envelope undergoes more active remodeling than the trabecular envelope, we have developed a computerized semiautomatic method allowing measurements in real value of bone turnover on subcortical surfaces of bone as well as on trabecular bone. In 33 osteoporotic women, se-

TABLE 3. *Linear correlations between serum BGP and other biochemical or histologic indices of bone turnover in postmenopausal osteoporosis*

Parameters	N	r	P
Biochemistry			
Serum alkaline phosphatase	25	0.03	NS
Urinary hydroxyproline	25	0.21	NS
Trabecular bone histology			
Osteoid surfaces	33	0.74	0.001
Osteoid volume	33	0.71	0.01
Total tetracycline-labelled surfaces	28	0.70	0.001
Bone formation rate	28	0.70	0.001
Resorption surfaces	33	0.27	NS
Osteoclast number	33	0.35	NS
Trabecular + endosteal bone			
Osteoid surfaces	33	0.77	0.001
Osteoid volume	33	0.75	0.001
Total tetracycline-labelled surfaces	28	0.69	0.001
Bone formation rate	28	0.76	0.001
Osteoclast number	33	0.19	NS

rum osteocalcin was significantly correlated with the osteoid parameters (r = 0.56 to 0.68) and with the bone formation rate derived from the tetracycline labelled surfaces (r = 0.75, p < 0.001), but not with bone resorption. When the remodeling activity of the trabecular and the endosteal bone were pooled, the correlation between serum osteocalcin and bone formation was improved (Table 3), an expected finding as serum osteocalcin reflects the osteoblastic activity of the entire skeleton.

Corticosteroid-induced osteoporosis is another situation where serum osteocalcin provides information about the level of bone formation. In 30 patients on chronic corticosteroid treatment, serum osteocalcin was significantly decreased (4.2 ± 2.7 ng/ml vs 6.4 ± 2.2 ng/ml in age-matched controls, p < 0.001), despite an increased bone resorption assessed by urinary hydroxyproline. Interestingly, serum osteocalcin was negatively correlated with the daily dose of prednisone (r = − 0.57, p < 0.001) but not with the cumulative dose previously received, indicating that circulating osteocalcin reflects the instantaneous effect of steroids (Table 4). In 12 of these patients who had nontraumatic vertebral fractures and an iliac crest biopsy, serum osteocalcin was correlated with the osteoid surfaces (r = 0.82), the osteoid volume (r = 0.60) but not with the resorption surfaces (r = 0.27). Thus, serum osteocalcin reflects bone formation whether bone turnover is low, normal or high. The specificity of circulating osteocalcin levels to reflect bone formation has recently been confirmed by

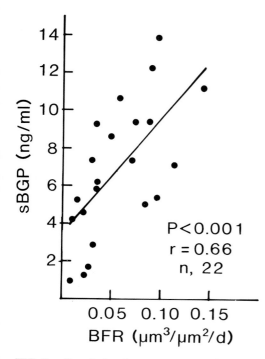

FIG 1. Correlation between serum BGP and the tetracycline based bone formation rate (BFR) in untreated patients with postmenopausal osteoporosis.

TABLE 4. *Serum BGP in corticosteroid-treated patients according to the daily dose of prednisone*

N	Prednisone dose (mg/day)	B G P (ng/ml)
3	60	0.6 ± 0.1[a]
6	30	2.0 ± 0.7[a]
11	10–20	5.5 ± 2.7
10	3–10	5.3 ± 2.1
30	3–60	4.2 ± 2.7[a]

[a]p < 0.01–0.001 vs controls.

Riggs et al. (92) who showed that a continuous 24-hr intravenous infusion of the 1 to 34 synthetic fragment of human parathyroid hormone induced a significant decrease of serum osteocalcin despite a significant 69% increase of urinary hydroxyproline in 18 normal women.

Effects of Treatment of Osteoporosis on Serum Osteocalcin

Serum osteocalcin decreases after calcitonin treatment in Paget's disease of bone (12), decreases after parathyroidectomy in primary hyperparathyroidism (12,16) and increases in patients with rickets after treatment with 1,25-dihydroxyvitamin D (34). In contrast, few data are available on osteocalcin variations in osteoporosis after treatment. We have shown that a short-term treatment (4 months) with sodium fluoride, a potent stimulator of osteoblastic activity, induces a slight but significant increase of serum osteocalcin (15). In 5 patients with corticosteroid induced osteoporosis treated for 10 to 19 months with sodium fluoride, we found a marked increase of serum osteocalcin from 3.3 ± 1.2 to 7.2 ± 2.2 ng/ml ($p < 0.01$), with no change of serum alkaline phosphatase (Fig. 2). Serum osteocalcin also increased in 13 osteoporotic women from 3.9 ± 0.6 ng/ml to 6.4 ± 0.9 ng/ml after a 2 week treatment with calcitriol at a daily dose of 2 μg/day (117). A short administration of calcitriol (2 days) induces an increase of serum osteocalcin in osteoporotic patients which is of greater magnitude than in pre- or postmenopausal normal women (24). These data confirm the experimental observation that osteocalcin synthesis is dependent on vitamin D and suggest that a calcitriol challenge might be an interesting test to evaluate the osteoblastic activity assessed by serum osteocalcin levels.

An ideal marker of bone formation would be a bone matrix constituent specifically synthesized by osteoblasts at a rate proportional to collagen synthesis, with a fraction released into the circulation proportional to the fraction incorporated into the matrix. If this substance is degraded during resorption into small fragments and if its metabolic clearance is known, measurement of the intact substance in serum should be an accurate marker of bone formation (76). None of the currently available markers of bone formation meet all these criteria but osteocalcin is the most satisfactory. It is specific for osteoblasts, present in serum and in bone matrix and the lack of correlation with bone resorption suggest that it is degraded into nonimmunoreactive fragments during the pro-

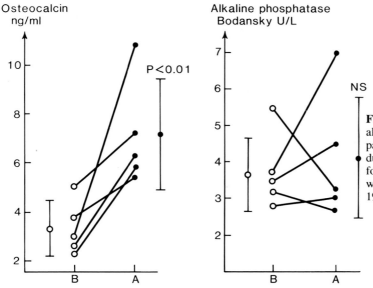

FIG. 2. Serum osteocalcin and alkaline phosphatase values in 5 patients with corticosteroid-induced vertebral osteoporosis before (**B**) and after (**A**) treatment with sodium fluoride for 10 to 19 months.

cess of resorption. Indirect calculations suggest that about 30% of osteocalcin synthesized is incorporated into bone matrix and 70% released into the circulation but there is not direct evidence for it. Correlation with histology suggest that serum osteocalcin levels closely follow the rate of bone formation in diseases characterized by a modification of bone turnover, but this might not be the case where the texture of the bone is not normal, i.e., nonlamellar. Furthermore, we need more information about the volume of distribution and the metabolic clearance of the substance. Nevertheless, serum osteocalcin appears to be a specific and sensitive marker of osteoblastic bone formation in osteoporosis. In contrast to serum alkaline phosphatase, its measurement can detect a decrease of bone formation, and a mild increase. Serum osteocalcin should therefore be useful in the investigation of osteoporosis and for monitoring the effects of treatments which modulate bone formation. Until the data are available, one should be cautious because some treatments which modify the composition of bone, such as sodium fluoride that induces the formation of fluoroapatite, might modify the fraction of osteocalcin released into the circulation and the fraction incorporated into bone. It also should be kept in mind that circulating osteocalcin will reflect the instantaneous level of osteoblastic activity at the skeleton level and not necessarily the cumulative effect of a treatment over a long period of time.

Other Markers of Bone Formation

Serum Procollagen I Carboxyterminal Extension Peptide

Collagens are synthesized intracellularly as precursor molecules, procollagens which include an aminoterminal and a carboxyterminal globular extension. During the extracellular processing of collagen, there is a cleavage of these extension peptides prior to the fibril formation (90). The carboxyterminal peptide cleaved from type I procollagen (pcoll-I-C), which is predominant in bone is stabilized by interchain disulfide bonds as a molecule of approximately 100.000 daltons. This molecule circulates in blood where it can be measured by radioimmunoassay (109). Because this extension peptide is produced by the osteoblasts at a rate which is equimolar with the rate of bone collagen synthesis, and because it is not incorporated into bone matrix, serum level of pcoll-I-C might be a valuable marker of bone formation. Increased serum levels of pcoll-I-C have been reported in Paget's disease of bone (101,110) but values were correlated with both serum alkaline phosphatase and urinary hydroxyproline. After treatment with dichloromethylene diphosphonate, a potent inhibitor of bone resorption serum pcoll-I-C decreased to normal values in the same patients (101). Thus, levels of pcoll-I-C could reflect bone formation, bone resorption, or a combination of the two. The fact that a single dose of 30 mg of prednisone suppresses the serum level of pcoll-I-C without decreasing urinary hydroxyproline excretion, suggests that serum pcoll-I-C reflects bone formation and not resorption (102). Simon et al. have correlated serum pcoll-I-C with bone histomorphometry in a heterogenous population comprising normal individuals, patients with so-called radiographic osteopenia and patients with osteoporosis. Serum pcoll-I-C was lower in "osteopenic" patients than in normals (53.7 ± 25.2 vs 87.9 ± 40.7 ng/ml) but the two groups were not matched for age. There was a weak correlation between serum pcoll-I-C and the bone formation rate with an r value ranging from 0.36 to 0.45. Correlations with bone resorption were not mentioned (103). These data are rather disappointing but it should be noted that serum pcoll-I-C might be influenced by its rate of metabolic clearance which is unknown. Obviously, more data are necessary to precisely estimate the value of pcoll-I-C measurement in assessing the bone-remodeling activity in osteoporosis.

Urinary Excretion of Nondialyzable Hydroxyproline

The amino-terminus of type I procollagen consists of a short collagen-type helical region containing hydroxyproline and of noncollagenous regions containing intrachain, but not interchain, disulfide bonds (90). During the processing of procollagen, the amino-terminal extension peptide is cleaved and probably released into the circulation. Several lines of evidence indicate that the nondialyzable polypeptides containing hydroxyproline excreted in the urine derive mainly from the breakdown of newly synthesized collagens arising from these aminoterminal extension peptides (38,56). Nondialyzable urinary hydroxyproline consists of heterogenous peptides with an average molecular weight of 5,000 and represents about 10% of the total excretion of hydroxyproline in urine. Thus, fractionation of urinary hydroxyproline into dialyzable and nondialyzable forms might give some information about the rate of bone formation, but these measurements lack sensibility because they are not specific for bone metabolism.

BIOCHEMICAL MARKERS OF BONE RESORPTION

Hydroxyproline

Hydroxyproline is found almost exclusively in collagens and represents about 13% of the aminoacid content of the molecule (89). Hydroxyproline is derived from proline by a post-translational hydroxylation occuring within the peptide chain. Because free hydroxyproline released during degradation of collagen cannot be reutilized in collagen synthesis, most of the endogenous hydroxyproline present in biologic fluids is derived from the degradation of various forms of collagen. As half of human collagen resides in bone where its turnover is probably faster than in soft tissues, excretion of hydroxyproline in urine is regarded as a marker of bone resorption. Actually, the relationship of the urinary hydroxyproline to the metabolism of collagen is more complex. Hydroxyproline is present in biologic fluids in different forms. About 90% of the hydroxyproline released by the breakdown of collagen in the tis-

sues, and especially during bone resorption, is degraded to the free aminoacid which circulates in plasma, is filtered and almost entirely reabsorbed by the kidney. It is eventually completely oxidized in the liver and degraded to carbon dioxide and urea (49). About 10% of the hydroxyproline released by the breakdown of collagen circulates in the peptide-bound form and these peptides containing hydroxyproline are filtered and excreted in urine without any further metabolism. Thus, the urinary total hydroxyproline represents only about 10% of total collagen catabolism. Hydroxyproline is present in urine under three forms: free hydroxyproline, hydroxyproline-containing small peptides that are dialyzable and represent over 90% of the total urinary excretion of this aminoacid, and a small amount of nondialyzable polypeptides containing hydroxyproline (89). These polypeptides appear to be derived mainly from the breakdown of newly synthesized collagens and therefore nondialyzable urinary hydroxyproline seems to be a marker of bone formation and not resorption (see above). Most studies were performed with measuring total hydroxyproline in urine, thus reflecting mainly bone resorption. Hydroxyproline can also be measured in plasma where it circulates in different forms (protein-bound, peptide-bound, and free). Because of the low levels, plasma hydroxyproline measurement is not a very sensitive index of bone metabolism and is restricted to uremic patients (10).

Urinary Hydroxyproline and Aging

After acid hydrolysis of a urine sample, hydroxyproline is measured by colorimetry after oxidation by the chloramine-T (50). The normal values for hydroxyproline excretion are dependent on dietary intake of hydroxyproline, on sampling time, body size, sex and age. Because dietary collagen affects the 24-hr urinary excretion of total hydroxyproline, patients are usually placed on a low gelatin diet for 48 hr before the first urine collection. The excretion after a 12-hr fast does not seem to be influenced by the previous day's diet and another alternative is to assess bone resorption from hydroxyproline measurement in the fasting urine collected over 2 hr ("spot" technique) (75). Urinary total hydroxyproline excretion follows a circadian rhythm with peak excretion during the night, suggesting increased bone resorption during the night (65). Because urinary hydroxyproline depends on body size and on glomerular filtration rate, indirect correction has been performed using body weight, body surface area, the 24-hr creatinine excretion, the glomerular filtration rate and recently bone mass assessed by the bone mineral content of the forearm (20,45,75,89,95). These corrections are especially relevant when one wants to assess the effect of age on urinary excretion of hydroxyproline, because both the glomerular function and bone mass decrease with aging. In contrast to the uncorrected excretion of hydroxyproline which is either constant or decreases with aging (95), the hydroxyproline: creatinine ratio has been found to be higher in elderly individuals than in young adults and is higher in old women than in old men (42,115). Also, bilateral oophorectomy is followed by a rise of urinary calcium and 24-hr urinary hydroxyproline which reflects an increase in the rate of resorption. We have measured urinary total hydroxyproline in 174 healthy women aged 30 to 94 years and data were expressed corrected for the glomerular filtration rate (assessed by the creatinine clearance) and for the body size derived from height and weight (20). Urinary hydroxyproline increased with aging (r = 0.29, p < 0.001) from 24 ± 2.3 mg/dl GFR in the fourth decade to 35 ± 3.2 mg/dl GFR in the tenth decade. By correcting the hydroxyproline: creatinine ratio with the bone mineral content of the forearm, Myldstrup (45) also reported an increase with age in females after menopause but not in men. These data suggest that the excretion of hydroxyproline per unit of volume of bone increases with aging, at least in women but it is not clear if this increase is limited or not to the decade following menopause. Further studies correcting hydroxyproline excretion by bone mass evaluated by dual photon absorptiometry of the

spine and of the total skeleton should be performed to clarify this issue.

Urinary Hydroxyproline in Osteoporosis

The mean value of urinary total hydroxyproline has been found to be normal in most studies (4,31,69,114) as is the case with most biochemical parameters in postmenopausal osteoporosis. However, analysis of individual values show that up to 30% of the patients can have values above the normal range (31). Increased urinary hydroxyproline appears to be more frequent in patients with increased serum immunoreactive parathyroid hormone (46), a small subset of osteoporotic patients with increased bone turnover (111). There are few studies correlating urinary hydroxyproline with more direct measurements of bone resorption (i.e., calcium kinetics and bone histomorphometry) in osteoporosis. In a small and heterogenous group of osteoporotic patients, Klein et al. (52) found a good correlation between urinary hydroxyproline and calcium resorption rate before and after treatment with calcium and/or steroids. In 34 untreated women with postmenopausal osteoporosis, all of them having crush fractures, Gallagher et al. (69) reported a linear correlation (r = 0.59, (p < 0.001) between urinary hydroxyproline and bone resorption rate calculated from the difference between the mineralization rate and the calcium balance. The linear correlations calculated from the individual values of 15 untreated osteoporotic women reported by Lauffenburger et al. (58) indicate that urinary hydroxyproline is correlated with kinetically determined bone resorption (r = 0.77) but also with calcium accretion (r = 0.82). In contrast, urinary hydroxyproline was negatively correlated with both the osteoclast count (r = − 0.22, NS) and the trabecular resorption surfaces (r = − 0.53, p < 0.05) on iliac crest biopsies (58). White et al. (113) found in 26 untreated osteoporotic patients that urinary hydroxyproline was negatively correlated with the osteoclastic resorption surface (r = − 0.40, p < 0.05) but not with the osteoclast count (r = − 0.11) or the total resorption surfaces (r = − 0.17). Furthermore, hydroxyproline excretion was not different in 15 patients with histologically defined active osteoporosis and in 5 patients with inactive osteoporosis (21.9 ± 1.8 mg/g creatinine vs 25.6 ± 7.0 mg/g creatinine, respectively, NS). When comparing urinary excretion of hydroxyproline with bone resorption measured on trabecular bone of iliac biopsy in 33 untreated patients with postmenopausal osteoporosis, we could not find any significant correlation. The fact that hydroxyproline excretion seems to correlate reasonably well with bone resorption of the skeleton determined by calcium kinetics but not with bone resorption of the trabecular envelope determined by histomorphometry, needs to be explained. Bone histomorphometry is hindered by the lack of an accurate technique measuring bone resorption and this might explain part of the discrepancy. Also, trabecular bone resorption may not be representative of total bone resorption. Cortical bone represents 80% of the entire skeleton and bone resorption of the subcortical endosteal envelope appears to increase with aging (116) and to be more active than trabecular resorption in patients with osteoporosis (111,114).

Other Markers of Bone Resorption

Urinary Hydroxylysine Glycoside

Hydroxylysine is another aminoacid unique to collagen and proteins containing collagen-like sequences. Like hydroxyproline, hydroxylysine is not reutilized for collagen biosynthesis and although it is much less abundant than hydroxyproline, it is a potential marker of collagen degradation. Hydroxylysine is present in part as galactosylhydroxylysine and in part as glucosylgalactosylhydroxylysine. The relative proportion and total content of the two glycosylated hydroxylysines are different for different collagens, and their ratio is markedly different in bone and skin (79). Hydroxylysine glycosides are excreted in urine and they seem to be less metabolized than hydroxyproline

(11,99). For these reasons, the ratio of glucosylgalactosylhydroxylysine to galactosylhydroxylysine excretion in urine might be a sensitive marker of collagen degradation and could provide information about the origin of the collagen breakdown. Consistent data have been obtained in patients with Paget's disease of bone before and after treatment with antiresorptive agents (55) but no data are available in osteoporosis. Hydroxylysine glycosides determination require an automatic amino acid analyser which limits the use of this measurement.

Plasma Tartrate-Resistant Acid Phosphatase

Acid phosphatase is an enzyme whose chemical role is similar to that of alkaline phosphatase, but it functions at a lower pH. Acid phosphatase is a lysosomal enzyme that is mainly present in bone, prostate, platelets, erythrocytes and the spleen. These different isoenzymes can be separated by electrophoretic methods which lack sensitivity and specificity. The bone acid phosphatase is resistant to L (+)-tartrate, whereas the prostatic isoenzyme is inhibited, a pattern which is used for the diagnosis of prostatic cancer (59). Acid phosphatase circulates in blood in much lower concentrations than alkaline phosphatases, with higher activity in serum than in plasma because of the release of platelet phosphatase activity during the clotting process.

In normal plasma, tartrate-resistant acid phosphatase corresponds to plasma isoenzyme 5 which may originate from bone. Osteoclasts contain a tartrate-resistant acid phosphatase which is released into the circulation (67) and that probably accounts for the high plasma levels found in Paget's disease of bone. In 46 patients with primary hyperparathyroidism, Stepan et al. (107) found increased levels of tartrate-resistant acid phosphatase, with a mean 5-fold increase above the normal mean. Individual values were correlated with urinary hydroxyproline and with serum immunoreactive parathyroid hormone. Unfortunately, no data are available on measurements of plasma tartrate–resistant acid phosphatase in osteoporosis. The development in the future of radio-immunoassays using antisera or monoclonal antibodies specifically directed against the bone isoenzyme should be valuable to assess the ability of plasma acid phosphatase to predict osteoclastic bone resorption in osteoporosis.

CONCLUSIONS

There is not yet an ideal marker of bone formation but circulating osteocalcin is the most satisfactory at the present time. Serum level of the carboxyterminal extension of procollagen I should be a valuable marker but needs to be validated in osteoporosis. The identification of new bone-specific proteins will lead in the near future to the development of a battery of radio-immunoassays. The circulating levels of these proteins are likely to reflect different events of bone metabolism at the cell and the tissue level and should shed new light on the mechanisms of bone remodeling. Because of its hydroxyapatite and collagen-binding properties, and because its concentration is decreased in the bone of calves affected with a variety of osteogenesis imperfecta (See Chapter 6, 7, *this volume*), osteonectin is an interesting potential marker of bone metabolism in osteoporosis. Using a polyclonal antiserum raised against purified bovine osteonectin, we have developed a radioimmunoassay for human osteonectin and we have shown that osteonectin is present in the serum (62). The recent demonstration that human platelets contain significant amounts of osteonectin that are secreted during thrombin stimulation, thus contributing largely to the levels detected in serum (105), indicate that one should be cautious in interpreting circulating levels of a given bone protein.

Available markers of bone resorption are not satisfactory. An ideal marker would be a bone specific matrix constituent released into the circulation during resorption without being degraded by the osteoclasts. Unfortunately, what we know about bone collagen metabolism suggests that most, if not all, bone matrix constituants released during osteoclastic resorption may be degraded into small fragments. Another alternative is to measure an enzyme that would be specific for the osteoclasts, released into the circulation at a rate proportional to their activity and measurable in serum with a specific assay. The future development of monoclonal antibodies to the bone acid phosphatase and to other osteoclast-specific enzymes may allow osteoclast function to be estimated indirectly.

Bone histomorphometry is a valuable tool to validate new biochemical markers but it should be remembered that both techniques reflect bone metabolism at a different level. Circulating markers reflect the osteoblastic (or the osteoclastic) activity of the whole skeleton and depend both on the number and on the activity of bone cells. Conversely, bone histomorphometry has been usually limited to trabecular bone remodeling measured on a limited area of the ilium. Thus, the correlation between serum osteocalcin and bone formation can be improved by taking into account both the trabecular and the subcortical endosteal envelopes, which may have different remodeling rates. Moreover, if bone loss in osteoporosis results from the combination of increased bone resorption at the subcortical endosteal surface and decreased bone formation at the trabecular level, circulating markers might be normal as they reflect the summated turnover of all the skeleton envelopes. Furthermore, circulating markers also take into account bone turnover of the appendicular, and mainly cortical, skeleton that may exhibit a turnover different from the axial skeleton (99). Another aspect to bear in mind when interpretating in vivo measurements of bone turnover is the differential effect of hormones and agents at the cell and at the tissue level.

For example, parathyroid hormone decreases collagen and osteocalcin synthesis by bone cells *in vitro* but hyperparathyroidism is associated with increased serum osteocalcin and urinary hydroxyproline because of the marked increase of bone cell recruitment, regardless of the individual cell activity.

The combination of available and new markers of bone remodeling along with bone histo-morphometry and radiocalcium kinetics should be able to refine the concept of heterogeneity of bone turnover in osteoporosis and to determine whether the prominent feature is related to bone formation, bone resorption, or both, according to the different skeletal envelopes.

Addendum: This chapter was written in November 1985 and is reflective of research to that date.

REFERENCES

1. Anderson, M.C., and Reynolds, J.J. (1973): Pyro-phosphate stimulation of calcium uptake into cultured embryonic bones. Fine structure of matrix vesicles and their role in calcification. *Devel. Biol.*, 34:211–215.
2. Beresford, J.N., Gallagher, J.A., Poser, J.W., and Russell, R.G.G. (1984): Production of human bone cells in vitro. Effects of 1.25(OH)$_2$D$_3$, 24, 25(OH)$_2$D$_3$, parathyroid hormone and glucocorticoids. *Metab. Bone Dis. Rel. Res.*, 5:229–234.
3. Birkett, D.J., Conyers, R.A.J., Neale, F.C., Posen, S., and Brudenell-Woods, J. (1967): Action of urea on human alkaline phosphatases with a description of some automated techniques for the study of enzyme kinetics. *Arch. Biochem. Biophys.*, 124:470–479.
4. Brown, J.P., Delmas, P.D., Malaval, L., Edouard, C., Chapuy, M.C., and Meunier, P.J. (1984): Serum bone Gla-Protein: A specific marker for bone formation in postmenopausal osteoporosis. *Lancet*, i, 1091–1093.
5. Brydon, W.G., Crofton, P.M., Smith, A.F., Barr, D.G.D., and Markness, R.A. (1975): Hypophosphatasia: Enzyme studies in cultured cells and tissues. *Biochem. Soc. Trans.* 3:927–929.
6. Catherwood, B.D., Marcus, R., Madvig, P., and Chelling, A.J. (1985): Determinants of bone gamma-carboxyglutamic acid-containing protein in plasma of healthy aging subjects. *Bone*, 6:9–13.
7. Clark, L.C., and Beck, E. (1950): Plasma alkaline phosphatase activity. I. Normative data for growing children. *J. Pediat.*, 36:335–343.
8. Clubb, J.S., Neale, F.C., and Posen, S. (1965): The behavior of infused placental alkaline phosphatase in human subjects. *J. Lab. Clin. Med.*, 66:493–507.
9. Crilly, R.G., Jones, M.M., Horsman, A., and Nordin, B.E.C. (1980): Rise in plasma alkaline phosphatase at the menopause. *Clin. Science*, 58:341–342.
10. Cundy, T., Bartlett, M., Bishop, M., Earnshaw, M., Smith, R., and Kanis, J.A. (1983): Plasma hydroxyproline in uremia: Relationship with histologic and biochemical indices of bone turnover. *Metab. Bone Dis. Rel. Res.*, 4:297–303.
11. Cunningham, L.W., Ford, J.D., and Segrest, J.P. (1967): The violation of identical hydroxylysyl gly-cosides from hydrolysates of soluble collagen and from human urine. *J. Biol. Chem.*, 242:2570–2571.
12. Deftos, L.J., Parthemore, J.G., and Price, P.A. (1982): Changes in plasma bone gla-protein during treatment of bone disease. *Calcif. Tissue Int.*, 34:121–124.
13. Delmas, P.D. (1984): The gla-containing protein of bone. In: *Marker Proteins in Inflammation*, edited by P. Arnaud, J. Bienvenu, and P. Laurent, Volume II, pp. 281–294. Walter de Gruyter, Berlin-New York.
14. Delmas, P.D. (1986): Bone gla-protein (osteocalcin): a specific marker for the study of metabolic bone diseases. In: *Fifth International Congress on Calciotropic Hormones and Calcium Metabolism*, edited by M. Cecchettin and G. Segre, pp. 19–28. ICS 679. Elsevier Science, Amsterdam.
15. Delmas, P.D., Casez, J.P., Boivin, G.Y., Chapuy, M.C., Valentin-Opran, A., Edouard, C., and Meunier, P.J. (1984): In: *Osteoporosis*, edited by C. Christiansen, C.D. Arnaud, B.E.C. Nordin, A.M. Parfitt, W.A. Peck, and B.L. Riggs, pp. 581–586. Aalborg Stiftsbogtrykkeri, Glostrup, Denmark.
16. Delmas, P.D., Demiaux, B., Malaval, L., Capuy, M.D., Edouard, C., and Meunier, P.J. (1986): Serum bone gla-protein (osteocalcin) in primary hyperparathyroidism and in malignant hypercalcemia. Comparison with bone histomorphometry. *J. Clin. Invest.*, 77:985–991.
17. Delmas, P.D., Demiaux, B., Malaval, L., Chapuy, M.C., and Meunier, P.J. (1986): Serum bone gla-protein is not a sensitive marker of bone turnover in Paget's disease of bone. *Calcif. Tissue Int.*, 38:60–61.
18. Delmas, P.D., Malaval, L., Arlot, M.D., and Meunier, P.J. (1985): Serum bone gla-protein compared to bone histomorphometry in endocrine diseases. *Bone*, 6:329–341.
19. Delmas, P.D., Stenner, D.D., Romberg, R.W., Riggs, B.L., and Mann, K.G. (1984): Immuno-chemical studies of conformational alterations in bone gla-containing protein. *Biochemistry*, 23:4720–4725.
20. Delmas, P.D., Stenner, D., Wahner, H.W., Mann, K.G., and Riggs, B.L. (1983): Serum bone gla protein increases with aging in normal women: implications for the mechanism of age-related bone loss. *J. Clin. Invest.*, 71:1316–1321.
21. Delmas, P.D., Tracy, R.P., Riggs, B.L., and Mann, K.G. (1984): Identification of the non collagenous proteins of bovine bone by two-dimensional gel electrophoresis. *Calcif. Tissue Int.*, 36:308–316.
22. Delmas, P.D., Wilson, D.M., Mann, K.G., and Riggs, B.L. (1983): Effect of renal function on plasma levels of bone gla-protein. *J. Clin. Endocrinol. Metab.*, 57:1028–1030.
23. Delmas, P.D., Wahner, H.W., Mann, K.G., and Riggs, B.L. (1983): Assessment of bone turnover in postmenopausal osteoporosis by measurement of serum bone gla-protein. *J. Lab. Clin. Med.*, 102:470–476.
24. Duda, R.J. Jr., Mann, K.G., and Riggs, B.L.

(1985) Abstract: Calcitriol stimulation test for osteoblast function. Results in postmenopausal osteoporosis. *Seventh Annual Metting, American Society for Bone and Mineral Research*, p. 129. Washington D.C., June 1985.

25. Epstein, S., Posen, J., Mc Clintock, R., Johnston, C.C. Jr., Bryce, G., and Hui, S. (1984): Differences in serum bone gla-protein with age and sex. *Lancet* i:307–310.

26. Farley, Jr., Chesnut, C.J., and Baylink, D.J. (1981): Improved method for quantitative determination in serum alkaline phosphatase of skeletal origin. *Clin. Chem.* 27:2002–2007.

27. Fishman, W., and Ghosh, N. (1967): Isoenzyme of human alkaline phosphatase. *Adv. Clin. Chem.* 10:255–267.

28. Fleish, H., Russell, R.G.G., and Strauman, F. (1966): Effects of pyrophosphate on hydroxyapatite and its implications in calcium homeostasis. *Nature*, 212:901–903.

29. Fogelman, I., Poser, J.W., Smith, M.L., Hart, D.M., and Bevan, J.A. (1984): Alterations in skeletal metabolism following oophorectomy. In: *Osteoporosis*. edited by C. Christiansen, C.C. Arnaud, B.E.C. Nordin, A.M. Parfitt, W.A. Peck, and B.L. Riggs, pp. 519–522. Aalborg Stiftsbogtrykkeri, Glostrup, Denmark.

30. Frost, H.M. (1963): Bone remodelling dynamics. C.C. Thomas, Springfield.

31. Gallagher, J.C., Aaron, J., Horsman, A., Marshall, D.H., Wilkinson, R., and Nordin, B.E.C. (1973): The crush fracture syndrome in postmenopausal women. *Clinic. Endocrinol. Metabol.* 2:293–305.

32. Gallagher, J.C., Young, M.M., and Nordin, B.E.C. (1972): Effects of artificial menopause on plasma and urine calcium and phosphate. *Clin. Endocrinol.*, 1:57–64.

33. Gallop, P.M., Lian, J.B., and Hauschka, P.V. (1980): Carboxylated calcium-binding proteins and vitamin K. *New Engl. J. Med.*, 302:1460–1466.

34. Gunberg, C.M., Cole, D.E.G., Lian, J.B., Reade, T.M., and Gallop, P.M. (1983): Serum osteocalcin in the treatment of inherited rickets with 1,25-dihydroxyvitamin D₃. *J. Clin. Endocrinol. Metab.*, 56:1063–1067.

35. Gunberg, C.M., Lian, J.B., and Gallop, P.M. (1983): Measurements of γ-carboxyglutamate and circulating osteocalcin in normal children and adults. *Clin. Chim. Acta*, 128:1–8.

36. Gunberg, C.M., Lian, J.M., Gallop, P.M., and Steinberg, J.J. (1983) Urinary γ-carboxyglutamic acid and serum osteocalcin as bone markers: studies in osteoporosis and Paget's disease. *J. Clin. Endocrinol. Metab.*, 57:1221–1225.

37. Gunberg, C.M., Wilson, P.S., Gallop, P.M., and Parfitt, A.M. (1985): Determination of osteocalcin in human serum: Results with two kits compared with those by a well-characterized assay. *Clin. Chem.*, 31:1720–1723.

38. Haddad, J.G., Courant, S., and Avioli, L.V. (1970): Non dialyzable urinary hydroxyproline as an index of bone collagen formation. *J. Clin. Endocrinol.*, 30:282–287.

39. Hauschka, P.V., and Carr, S.A. (1982): Calcium-dependent α-helical structure in osteocalcin. *Biochemistry*, 21:2538–2547.

40. Hauschka, P.V., Frankel, J., Demuth, R., and Gunberg, C.M. (1983): Presence of osteocalcin and related higher molecular weight 4-carboxyglutamic acid-containing proteins in developing bone. *J. Biol. Chem.*, 258:176–182.

41. Hauschka, P.V., Lian, J.B., and Gallop, P.M. (1975): Direct identification of the calcium-binding amino acid, γ-carboxyglutamate, in mineralized tissue. *Proc. Natl. Acad. Sci.* (USA), 72:3925–3929.

42. Hoogkinson, A., and Thompson, T. (1982): Measurement of the fasting urinary hydroxyproline: creatinine ratio in normal adults and its variations with age and sex. *J. Clin. Pathol.*, 35:807–811.

43. Hulth, A.G., Nilsson, B.E., and Westlin, N.E. (1979): Alkaline phosphatase in women with osteoporosis. *Acta Med. Scand.*, 206–201.

44. Hunsberger, A. Jr., and Furguson, L.K. (1932): Variations of phosphatase and inorganic phosphorus in serum during fracture repair. *Arch. Surg.*, 24:1052–1055.

45. Hyldstrup, L., Mc Nair, P., Jensen, G.F., Nielsen, H.R., and Transbol, I. (1984): Bone mass as referent for urinary hydroxyproline excretion: age and sex-related changes in 125 normals and in primary hyperparathyroidism. *Calcif. Tissue Int.*, 36:639–644.

46. Joly, R., Chapuy, M.C., and Alexandre, C., Meunier, P.J. (1980): Osteoporoses à haut niveau de remodelage et fonction parathyroïdienne. *Pathol. Biol.* 28:417–424.

47. Kay, H.D. (1930): Plasma phosphatase. The enzyme in disease, particularly in bone disease. Part. 2. *J. Biol. Chem.*, 89:249–256.

48. Keating, F.R., Jones, J.D., Elveback, L.R., and Randall, R.V. (1969): The relation of age and sex to distribution of value in healthy adults of serum calcium, inorganic phosphorus, magnesium, alkaline phosphatase, total proteins, albumin, and blood urea. *J. Lab. Clin. Med.*, 73:825–834.

49. Kivirikko, K.I. (1983): Excretion of urinary hydroxyproline peptide: in the assessment of bone collagen deposition and resorption. In: *Clinical Disorders of Bone and Mineral Metabolism*, edited by B. Frame and J.T. Potts, pp. 105–107. Excerpta Medica, Amsterdam.

50. Kivirikko, K.I., Laitinen, O., and Prockop, D.J. (1967): Modifications of a specific assay for hydroxyproline in urine. *Anal. Biochem.*, 17:249–255.

51. Kleerekoper, M., Horne, M., Cornish, C.J., and Posen, S. (1970): Serum alkaline phosphatase after fat ingestion. *Clin. Sci.*, 38:339–345.

52. Klein, L., Lafferty, F.W., Pearson, O.H., and Curtiss, P.J. (1964): Correlation of urinary hydroxyproline, serum alkaline phosphatase and skeletal calcium turnover. *Metabolism*, 13:272–284.

53. Klein, B., Read, P.A., and Babson, A.L. (1960): Rapid method for the quantitative determination of serum alkaline phosphatase. *Clin. Chem.*, 6:269–275.

54. Krabbe, S., Christiansen, C., Rodbro, P., and Transbol, I. (1980): Pubertal growth as reflected by simultaneous change in bone mineral content and

serum alkaline phosphatase. *Acta Pediatr. Scand.*, 69:49–52.

55. Krane, S.M., Kantrowith, F.G., Byrne, M., Pinnell, S.R., and Singer, F.R. (1977): Urinary excretion of hydroxylysine and its glycosides as an index of collagen degradation. *J. Clin. Invest.*, 59:819–827.

56. Krane, S.M., Munoz, A.J., and Harris, E.D. (1970): Urinary polypeptides related to collagen synthesis. *J. Clin. Invest.*, 49:716–729.

57. Langman, M.J.S., Leuthold, E., Robson, E.B., Harris, J., Luffman, J.E., and Harris, H. (1966): Influence of diet on the intestinal component of serum alkaline phosphatase in people of different ABO blood groups and secretor status. *Nature* (Lond.), 212:41–43.

58. Leuffenburger, T., Olah, A.J., Dambacher, M.A., Guncaga, J., Lentner, C., and Haas, H.G. (1977): Bone remodelling and calcium metabolism: A correlated histomorphometric, calcium kinetic and biochemical study in patients with osteoporosis and Paget's disease. *Metabolism*, 26:589–606.

59. Li, C.Y., Chuda, R.A., Lam, W.K.W., and Yam, L.T. (1973): Acid phosphatase in human plasma. *J. Lab. Clin. Med.*, 82:446–460.

60. Lian, J.B., and Friedman, P.A. (1978): The vitamin K. dependent synthesis of γ-carboxyglutamic acid by bone microsomes. *J. Biol. Chem.*, 253:6623–6626.

61. Lian, J.B., Tassinari, M., and Glowacki, J. (1984): Resorption of implanted bone prepared from normal and warfarin-treated rats. *J. Clin. Invest.*, 73:1223–1226.

62. Malaval, L., Delmas, P.D., and Meunier, P.J. (1985): Measurement of serum osteonectin by radioimmunoassay. *Seventh Annual Meeting, American Society for Bone and Mineral Research*, Washington D.C., June 1985.

63. Malluche, H.H., Faugere, M.C., Fanti, P., and Price, P.D. (1983): Bone gla-protein, a biochemical index of bone formation and mineralization in uremic patients. *Calcif. Tissue Int.*, 35:(Suppl.) A146.

64. Malone, J.D., Teitelbaum, S.L., Griffin, G.L., Senior, R.M., and Kahn, A.J. (1982): Recruitment of osteoclast precursors by purified bone matrix constituents. *J. Cell. Biol.*, 92:227–230.

65. Maltallen, C.C. (1970): Circadian rhythm of urinary total and free hydroxyproline excretion and its relation to creatinine ratio. *J. Lab. Clin. Med.*, 75:11–18.

66. McComb, R.B., Bowers, G.H., Jr., and Posen, S. (1979): *Alkaline Phosphatase*. Plenum Press, New York.

67. Minkin, C. (1982): Bone acid phosphatase: tartrate-resistant acid phosphatase as a marker of osteoclast function. *Calc. Tissue Int.*, 34:285–290.

68. Morgenstern, S., Kessler, G., Auerbach, J., Flor, R.V., and Klein, B. (1965): An automated p-nitrophenylphosphate serum alkaline phosphatase procedure for the auto-analyzer. *Clin. Chem.*, 11:876–888.

69. Moskowith, R.V., Klein, L., and Katz, D. (1965): Urinary hydroxyproline levels in an aged population. A study of non osteoporotic and osteoporotic patients. *Arthritis and Rheum.*, 8:61–68.

70. Moss, D.W. (1982): Alkaline phosphatase isoenzymes. *Clin. Chem.*, 28:2007–2016.

71. Moss, D.W., Campbell, D.M., Anagnostou-Kakaras, E., and King, E.J. (1961): Characterization of tissue alkaline phosphatases and their partial purification by starch-gel electrophoresis. *Biochem. J.*, 81:441–447.

72. Moss, D.V., and King, E.J. (1962): Properties of alkaline-phosphatase fractions separated by starch-gel electrophoresis. *Biochem. J.*, 84:192–195.

73. Nishimoto, S.K., and Price, P.A. (1980): Secretion of the vitamin K dependent protein of bone by rat osteosarcoma cells. *J. Biol. Chem.*, 255:6529–6583.

74. Nishimoto, S.K., and Price, P.A. (1979): Proof that the γ-carboxyglutamic acid-containing bone protein is synthesized in calf bone. *J. Biol. Chem.*, 254:437–441.

75. Nordin, B.E.C., Horsman, A., and Aaron, J. (1976): Diagnostic procedures. In: *Calcium, Phosphate and Magnesium Metabolism. Clinical Physiology and Diagnostic Procedures*, edited by B.E.C. Nordin, pp. 469–524. Churchill Livingstone, New York.

76. Parfitt, A.M., and Kleerekoper, M. (1984): Diagnostic value of bone histomorphometry and comparison of histologic measurements and biochemical indices of bone remodeling. In: *Osteoporosis*, edited by C. Christiansen, C.D. Arnaud, B.E.C. Nordin, A.M. Parfitt, W.A. Peck, and B.L. Riggs. pp. 111–120. Aalborg Stiftsbogtrykkeri, Glostrup, Denmark.

77. Patterson-Allen, P., Brautigam, C.E., Grindeland, R.E., Asling, C.W., and Callahan, P.X. (1982): A specific radioimmunoassay for osteocalcin with advantageous species crossreactivity. *Anal. Biochem.*, 120:1–7.

78. Peach, H., Compston, J.E., Vedi, S., and Horton, L.W.L. (1982): Value of plasma calcium, phosphate, and alkaline phosphatase measurements in the diagnosis of histological osteomalacia. *J. Clin. Pathol.*, 35:625–630.

79. Pinnell, S.R., Fox, R., and Krane, S.M. (1971): Human collagens: differences in glycosylated hydroxylysines in skin and bone. *Biochim. Biophys. Acta.*, 229:119–122.

80. Posen, S., Cornish, C., and Kleerekoper, M. (1977): Alkaline phosphatase and metabolic bone disorders. In: *Metabolic Bone Disease*, edited by L.V. Avioli, and S.M., Krane, pp. 141–181. Academic Press, New York.

81. Posen, S., and Grunstein, H.S. (1982): Turnover rates of skeletal alkaline phosphatase in human. *Clin. Chem.*, 28:153–154.

82. Poser, J.W., Esch, F.S., Ling, N.C., and Price, P.A. (1980): Isolation and sequence of the vitamin K-dependent protein from human bone. Undercarboxylation of the first glutamic acid residue. *J. Biol. Chem.*, 255:8685–8691.

83. Price, P. (1983): Osteocalcin. In: *Bone and Mineral Research*, edited by W.A. Peck, pp. 157–190. Excerpta Medica, Amsterdam.

84. Price, P.A., and Baukol, S.A. (1980): 1,25-dihydroxyvitamin D₃ increases synthesis of the vitamin K-dependent bone protein by osteosarcoma cells. *J. Biol. Chem.*, 255:11660–11663.

85. Price, P.A., and Nishimoto, S.K. (1980): Radioimmunoassay for the vitamin K-dependent protein of bone and its discovery in plasma. *Proc. Natl. Acad. Sci.* (U.S.A.), 77:2234–2238.

86. Price, P.A., Otsuka, A.S., Poser, J.W., Kristaponis, J., and Raman, N. (1976): Characterization of a γ-carboxyglutamic acid containing protein from bone. *Proc. Natl. Acad. Sci.* (U.S.A), 73:1447–1451.

87. Price, P.A., Parthemore, J.G., and Deftos, L.J. (1980): New biochemical marker for bone metabolism. *J. Clin. Invest.*, 66:878–883.

88. Price, P.A., Williamson, M.K., and Lothringer, J.W. (1981): Origin of the vitamin K-dependent bone protein found in plasma and its clearance by kidney and bone. *J. Biol. Chem.*, 256:12760–12766.

89. Prockop, O.J., Kivirikko, K.I. (1968): Hydroxyproline and the metabolism of collagen. In: *Treatise on Collagen*, Vol. 2, A.B.S., edited by B.S. Gould, pp. 215–246. Academic Press, New York.

90. Prockop, D.J., Kivirikko, K.I., Tuderman, K., and Guzman, N.A. (1979): The biosynthesis of collagen and its disorders. *N. Engl. J. Med.*, 301:13–23.

91. Rasmussen, H. (1983): Hypophosphatasia. In: *Metabolic Basis of Inherited Disease, 5th ed.*, edited by J.B. Stanbury, J.B. Wyngaarden, D.S. Fredrickson, J.L. Goldstein, M.S. Brown, pp. 1497–1507. McGraw-Hill Book Company, New York.

92. Riggs, B.L., Tsai, K.S., and Mann, K.G. (1984): Evidence that serum bone gla-protein is a measure of bone formation but not of bone resorption. *Calcif. Tissue Int.*, 36:497. (Abstr.)

93. Roberts, W.M. (1930): Variations in the phosphatase activity of the blood in disease. *Br. J. Exp. Pathol.*, 11:90–95.

94. Robinson, R. (1932): *The Significance of Phosphoric Esters in Metabolism*. New York University Press, New York.

95. Saleh, A.E.C., and Coenegrach, T. (1968): The influence of age and weight on the urinary excretion of hydroxyproline and calcium. *Clin. Chim. Acta.*, 21:445–452.

96. Schiele, F., Henny, J., Hitz, J., Petitclerc, C., Gueguen, R., and Siest, G. (1983): Total bone and liver alkaline phosphatase in plasma: biological variations and reference limits. *Clin. Chem.*, 29:634–641.

97. Seargeant, L.E., and Stinson, R.A. (1979): Evidence that three structural genes code for human alkaline phosphatases. *Nature* (Lond.), 281:152–154.

98. Seeman, E., Wahner, H.W., Offord, K.P., Kumar, R., Johnson, W.J., and Riggs, B.L. (1982): Differential effects of endocrine dysfunction on the axial and the appendicular skeleton. *J. Clin. Invest.*, 69:1302–1309.

99. Segrest, J.P., and Cunningham, L.W. (1970): Variations in human urinary O-hydroxylysyl glycoside levels and their relationship to collagen metab-

olism. *J. Clin. Invest.*, 49:1497–1509.

100. Shifrin, L.Z. (1970): Correlations of serum alkaline phosphatase with bone formation rates. *Clin. Orthop. Rel. Res.*, 70:212–215.

101. Simon, L.S., Krane, S.M., Wortman, P.D., Krane, L.M., and Kovitz, K.L. (1984): Serum levels of type I and III procollagen fragments in Paget's disease of bone. *J. Clin. Endocrinol. Metab.*, 58:110–120.

102. Simon, L.S., and Krane, S.M.K. (1983): Procollagen extension peptides as markers of collagen synthesis. In: *Clinical Disorders of Bone and Mineral Metabolism*, edited by B. Frame and J.T. Potts Jr., pp. 108–111. Excerpta Medica, Amsterdam.

103. Simon, L.S., Parfitt, A.M., Villanueva, A.R., and Krane, S.M. (1984): Procollagen type I carboxy terminal extension peptide (p Coll-I-C) in serum as a marker of collagen synthesis: correlation with iliac trabecular bone formation rate. *Calcif. Tissue Int.*, 36:498. (Abstr.)

104. Slovik, D.M., Gundberg, C.M., Neer, R.M., and Lian, J.B. (1984): Clinical evaluation of bone turnover by serum osteocalcin measurements in a hospital setting. *J. Clin. Endocrinol. Metab.*, 59:228–230.

105. Stenner, D.D., Tracy, R.P., Riggs, B.L., and Mann, K.G. (1987): Human platelets contain and secrete osteonectin, a major protein of mineralized bone. *Proc. Natl. Acad. Sci.* (U.S.A.), (in press).

106. Stepan, J., Pacovsky, V., Horn, V., Silinkova-Malkova, E., Vokrouhlicka, O., Konopasek, B., Formankova, J., Hrba, J., and Marek, J. (1978): Relationship of the activity of the bone isoenzyme of serum alkaline phosphatase to urinary hydroxyproline excretion in metabolic and neoplastic diseases. *Eur. J. Clin. Invest.*, 8:373–377.

107. Stepan, J.J., Silinkova-Malkova, E., Havrenek, T., Formankova, J., Zicmova, M., Lacmmanova, J., Strakova, M., Broulik, P., and Pacovsky, V. (1983): Relationship of plasma tartrate resistant acid phosphatase to the bone isoenzyme of serum alkaline phosphatase in hyperparathyroidism. *Clin. Chim. Acta*, 133:189–200.

108. Stock, J.L., Coderre, J.A., and Mallette, L.E. (1985): Effects of a short course of estrogen on mineral metabolism in postmenopausal women. *J. Clin. Endocrinol. Metab.*, 61:595–600.

109. Taubman, M.B., Goldberg, B., and Smerr, C.J. (1974): Radioimmunoassay for human procollagen, *Science*, 186:1115–1118.

110. Taubman, M.B., Kammerman, S., and Goldberg, B. (1976): Radioimmunoassay of procollagen in serum of patients with Paget's disease of bone. *Proc. Soc. Exp. Biol. Med.*, 152:284–290.

111. Teitelbaum, S.L., Rosenberg, E.M., Richardson, C.A., and Avioli, L. (1976): Histological studies of bone from normocalcemic postmenopausal osteoporotic patients with increased circulating parathyroid hormone. *J. Clin. Endocrin. Metab.*, 42:537–543.

112. Termine, J.D., Belcourt, A.B., Conn, K.M., and Kleinman, H.K. (1981): Mineral and collagen-binding proteins of fetal calf bone. *J. Biol. Chem.*, 256:10403–10408.

113. Walton, R.J., Preston, C.J., Russell, R.G.G., and Kanis, J.A. (1975): An estimate of the turnover rate of bone-derived plasma alkaline phosphatase in Paget's disease. *Clin. Chim. Acta.*, 63:227–229.

114. White, M.P., Bergfeld, M.A., Murphy, W.A., Avioli, L.V., and Teitelbaum. S.L. (1982): Postmenopausal osteoporosis. A heterogenous disorder as assessed by histomorphometric analysis of iliac crest bone from untreated patients. *Amer. J. Med.*, 72:193–202.

115. Williams, C.B., and Windsor, A.C.M. (1971): The use of the hydroxyproline-creatinine ratio in elderly patients. *Geront. Clin.*, 13:277–284.

116. Wu, K., Jett, S., and Frost, H.M. (1967): Bone resorption rates in rib in physiological, senile and postmenopausal osteoporosis. *J. Lab. Clin. Med.*, 69:810–818.

117. Zerwekh, J.E., Sakhaee, K., and Cyc, P.A.K. (1985): Short-term 1,25 dihydroxyvitamin D_3 administration raises serum osteocalcin in patients with postmenopausal osteoporosis. *J. Clin. Endocrinol. Metab.*, 60:615–617.

Osteoporosis: Etiology, Diagnosis, and
Management, edited by B. Lawrence Riggs and
L. Joseph Melton, III. Raven Press, New York
© 1988.

11

Assessment of Bone Turnover by Histomorphometry in Osteoporosis

Pierre J. Meunier

INSERM Unit 234, Faculté Alexis Carrel, 69008 Lyon, France

Osteoporosis can be anatomically defined as a rarefaction of calcified bone tissue within the periosteal envelope of bones to such a degree that the skeleton is then unable to sustain body weight. The fracture threshold is reached and nontraumatic vertebral collapses and/or long bone fractures occur. This definition suggests that in osteoporosis the first information needed is an estimate of the amount of bone in the patient's body. Noninvasive methods of measurement of the bone mineral content are able to provide this information from different sites of the skeleton.

The pathophysiologic mechanism underlying the bone loss in the osteoporotic is characterized by an abnormal accentuation of the physiologic disequilibrium between bone resorption and bone formation that normally leads to age-related osteopenia. Although it might seem that all osteoporotic status should result from the same kinds of imbalance, the osteoporotic syndrome is characterized by anatomic and histopathogenetic heterogeneity, with different disturbances in bone remodeling, at the organ, tissue, and cell levels, leading to the same clinical syndrome. Neither noninvasive methods of measurement of bone density, nor the evaluation of circulating markers of bone turnover are able to evaluate the disturbances in bone remodeling capable of inducing the negative

bone tissue balance responsible for osteoporosis. In contrast, *bone histomorphometry* is the only method which gives access to a direct and precise analysis of the static and dynamic cellular and tissue abnormalities and in particular to the measurements made at the intermediary level of organization of bone, i.e., the osteon in cortical bone and the trabecular basic structural unit (see Chapter 2, *this volume*).

In the last two decades, the field of bone histomorphometry has markedly progressed and now serves two main needs in osteoporotic states: the diagnosis of bone disease and research devoted to achieving a better understanding of the pathophysiology of osteoporosis and of the evaluation of histologic effects of its new therapeutic approaches. The tetracycline double-labelling procedure which has permitted the introduction of the dimension of time into the quantitative analysis has markedly contributed to the recent advances in this field. In addition, the quantal concept of bone remodeling, detailed in Chapter 2, fully justifies the quantitative approach permitted by bone histomorphometry.

METHODOLOGY

Bone histomorphometry demands strict methodologic conditions, because an unequivocal qualitative identification and description of the parameter to be measured is pivotal to any quantitative analysis. Thus bone biopsy techniques yielding a well-preserved tissue sample and histologic methods allowing discretely measured variables are two prerequisites for an accurate bone histomorphometry in osteoporotic states.

Bone Biopsy

Iliac biopsy is now universally used. It requires local anesthesia not only of external but also of the internal periosteum, and a 1 cm long skin and muscle incision. It creates minimal pain, provides a large area of spongy bone, and is safe. The results of a multicenter survey on the side effects of 14,810 iliac biopsies have been reported by Duncan (12). Nine thousand and thirty were obtained by the transiliac horizontal approach through the iliac crest. An overall incidence of complications of 0.52% was found. The most common problems were hematomas (0.24%), pain for 7 or more days (0.11%), femoral neuropathy (0.09%), and skin infection (0.07%). The first condition for a valid analysis of iliac bone biopsy in osteoporosis is to get a complete, noncompressed and unbroken core. The risk of having a poor sample is doubled when the operator is inexperienced (12):16.7% of poor biopsies in the latter case against only 8.8% in experienced hands.

In the iliac bone, the bone biopsy may be obtained either by a vertical approach, as described first by Sacker and Nordin (42), or by a *horizontal* transiliac method, as described by Bordier et al. (2). The latter method gives a sample with cortex at both ends which is a representative volume of iliac bone in its entirety, i.e., as an organ, and permits the measurement of trabecular and cortical parameters as well as of the total bone density (4) or core volume, expressed in percent (Fig. 1). The transiliac biopsy is taken from an area situated 2 cm behind the anterosuperior iliac spine and 2 cm below the summit of the iliac crest.

Jowsey has shown that a trephine having a 5 mm inner diameter was responsible for a large sampling variation in measurements on microradiographs of parameters reflecting the amount of bone (16), and Jameshidi's needle, because of its small size, is not recommended for the histomorphometric analysis of biopsies taken in osteoporotic patients.

Preparation of Bone Sections

It is essential that bone cores be processed without prior decalcification. The most used fixatives are 70% ethanol, absolute methanol or 10% formalin at pH 7.0. Formalin, however, causes more fading of the tetracycline labels than alcoholic fixatives do. Embedding bone samples in plastic monomers provides blocks of the same hardness as the bone, and methylmetacrylate is the most convenient plastic. Nonconsecutive serial sections, 4 to 20 μm thick, are cut with specially designed microtomes with carbide-edged, diamond or glass knives. Some laboratories dissolve the plastic before staining, while others do not in order to preserve the architecture of the sections, particularly fragile in osteoporosis.

The only prerequisite in the staining procedure is to use a method that allows an unequivocal identification of osteoid and bone cells. In our hands, solochrome cyanin R, in 1% aqueous solution, is a reliable osteoid stain, having the same discriminant capacity as Von Kossa's process which is classically recognized as the reference method (28). Solochrome cyanin is also very convenient for measuring bone volume parameters by using automated image-analyzing computers, because it produces a clear contrast between dark-stained calcified bone tissue and almost unstained marrow spaces or Haversian canals. In contrast, the widely used Goldner's process underestimates both osteoid volume and osteoid surfaces (18,28), but is excellent for evaluating resorption parameters giving a good discrimination of osteoclasts and of resorption cavities. Toluidine blue offers a good visualization of osteoblastic cells and has been shown by Bordier and Tun Chot (3) to be useful for the determi-

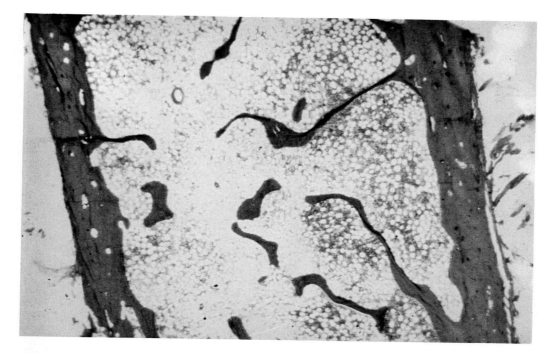

FIG. 1. Section of an undecalcified transiliac specimen in a case of trabecular osteoporosis with a marked atrophy of spongy bone. Stain: Goldner's method, 12x.

nation of the calcification front, that appears as a granular metachromatic dark line at the osteoid calcified bone interface and indicates an active mineralization process. Unfortunately, the reproducibility of this calcification front is rather poor, and the measurement of the front's extent does not disclose the osteoid calcification rate or the osteoid appositional rate which can be obtained only from the tetracycline multiple-labelling method (3).

This analysis of tetracycline double-labelling is possible in osteoporotic patients, as a routine procedure, on unstained bone sections. A convenient labelling protocol to use prior to transiliac biopsy consists of giving about 10 mg/kg/day of demethylchlortetracycline (DMC) or tetracycline hydrochloride (THC) orally for 2 days, no medication for 10 to 12 days, and DMC or THC again for 2 or 4 days. The bone biopsy must be taken not before 2 days after the end of the second labelling period (Fig. 2).

Measurements and Histomorphometric Parameters

The manual point-counting method or image-analyzing computers may be used for histologic measurements that must be performed on several nonconsecutive sections of the bone core (16 in our laboratory) and not on only one single section because of the intersection variation. The point-counting method consists of projecting integrating grids over the section of bone biopsy. The percentage of hits overlying a structure or the number of intersections between the grid and the bone perimeters are accurate estimates of the volumetric or surface density of the analyzed component (43). This method, requiring analysis of a large number of fields, is tedious and time-consuming.

Methods using fully automated or semi-automated image-analyzing computers (27) considerably reduce analysis time. The fully automated devices include a TV camera and the

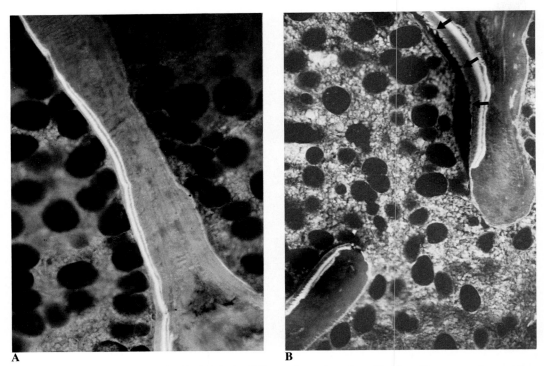

FIG. 2.   A, B. Tetracycline double-labels in different formation sites. **B:** The silhouettes of osteoblasts (*arrows*) lining the osteoid seam are visible (unstained undecalcified bone under fluorescence).

projection of the histologic image on a screen where the different components are measured according to their levels of gray. They are well-suited to the measurement of bone volume or density, but not for the evaluation of remodeling surfaces or dynamic parameters that have to be identified qualitatively before their quantitation. These computers are unable to recognize sectioning or staining artifacts.

Semi-automated image analyzers (21) combine the advantages of discriminatory input by an investigator with reduced evaluation time stemming from computer analysis and calculations. The image of a luminous cursor moved on a digitizing table is projected in the optical system of a microscope equipped with a drawing tube. The operator chooses and traces all histologic details to be quantified by moving the cursor on the platen (Fig. 3).

Static Parameters Expressing the Amount of Bone

Trabecular bone volume (Tb/BV, %), or volumetric density of trabecular bone, which is the percentage of bone tissue present between the two subcortical envelopes. This parameter includes calcified bone and osteoid. It is measurable either by point-counting or with a fully automated image-analyzing computer. The intraobserver and interobserver errors, both expressed by the intrapair coefficient of variation

$$CV = \frac{\sqrt{\sum \frac{d2}{2n}}}{M} \times 100$$

in which *d* is the difference between two measurements, *n* is the number of biopsies

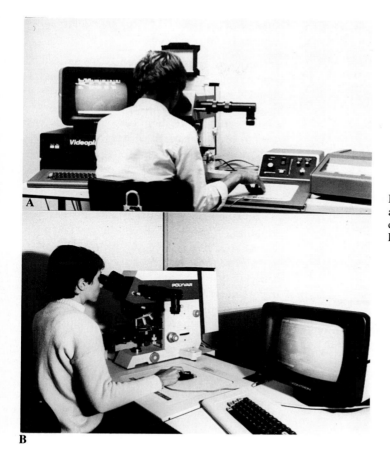

FIG. 3. Semiautomated image analyzing computers including a digitizing tablet. **A:** Videoplan. **B:** IBAS 1.

and M the overall mean value of the mean of two measurements, are respectively 1.8 and 2.1% with the computerized method and 2.0 and 2.2% with the manual measurement method of trabecular bone volume (6). In 38 biopsies from 19 osteoporotic patients, all having at least one vertebral collapse, the intrapair CV between parameter values obtained with both the manual point-counting method and the computerized method (Quantimet 720) was 7.4%. A highly significant correlation between manual and automatic method was found (r = 0.95, p < 0.001). Other authors who compared manual and automatic methods found a significant correlation (11) and a low variation (20) between both methods. The automatic method is preferable for Tb/BV measurements because it is the fastest one. In order to evaluate the intersample variation for Tb/BV in osteoporosis, Chavassieux in our laboratory (7) has analyzed two complete contiguous transiliac bone biopsies in 19 osteoporotic patients. The intrapair coefficient of variation (CV) was 13.4% and the confidence interval for one subject was 29%, but only 10% for a group of 10 osteoporosis and 7% for a group of 20 patients. Thus, if two successive iliac biopsies are taken in one patient or in one group of patients, the value of Tb/BV on the second biopsy must be out of the above ranges to say that the second biopsy significantly differs from the first one at a risk of 5%. The minimum detectable difference in groups of 10 or 20 patients is lower in osteoporosis than in controls (11).

These variations were much more important if one of the iliac biopsies was taken at more than 1.5 cm from the recommended site (1,24). These differences seem to be in relation to the architectural organization of trabeculae, iliac crest not being perfectly anisotropic (46). In addition, one single thick trabecula can widely modify Tb/BV value (46).

Total bone density or core volume (Tt/CV, %) represents the percentage of the total volume of the bone as an organ, occupied by bone matrix, from periosteum to periosteum, thus including cortices and spongy bone (9,4).

Mean thickness of the iliac cortices (Ct.Th, μm), is easy to measure on internal and external cortices.

Main Bone Formation Parameters

Trabecular osteoid volume (Tb/OV, %), represents the fraction of bone tissue within subcortical envelopes occupied by osteoid.

Trabecular osteoid surfaces (Tb/OS, %) is the percentage of total trabecular surfaces covered with osteoid.

Trabecular osteoid thickness (Tb/O.Th, μm) can be measured directly with a micrometer or a semiautomated image analyzer. The direct measurement can be replaced by calculation of the osteoid seam thickness index (TIOS), which is the ratio Tb/OV ÷ Tb/OS × 100 (28), and in metabolic bone disease is closely correlated with the true osteoid seam width (27).

Calcification rate or mineral apposition rate (MAr, μ/day) is the rate of progression of the calcification front labelled twice by tetracycline (13).

Main Bone Resorption Parameters

Trabecular resorption surfaces or eroded surfaces (Tb/ES, %) are the percentage of total trabecular surfaces created, i.e., where osteoclastic resorption is continuing or where resorption has ceased but where the osteoblasts have not yet started to refill Howship's lucunae.

Number of osteoclasts (N Oc) per square millimeter of bone section.

The above parameters (reflecting trabecular bone remodeling) are those used most often for clinical histomorphometry of osteoporosis for a diagnostic purpose. The intermethod and intersample variations of these parameters in osteoporosis are summarized in Table 1 (6,7), expressed as the intrapair coefficients of variation. The confidence intervals for each parameter in a single patient and groups of 10 and 20 osteoporotics are also shown in this table and define the limits of the intersample variation, in case of a second biopsy taken after therapy. For osteoid parameters, there are large variations for one patient and groups, particularly for osteoid volume. They are less important for trabecular resorption surfaces and in osteoporosis the variation for this parameter is lower than those previously published in controls (11,22,25).

Parameter Measured at the Basic Structure Unit Level: Wall Thickness of Trabecular Packet

This completed bone packet is bound on one side by the bone/marrow interface, and on the other by the scalloped cement line which represents the limits of the preceding resorption phase. The average distance between this cement line and the surface of the completed packet is the wall thickness (W.Th., μm) which is measured under polarized light (Fig. 4). This parameter provides a direct indication of the amount of bone formed during the osteoblastic phase of the basic multicellular unit.

BONE HISTOMORPHOMETRIC FINDINGS IN OSTEOPOROSIS

Histomorphometric findings are the basis of diagnosis value of bone biopsy in osteoporosis, of the demonstration of the histologic heterogeneity of osteoporotic syndromes, and of the value of bone histomorphometry as a research tool for the evaluation of curative treatments in osteoporosis as a disease. These data should be

TABLE 1. *Intermethod and intersample variations of parameters reflecting trabecular remodeling (19 osteoporotic patients). Interval confidence for 1,10 and 20 patients defining the limits of the intersample variation*

	Intermethod variation[a]	Intersample variation[b]			
	Intrapair coefficient of variation (%)	Intrapair coefficient of variation (%)	Interval confidence (%)		
			n:1	n:10	n:20
Trabecular osteoid volume (Tb/OV, %)	33.9	36.5	79	27	19
Trabecular osteoid surfaces (Tb/OS, %)	20.4	19.8	42	14	10
Thickness index of osteoid seams (TIOS)	20.1	22.3	46	16	11
Trabecular resorption surfaces (Tb/ES, %)	19.1	16.0	28	10	7
Mineral appositional rate (MAr, /μm/day)	nm[c]	7.0	nm[c]	nm[c]	nm[c]

[a]Manual point-counting method versus semi automatic method (Videoplan).
[b]Between two contiguous transiliac biopsies.
[c]nm, nonmeasured.

interpreted as a function of the age-related changes in bone mass and bone remodeling.

Age-related Changes in Bone Mass and Bone Remodeling

Age-related bone loss is universal, and histomorphometric studies in control subjects have clearly shown that decrease in trabecular bone volume is a phenomenon that occurs with age (8). Tb/BV decrease varies in men and women not only in magnitude, but also in its pattern, with a transient accelerated phase that occurs in women after menopause (32). There is, however, in females a significant trabecular bone loss before menopause (23). The acceleration of bone turnover responsible for the postmenopausal bone loss has been described in detail in Chapter 2. The mean wall thickness of the trabecular basic structure units decreases significantly with age (17), but mineral apposition rate and osteoid apposition rate, identical in control subjects, are constant with age (24,33). The mean "lifespan" of the active osteoblast population in a remodeling focus, or formation period, can be calculated by dividing W. Th., expressed in microns, by the osteoid apposition rate (OAr), expressed in μ/day. Since wall thickness decreases with age

whereas OAr is constant, it can be deduced that the formation period, i.e., the duration of activity of differentiated osteoblasts, *decreases with age* in normal subjects. This change seems to be a fundamental characteristic of bone ageing. The age-related decrease of wall thickness suggests that, with increasing age, the osteoblast population becomes progressively less able to reconstitute previously resorbed bone, leading to a net decrease of bone formation, i.e., a bone formation deficit in the individual bone remodeling units (BRU). Any increase in BRU birthrate will multiply these individual deficits and will accelerate bone loss (36). Thus, any hyperremodeling due to an increased activation frequency of the basic multicellular unit magnifies the bone tissue imbalance at the organ-level. Thyrotoxicosis (26) and primary or secondary hyperparathyroidism (31), as well as the high remodeling subset of idiopathic or postmenopausal osteoporosis are associated with such a disorder.

Bone Histomorphometry and Diagnosis of Trabecular Osteoporosis with Crush Fracture

For osteoporotic patients suffering from a crush fracture syndrome due to a primary os-

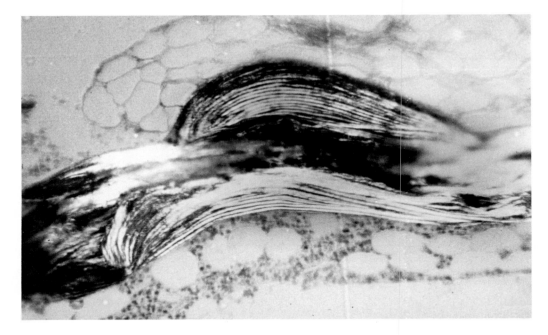

FIG. 4.   Trabecular packets (TP) in polarized light. Undecalcified bone. Stain Solochrome cyanin R. 400x.

teoporosis, the most discriminative parameter between these patients and age- and sex-matched controls is Tb/BV, because Tb/BV differs to a greater degree than Tt/CV between controls and osteoporotics (4). This is not surprising since the vertebral bodies are more than 90% spongy bone.

When 154 patients (106 females and 48 males), suffering from apparently idiopathic osteoporosis with at least one crushed vertebra were compared to 285 autopsied control subjects who suffered violent deaths, the individual values for Tb/BV were found to overlap the area of the mean control values (± one standard deviation) in 17% of males and 22% of females (29). None of the clinically diagnosed osteoporotics had a Tb/BV higher than 16% (Fig. 5). These data show the limited validity of measurements of Tb/BV for the diagnosis of trabecular osteoporosis in an individual patient.

The mean value for Tb/BV, computed in both sexes for each 10-year division of age in the osteoporotic population, are very similar (Table 2). This demonstrates at the same time the homogeneity of the group in terms of trabecular rarefaction and the validity of the fracture threshold concept, because at any age, in both sexes, the critical amount of trabecular bone is about the same. The vertebral fracture risk seems to appear for a Tb/BV of 16% and to increase when Tb/BV decreases from 16 to about 10%. Below this figure the vertebral collapses seem to be unavoidable.

Histomorphometric analysis of bone biopsy is used in another important way in the diagnosis of an osteoporotic syndrome with vertebral fractures: to expressly exclude *osteomalacia*. This exclusion of osteomalacia is important in cases in which the biochemical signs of the disease are uncertain. In 8 of 162 patients (5%) with a typical crush fracture syndrome and normal serum calcium, phosphorus and alkaline phosphatase levels, we found clearcut histologic signs of osteomalacia, including abnormally thick osteoid seams and a low mineral apposition rate. When we considered separately the calcified bone volume in 39 females with osteomalacia, by substracting the osteoid

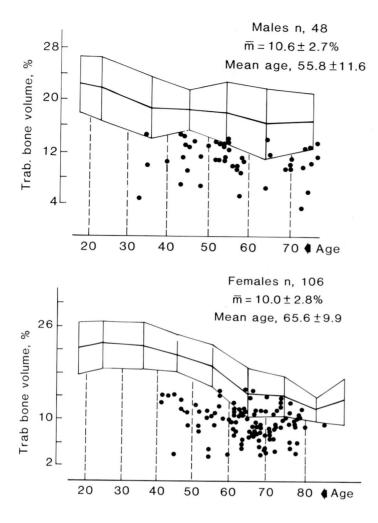

Males n, 48
$\bar{m} = 10.6 \pm 2.7\%$
Mean age, 55.8 ± 11.6

Females n, 106
$\bar{m} = 10.0 \pm 2.8\%$
Mean age, 65.6 ± 9.9

FIG. 5. A, B. Individual values of iliac trabecular bone volume (Tb/TV) in 154 osteoporotic patients, (**A**:48 males; **B**:106 females) all having at least one crushed vertebra, compared to mean values of Tb/BV in 285 autopsied controls. (176 males and 109 females).

volume from the total trabecular bone volume, we found 25 patients with a reduced calcified bone volume, which explains why crushed vertebrae in osteomalacia are not rare (30).

Bone Histomorphometry and Heterogeneity of Fracture Syndromes

Bone histomorphometry has permitted the demonstration of a double heterogeneity in osteoporotic states: an anatomic heterogeneity between osteoporosis with vertebral crush fractures and osteoporosis responsible for hip fractures, and a heterogeneity of remodeling levels in osteoporotic patients with trabecular osteoporosis and vertebral crush fractures.

Anatomical Profiles

It has been suggested (40) that fracture syndromes with vertebral fractures and with hip fractures may represent different sorts of bone loss which may be caused by different mechanisms: Type I osteoporosis is characterized by a deficit in spinal trabecular bone and by crush fracture syndrome. In contrast, type II osteoporosis is characterized by a dominant loss of cortical bone and by hip fractures. These dis-

TABLE 2. *Mean trabecular bone volume for each ten years of age in 154 osteoporotic patients, all having at least one vertebral crush fracture*

	Mean age	Trabecular bone volume (Tb/TV)					
		30–39	40–49	50–59	60–69	70–79	80–89
106 females	65.6 ± 9.9		12.0 ± 3.3	10.4 ± 2.9	9.9 ± 2.9	9.7 ± 2.9	9.8 ± 1.3
48 males	55.8 ± 11.6	9.9 ± 2.7	11.2 ± 2.8	11.2 ± 2.1	10.3 ± 2.9	10.2 ± 3.1	

tinctions between the syndromes were based on noninvasive measurements of bone mass at the different sites of fracture, as well as differences in the fracture pattern seen with aging (41). In cooperation with Johnston from Indiana University, we have recently had the opportunity to evaluate and to compare patients with early crush fracture disease and hip fractures using histomorphometric analysis of transiliac bone biopsies (14). Thirty two female patients with a recent vertebral crush fracture syndrome (mean age: 65.1 ± 5.4) and 27 patients who suffered in the last two days from a hip fracture (mean age: 83.6 ± 8.9) underwent an iliac bone biopsy under local anesthesia on the fourth day following the end of second tetracycline-labelling in the former group, and during the surgical procedure for the latter one. In order to obtain data on mineral apposition rate in these patients with femoral neck fracture, a part of the population of the residential home was labelled each year with tetracycline, and in 21 of the 27 hip fracture patients data on mineral apposition rate were available. Tb/BV was found significantly lower in patients with vertebral crush fracture than in those with hip fractures. In contrast, the thickness of the cortices was found significantly reduced in those with hip fractures, compared with vertebral crush fracture patients (Table 3). There was no difference between the two groups for trabecular osteoid volume, trabecular osteoid surface, trabecular resorption surfaces (or eroded surfaces), or thickness index of osteoid seams. The number of osteoclasts per mm^2 was significantly increased in patients with hip fractures. There was no significant difference in the mineral apposition rates between the two groups. Biochemically, serum parathyroid hormone was significantly increased above that expected in normals of similar age for the hip fracture group, and serum calcium was significantly lower in this group than in patients with vertebral crush fracture.

Three of the patients who presented with hip fractures were found on iliac biopsies to have definite evidence of osteomalacia, with an additional one probably having this disorder. They were excluded from the above histomorphometric study and they represent 13% of patients (4 out of 31). No detailed biochemical data were available on these osteomalacic patients. Figures 6A and B, are representative photomicrographs of the two fracture types.

These histomorphometric data are in general agreement with the hypothesis that patients with early postmenopausal vertebral crush fractures and those with later hip fractures represent two different populations. Crush fractures occur in women who have a more significant early deficit in trabecular bone, and our patients show a somewhat similar deficit in trabecular bone measured on transiliac biopsies (mean deviation Z–score of − 1.26) to those studied at the Mayo Clinic using dual photon absorptiometry (39) for measurement of vertebral bone mass (mean deviation Z–score of − 1.31). In contrast, the patients with hip fractures had an increased Tb/TV compared to values expected for age (14). Lips (19) also found no reduction in Tb/BV in 55 patients with cortical femoral neck fractures as compared to controls, but found a lower Tb/TV in 70 patients with trochanteric fractures. The sig-

Table 3. *Histomorphometric parameter values. Comparison between patients with vertebral crush fracture and those with hip fractures*

	Vertebral crush fracture		Hip fracture		
	n		n		P
Trabecular bone volume (%)	27	12.0 ± 4.4^a	25	14.8 ± 3.6	.01
Thickness of cortices (μm)	32	823 ± 468	27	436 ± 231	< .001
Trabecular osteoid volume (%)	31	3.3 ± 1.9	25	3.7 ± 2.0	.51
Trabecular osteoid surface (%)	31	23.2 ± 11.7	25	23.2 ± 9.9	.99
Thickness index of osteoid seams	31	14.4 ± 4.6	25	15.5 ± 4.2	.34
Trabecular eroded surfaces (%)	31	5.7 ± 2.9	27	6.6 ± 3.4	.33
Number of osteoclasts/mm^2	26	$.24 \pm .16$	26	$.39 \pm .31$	.30
Mineral apposition rate (μm/day) in trabecular bone	26	$.63 \pm .14$	19	$.62 \pm .10$	.64

^{a}mean $\pm$ SD.

nificant increase in the number of osteoclasts in our hip fracture population was also found in Lips' study (19).

Histological Heterogeneity of Trabecular (Type I) Osteoporosis

Bone histomorphometry is the most precise tool for assessing the turnover of trabecular bone remodeling in type I osteoporosis, and for determining whether its histopathogenetic mechanisms are single or multiple. In 109 osteoporotic patients whose bones were double-labelled with tetracycline, we found that 34 patients (31%) had eroded surfaces higher than 2 standard-deviations above the normal mean of 130 control subjects ($3.6 \pm 1.1\%$) evaluated by Courpron (8). These 34 patients had at the same time abnormally extended osteoid surfaces, and we considered them as having a "high remodeling osteoporosis" (29) (Fig. 7). On the basis of increased trabecular osteoblastic osteoid surface, osteoid volume, and osteoid appositional rate, Whyte (47) and Teitlebaum (44), have confirmed this histological heterogeneity of post-menopausal osteoporosis and have distinguished between "active" and "inactive" osteoporosis. Parfitt (35) has found in Michigan only a few patients (less than 10%) with an increased trabecular turnover. In order to determine whether this increase in re-

modeling surfaces was due to an increase in the "lifespan" of the bone cells or to an increase in the "birthrate" of new basic multicellular units, we measured the osteoid appositional rate from the tetracycline double-labelling (29). In our 109 osteoporotic patients, we found 28 patients with an OAr lower than the normal mean ($.72 \pm .12$ μ/day) minus 2 SD. In five cases, this "osteoblastic depression" was associated with overextensive remodeling surfaces, and in these cases the increase in remodeling surfaces was very likely due to an increased duration in the time to completion of the trabecular basic structure unit. However, in 23 cases (21% of patients), the high remodeling was certainly due to an increase in the activation frequency of the basic multicellular units. In 52 patients (48%) no significant abnormality in remodeling surfaces or osteoid appositional rate was found at the time of the biopsy. In this group, the mean wall thickness of trabecular packets was found reduced as compared to age and sex-matched control subjects (10). This suggests that decreased bone formation and more specifically a reduced formation period was a major contributor of the bone loss in these patients. This histodynamic heterogeneity of trabecular osteoporosis demonstrated in cross-sectional studies could be due to a within-patient longitudinal fluctuation if the disease is phasic in nature.

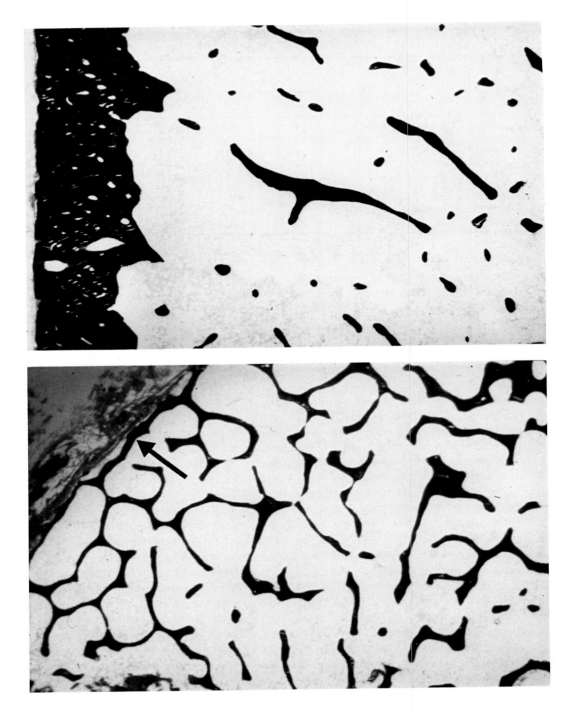

FIG. 6.   A, B. Comparison between transiliac bone biopsies from a 62-year-old female with trabecular or type I osteoporosis (**A**) and a 80-year-old female with cortical or type II osteoporosis responsible for a femoral neck fracture (**B**). In A there is a marked atrophy of trabecular bone, but a thick and compact iliac cortex. In B trabeculae are numerous and iliac cortex is very thin (*arrow*). Stain: Solochrome cyanin R, 25x.

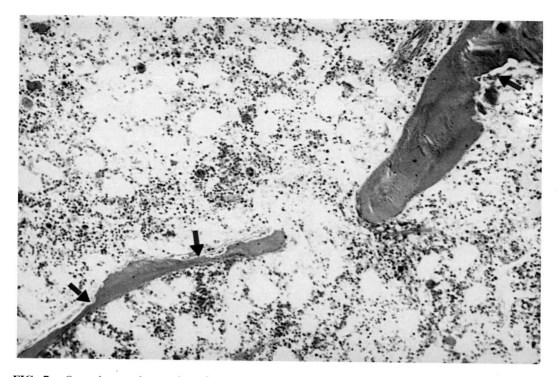

FIG. 7. Osteoclasts and extension of eroded surfaces (*arrows*) in a case of high remodeling trabecular osteoporosis. Iliac bone biopsy. Stain: Goldner's method, 100x .

This cannot be excluded, although in our study (29) the mean ages of patients were very close in the three subsets. When a "high remodeling," or a profile of "active" or of high turnover osteoporosis is discovered in apparently idiopathic osteoporosis, a search should be made for an occult endocrine disturbance. In a group of 21 osteoporotic patients exhibiting the histologic signs of high remodeling, we found 8 patients with an increased immunoreactive parathyroid hormone level (15), and in 7 patients we found an unexpected and mild thyrotoxicosis, due in most cases to a toxic adenoma, underlying a high remodeling osteoporosis (31).

Bone Histomorphometry and Evaluation of Treatments

The detection by using dynamic histomorphometry of histopathogenetic mechanisms involved in patients suffering from osteoporosis is pertinent to the selection of the best therapeutic regime to be used. Theoretically, patients with high turnover osteoporosis should be treated intermittently by agents capable of reducing the differentiation of osteoclasts or the duration of the osteoclast activity, without depressing the osteoblastic activity. Calcitonin and diphosphonates seem capable of fulfilling this purpose, but the efficacy of this strategy has still to be proven by prospective controlled studies. In other situations, when the major mechanism involved is a defect in bone formation, agents capable of increasing the number and/or the individual cellular activity of the osteoblasts seem more appropriate. Fluoride is the most potent agent for promoting osteoblastic activity (5).

Bone histomorphometry is a most valuable tool in assessing the efficacy of agents used for a curative treatment of patients with trabecular osteoporosis responsible for vertebral crush fractures. This approach is not justified for ethical reasons in the evaluation of the preventive drugs. Illustrative of this application to curative therapies are studies of the effects of synthetic human parathyroid hormone fragment (37), of combined intermittent calcitonin and constant oral phosphate (38), and of fluoride (5). For the evaluation of the anabolic effect on trabecular bone mass of fluoride, we used static and dynamic bone histomorphometry to evaluate the magnitude of the gain in trabecular bone and also to better define the mechanisms underlying this gain. In 61 patients, all having at least one vertebral collapse due to postmenopausal osteoporosis and treated for 2 years with 50 mg/day of sodium fluoride, 1 g of elemental calcium and 8,000 IU per day of vitamin D^2, two transiliac biopsies were taken, once before and once after, on the opposite side, the two-year treatment (34). The most striking histomorphometric change was a marked increase in the osteoid surfaces, a mean 2.0-fold increment appearing at the end of the treatment. A small (1.2-fold), insignificant increase in resorption surfaces was also noted, indicating an imbalance of coupling in favor of bone formation. This imbalance resulted in a marked increase in trabecular bone volume, from $9.5 \pm 3.0\%$ to $16.0 \pm 6.5\%$. This represents a mean increase corresponding to 68% of the pretreatment value, largely beyond the confidence interval for intersample variation. In polarized light there was no woven bone, and no periosteocytic mineralization defects were seen with any staining process. Identical histomorphometric changes were found in 15 osteoporotic male patients with primary masculine osteoporosis treated identically for 2 years. The histologic response to treatment was, however heterogenous and 20 out of 61 patients (33%) with postmenopausal osteoporosis had an increase in trabecular bone volume lower than 30%, i.e., lower than the confidence interval for intersample variation in a single subject (see Table 1). The percentage of histologic nonresponders was not significantly different in the three subsets of osteoporosis: 36% in patients with high remodeling osteoporosis, 35% in patients with normal remodeling and 20% in patients with osteoblastic depression. In the

latter group, however, the histologic response tended to be better. In responders the mean wall thickness of trabecular packets was found to be increased by the treatment. Because the osteoid appositional rate was unchanged, this suggests that the formation period or lifespan of the active osteoblasts was increased by fluoride therapy. Iliac cortical thickness was not changed after treatment, in all three subsets of patients (34).

CONCLUSIONS

If one takes into account the confidence intervals defining the limit of the intersample variation, histomorphometric analysis of undecalcified transiliac bone biopsy is a reliable method for the diagnosis and for the analysis of the pathophysiologic mechanisms of osteoporotic states. Bone histomorphometry is the only method capable of unequivocally diagnosing osteomalacia and to exclude this disorder in a patient with a vertebral crush fracture syndrome. It is the only method for a precise identification of the remodeling disturbances underlying the bone loss in a given osteoporotic patient. For clinical practice, the particular findings that make transiliac bone biopsy necessary are a rapid worsening of osteoporosis with several crush fractures occurring in a short period of time, "juvenile" osteoporosis with a first crush fracture before 55 years, and any unclear biochemical abnormality in serum or urine parameters reflecting bone metabolism. Bone histomorphometry is also a useful research tool in osteoporosis because it provides the unique possibility of giving access to the intermediary level of organization of bone for a precise evaluation of the osteoblastic function, and of evaluating the effects of treatments at the bone tissue and bone cell levels.

ACKNOWLEDGMENTS

I would like to express my appreciation for the cooperation of Dr. P. Courpron, Mrs. C. Edouard, Dr. A.J. Darby, Dr. M. Arlot, Dr. D. Briancon, Dr. P. Chavassieux, Dr. S. Charhon, and Dr. K. Galus. I wish to thank Miss J. Rochet for preparation of the manuscript.

REFERENCES

1. Bergot, C., Laval-Jeantet, A.M., and Laval-Jeantet, M. (1978): Etude critique des variations de la mesure de la masse osseuse par biopsie iliaque. *Rev. Rhum.*, 5:317–324.

2. Bordier, P., Matrajt, H., Miravet, L., and Hioco, D. (1964): Mesure histologique de la masse et de la résorption des travées osseuses. *Pathologie-Biologie*, 12:1238–1243.

3. Bordier, P.J., and Tun Chot, S. (1972): Quantitative histology of metabolic bone disease. *Clin. Endocrinol. Metab.* 1:197–215.

4. Boyce, B.F., Courpron, P., and Meunier, P.J. (1978): Amount of bone in osteoporosis and physiological senile osteopenia. Comparison of two histomorphometric parameters. *Metab. Bone Dis. Rel. Res.*, 1:35–38.

5. Briancon, D., and Meunier, P.J. (1981): Treatment of osteoporosis with fluoride, calcium and vitamin D. *Orthop. Clin. North Am.*, 3:629–648.

6. Chavassieux, P.M., Arlot, M.E., and Meunier, P.J. (1985): Intermethod variation in bone histomorphometry: comparison between manual and computerized methods applied to iliac bone biopsies. *Bone*, 6:221–229.

7. Chavassieux, P.M., Arlot, M.E., and Meunier, P.J. (1985): Intersample variation in bone histomorphometry: comparison between parameter values measured on two contiguous transiliac bone biopsies. *Calcif. Tissue Int.*, 37:345–350.

8. Courpron, P., Meunier, P., Edouard, C., Bringuier, J.P., and Vignon, G. (1973): Données histologiques quantitatives sur le vieillissement osseux humain. *Rev. Rhum.*, 40:469–483.

9. Courpron, P., Meunier, P.J., Bressot, C., and Ginoux, J.M. (1977): Amount of bone in iliac crest biopsy. In: *Bone Histomorphometry 1976*, edited by P.J. Meunier, pp. 39–53. Société Nouvelle Imprimerie Fournie, Toulouse.

10. Darby, A.J., and Meunier, P.J. (1981): Mean wall thickness and formation periods of trabecular bone packets in idiopathic osteoporosis. *Calcif. Tissue Int.*, 33:199–204.

11. De Vernejoul, M.C., Kuntz, D., Miravet, L., Goutallier, D. and Ryckewaert, A. (1981): Bone histomorphometry reproductibility in normal patients. *Calcif. Tissue Res.*, 33:369–374.

12. Duncan, H., Rao, S.D., and Parfitt, A.M. (1981): Complications of bone biopsies. In: *Bone Histomorphometry 1980*, edited by W.S.S. Jee and A.M. Parfitt, pp. 483–486. Armour Montagu, Paris.

13. Frost, H.M. (1969): Tetracycline based histological analysis of bone remodeling. *Calcif. Tissue Res.*, 3:211–237.

14. Johnston, C.C., Norton, J., Khairi, M.R.A., Kernek, C., Edouard, C., Arlot, M., and Meunier, P.J. (1985): Heterogeneity of fracture syndromes in postmenopausal women. *J. Clin. Endocrinol. Metab.*, 61:551–556.

15. Joly, R., Chapuy, M.C., Alexandre, C., and Meunier, P.J. (1980): Ostéoporoses à haut niveau de remodelage et fonction parathyroidienne. *Pathologie-Biologie*, 28:417–424.

16. Jowsey, J. (1977): *The Bone Biopsy*. Plenum Medical Book Company, New York, London.

17. Lips, P., Courpron, P., and Meunier, P.J. (1978): Mean wall thickness of trabecular bone packets in the human iliac crest: changes with age. *Calcif. Tissue Res.*, 26:13–17.

18. Lips, P. (1982): Metabolic causes and prevention of femoral neck fractures. Ph. D. Thesis. Free University of Amsterdam, Rodopi, Amsterdam.

19. Lips, P., Netelenbos, J.C., Jongen, M.J.M., Van Ginkel, F.C., Althuis, A.L., Van Schaik, C.L., Van der Viggh, W.J.F., Vermeiden, J.P.W., and Van der Meer, C. (1982): Histomorphometric profile and vitamin D status in patients with femoral neck fracture. *Metab. Bone Dis. Rel. Res.*, 4:85–89.

20. Malluche, H.H., Sherman, D., Manaka, R., and Massry, S.G. (1981): Comparison between different histomorphometric methods. In: *Bone Histomorphometry 1980*, edited by W.S.S. Jee and A.M. Parfitt, pp. 449–451, Armour Montagu, Paris.

21. Malluche, H.H., Sherman, D., Meyer, W., and Massry, S.G. (1982): A new semiautomatic method for quantitative static and dynamic bone histology. *Calcif. Tissue Res.*, 34:439–448.

22. Malluche, H.H., Meyer, W., Sherman, D., and Massry, S.G. (1982): Quantitative bone histology in 84 normal American subjects. Micromorphometric analysis and evaluation of variance in iliac bone. *Calcif. Tissue Int.*, 34:449–455.

23. Marcus, R., Kosek, J., Pfefferbaum, A., and Horning, S. (1983): Age-related loss of trabecular bone in premenopausal women: a biopsy study. *Calcif. Tissue Int.*, 35:406–409.

24. Melsen, F., Melsen, B., and Mosekilde, L. (1978): An evaluation of the quantitative parameters applied in bone histology. *Acta Pathol. Microbiol. Scand.* (sect. A), 86:63–69.

25. Melsen, F., and Mosekilde, L. (1978): Tetracycline double-labeling of trabecular bone in 41 normal adults. *Calcif. Tissue Res.*, 26:99–102.

26. Meunier, P.J., Bianchi, G.S., Edouard, C., Bernard, J.C., Courpron, P., and Vignon, G. (1972): Bony manifestations of thyrotoxicosis. *Orthop. Clin. North Am.*, 3:745–774.

27. Meunier, P. (1973): Use of an image-analyzing computer for bone morphometry. In: *Clinical Aspects of Metabolic Bone Disease*, edited by B. Frame, A.M. Parfitt, and H. Duncan. pp. 148–151. Excerpta Medica, Amsterdam.

28. Meunier, P.J., Edouard, C., Courpron, P., and Toussaint, F. (1975): Morphometric analysis of osteoid in iliac trabecular bone. In: *Vitamin D and Problems related to Uremic Bone Disease*, edited by A.W. Norman, K. Schaefer, H.G. Grigoleit, D.V. Herrath, and E. Ritz. pp. 149–155. Walter de Gruyter, Berlin, New York.

29. Meunier, P.J., Sellami, S., Briancon, D., and Edouard, C. (1981): Histological heterogeneity of apparently idiopathic osteoporosis. In: *Osteoporosis. Recent Advances in Pathogenesis and Treatment*, edited by H.F. De Luca, H. Frost, W.S.S. Jee, C. Johnston and A.M. Parfitt. pp. 293–301, University Park Press, Baltimore.

30. Meunier, P.J. (1981): Bone biopsy in diagnosis of metabolic bone disease. In: *Hormonal Control of*

Calcium Metabolism, edited by D.V. Cohn, R.V. Talmage, and J.L. Mathews, pp. 109–117, Excerpta Medica, Amsterdam.

31. Meunier, P.J., and Bressot, C. (1982): Endocrine influences on bone cells and bone remodeling evaluated by clinical histomorphometry. In: *Endocrinology of Calcium Metabolism*, edited by J.A. Parsons, pp. 445–465, Raven Press, New York.

32. Meunier, P., Courpron, P., Edouard, C., Bernard, J., Bringuier, J., and Vignon, G. (1973): Physiological senile involution and pathological rarefaction of bone: quantitative and comparative histological data. *Clin. Endocrinol. Metab.*, 2:239–256.

33. Meunier, P.J., Courpron, P., Edouard, C., Alexandre, C., Bressot, C., Lips, P., and Boyce, B.F. (1979): Bone histomorphometry in osteoporotic states. In: *Osteoporosis II*, edited by U.S. Barzel, pp. 27–47. Grune and Stratton, New York.

34. Meunier, P.J. (1986): Treatment of trabecular osteoporosis with sodium fluoride. *Program and Abstracts, Endocrine Society, 68th Annual Meeting*. p. 23.

35. Parfitt, A.M., and Kleerekoper, M. (1984): Diagnostic value of bone histomorphometry and comparison of histologic measurements and biochemical indices of bone remodeling. In: *Osteoporosis. Proceedings of Copenhagen International Symposium on Osteoporosis*, edited by C. Christiansen, C.D. Arnaud, B.E.C. Nordin, A.M. Parfitt, W.A. Peck, and B.L. Riggs. pp. 111–120, Aalborg Stiftsbogtrykkeri, Glostrup, Denmark.

36. Parfitt, A.M. (1982): The coupling of bone resorption to bone formation: a critical analysis of the concept and of its relevance to the pathogenesis of osteoporosis. *Metab. Bone Dis. Rel. Res.*, 4:1–6.

37. Parsons, J.A., Meunier, P.J., Neer, R.M., Podbesek, R., and Reeve, J. (1981): Effects of synthetic human parathyroid hormone fragment (hPTH 1-34) on bone mass and bone mineral metabolism. In: *Osteoporosis. Recent Advances in Pathogenesis and Treatment*, edited by H.F. De Luca, H. Frost, W.S.S. Jee, C. Johnston, and A.M. Parfitt. pp. 457–465. University Park Press, Baltimore.

38. Rasmussen, H., Bordier, P., Marie, P., Auquier, L., Eisenger, J.B., Kuntz, D., Caulin, F., Argemi, B., Gueris, J., and Jullien, A. (1980): *Metab. Bone Dis. Rel. Res.*, 2:107–111.

39. Riggs, B.L., Wahner, H.W., Seeman, E., Offord, K.P., Dunn, W.L., Mazess, R.B., Johnson, K.A., and Melton, L.J., III (1982): Changes in bone mineral density of the proximal femur and spine with aging. *J. Clin. Invest.*, 70:716–723.

40. Riggs, B.L., and Melton, L.J., III (1983): Evidence of two distinct syndromes of involutional osteoporosis. *Am. J. Med.*, 75:899–901.

41. Riggs, B.L., and Melton, L.J., III (1986): Involutional osteoporosis. *N. Engl. J. Med.*, 314:1676–1686.

42. Sacker, L.S., and Nordin, B.E.C. (1954): A sample bone biopsy needle. *Lancet*, i:347.

43. Schenk, R.K., Merz, W.A., and Müller, J.A. (1969): A quantitative histological study of bone resorption in human cancellous bone. *Acta Anatomica (Basel)*, 74:44–53.

44. Teitlebaum, S.L., Bergfeld, M.A., Avioli, L.V., and Whyte, M.P. (1981): Failure of routine biochemical studies to predict the histological heterogeneity of untreated postmenopausal osteoporosis. In: *Osteoporosis. Recent Advances in Pathogenesis and Treatment*, edited by H.F. De Luca, H. Frost W.S.S. Jee, C. Johnston, and A.M. Parfitt, pp. 303–309. University Park Press, Baltimore.

45. Vedi, S., and Compston, J.E. (1984): Direct and indirect measurements of osteoid seam width in human iliac crest biopsies. *Metab. Bone Dis. Rel. Res.*, 5:269–274.

46. Whitehouse, W.J. (1974): The quantitative morphology of anisotropic trabecular bone. *J. Microsc.*, 101:153–168.

47. Whyte, M.P., Bergfeld, M.A., Murphy, W.A., Avioli, L.V., and Teitlebaum, S.L. (1982): Postmenopausal osteoporosis. A heterogeneous disorder as assessed by histomorphometric analysis of iliac crest bone from untreated patients. *Am. J. Med.*, 72:193–201.

Osteoporosis: Etiology, Diagnosis, and Management, edited by B. Lawrence Riggs and L. Joseph Melton, III. Raven Press, New York © 1988.

12

Sex Steroids In The Pathogenesis and Prevention Of Osteoporosis

Robert Lindsay

Regional Bone Center, Helen Hayes Hospital, New York State Department of Health, West Haverstraw, New York 10993

The realization that osteoporosis is a condition that is significantly more common among the female population and the postmenopausal group in particular, suggests a cause and effect relationship between the bone disease and the changes that occur in sex steroids as women age. This potential relationship has been hotly debated since Albright's classic description of the clinical presentation of the disorder (7). Data obtained in many centers since that time have confirmed that fractures are significantly more common among aging women than among males of similar age (81), although this is not necessarily true in all societies (45). Since the relative sex ratios of each of the more common fractures associated with osteoporosis differ markedly, it may be that sex steroids, and estrogens in particular, exert variable effects on different areas of the skeleton and indeed it is entirely possible that areas of the skeleton may be independent of sex hormone influence. This chapter reviews the evidence for a cause and effect relationship between sex steroids and osteoporosis, and examines the role of therapy with sex steroids in the prevention of the disorder.

As early as 1882, Bruns had noted that fractures of the proximal femur were more fre-quent in women than in men, after middle age (32). However, much earlier evidence of the existence of osteoporosis and its sexual dichotomy in presentation, exists in the literature (140). The concept that osteoporosis was consequent upon ovarian failure belongs to Fuller Albright (6–8). As Albright noted, there appears to be a greater percentage of osteoporotic women who have had oophorectomy than would be expected (7). More recent examination, however, has confirmed that the sexual dichotomy in bone mass, and loss existed in previous centuries (11), and in most ethnic groups today (79,80) (Fig. 1).

Nonetheless, the concept that spinal osteoporosis was consequent upon loss of ovarian function remained in doubt until new methods of skeletal quantification became available, and is still argued. Donaldson and Nassim (64), for example, had challenged Albright's conclusion since they were unable to demonstrate a significant degree of spinal osteoporosis in a large group of women who had undergone oophorectomy. Thus, other theories for the high prevalence of fracture syndromes have been proposed.

Early cross-sectional studies, using radiogrammetric methods of estimating skeletal

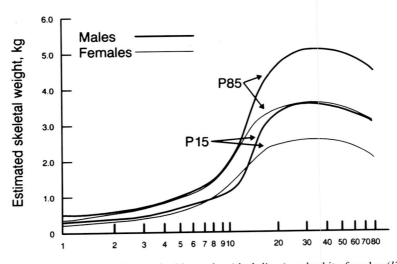

FIG. 1. Comparative skeletal weights of white males (*dark lines*) and white females (*light lines*). From Garn et al., ref 79, with permission.

mineral, suggested a disproportionate fall in bone mass among women after the fifth decade, in comparison to that observed among men (19,156). The same groups further demonstrated a temporal relationship between the onset of this process of bone loss and the menopause (157,169). Similar results were obtained when newer quantitative techniques were applied to peripheral cortical bone (the radius) and the spine (41,110,159).

Such cross-sectional data have now been reproduced using a wide variety of different techniques. Most have confirmed that bone loss is accelerated in the postmenopausal phase of life (23,41,54,59,78,80,110,121,125,145, 153,154,157,158,169,202). However, not all such cross-sectional studies have been able to demonstrate an acceleration of the decline in bone mass with age at the time of the menopause (13,122,189,217). One more recent study has suggested that there may be different patterns of bone loss at different sites in the skeleton, with linear loss occurring in the spine from about age 20 years, while a postmenopausal acceleration of loss is evident only in the peripheral bone of the radius (189). However, data obtained using a quantitative computerized tomography (CT) technique suggest that the age-related changes in vertebral trabecular bone are similar to those observed in pe-

ripheral cortical bone (41), and our own data support this concept (Fig. 2), with axial bone loss becoming evident after the age of 40 years. Thus these more recent techniques suggest that some significant premenopausal bone loss may take place (115), perhaps related to the gradual failure of ovarian function that precedes the overt menopause.

The only prospective study examining bone mass in both pre- and postmenopausal women confirms the presence of premenopausal loss of bone, and failed to find a postmenopausal acceleration of loss within the axial skeleton (184). The conflicting nature of these cross-sectional studies, and the dichotomy of behavior between the axial and peripheral skeleton in this one longitudinal study, suggests the necessity for more detailed examination of the problem. Clearly, if differences exist in rates of loss between different skeletal sites, then the relative estrogen (or sex steroid) sensitivity of these different sites requires each to be examined in detail.

THE CLIMACTERIC

Changes in the Skeleton

The cross-sectional data reviewed above, generally suggest that the onset of bone loss

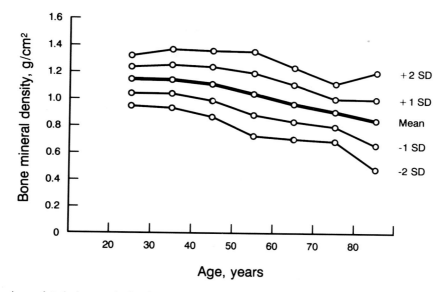

FIG. 2. Age related changes in lumbar mineral areal density (g/cm²) measured by dual photon absorptiometry in 400 normal white females.

occurs after the fourth decade with a definite increase in the rate of loss occurring around the time of menopause (115). As indicated, not all of the data in the literature confirm this, however, and it has been suggested that different regions in the skeleton may have variable responses to the lifestyle, nutritional, and endocrine changes which occur with age. The available data suggest that the sex difference in fracture (1:13M:F), than for all other osteoporotic fractures. It perhaps would be surprising if the vertebrae did not show significant sensi- if the vertebrae did not show significant sensitivity to ovarian failure. In an elegant study to examine this hypothesis (183), Richelson evaluated bone mass in 14 women who had premenopausal oophorectomy, on average 20 years prior to the average age of menopause. The measured bone mineral at all sites (radius, spine, and hip) was significantly less than would be expected for their age, and equivalent to the bone mass at the same sites in women who were some 20 years older and who had gone through a normal menopause at the expected age. The conclusion of the authors was that estrogen deficiency and not aging was the predominant cause of bone loss during the first two decades after menopause.

These data are consistent with kinetic changes observed across the menopause (96,97). Our own prospective data, examining bone mass after oophorectomy, confirm the concept that there is an acceleration of bone loss during the first few years after oophorectomy (Fig. 3). While the exact period of acceleration could not be evaluated for individual patients, on average, this acceleration was evident for the first 4 to 6 years after oophorectomy. Clearly in this circumstance, the acceleration of bone loss is exaggerated by the sudden termination of ovarian function in this group of premenopausal women, and this may explain some of the problems in identifying an *obvious* acceleration of bone loss immediately following the much more gradual process of the natural climacteric (115).

Finally it is still not clear whether or not the rate of bone loss in postmenopausal women varies significantly such that there is a subgroup of so-called "fast losers." Few prospective studies have examined this issue. In an early study of the effects of endogenous sex steroid production we demonstrated that the rate of loss of peripheral bone was closely related to the endogenous supply of estrogen (Fig. 4), which in the postmenopausal popula-

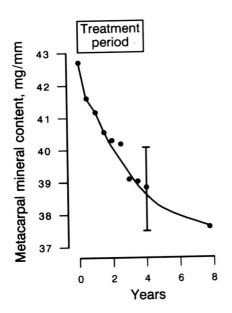

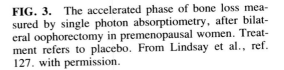

FIG. 3. The accelerated phase of bone loss measured by single photon absorptiometry, after bilateral oophorectomy in premenopausal women. Treatment refers to placebo. From Lindsay et al., ref. 127. with permission.

tion comes primarily from peripheral conversion of adrenal androgens occurring primarily in fat (198) (Fig. 5). Thus, not only is there a relationship between estrogen and bone loss, but by careful investigation we were also able to demonstrate a relationship between adrenal "tone" and rate of loss of bone (132,147). Studies by other groups have confirmed both findings (30,53,170). However, we could not demonstrate the converse, that is a difference in adrenal function in fast versus slow losers, suggesting that the peripheral conversion step to estrogen is a mandatory and necessary one before the skeletal effects can be obtained (147). Significant alterations in the circulating levels of many steroids occur after menopause (Table 1) (3,148), and it still remains conceivable that changes in other sex steroids of ovarian origin, perhaps androgens, can also interfere with skeletal homeostasis at this point in life. The effects of cigarette consumption, one of the risk factors associated with osteoporosis (56), may potentially be mediated through effects on estrogen metabolism. Women who

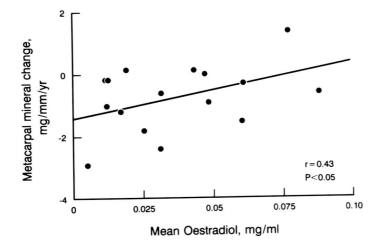

FIG. 4. Relationship of the rate of early post-oophorectomy bone loss (by SPA) to average circulating estradiol level, measured monthly for 2 years. From Lindsay et al., ref. 134, with permission.

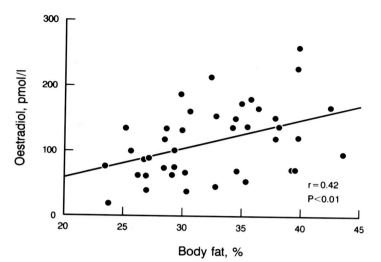

FIG. 5. Relationship between circulating estrogen in oophorectomized women and percent body fat, calculated from height and weight. From Lindsay et al., ref. 134, with permission.

smoke are reported to have an earlier menopause than those who do not (10,123) and cigarette consumption may lower estrogen levels in both premenopausal and postmenopausal women (111,143).

When the circulating levels of sex steroids are examined in patients who have presented with fracture, these are generally not different from those found in control populations (57,185), although again the findings are not universal (149). Since most patients with fracture syndromes present with evidence of low or normal bone turnover (174), and the phenomenon of rapid bone loss precedes fracture by perhaps many years, it is not surprising that these discrepancies exist. It is naive to expect earlier menopause than those who do not (10,123) and cigarette consumption may lower estrogen levels in both premenopausal and postmenopausal women (111,143).

that the relatively subtle differences in plasma hormone levels, found at the height of the changes in mineral homeostasis, will persist after the process is complete, especially if a cause and effect relationship is assumed.

Finally there is conflicting evidence regarding the status of estrogen receptors in other organs, more traditionally associated with sex steroid action, in postmenopausal osteoporosis in uterine tissue. In an assessment of estrogen recepter activity, one study concluded that since osteoporotic patients had similar concentrations of uterine estrogen receptors, there was no support for a defect in estrogen binding as a cause of low bone mass (58). However in a study of estrogen binding in vaginal epithelium, the uptake of ^{3}H-estradiol was significantly less in osteoporotic individuals (21). Thus, the question of inadequate estrogen action, by virtue of low receptor number or inefficient binding to adequate receptor concentration, as a cause of bone loss requires reevaluation.

Prospective Changes in Bone Mass

In our initial experiments, we examined bone mass in women 3 years after oophorectomy, and compared those results to the same measures in an aged matched group of women who had had hysterectomy with ovarian conservation, also three years previously, and in

TABLE 1. *Comparison of patients treated with synthetic estrogen versus placebo-treated groups*

	Premenopausal	Postmenopausal
Estradiol	0.05 +/− 0.005	0.013 +/− 0.001
Estrone	0.08 +/− 0.01	0.06 +/− 0.01
Testosterone	0.31 +/− 0.02	0.25 +/− 0.03 (NS)
Dihydrotesterone	0.29 +/− 0.02	0.15 +/− 0.02
Androstenedione	1.9 +/− 0.1	0.5 +/− 0.04

After Abraham & Maroulis, ref. 3.

whom ovarian function could still be detected. This simple experiment confirmed that the loss of ovarian function was associated with a reduction in bone mass that was independent of the effects of age. A more detailed prospective study (5), from the time of oophorectomy, demonstrated the marked variability in rates of bone loss at that time of life (Fig. 6). The calculated accelerated phase of bone loss was noted to be exponential with time, with a half life of 1.5 years. We could not demonstrate a bimodal distribution of bone loss within that specific population, a finding supported by data from at least one other center (208), although others have demonstrated such a distribution in a postmenopausal population (53).

Biochemical Changes

Cross-sectional data suggest subtle but profound changes in the biochemistry of mineral homeostasis at the time of menopause or castration and are confirmed by longitudinal data (Fig. 7). Serum calcium and phosphate both increase within the normal range, and the urinary excretion of both ions increases concomi-

tantly (68). Higher levels of serum alkaline phosphatase and in the uninary excretion of hydroxyproline indicate an increase in the rate of bone remodeling that accompanies those ionic changes. The relationship between serum and urine calcium does not change significantly, perhaps suggesting no change in the renal handling of calcium. Direct and kinetic evidence suggests that the absorption efficiency for calcium across the intestine declines at this point in life (95,96). Assuming that calcium supply does not change, this suggests that the precarious calcium balance status will be exacerbated by the overall decreased efficiency in the handling of calcium that must occur.

Menopausal Changes in Sex Steroids

Through the climacteric years women gradually progress from a situation in which there is a regular cyclic behavior of the ovary with wide fluctuations in the circulating levels of all sex steroids, to one in which there is a relatively low rate of production of sex steroids with consequent low circulating levels. The reduction in circulating estrogen levels is about

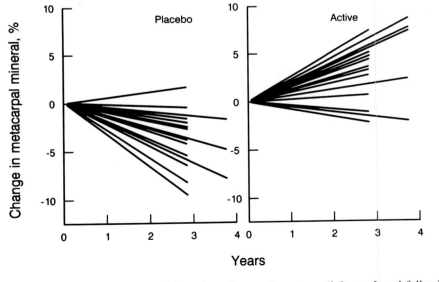

FIG. 6. Variability in rates of bone loss after oophorectomy (*left panel*) and following estrogen therapy (*right*). Each line is calculated regression line for one patient, with a minimum of seven measurements throughout 3 years.

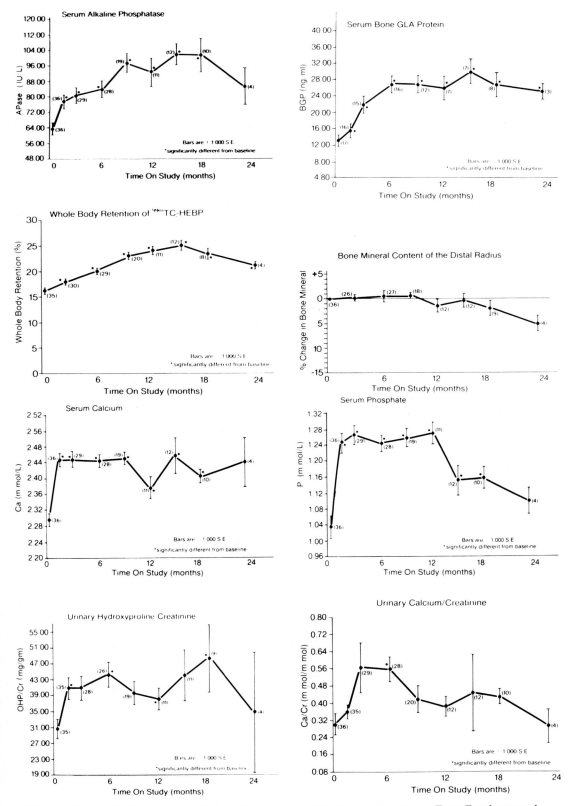

FIG. 7. Changes in biochemistry of mineral homeostatis following oophorectomy. From Fogelman et al., ref. 68, with permission.

80% and ceases to be cyclic (160) with average estradiol levels between 5 to 25 pg/ml. Estrone levels are somewhat higher than estradiol levels in the postmenopause, in contrast to the premenopause, although the importance of this ratio change is not entirely clear. In general, oophorectomized women have similar sex steroid profiles to naturally postmenopausal women, with absolute circulating levels of estrogen similar or only slightly lower.

Ovarian failure clearly begins at a considerably earlier age than that of the overt menopause, with increasing incidence of irregular cycles and anovulation after age 35 years, perhaps corresponding to the age of onset of bone loss (115). With the reduced production of ovarian estrogen the major source of circulating hormone becomes, at least indirectly, the adrenal gland. Androgens synthesized by the adrenal are converted peripherally to estrogen. The major site of conversion is fatty tissue (73,132,171,224). Thus the conversion rate of androstenedione to estrone increases with weight, and also with age (98,141). It is entirely possible that some of the protective effect of obesity for osteoporosis is related to this phenomenon, since in the immediate post-oophorectomized women and in postmenopausal women there is a negative relationship between urine calcium, hydroxyproline and circulating levels of estrogen, that in turn correlate positively with obesity (73,132). This and the changes in mineral homeostasis outlined below which follow memopause, suggest very strongly that there is a cause and effect relationship between ovarian failure and bone loss.

Bone Turnover

The elegant studies of Heaney et al. (97), suggest that the onset of the menopause is associated with a 20% increase in bone resorption and a 15% increase in bone formation. The large observed increment in bone resorption increases the dificit between formation and resorption at menopause, with a new average imbalance equivalent to 40 mg calcium per day. The net removal of calcium from the skeleton is associated with a decline in calcium absorption efficiency and increase in urinary excretion of calcium. From those studies, it is not clear which of these processes are cause and which are effect. However, when net intestinal calcium absorption is related to urinary calcium, a positive relationship is found, suggesting that external factors controlling calcium balance setting cause the bone loss rather than the converse (94). Although these changes are quite small they clearly are sufficient to account for the average rate of bone loss in this population. Their subtlety (being within the range of physiologic norm) perhaps suggests some of the apparent difficulty that others have had in observing the effects and determining the cause. However, newer data, obtained by examining bone turnover by a quantitative nuclear medicine technique, have demonstrated an increase in uptake of technetium ($^{99}T_m$)-labelled diphosphonate following oophorectomy, thought to be compatible with increased skeletal metabolism and turnover (68). The effect appears to peak after 1 to 2 years (Fig. 7), relating well to the changes in bone mass that we have observed from oophorectomy. The same group and others have also demonstrated increases in circulating BGP for the two years of their post-oophorectomy follow-up, compatible also with increased turnover. These data might be considered to be consistent with the decline in circulating calcitonin levels observed by one group following castration (233), with no consistent changes evident in PTH or 1,25-$(OH)_2D_3$.

"Premenopausal" Amenorrhea

It is logical that, if a natural menopause associated with reduced estrogen levels results in increased loss of skeletal mass, then other states of estrogen deficiency should produce a similar effect that is independent of age. Such a conclusion is also suggested by the effects of premature ovarian failure or oophorectomy (183). Hypothalamic amenorrhea produces an estrogen-deficient state and is common among female athletes, particularly runners (193). Several groups have now demonstrated a significant reduction in bone mineral density among women athletes with prolonged amenorrheic states (42,64,85,124,137,151). This association is persuasive, but does not rule out the possibility that light-boned individuals are predisposed to become elite athletes, thence amenorrheic. However, amenorrhea resulting from hyperprolactinemia also results in reduced bone mineral (42,119). Thus, periods of reduced ovarian function prior to the climacteric appear to be prejudicial to bone mass. Prospective studies are required to determine if young athletes actually lose bone when amenorrhea ensues. A more detailed follow-up of the same patients suggests that the effect is exacerbated by dietary calcium deficiency (C.H. Chesnut, personal communication, 1986) highlighting the interaction of calcium and activity noted in our study of eumenorrheic young women (116).

It appears from these data that there is a significant, but subtle, increase in bone remodeling after loss of ovarian function. The Frost hypothesis linking bone formation and bone resorption in a tightly-coupled system (72) requires that in any circumstance in which bone turnover is changed, the alterations in resorption and formation should be similar. Turnover within the skeleton can be changed by increasing the rate of activation of remodeling cycles, and hence creating more cycles in force at any single point in time, and by changing the activity of the cell populations within each group of remodeling cells. Parfitt has calculated the likely contribution of each of these and concludes that 50 to 60% of the increase in turnover results from more frequent activation of remodeling sites, and the remainder from increased cellular activity (175). Since in the premenopausal phase of life, there is already an imbalance between osteoblast and osteoclast activity, either mechanism could exacerbate this inequality. It seems likely that both do and that there is increased avidity of individual osteoclasts for bone in situations of estrogen deprivation.

TURNER'S SYNDROME

Osteoporosis is quoted as occurring in most, if not all patients with Turner's syndrome (ovarian agenesis) and can be associated with vertebral collapse and protrusio acetabuli (22,65). Reductions in cortical thickness before age 11 years has been shown, suggesting that not all of the problem was related to estrogen insufficiency (20), although it has been suggested that a relative estrogen deficiency may be present in these patients during childhood (55). However, there was in the same study, a further reduction in cortical width up to age 25 years, while those on estrogen had significantly higher cortical thickness. Other studies have failed to confirm the reduction in bone among the younger population (177), although it seems likely that the delay in skeletal maturation associated with the XO state is accompanied by some delay in obtaining adult skeletal status that might account for the apparent reduction in mineral (196). In general, younger patients (<30 years) with Turner's syndrome show about a 25% reduction in bone mass. Iliac crest biopsy suggests high turnover and alkaline phosphatase can be elevated (31). Estrogen therapy appears to improve the skeletal status significantly, but no biopsy or fracture data are available for this population.

HYPERESTROGENIC STATES

If reduced ovarian function is detrimental to skeletal health, one can ask whether or not hyperestrogenic states can improve skeletal status, particularly in premenopausal women. Some data suggest that pregnancy may reduce the risk of subsequent osteoporosis (126,136). More recently, we have evaluated the role of a variety of risk factors in determining bone mass among postmenopausal women (136). We compared two groups of women who were found to have axial bone mass either greater than or less than 2 SD from the average for their age and sex. In this preliminary study, those with high bone mass were more obese, and had a significantly greater number of pregnancies. Curiously, they had also lactated for a significantly longer period of time.

In addition to pregnancy, use of the contraceptive may cause some small increase in axial bone mass (116), or peripheral bone mass (84), although we think this effect is not maintained.

ESTROGENS

Effects of Replacement

The introduction of estrogen treatment in the early postmenopausal years seems a logical approach for those at risk of osteoporosis, if indeed the primary defect inducing bone loss is ovarian failure. To test this hypothesis we began a series of studies some 20 years ago designed to evaluate the effects of estrogen in the prevention of bone loss.

We utilized our oophorectomized population, described above, to examine the effects of estrogen therapy in a formal controlled double-blind study. In three groups of patients, followed from 6 weeks, 3 years, or 6 years after oophorectomy, estrogen (mestranol 24 mg/day) significantly retarded bone loss (129,133). The effects of estrogen were clearly evident, independently of the point at which intervention was begun (1). However, since the effect was primarily reduction in the rate of bone loss, the earlier treatment was begun, the more beneficial the effect, since bone mass was maintained at a higher level. Some small improvement in bone mass was evident if estrogen therapy was initiated during the rapid phase of bone loss (129) (Fig. 8). The increase of cortical bone mass was only some 2 to 4%, which is the amount that might be expected if therapy were introduced during that period of excessive osteoclast activity which had produced a consequent increase in the temporary deficit in bone, but osteoblasts had yet to fill the resorption cavities. At that point reduction in the activity of osteoclasts, with no immediate effect on the rate of bone formation (187), would result in a period of positive balance within the skeleton and an increase in the total mass. The effects of estrogen appear to continue for as long as they are administered. In

this study we were able to demonstrate the effects for at least 10 years (133). A slight decrement in bone mass in the estrogen treated group at that time, led us to suggest that we were observing estrogen independent and perhaps age dependent increase in the rate of loss. At this point the phenomena associated with type II osteoporosis (186) could conceivably be beginning to operate although we have not specifically investigated this point.

Withdrawal of estrogen therapy results, in our population in an increase in the rate of bone loss (127). In the four years following estrogen removal the rate of bone loss was exactly equal to that following oophorectomy (127). These data have been confirmed in one other center (106). In a further evaluation of this issue, Christiansen (51) has also demonstrated resumption of bone loss following estrogen removal. However, in that study estrogen therapy was only of 2 years' duration and therefore the control group were still in the rapid phase of bone loss. Thus, since the rate of bone loss after estrogen withdrawal exactly paralleled this, despite assumptions to the contrary, these data from all groups are in fundamental agreement. Therefore, each year of estrogen treatment, if initiated at menopause or oophorectomy, will buy another year before bone loss begins and presumably will reduce the time that any individual will spend below the theoretical fracture threshold. This clearly will reduce fracture incidence overall, even if estrogens are used only for comparatively short periods.

The bone loss phenomenon in the immediate postmenopausal phase of life is exquisitely sensitive to estrogen. To test the dose response relationship we evaluated the effects of varying doses of conjugated equine estrogens on bone loss over a two year period. Some reduction in loss was evident at a dose of 0.3 mg/day, and the maximum protective effect was seen at 0.625 mg/day (Fig. 9) (135). In all the studies we have conducted, reduction in the rate of bone loss is evident with all estrogenic compounds if they are given in adequate amounts. Estriol, a particularly weak estrogen does not appear to affect skeletal homeostasis until

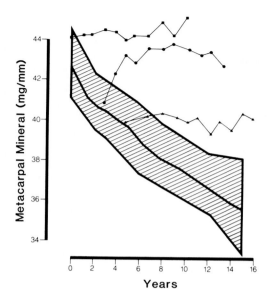

FIG. 8. Changes in bone mass by SPA in placebo-treated patients (hatched area: mean +/− SD) and in 3 groups of estrogen treated patients, part of our original double-blind study.

given in multiple daily doses to provide more than 8 to 12 mg/day (128).

The biochemical effects following estrogen treatment are exactly the converse of those occurring after menopause or oophorectomy (240). Serum calcium and phosphate fall slightly; urine calcium and hydroxyproline also fall; and alkaline phosphatase activity in serum is also reduced. The change in urine phosphate, a reduction in $TmPO_4/GFR$ suggests

increase in parathyroid hormone activity at the level of the kidney, and we have also seen an increase in urinary cAMP excretion in estrogen-treated patients (130). The changes in calcium balance which occur at menopause are reversed by the introduction of estrogen (96,150).

Studies involving the use of estrogen for prevention of osteoporosis have been performed by a number of other groups, particu-

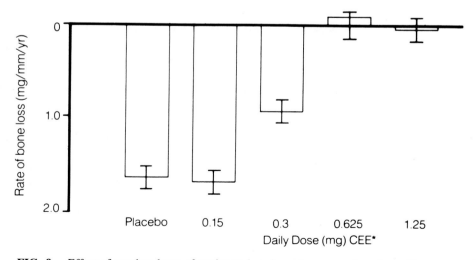

FIG. 9. Effect of varying doses of conjugated equine estrogens on bone loss. Five groups of patients were treated randomly with either placebo or one of 4 different daily doses of equine estrogen. From Lindsay et al., ref. 135, with permission.

larly since bone mass measurements have become available. Early results from the U.S.A. and U.K. confirmed our findings by demonstrating reduction in bone loss in women who had undergone a natural menopause (104,181) More recent studies have confirmed these data (50,83,105,166). These published data confirm the conclusions drawn by some early workers, who examined the skeletal effects of estrogen prior to the availability of bone mass measurements (6,34,101). From a variety of techniques and experimental designs, we are led to the conclusion that estrogen prevents postmenopausal osteoporosis.

Several retrospective studies have examined the question of fracture frequency following estrogen use. The majority have evaluated the prevalence of estrogen exposure among individuals with hip fracture and compared it to that in a control population. In each case, estrogen exposure is associated with a significant reduction in hip fracture frequency (66,109, 120,231). The consensus of the available data suggests that estrogen prescribed early in the postmenopause for a minimum of 5 years will result in an approximate reduction of 50% in hip fracture frequency. That is, hip fracture frequency among women would be reduced to that currently experienced among men. If that were the case at other sites of fracture, then we could expect 90% reduction in vertebral crush fracture, a figure suggested by our prospective data (133).

Interactions

It is clear that not all postmenopausal women need be prescribed estrogen therapy to prevent osteoporosis. For those who do require preventive therapy, the minimum dose that provides effective prevention should be used. The initial step must be elimination of those risk factors that are amenable to such an approach. Our next step is provision of adequate calcium intake, assumed from Heaney's data (95) to be a total intake of 1.5 g/day elemental calcium. Advice is also given on activity types and levels. Since there appears to be a definite interaction between calcium and estrogen (96),

it is entirely possible that this interaction will allow a lower estrogen dose in the calcium replete woman. That is to say that since the women obtaining 1 to 1.5 g calcium/day will be closer to calcium balance than women on an average intake of calcium, a lower estrogen dose may be required to achieve good balance or prevent bone loss, since the improvement in calcium efficiency required will be significantly less. One study suggests that this concept may be correct. In a small group of women treated with 0.3 mg conjugated equine estrogen and calcium supplementation to give a total intake of 1.5 g/day, bone loss was prevented for the two years of the study (82). In comparison, double this estrogen dose appears to be the minimum effective dose in calcium-depleted women (135).

Other Steroids

The effects of estrogens are not unique to that class of compound. Recent data suggest that certain progestogens and anabolic agents will produce similar effects. In our initial studies we demonstrated that a depot progestogen will reduce bone loss (131). More recently we also demonstrated that oral norethindrone in a daily dose of 5 mg effectively retards bone loss (2). Other studies have shown that progestogens can reduce urine calcium and perhaps also urine hydroxyproline, suggesting that inhibition of bone resorption is the mechanism of skeletal preservation. However, in vitro data suggest that progestogens may increase bone formation (221). One study examining the short term effects of combination treatment has suggested that the biochemical consequences of progestogen addition demonstrate that the anabolic effect is present in vivo (52). This requires more detailed investigation.

Anabolic agents or androgens were suggested by Albright (6) as potential therapeutically useful agents in osteoporosis, since those would also reverse the negative calcium balance status of affected patients. In a long-term follow up study of the effectiveness of androgens and estrogens, Gordan (87) noted that androgens were not well-tolerated because of their masculinizing effects. Only a few of the original patients remained on therapy for more than two years and prevention of recurrent fractures was not evident. More recently, Chesnut (49) examined the effects of stanozolol and found a small but significant increment in total body calcium during the two years of treatment (238). Some *in vitro* evidence suggests that anabolic agents may stimulate bone formation (221).

Mode of Action

The precise mechanism by which estrogens exert their effects on the skeleton has been the subject of much discussion, and is even today not at all clear.

In original observations on the effects of various sex steroids on bone in osteoporosis, Albright (6) noted the marked reduction in calcium excretion (both urinary and fecal) and the temporary improvement in calcium balance observed following estrogen therapy. In this publication, Albright also noted the generally satisfactory long-term response of patients with established osteoporosis to estrogen therapy. This finding was later confirmed in a review of patients treated with estrogen over a 25-year period, some of whom were Albright's original patients (101,227). The increase in calcium absorption and decrease in urinary calcium noted by Albright was the first demonstration of the increase in the efficiency with which estrogen replete individuals can handle dietary calcium. Alkaline phosphatase activity did not increase, contrary to Albright's expectation, and suggested a lack of effect on the osteoblast population, later confirmed (187,188) histologically. Despite these early observations, and the confirmatory evidence that estrogen prevented bone loss (59) there was little advance in determining the mechanism of estrogen effect until recently. Such early results showing urinary calcium excretion (6,197,239) and the fall in serum calcium concentration (25,110,176) were originally thought to be caused by an increase in skeletal resistance to the effects of

parathyroid hormone. The concept was more carefully developed by Heaney (93) who synthesized the available evidence into a "unified" hypothesis of the pathogenesis of the disease. This explanation failed to evaluate the information afforded by some of the other biochemical effects of estrogen administration. A well documented fall in serum phosphorus always occurs after estrogen administration (25, 129,168,176,182) and a marked reduction in the tubular maximum for phosphate excretion is also seen (129,168). These effects are consistent with a decrease in either growth hormone secretion, or an increase in the secretion and renal effects of parathyroid hormone. The biochemical effects on urine phosphorus and calcium continue even if estrogens are prescribed for many years (133). The final conclusions from this early work were therefore somewhat conflicting, with, on the one hand, evidence supporting an increase in skeletal resistance (172) to PTH but an increase in renal activity of PTH, which would also be consistent with the decreased secretion of calcium in urine.

These somewhat inconsistent results led to a search for estrogen receptors in bone. Initial results were thought to be positive (222), but a more careful evaluation of the issue led to the conclusion that the protein binding estrogen in skeletal tissue is in fact α-fetoprotein and that true estrogen receptors are not present in bone (47). Other proteins capable of binding estrogen can also be identified in bone (204), but there is no evidence that these glycoproteins can act as true receptors. Mononuclear cells in marrow have been identified that appear to have true receptors for estrogen, but their role in estrogen action on the skeleton is unclear. On the other hand, receptors for glucocorticoids have clearly been found in bone (146). There appears to be no estrogen interaction with these steroid receptors, although progestogens do cross-react at higher than physiological concentrations. Direct inhibition of bone resorption *in vitro* using meaningful concentrations of estrogen has never been shown satisfactorily (43,139).

Such difficulties in defining a direct effect of estrogen on the skeleton have led to attempts to explain the action of estrogen using the biochemical changes in serum as a key. It has been demonstrated in several laboratories that circulating calcitonin levels are lower in women than in men at all ages (24,60,102). It has also been suggested that osteoporosis can be associated with deficiency of calcitonin (161,205,209). However patients who have undergone total thyroidectomy are not necessarily more at risk of osteoporosis than others (216), although extrathyroidal sources of calcitonin may be sufficient in such circumstances to be physiologically important (74). Curiously, calcitonin levels appear to be increased in women during times of calcium stress such as growth, pregnancy and lactation (192,207). These are mostly times at which excessive resorption of the skeleton might beneficially be prevented, since probably the major biologic action of calcitonin is inhibition of osteoclast function and reduction of bone resorption (12,46,71). These findings and the suggestion of lower calcitonin levels after menopause, together with a reduced responsiveness to its secretagogue (205), led to the suggestion that the sex steroids may play a role in the control of calcitonin secretion (102). Subsequent evidence from the same group supported that concept (206). Indeed, it makes an attractive hypothesis, for if the primary effect of estrogen were to stimulate calcitonin production, the sequelae could explain much of the biochemical changes following estrogen administration. Additionally, racial differences in calcitonin might (or might not) explain the resistance of black races to osteoporosis (165,208). However, not all of the evidence supports this concept. Castration has been reported to increase calcitonin levels in one study (206) and in another, no differences in circulating levels were found after menopause (48), although the same group demonstrated a reduction in calcitonin reserve (215) in patients with established osteoporosis. In another study, estrogen therapy in elderly women had no effect on basal calcitonin levels but markedly augmented the response to calcium (164). On the other hand,

Tiegs et al. (216) could find no evidence for calcitonin deficiency in patients with established osteoporosis and demonstrated that patients with osteoporosis who had previously undergone thyroidectomy had less of a reduction in bone mass than intact patients with osteoporosis, even though the latter group had no calcitonin response to intravenous calcium. Much of the controversy results from the difficulty with radioimmunoassay techniques for calcitonin (99). Measurement of normal circulating levels in women stretches the sensitivity of the available assays, and one group have reported that the monomeric form of calcitonin, present in even lower concentrations, may be the more relevant measurement (99), a suggestion others have rejected (205). Finally, classical estrogen receptors have not been demonstrated in the C-cells of the thyroid (229), although it has been suggested that estrogen directly stimulates the secretion of calcitonin (89). While resolution of these issues is awaited, this proposed mechanism for estrogen action must be considered a hypothesis despite its obvious attractions.

The putative increase in calcitonin secretion might be expected to produce a series of biochemical effects, if indeed there were to result a decline in rate of bone resorption. The reduced flow of calcium from bone to blood would lead to a small fall in serum calcium, that is observed (129), and presumably mild secondary increase in PTH secretion. Several groups have indeed found increases in circulating immunoreactive PTH after estrogen administration to postmenopausal patients (75,188,206). Others have failed to demonstrate a change in circulating PTH with estrogens (206,223). In the most recent rigorous test of this phenomenon (211), a short course of ethinylestradiol resulted in a fall in serum PTH in three out of four assays used, and no change in the fourth, perhaps amply demonstrating the problems with immunoassay systems for PTH. This final study could not demonstrate the reduction in $TmPO_4$ that had previously been shown to be induced by estrogen (129,170) and was assumed to result from increased PTH activity. Indeed estrogen appears to increase urinary excretion of cyclic AMP, again assumed to be a PTH induced phenomenon (130). The increments in $1,25(OH)_2D_3$ that result from the oral estrogen administration (211,233) may in fact simply be the result of increased hepatic synthesis of the carrier protein for vitamin D, so-called D binding protein (27). Balance data suggest that estrogens improve the efficiency of calcium absorption across the intestine (96), assumed to be a vitamin D-dependent effect. Formal absorption tests have confirmed this (40,75). If the increments in circulating $1,25(OH)_2D_3$ consequent on estrogen therapy are in fact due to changes in D-binding protein, it is difficult to perceive how improvements in absorption efficiency can be obtained. As Heaney has shown, the net effect of loss of ovarian function is a loss of efficiency in handling available calcium from the diet, that is restored by estrogen replacement.

However, estrogens clearly inhibit bone resorption *in vivo* and formation, documented both biochemically (104,129,133) and histologically (187). A net positive effect on bone balance is assumed to result from the early inhibition of resorption, independent of the mechanism, and a much later, by months at least, reduction in formation (187). More recent evidence suggests an earlier effect on formation when this is measured biochemically. Serum levels of bone GLA-protein, a marker for formation (180,230), fall quickly after estrogen administration (211), although that simply could be an expression of reduced skeletal turnover (61). Therefore the mechanism of estrogen action remains obscure. It remains entirely conceivable that estrogens act on a small population of cells, perhaps in marrow, that remain to be identified, and that their effects are mediated through the myriad of paracrine factors that mediate signalling in bone. Estrogens do have significant effects on other connective tissues, apparently preventing the reduction in skin thickness that follows the menopause (28). Others have demonstrated a variety of effects in various tissues. In particular, the metabolism of collagen has been extensively studied in dermis (100,117,201), uterus (17,67,117), as well as bone (100,201). Estrogens not only influence collagen production, but also stimulate lysyl oxidase and maturation of collagen in mouse bone.

Side-Effects

It is now generally accepted that unopposed estrogen therapy increases the risk of endometrial cancer. The data suggest that the magnitude of the increase in risk is somewhere between 1.7 to 20 times (88,107,113,142,144, 231,241). The effects are dependent on both dose and duration of treatment. However, the reports have been criticized, with suggestions that they magnify the problem because of detection bias and failure to take into account the prevailing natural incidence of the disease (77). Additionally, it has been suggested that the cancer induced under the influence of estrogen therapy may be more benign than the normal behavior of endometrial malignancies. Nonetheless, there is a clear increase in risk and more recent evidence suggests that the risk may continue after cessation of therapy (195). It is important, however, to note that obesity is also associated with a 3 to 9 fold increase in risk (91), presumably because obese individuals have higher endogenous estrogen levels than their slim counterparts (112,132). The consequence of this association between estrogen and endometrial malignancy has been the increasing use of progestogen in prescription regimens. Progestogen reduces the number of estrogen receptors in the endometrium (108,234), as well as exerting profound biochemical changes in the tissue (235). In several studies which have examined the effects of progestogen, given cyclically in an estrogen regimen, the incidence of hyperplasia and cancer was either not changed or significantly decreased (14,33,39,75,76,92,167,213,235). Indeed, reversal of abnormal hyperplastic changes by progestogen administration reinforces the concept that progestogens exert a protective effect (76,235).

A greater controversy surrounds the issue of estrogen use and breast cancer. The incidence, morbidity and mortality of breast cancer are so significantly greater than for endometrial cancer that a relationship between estrogen use and breast cancer would have potentially much more serious consequences. However, a relationship has been difficult to prove (29,77,103, 114,191). The general consensus appears to suggest that with two such common situations as breast cancer and estrogen treatment, if a significant relationship existed, it should have been fairly easy to find (173). However, we regard the previous occurrence of a breast cancer as an absolute contraindication to therapy with estrogen, while a previous endometrial malignancy, especially if more than three years previously, is only a relative contraindication. The occurrence of high circulating prolactin levels in situations of high unopposed estrogen activity have suggested a role for prolactin in the genesis of breast cancer. Prolactin does stimulate the growth of tumor tissue in culture (36). However, estrogen therapy at the relatively low doses required to protect against bone loss, does not alter circulating prolactin levels (18).

Estrogens are potent stimulators of hepatic protein synthesis. As a result, increments in circulating proteins of hepatic origin have been reported after estrogen use (152). The most important of these are several of the coagulation factors, since it has been thought that increases in circulating levels of factors VII, VIII, and X might predispose to thromboembolic disease among the aging population. While synthetic estrogens are associated with changes in all factors (155), much more modest increases are evident after the use of compounds approximating more closely to naturally occurring estrogens that appear to exert lesser effects on the liver. Increases in plasminogen and angiotensin converting enzyme have also been reported. Despite such biochemical changes, there is currently no evidence to suggest that estrogens are associated with an increased incidence of thromboembolic disease or hypertension (92,155,167). In our prospective studies those patients treated with synthetic estrogen, arguably the worst scenario, had average blood pressures lower than the placebo-treated group (155) (Table 2).

TABLE 2. *Risk factors associated with osteoporosis*[a]

Female sex
Caucasian or Asiatic ethnicity
Positive family history
Low calcium intake (lifelong)
Early menopause (or oophorectomy)
Sedentary lifestyle
Nulliparity
Alcohol abuse
High sodium intake
Cigarette smoking
High caffeine intake
High protein intake
High phosphate intake
Secondary causes of bone loss (steroids, hyperthyroidism)

[a]Roughly arranged in descending order of importance.

Other Effects

Concerns about side effects of long-term therapy, which perhaps should not have been unexpected, has resulted in a number of studies that have examined the potential risks and benefits of therapy with estrogen for postmenopausal women. These have been reviewed in the literature and it is not the function of this chapter to review such general effects (37,77, 163,219). However, it is worth drawing attention to the preliminary, and as yet circumstantial evidence that estrogen therapy may improve the risk of other disorders as well as osteoporosis. Reductions in all-cause mortality have been found with estrogen use (35,38) probably related primarily to reduction in death due to heart disease (4,15,178,190,214). Such a biological effect of estrogen is plausible as exogenous estrogen has been shown to increase HDL-2 levels (226), high levels of which are associated with protection against ischemic heart disease (162). In the Lipid Research Study (225), mean serum tryglyceride rose by 26%, total serum cholesterol fell by 4%, HDL-cholesterol increased by 10%, while LDL-cholesterol fell by 11%. Larger changes in the cholesterol fractions have been reported (228). However, not all studies have shown a positive effect of estrogen on cardiovascular disease (236) and the issue requires detailed study.

In that review of data from the Framingham

study, it was suggested that estrogens had significant detrimental effects on cardiovascular morbidity, including an increased incidence of stroke among non-smokers. There was a 50% increase in risk of cardiovascular morbidity and a two-fold increased risk of cerebrovascular disease. These data clearly conflict with those of other studies quoted above, which in general suggested a 50% *reduction* in risk of cardiovascular disease (15). The reasons for discrepancy between these studies and that from the Framingham database are not immediately clear. Differences in analytic techniques exist and perhaps account for some of the discrepancy, but this appears, at least superficially, to be insufficient by itself. As a general issue it is of concern that epidemiologic studies can produce such widely different conclusions.

Recently, a negative relationship between the onset of rheumatoid arthritis and previous use of estrogens as replacement therapy was reported from the Netherlands (220), similar to an effect previously suggested for the oral contraceptive (257). Pregnancy has also been reported to improve the symptoms of rheumathoid arthritis (218). Again however, negative data are available from the literature (138) and the issue is far from decided. If the effect is real, it is entirely possible that this is mediated through estrogen interaction with the immune system since estrogens are known to modulate both T cell and macrophage activity (90).

OSTEOPOROSIS IN MEN

No examination of the effects of sex steroids on bone would be complete without evaluation of their role in osteoporosis among the male population. Since osteoporotic fractures are significantly but variably more common among women than men (194), the difference is often assumed, although far from completely proven, to be due to menopause. The documented effects of estrogen withdrawal at this time, together with the observed prevention of bone loss by reintroduction of estrogen, of course support this hypothesis, and lead to the conclusion that the fracture differences be-

tween the sexes are, therefore, consequent upon menopause. If effects of sex hormones are indeed so overwhelming, one might expect that in situations in which sex hormone production is reduced in men, there will be significant, if not dramatic consequences for the skeleton.

That testicular failure leads to increased frequency of osteoporotic fractures was an original suggestion of Fuller Albright (8). One more recent study, evaluated 105 men with vertebral fractures, and used men presenting with Paget's disease as a control population. Of importance in the development of osteoporosis in that population were underlying disease (with cortisol administration) and gastrectomy. Hypogonadism was present in 7 by biochemistry, and in further 12 by history, although with normal testosterone levels. Alcohol and cigarette consumption was also higher in the osteoporotic group, findings supported by other studies (203). Alcohol has multiple biochemical effects which might interfere with skeletal homeostasis, but also reduces circulating levels of testosterone, both in the short and longer term (9,86), and might therefore contribute to the effects of relative hypogonadism.

In a more structured study to test the same hypothesis, Greenspan et al. (242) evaluated bone mass in 18 men who had prolactin-secreting pituitary tumors. Bone mass in both the axial and peripheral skeleton was reduced in the hyperprolactinemic group, all except one of whom were hypogonadal when originally seen, hypogonadism being as common in the male with such microadenomata as in the female (44). An increase in bone mass was seen after serum testosterone was corrected (210). Marked histological improvement in transilial biopsy appearance had been reported previously in a hypogonadal male treated with testosterone (16). Thus, since hypogonadism among the elderly population of males is a subtle and often missed diagnosis, it would seem likely that this will contribute to the incidence of osteoporotic fracture in this population (70). Curiously one report suggests that calcitonin levels may be lower in male osteoporotic subjects (69), and shows a linear relationship between circulating calcitonin and testosterone. While this is of interest since a role for calcitonin in the mechanism of estrogen action on bone is being debated, it requires further study.

In contrast, osteoporosis among young men may have a completely different etiology, and a significant proportion of these cases have underlying renal lithiasis (26,179). More recent data suggest that here alcohol may also play a pathogenetic role (62) as may cigarette consumption. The role of hypogonadism in that series of patients was not stressed. However, in view of the effects of alcohol on testicular function, the particular issue should be re-evaluated. Nonetheless the relationship, in non-alcoholics, between nephrolithiasis and osteoporosis seems real, though the combination is a comparatively rare occurrence.

In Klinefelter's syndrome, also associated with hypogonadism, there is reported to be high incidence of low bone mass (199) and osteoporosis. This has been inadequately studied thus far, and the relationship of osteoporosis to the genetic defect or the resultant hypogonadism is not clear. As noted, in gonadal agenesis in females the skeletal problem may precede the normal age of puberty, and not totally be dependent on the adult hypogonadal state.

Addendum

Two recent studies reported at the 1987 meeting of the American Society for Bone and Mineral Research have provided strong evidence that bone cells do indeed contain estrogen receptors. (*J. Bone Mineral Res.*, 2:(Suppl. 1), June 1987, Abstr. 237,238). Komm et al. found that a rat osteogenic sarcoma cell line showed specific binding to [^{125}I] 17β-estradiol and the cytosol contained an mRNA to estrogen receptor. Ericksen et al. showed that cultured osteoblast-like cells from normal human bone cells had specific binding of [^{3}H]17β-estradiol using a new assay for functional estrogen receptors. Also, estrogen treatment *in vitro* induced the formation of progesterone receptors, one of the most characteristic biologic responses of target tissues to estrogen action. Collectively, these data suggest that cells of the osteoblast lineage respond to estrogen di-

rectly through a classical receptor mediated mechanism and that bone may be a typical target tissue for estrogen, similar to endometrium and breast acinar tissue. If so, this provides a strong rationale for using estrogen replacement therapy for maintaining bone cell health in postmenopausal women. *(Editor's note)*

REFERENCES

1. Abdalla, H., Hart, D.M., and Lindsay, R. (1984): Differential bone loss and effects of long-term estrogen therapy according to time of introduction of therapy after oophorectomy. In: *Osteoporosis*, edited by C. Christiansen, et al., pp. 621-624. Aalborg Stiftsbogtrykkeri, Glostrup, Denmark.
2. Abdalla, H., Hart, D.M., Lindsay, R., Leggate, I., and Hooke, A. (1985): Prevention of bone loss in postmenopausal women by norethisterone. *Obstet. Gynecol.*, 6:789–792.
3. Abraham, G.E., and Maroulis, G.B. (1975): Effect of exogenous estrogens on serum pregnenolone, cortisol, and androgens in postmenopausal women. *Obstet. Gynecol.*, 45:271–274.
4. Adam, S., Williams, V., and Vessey, M.P. (1981): Cardiovascular disease and hormone replacement treatment: A pilot case-control study. *Brit. Med. J.*, 282:1277–1278.
5. Aitken, J.M., Hart, D.M., Anderson, J.B., Lindsay, R., and Smith, D.A. (1973): Osteoporosis after oophorectomy for non-malignant disease. *Brit. Med. J.*, i:325–328.
6. Albright, F. (1947): The effect of hormones on osteogenesis in man. *Recent Prog. Horm. Res.*, 1:293–353.
7. Albright, F., Bloomberg, F., and Smith, P.H. (1940): Postmenopausal osteoporosis. *Trans. Assoc. Am. Phys.*, 55:298–305.
8. Albright, F., and Reifenstein, E.C., Jr. (1948): Metabolic bone disease: osteoporosis. In: *The Parathyroid Glands and Metabolic Bone Disease*, edited by F. Albright, and E.C. Reifenstein, pp. 145–204. Williams & Wilkins, Baltimore.
9. Anderson, R.A., Willis, B.R., Oswald, C., Reddy, J.M., Boyle, S.A., and Zanneveld, L.J.D. (1980): Hormonal imbalance and changes in testicular morphology induced by chronic ingestion of ethanol. *Biochem. Pharmacol.*, 29:1409–1419.
10. Anderson, F.S., Transbol, I., and Christiansen, C. (1982) Is cigarette smoking a promotor of the menopause? *Acta Med. Scand.*, 212:137–139. (1968).
11. Armelagos, G.J. (1968): Disease in Ancient Nubia. Changes in disease patterns from 350 B.C. to A.D. 1400 demonstrate the interaction of biology and culture. *Science*, 163:255–259.
12. Arnett, T., and Dempster, D. (1986): Effect of pH on bone resorption by rat osteoclasts in vitro. *Endocrinology*, 119:119–124.
13. Arnold, J.S., Bartley, M.H., Tont, S.A., and Jenkins, D.P. (1966): Skeletal changes in aging and disease. *Clin. Orthop. Rel. Res.*, 49:17–38.
14. Aylward, M., Maddock, J., Parker, A., Protheroe,

D.A. and Ward, A. (1978): Endometrial factors under treatment with oestrogen and oestrogen/ progestogen combinations. *Postgrad. Med. J.*, 54(2):74–81.

15. Bain, C., Willet, W., Hennekins, C.H., et al. (1981): Use of postmenopausal hormones and risk of myocardial infarction. *Circulation*, 64:42–46.

16. Baran, D.T., Bergfeld, M.A., Teitelbaum, S.L., and Avioli, L.V. (1976): Effect of testosterone therapy on bone formation in an osteoporotic hypogonadal male. *Calcif. Tiss. Res.*, 26:103–106.

17. Barker, K.L.H., and Warren J.C. (1966): Estrogen control of carbohydrate metabolism in the rat uterus: pathways of glucose metabolism. *Endocrinology*, 78:1205–1212.

18. Barlow, D.H., Beastall, G.H., Abdalla, H.I., Elias-Jones, J., Lindsay, R., and Hart, D.M. (1985): Effect of long-term hormone replacement on plasma prolactin concentrations in women after oophorectomy. *Brit. Med. J.*, 290:589–591.

19. Barnett, E., and Nordin, B.E.C. (1960): The radiological diagnosis of osteoporosis: a new approach. *Clin. Radiol.*, ii:166–174.

20. Barr, D.G. (1974): Bone deficiency in Turner's syndrome measured by metacarpal dimensions. *Arch. Dis. Child*, 49(10):821–822.

21. Bartizal, F.J., Coulam, C.B., Gaffey, T.A., Ryan, R.J., and Riggs, B.L. (1976): Impaired binding of ostradiol to vaginal mucosal cells in postmenopausal osteoporosis. *Calcif. Tiss. Res.*, 21:412–416.

22. Beals, R.K. (1973): Orthopedic aspects of the XO (Turner's) Syndrome. *Clin. Orthop. Rel. Res.*, 97:19–30.

23. Bloom, R.A., and Laws, J.W. (1970): Humeral cortical thickness as an index of osteoporosis in women. *Brit. J. Radiol.*, 43:522–527.

24. Body, J.J., and Heath, H., III. (1983): Effects of age, sex, calcium and total thyroidectomy on circulating monomeric calcitonin concentrations. *Calcif. Tiss. Res.*, 35(6):A45.

25. Bogdonoff, M.D., Shock, N.W., and Parsons, J. (1954): The effects of stilbestrol on the retention of nitrogen, calcium, phosphorus and potassium in aged males with and without osteoporosis. *J. Gerontol.*, 9:262–275.

26. Bordier, P.J., Mirouet, L., and Hcoco, D. (1973): Young adult osteoporosis. *Clin. Endocrinol, Metab.*, 2:277–292.

27. Bouillon, R., Van Assche, F., Van Baelen, H., Heynes, W., and DeMoor, P. (1981): Influence of the vitamin D-binding protein on the serum concentrations of 1, 25-dihydroxyvitamin D₃. Significance of the free 1,25-dihydroxyvitamin D₃ concentration. *J. Clin. Invest.*, 67(3):589–596.

28. Brincat, M., Moniz, C.J., Studd, J.W.W., Darby, A., Magos, A., Embure, Y., and Vers, I.E. (1985): Long-term effect of the memopause and sex hormones on skin thickness. *Brit. J. Obstet. Gynecol.*, 92:256–259.

29. Brinton, L.A., Hoover, R.N., Sziclo, M., et al. (1981): Menopausal estrogen use and risk of breast cancer. *Cancer*, 47:2517–2522.

30. Brody, S., Carlstrom, K., Lagrelius, A., Lunell, N.O., and Rosenborg, L. (1982): Adrenocortical

31. Brown, D.M., Jowsey, J., Bradford, D.S., and Brincra, T. (1974): Osteoporosis in ovarian dysgenesis. *J. Pediatr.*, 84:816–820.'

32. Bruns, P. (1882): Die allgemeine hehre von den Knockenbruchen, *Deutsche Chwurgie*, 27:1–400.

33. Budoff, P.W., and Sommers, S.C. (1979): Estrogen progesterone therapy in postmenopausal women. *J. Reprod. Med.*, 22:241–247.

34. Burch, J.C., Byrd, B.F., and Vaughn, W.K. (1974): The effects of long-term estrogen on hysterectomized women. *Am. J. Obstet. Gynecol.*, 118:778–782.

35. Burch, J.C., Byrd, B.F., and Vaughn, W.K. (1975): Effects of long-term estrogen administration to women following hysterectomy. *Front Horm. Res.*, 3:208–214.

36. Burke, R.E., and Gaffney, E.V. (1978): Prolactin can stimulate general protein synthesis in human breast cancer cells (MCF7) in long-term culture. *Life Sci.*, 23:901–906.

37. Bush, T.L., and Barrett-Connor, E. (1985): Noncontraceptive estrogen use and cardiovascular disease. *Epidemiol. Rev.*, 7:80–104.

38. Bush, T.L., Cowan, L.D., Barrett-Connor, E., Criqui, M.H., Kason, J.M., Wallace R.B., Tyroler, A., and Rifkind, B.M. (1983): Estrogen use and all-cause mortality. *J. Am. Med. Assoc.*, 249:903–906.

39. Campbell, S., McQueen, J., Minardi, J., and Whitehead, M.I. (1978): The modifying effect of progestogen on the response of the postmenopausal endometrium to exogenous oestrogens. *Postgrad. Med. J.*, 54:59–64.

40. Cannigia, A., Gennasi, C., Borella, G., Benant, M., Cesari, L., Paggi, C., and Escobar, C. (1970): Intestinal absorption of calcium -47 after treatment with oral estrogen and gestagen in senile osteoporosis. *Brit. Med. J.*, 4:30–32.

41. Cann, C.E., Genant, H.K., Kolb, F.O., and Ettinger, B. (1985): Qualitative computed tomography for prediction of vertebral fracture risk. *Bone*, 6:1–7.

42. Cann, C.E., Martin, M.C., and Genant, H.K. (1984): Decreased spinal mineral content in amenorrheic women. *J. Am. Med. Assoc.*, 251:626–629.

43. Caputo, C.B., Meadows, D., and Raisz, L.G. (1976): Failure of estrogens and androgens to inhibit bone resorption in tissue culture. *Endocrinology*, 98:1065–1068.

44. Carter, J.N., Tyson, J.E., Tolis, G., VanVliet, S., Faiman, C., and Friesen, H.G. (1981): Prolactin secreting tumors and hypogonadism in 22 men. *N. Engl. J. Med.*, 299:847–852.

45. Chalmers, J., and Ho, K.C. (1970): Geographical variations in senile osteoporosis: the association with physical activity. *J. Bone Joint Surg.*, 52B:667–675.

46. Chambers, T.J., and Moore, A. (1978): The sensitivity of insolated osteoclasts to morphological transformation by calcitonin. *J. Clin. Endocrinol. Metab.*, 57:819–824.

47. Chen, T.L., and Feldman, D. (1978): Distinction

between α-fetoprotein and intracellular estrogen receptors: evidence against presence of estradiol receptors in rat bone. *Endocrinology*, 102:236–240.

48. Chesnut, C.H., III, Baylink, D.T., Sisom, K., Nelp, W.B., and Roos, B.A. (1980): Basal plasma immunoreactive calcitonin in postmenopausal osteoporosis. *Metabolism*, 29:559–562.

49. Chesnut, C.H., III, Ivey, J.L., Gruger, H.E., Mathews, M., Nelp, W.B., Sisom, K., Baylink, D.J. (1983): Stanozolol in postmenopausal osteoporosis: Therapeutic efficacy and possible mechanisms of action. *Metabolism*, 32:577–580.

50. Christiansen, C., Christiansen, M.S., McNair, P. (1980): Prevention of early postmenopausal bone loss: conducted 2-year study in 315 normal females. *Europ. J. Clin. Invest.*, 10:273–279.

51. Christiansen, C., Christiansen, M.S., and Transbol, I. (1981): Bone mass in postmenopausal women after withdrawal of estrogen/gestagen replacement therapy. *Lancet*, i:459–461.

52. Christiansen, C., Riis, B.T., Nilas, L., Rodbro, P., and Deftos, L. (1985): Uncoupling of bone formation and resorption by combined oestrogen and progestagen therapy in postmenopausal osteoporosis. *Lancet*, ii:800–801.

53. Christiansen, C., and Rodbro, P. (1983): Does postmenopausal bone loss respond to estrogen replacement therapy independent of bone loss rate. *Calcif. Tiss. Int.*, 35:720–722.

54. Cohn, S.H., Aloia, J.F., Vaswani, A.N., Zanzi, I., Vestsky, D., and Ellis, K.J. (1982): In: *Osteoporosis*, edited by J. Menczel, et al., pp 33–43, John Wiley & Sons Ltd., Chichester, 1982.

55. Conte, F.A., Grumbach, M.M., and Kaplan, S.L. (1975): A disphasic pattern of gonadotropin secretion in patients with the syndrome of gonadal dysgenesis. *J. Clin. Endocrinol. Metab.*, 40(4):670–674.

56. Daniell, H.W. (1976): Osteoporosis of the slender smoker. *Arch Intern. Med.*, 136:298–304.

57. Davidson, B.J., Riggs, B.L., Wahner, W.H., and Judd, H.L. (1983): Endogenous cortisol and sex steroids in patients with osteoporotic spinal fractures. *Obstet, Gynecol.*, 61:275–278.

58. Davidson, B.J., Riggs, B.L., Coulam, C.B., and Toft, D.O. (1980): Concentration of cylesolic estragen receptors in patients with postmenopausal osteoporosis. *Am. J. Obstet. Gynecol.*, 136:430–433.

59. Davis, M.E., Lanzl, L.H., and Cox, A.B. (1970): Detection, prevention and retardation of postmenopausal osteoporosis. *Obstet. Gynecol.*, 36:187–198.

60. Deftos, L.J., Weisman, M.H., and Williams, G.W. (1981): Influence of age and sex on plasma calcitonin in human beings. *N. Engl. J. Med.*, 302:1351–1353.

61. Delmas, P.D., Stenner, D., Wahner, H.W., Mann, K.G., Riggs, B.L. (1983): Increase in serum bone gamma-corboxyglutamic acid protein with aging in women: implications for the mechanism of age-related bone loss. *J. Clin. Invest.*, 71:1316–1321.

62. DeVernejoul, M.C., Bielakoh, T., Heire, M., Gueris, J., Hott, M., Modrowski, D., Kunitz, D., Miravet, L., and Ryckewaert A. (1983): Evidence

for defective osteoblastic function: A role for alcohol and tobacco consumption in osteoporosis in middle-aged men. *Clin. Orthop. Rel. Res.*, 179:107–115.

63. Donaldson, A., and Nassim, J.R. (1954): The artificial menopause with particular reference to the occurrence of spinal porosis. *Brit. Med. J.*, i:1228–1230.

64. Drinkwater, B.D., Nilson, K.L., and Chesnut, C.H., III (1984): Bone mineral content of amenorrheic and eumenorrheic athletes. *N. Eng. J. Med.*, 311:277–281.

65. Engel, E., and Forbes, A.P. (1965): Cytogenetic and clinical findings in 48 patients with congenitally defective or absent ovaries. *Medicine*, 44:135–164.

66. Ettinger, B., Genant, H.K., and Cann, C.E. (1985): Long-term estrogen therapy prevents bone loss and fracture. *Ann. Intern. Med.*, 102:319–324.

67. Fanstat, T. (1962): Hormonal burrs for collagen bundle generation in uterine stoma: extracellular studies of uterus. *Endocrinology*, 71:878–887.

68. Fogelman, I., Poser, J.W., Smith, M.L., Hart, D.M., and Bevan, J.A. (1984): Alterations in skeletal metabolism following oophorectomy. In: *Osteoporosis*, edited by C. Christiansen, et al., pp. 519–522. Aalborg Stiftsbogtrykkeri, Glostrup, Denmark.

69. Foresta, C., Busnardo, B., Ruzza, G., Zanattia, G., and Mioni, R. (1983): Lower calcitonin levels in young hypogonadic men with osteoporosis. *Horm. Metab. Res.*, 15:206–207.

70. Foresta, C., Ruzza, G., Mioni, R., et al. (1984): Osteoporosis and decline of gonadal function in the elderly male. *Horm. Res.*, 19:18–22.

71. Friedman, J., and Raisz, L.G. (1965): Thyrocalcitonin: inhibitor of bone resorption in tissue culture. *Science*, 150:1465–1466.

72. Frost, H.M. (1973): Bone remodeling and its relationship to metabolic bone disease. Charles C Thomas, Springfield, Ill.

73. Frumar, A., Moldsin, D., Geola, F., Shamamki, I., Talaryh, I., Deftos, L., and Judd, H. (1980): Relationship of fasting urinary calcium to circulatory estrogen and body weight in postmenopausal women. *J. Clin. Endocrinol.*, 50:70–75.

74. Galan, F.G., Rogers, R.M., and Girgis, S.I. (1981): Immunochemical characterization and distribution of calcitonin in the lizard. *Acta Endocrinol.*, 97:427–432.

75. Gallagher, J.C., Riggs, B.L., and DeLuca, H.F. (1980): Effect of estrogen on calcium absorption and serum vitamin D metabolites in postmenopausal osteoporosis. *J. Clin. Endocrinol. Metab.*, 51:1359–1364.

76. Gambrell, R.D. (1979): The role of hormones in the etiology of breast and endometrial cancer. *Acta Obstet. Gynecol. Scand.* (Suppl.), 88:73–81.

77. Gambrell, R.D. (1982): The menopause: Benefits and risks of estrogen-progesterone replacement therapy. *Fertil. Steril.*, 37:457–474.

78. Garn, S.M. (1981): The phenomenon of bone formation and bone loss. In: *Osteoporosis, Recent Advances in Pathogenesis and Treatment*. Edited by

H.F. DeLuca, et al., pp. 1–16. University Park Press, Baltimore.

79. Garn, S.M., Nagy, J.M., and Sandusky, S.T. (1972): Differential sexual dimorphism in bone parameters of subjects of European and African ancestry. *Am. J. Phys. Anthropol.*, 37:127–130.

80. Garn, S.M., Rohmann, C.G., and Wagner, B. Bone loss as a general phenomenon in man. *Fed. Proc.*, 26:1729–1736.

81. Garraway, W.M., Stauffer, R.N., Kurland, L.T., and O'Fallon, W.M. (1979): Limb fractures in a defined population. *Mayo Clin. Proc.*, 54:701–707.

82. Genant, H.K., Cann, C.E., and Ettinger, B. (1984): Quantitative computed tomography for spinal mineral assessment. In: *Osteoporosis*, edited by C.E. Christiansen, et al., pp. 65–72. Aalborg Stiftsbogtrykkeri, Glostrup, Denmark.

83. Genant, H.K., Cann, C.E., Ettinger, B., and Gordon, G.S. (1982): Quantitative computed tomography of vertebral spongiosa: a sensitive method for detecting early bone loss after oophorectomy. *Ann. Intern. Med.*, 97:699–705.

84. Goldsmith, N., and Johnston, J.O. (1975): Bone mineral: Effects of oral contraceptives, pregnancy and lactation. *J. Bone Joint Surg.*, 57A:657–668.

85. Gonzalez, E.R. (1982): Premature bone loss found in some nonmenstruating sportswomen. *J. Am. Med. Assoc.*, 248:513–514.

86. Gordon, G.G., Altman, K., Southren, A.L., Rubin, E, and Lieber, C.S. (1976): Effect of alcohol (eythanol) administration on sex-hormone metabolism in normal men. *N. Engl. J. Med.*, 295:793–797.

87. Gordan, G.S., Picchi, J., and Roof, B.S. Antifracture efficacy of long-term estrogens for osteoporosis. *Trans. Assoc. Am. Phys.*, 86:326–332.

88. Gray, L.A., Sr., Christopherson, W.M., and Hoover, R.N. (1977): Estrogens and endometrial carcinoma. *Obstet. Gynecol. Surg.*, 32(7):619–621.

89. Greenberg, C., Kirkreja, S.C., Bowser, E.N., Hargis, G.K., Henderson, W.T., and Williams, G.A. Effects of estradiol and progesterone on calcitonin secretion. *Endocrinology*, 118:2594–2598.

90. Grossman, J.C. (1984): Regulation of the immune system by sex steroids. *Endocrinol. Rev.*, 5:435–455.

91. Gusberg, S.B. (1976): The individual at high-risk for endometrial cancer. *Am. J. Ostet. Gynecol.*, 126:535–542.

92. Hammond, C.B., Jelovser, R., and Lee, K.L., (1979): Effects of long-term estrogen replacement therapy. II. Neoplasia. *Am. J. Obstet. Gynecol.*, 133:537–547.

93. Heaney, R.P. (1965): A unified concept of osteoporosis. *Am. J. Med.*, 39:377–380.

94. Heaney, R.P. (1986): Calcium, bone health, and osteoporosis. In: *Bone and Mineral Research, vol 4*, edited by W.A. Peck, pp. 255–301.

95. Heaney, R.P., Recker, R.R., and Saville, P.D. Calcium balance and calcium requirements in middle-aged women. *Am. J. Clin. Nutr.*, 30:1603–1611.

96. Heaney, R.P., Recker, R.R., and Saville, P.D. (1978): Menopausal changes in calcium balance

97. Heaney, R.P., Recker, R.R., and Saville, P.D. Menopausal changes in bone remodeling. *J. Lab. Clin. Med.*, 92:964–970.

98. Hemsell, D.L., Spodin, J.M., Brenner, P.F., Siiteri, P.K., and MacDonald, P.C. (1974): Plasma precursors of estrogen. II. Correlation of the extent of conversion of plasma androstenedione to estrone with age. *J. Clin. Endocrinol. Metab.*, 38:476–479.

99. Heath, H.H., III, and Sizemore, G.W. (1982): Radioimmunoassay for calcitonin. *Clin. Chem.*, 28:1219–1226.

100. Henneman, D.H. (1968): Effect of estrogen in vivo and in vitro collagen biosynthesis and maturation in old and young female guinea pigs. *Endocrinology*, 83:678–690.

101. Henneman, P.H., and Wallach, S. (1957): A review of the prolonged use of estrogens and androgens in postmenopausal and senile osteoporosis. *Arch. Intern. Med.*, 100:705–709.

102. Hillyard, C.J., Stevenson, J.C., and MacIntyre, I. (1978): Relative deficiency of plasma-calcitonin in women. *Lancet*, i:961–962.

103. Hoover, R., Gray, L.A., and Cole, P., et al. (1976): Menopausal estrogens and breast cancer. *N. Engl. J. Med.*, 295:401–405.

104. Horsman, A., Gallagher, J.C., Simpson, M., and Nordin, B.E.C. (1977): Prospective trial of estrogen and calcium in postmenopausal women. *Brit. Med. J.*, 2:789–792.

105. Horsman, A., James, M., and Francis, R. (1983): The effect of estrogen dose on postmenopausal bone loss. *N. Engl. J. Med.*, 309:1405–1407.

106. Horsman, A., Nordin, B.E., and Crilly, R.G. (1979): Effect on bone of withdrawal of oestrogen therapy. *Lancet*, ii:33.

107. Horwitz, R.I., and Feinstein, M.D. (1978): Alternative analytic methods for case-control studies of estrogens and endometrial cancer. *N. Engl. J. Med.*, 299(20):1089–1094.

108. Hsueh, A.J.W., Peck, E.J.W., and Clark, J.H. (1975): Progesterone antagonism of the oestrogen receptor and oestrogen-induced uterine growth. *Nature*, 254:337–339.

109. Hutchinson, T.A., Polansky, J.M., and Feinstein, A.R. (1979): Postmenopausal oestrogens protect against fracture of hip and distal radius. *Lancet*, ii:705–709.

110. Jasani, C., Nordin, B.E.C., Smith, D.A., and Swanson, I. (1965): Spinal osteoporosis and the menopause. *Proc. Roy. Soc. Med.*, 58:441–444.

111. Jensen, J., Christiansen, C., and Rodbro, P. (1985): Cigarette smoking, estrogens and bone loss during hormone replacement therapy early after menopause. *N. Engl. J. Med.*, 313:973–975.

112. Jensen, J., Riis, B.J., Hummer, L., and Christiansen, C. (1985): The effects of age and body composition on circulating serum oestrogens androstenedione after the menopause. *Brit. J. Obstet. Gynecol.*, 92:260–265.

113. Jick, H., Watkins, R.N., Hunter, J.R., Dinan, B.J., Madsen, S., Rothman, K.J., Walker, A.M. (1979): Replacement estrogens and endometrial

cancer. *N. Engl. J. Med.*, 300(5):218–222.

114. Jick, H., Watkins, R.W., and Hunter, T.R., et al. (1980): Replacement estrogen and breast cancer. *Am. J. Epidemiol.*, 112:586–594.

115. Johnston, C.C., Hui, S.L., Witt, R.M., Appledorn, R., Baker, R.S., and Longcope, C. (1985): Early menopausal changes in bone mass and sex steroids. *J. Clin. Endocrinol. Metab.*, 61:905–911.

116. Kanders, B., Lindsay, R., Dempster, D.W., Markhard, L., Valiquette, G. (1984): Determinants of bone mass in young healthy women. In: *Osteoporosis*, edited by C. Christiansen et al., pp. 337–340. Aalborg Stiftsbogtrykkeri, Glostrup, Denmark.

117. Kao, K.Y., Hitt, W.E., and McGavack, T.H. (1985): Connective tissue 13. Effect of estradiol benzoate upon collagen synthesis by sponge biopsy connective tissue. *Proc. Soc. Exp. Biol. Med.*, 119:364–367.

118. Kao, K.Y.T., Hitt, W.E., Bush, A.T., and MacGavack, T.H. (1964): Connective tissue XII. Stimulating effects of estrogens on collagen synthesis in rat uterine slices. *Proc. Soc. Exp. Biol. Med.*, 117:86–97.

119. Klibanski, A., Neer, R.M., Beitins, I.Z., Ridgway, C., Zervas, N.T., and MacArthur, J. (1980): Decreased bone density in hyperprolactenemic women. *N. Engl. J. Med.*, 303:1511–1514.

120. Kreiger, N., Kelsey, J.L., and Holford, T.R. (1982): An epidemiological study of hip fracture in postmenopausal women. *Am. J. Epidemiol.*, 116:141–148.

121. Krolner, B., and Nielsen, S.P. (1982): Bone mineral content of the lumbar spine in normal and osteoporotic women: cross sectional and longitudinal studies. *Clin. Sci.*, 62:329–336.

122. Leichter, I., Wermreb, A., Hazan, G., Loewinger, E., Robin, G.C., Steinberg, R., Mencyer, J., and Makin, M. (1981): The effect of age and sex on bone density, bone mineral content and cortical index. *Clin. Orthop. Rel. Res.*, 156:232–239.

123. Lindquist, O., and Bernstein, C. (1979): Menopausal age in relation to smoking. *Acta Med. Scand.*, 205:73–77.

124. Lindberg, J.S., Fears, W.B., and Hunt, M.M. (1984): Exercised induced amenorrhea and bone density. *Ann. Intern. Med.*, 101:647–649.

125. Lindsay, R. (1984): Osteoporosis and its relationship to estrogen. *Contemp. Obstet. Gynecol.*, 63:201–224.

126. Lindsay, R., Dempster, D.W., Clemens, T., Herrington, B., and Wilt, S. (1984): Incidence cost and risk factors of fracture of the proximal femur in the USA. In: *Osteoporosis*, edited by C., Christiansen, et al., pp. 311–316. Aalborg Stiftsbogtrykkeri, Glostrup, Denmark.

127. Lindsay, R., Hart, D.M., MacLean, A., Clark, A.C., Kraszowski, A., and Garwood, J. (1978): Bone response to termination of oestrogen treatment. *Lancet,* i:1325–1327.

128. Lindsay, R., Hart, D.M., MacLean, A., Garwood, J., Clark, A.C., and Kraszewski, A. (1979): Bone loss during oestriol therapy in postmenopausal women. *Maturitas*, 1:279–285.

129. Lindsay, R., Aitken, J.M., Anderson, J.B., Hart, D.M., MacDonald, E.B., and Clark, A.C. (1976): Long-term prevention of postmenopausal osteoporosis by oestrogen. *Lancet,* i:1038–1041.

130. Lindsay, R., and Sweeney, A. (1976): Urinary cyclic-AMP in osteoporosis. *Scott. Med. J.,* 21:231.

131. Lindsay, R., Hart, D.M., Purdie, P., Ferguson, M.M., Clark, A.C., and Kraszewski, A. (1978): Comparative effects of oestrogen and a progestogen on bone loss in postmenopausal women. *Clin. Sci. Mol. Med.*, 54:193–195.

132. Lindsay, R., Coutts, J.R.T., and Hart, D.M. (1977): The effect of endogenous oestrogen on plasma and mineral calcium and phosphate in oophorectomized women. *Clin. Endocrinol.*, 6:87–93.

133. Lindsay, R., Hart, D.M., Forrest, C., and Baird, C. (1980): Prevention of spinal osteoporosis in oophorectomized women. *Lancet*, ii:1151–1154.

134. Lindsay, R., Coutts, J.R.T., Sweeney, A., and Hart, D.M. Endogenous oestrogen and bone loss following oophorectomy. *Calcif. Tissue. Res.*, 22:213–216.

135. Lindsay, R., Hart, D.M., and Clark, D.M. (1984): The minimum effective dose of estrogen for prevention of postmenopausal bone loss. *Obstet. Gynecol.*, 63:759–763.

136. Lindsay, R., Herrington, B.S., and Tohme, J.F. (1986): Reproductive history and bone mass in women. *J. Bone Min. Res.*, 1 (Suppl. i):248.

137. Linnel, S.L., Stager, M.M., and Blue, P.W. Bone mineral content and menstrual regularity in female runners. *Med. Sci. Sports Exec.*, 16:343–348.

138. Linos, A., Washington, J.W., O'Fallon, W.M., et al. (1983): Case-control study of rheumatoid arthritis and prior use of oral contraceptives. *Lancet*, i:1299–1300.

139. Liskova, M. (1976): Influence of estrogens on bone resorption in organ culture. *Calcif. Tissue. Res.*, 22:207–218.

140. Little, K. (1973): *Bone Behavior*. Academic Press, London, N.Y.

141. Longcope, C., Jatee, W., and Griffing, G. (1981): Production rates of androgens and oestrogens in postmenopausal women. *Maturitas*, 3:215–223.

142. MacDonald, T.W., Annegers, J.F., O'Fallon, W.M., Dockerty, M.B., Malkasian, G.D., Jr., and Kurland, L.T. (1977): Exogenous estrogen and endometrial carcinoma: case-control and incidence study. *Am. J. Obstet. Gynecol.*, 127(6):572–580.

143. MacMahon, B., Trichopoulos, D., Cole, P., and Brown, T. (1982): Cigarette smoking and urinary estrogens. *N. Engl. J. Med.*, 307:1062–1065.

144. Mack, T.M., Pike, M.C., Henderson, B.E., Pfeffer, R.I., Gerkins, V.R., Arthur, M., and Brown, S.E. (1976): Estrogens and endometrial cancer in a retirement community. *N. Engl. J. Med.*, 294:1262–1267.

145. Madsen, M. (1977): Vertebral and peripheral bone mineral content by photon absorptiometry. *Invest. Radiol.*, 12:185–188.

146. Manologas, S.C., and Anderson, D.C. (1978): Detection of high affinity glucocorticoid binding in rat

bone. *J. Endocrinol.*, 36:379–380.

147. Manologas, S.C., Anderson, D.C., and Lindsay, R. (1979): Adrenal steroids and the development of osteoporosis in oophorectomised women. *Lancet*, ii:597–600.

148. Manwol, S.E., and Menan, K.M.J. (1977): Changes in reproductive hormone secretion during the climacteric and postmenopausal periods. *Clin. Obstet. Gynecol.*, 20:113–122.

149. Marshall, D.H., Crilly, R.C., and Nordin, B.E.C. (1959): Plasma androsteredione and oestrone levels in normal and osteoporotic postmenopausal women. *J. Am. Med. Assoc.*, 171:1637–1642.

150. Marshall, H., and Nordin, B.E.C. (1977): The effect of 1-hydroxy-alpha-vitamin D^3 with and without oestrogen on calcium balance in postmenopausal women. *Clin. Endocrinol.*, 7 (Suppl.):159s–168s.

151. Marcus, R., Cann, C., and Madvig, D. (1985): Menstrual function and bone mass in elite women distance runners. *Ann. Intern. Med.*, 102:158–163.

152. Maschak, C.A., and Lobo, R.A. (1985): Estrogen therapy and hypertension. *J. Reprod. Med.*, 30 (Suppl.):805–813.

153. Mazess, R.B. (1982): Advances in total body and regional bone mineral by dual-photon absorptiometry. In: *Osteoporosis*, edited by J. Menczel, et al., pp. 80–86. John Wiley & Sons Ltd., Chichester.

154. Maziere, B., Kuntz, D., and Dughesnay, M. (1982): In vivo analysis of bone calcium by local neutron activation of the hand in postmenopausal osteoporosis. In: *Osteoporosis*, edited by J. Menczel et al., pp. 117–125. John Wiley & Sons Ltd., Chichester.

155. McKay, Hart, D., Lindsay, R., and Purdie, D. (1978): Vascular complications of long-term oestrogen therapy. *Front. Horm. Res.*, 5:174–191.

156. Meema, H.E. (1962): The occurrence of cortical bone atrophy in old age and in osteoporosis. *J. Canad. Assoc. Radiol.*, 13:27–32.

157. Meema, H.E. (1963): Cortical bone atrophy and osteoporosis as a manifestation of aging. *Am. J. Roentgenol.*, 89:1287–1295.

158. Meema, H.E. (1966): Menopausal and aging changes in muscle mass and bone mineral content. *J. Bone Joint Surg.*, 48A:1138–1144.

159. Meema, H.E., Bunker, M.L., and Meema, S. (1965): Loss of compact bone due to menopause. *Obstet. Gynecol.*, 26:333–343.

160. Meldrum, D.R., Davidson, B., Taleryn, I., and Judd, H. (1981): Changes in circulatory steroids with aging in postmenopasual women. *Obstet. Gynecol.*, 57:624–628.

161. Milhaud, G., Benezech-Lefevre, M., and Mowkhtar, M.S. (1978): Deficient calcitonin response to calcium stimulation in postmenopausal osteoporosis. *Lancet*, i:475–478.

162. Miller, G.J., and Miller, M.E. (1975): Plasmahigh-density-lipoprotein concentration and development of ischemic heart disease. *Lancet*, 1:16–19.

163. Mishell, D.R., Jr. (1985): Estrogen replacement therapy: measuring benefit vs. cardiovascular risk. *J. Reprod. Med.*, 30 (Suppl.):795–826.

164. Morimoto, S., Tsuj, M., and Okada, Y. (1980): The effects of oestrogen on human calcitonin secretion after calcium infusion in elderly subjects. *Clin. Endocrinol.*, 13:135–143.

165. Mulder, H., Hackeng, W.H.L., and Silberbusch, J. (1979): Racial difference in serum calcitonin. *Lancet*, ii:154.

166. Nachtigall, L.E., Nachtigall, R.H., and Nachtigall, R.D. (1979): Estrogen replacement therapy I: a 10-year prospective study in the relationship to osteoporosis. *Obstet. Gynecol.*, 53:277.

167. Nachtigall, L.E., Nachtigall, R.H., and Nachtigall, R.D. (1979): Estrogen replacement therapy II: a prospective study in the relationship to carcinoma and cardiovascular and metabolic problems. *J. Obstet. Gynecol.*, 54(1):74–79.

168. Nassim, J.R., Saville, P.D., and Mulligan, L. (1956): Effect of stilboestrol on urinary phosphate excretion. *Clin. Sci.*, 15:367–371.

169. Nordin, B.E.C., MacGregor, J., and Smith, D.A. (1966): The incidence of osteoporosis in normal women: its relation to age and the menopause. *Quart J. Med.*, 137:25–38.

170. Nordin, B.E.C., Horsman, A., Aaron, J., and Gallagher, J.C. (1975): Postmenopausal bone loss. *Curr. Med. Res. Opin.*, (Suppl. 3) 3:28.

171. O'Dea, J.P., Wieland, R.G., Hallberg, M.C., Llesena, L.A., Zen, E.M., and Genuth, S.M. (1978): Effect of dietery weight loss on sex steroid binding, sex steroids and genodotrophins in obese postmenopausal women. *J. Lab. Clin. Med.*, 93:1007–1008.

172. Orimo, H., Fujima, T., and Yoshikawa, M. Increased sensitivity of bone to parathyroid hormone in oophorectomized rats. *Endocrinology*, 90:760–763.

173. Osteoporosis. (1984): NIH Consensus Development Conference. *J. Am. Med. Assoc.*, 252:799–802.

174. Parfitt, A.M., and Kleerekoper, A. (1984): Diagnostic value of bone histomorphometry and comparison of histologic measurements and biochemical indices of bone remodeling. In: *Osteoporosis*, edited by C. Christiansen, et al., pp. 111–120. Aalborg Stiftsbogtrykkeri, Glostrup, Denmark.

175. Parfitt, A.M. (1979): Quantum concept of bone remodeling and turnover: implications for the pathogenesis of osteoporosis. *Calcif. Tissue. Int.*, 28:1–5.

176. Parfitt, A.M. (1965): Changes in serum calcium and phosphorus during stilboestrol treatment of osteoporosis. *J. Bone Joint Surg.*, 47B:137–139.

177. Park, E. (1977): Cortical bone measurements in Turner's syndrome. *Am. J. Phys. Anthropol.*, 46(3):455–461.

178. Pfeffer, R.L., Kwaseki, T.T., and Charlston, S.K. Estrogen use and blood pressure in later life. *Am. J. Epidemiol.*, 110:469–474.

179. Perry, H.M., III, Fallon, M.D., Bergfeld, M., Teitelbaum, S.L., and Avioli, L.V. (1982): Osteoporosis in young men: a syndrome of hypercalciuria and accelerated bone turnover. *Arch. Intern. Med.*, 142:1295–1298.

180. Price, P.A., Parthemore, J.G., and Deftos, L.J. (1980): New chemical marker for bone metabolism. Measurement by radioimmunoassay of bone GLA protein in the plasma of normal subjects and pa-

tients with bone disease. *J. Clin. Invest.*, 66:878–883.

181. Recker, R.R., Saville, P.D., and Heaney, R.P. (1977): The effect of estrogens and calcium carbonate on bone loss in postmenopausal women. *Ann. Intern. Med.*, 87:649–655.

182. Reifenstein, E.C., Jr., and Albright, F. (1947): Metabolic effects of steroid hormones in osteoporosis. *J. Clin. Invest.*, 26:24–56.

183. Richelson, L.S., Wahner, H.W., Melton, L.J., and Riggs, B.L. (1984): Relative contributions of aging and estrogen deficiency to postmenopausal bone loss. *N. Engl. J. Med.*, 311:1273–1275.

184. Riggs, B.L., Wahner, H.W., Melton, L.J., III, Richelson, L.S., Judd, H.L., and Offord, K.P. (1985): Rates of bone loss in the appendicular and axial skeletons of women: evidence of substantial vertebral bone loss prior to menopause. *J. Clin. Invest.*, 77:1487–1491.

185. Riggs, B.L., Ryan, R.J., Wahner, H.W., Jiang, N.S., and Mattox, V.R. (1973): Serum concentrations of estrogen, testosterone and gonadotrophins in osteoporotic and non-osteoporotic women. *J. Clin. Endocrinol. Metab.*, 36:1097–1099.

186. Riggs, B.L. (1982): Evidence for etiologic heterogeneity of involutional osteoporosis. In: *Osteoporosis*, edited by J. Menczel, et al., pp. 3–14. John Wiley & Sons Ltd., Chichester.

187. Riggs, B.L., Jowsey, J., Kelly, P.J., Jones, J.D., and Maher, F.T. (1969): Effect of sex hormones on bone in primary osteoporosis. *J. Clin. Invest.*, 48:1065–1072.

188. Riggs, B.L., Jowsey, J., Goldsmith, R.S., Kelly, P.J., Hoffman, D.L., and Arnaud, C.D. (1972): Short- and long-term effects of estrogen and synthetic anabolic hormones in postmenopausal osteoporosis. *J. Clin. Invest.*, 51:1659–1663.

189. Riggs, B.L., Wahner, H.W., Dunn, W.L., Mazess, R.B., Offord, K.P., Melton, L.J., III. (1981): Differential changes in bone mineral density of the appendicular and axial skeleton with aging: relationship to spinal osteoporosis. *J. Clin. Invest.*, 67:328–335.

190. Ross, R.K., Paganini-Hin, A., Mack, T.M., et al. (1981): Menopausal oestrogen therapy and protection from death from ischemic heart disease. *Lancet*, i:858–860.

191. Ross, R.K., Paganini-Hin, A., and Gerkins, V.R., et al. (1980): A case control study of menopausal estrogen therapy and breast cancer. *JAMA*, 243:1635–1639.

192. Samaan, N.A., Anderson, G.D., and Adam-Mayne, M.E. (1975): Immunocreative calcitonin in the mother, neonate, child and adult. *Am. J. Obstet. Gynecol.*, 121:622–625.

193. Sanborn, C.F., Martin, B.J., and Wagner, W.W. (1982): Is athletic amenorrhea specific to runners. *Am. J. Obstet. Gynecol.*, 143:859–861.

194. Seeman, E., Melton, L.J., O'Fallon, W.M., and Riggs, B.L. (1983): Risk factors for spinal osteoporosis in men. *Am. J. Med.*, 75:977–983.

195. Shapiro, S., Kelly, J.P., Rosenberg, L., Kaufman, D.W., Helmrich, S.P., Rosenstein, N.B., Lewis, J.L., Jr., Knapp, R.C., Stalley, P.D., and Sethollandfeld, D. (1985): Risk of localized and widespread endometrial cancer in relation to recent and discontinued use of conjugated estrogens. *N. Engl. J. Med.*, 313:969–972.

196. Shore, R.M., Chesney, R.W., Mazess, R.B., Rose, P.G., Bergman, G.J. (1982): Skeletal demineralization in Turner's syndrome. *Calcif. Tissue. Int.*, 34:519–522.

197. Shorr, E. (1945): The possible usefulness of estrogens and aluminum hydroxide gels in the management of renal stone. *J. Urol.*, 53:507–520.

198. Siiteri, P.K. (1975): Postmenopausal oestrogen production. *Front. Horm. Res.*, 3:40–44.

199. Smith, D.A.S., and Walker, M.S. (1976): Changes in plasma steroids and bone density in Klinefelter's syndrome. *Calcif. Tissue. Res.*, 22(Suppl.):225–228.

200. Smith, D.M., Khairi, M.R.A., and Johnston, C.C. The loss of bone mineral with aging and its relationship to risk of fracture. *J. Clin. Invest.*, 56:311–318.

201. Smith, Q.T., and Allison, D.J. (1966): Studies on uterus, skin, and femur of rats treated with 17B-oestradiol benzoate for 1 to 20–21 days. *Acta Endocrinologica*, 53:598–610.

202. Solomon, L. (1979): Bone density in aging Caucasian and African populations. *Lancet*, i:1326–1330.

203. Spencer, H., Rubio, N., Rubio, E., Indreika, M., and Seitam, A. (1986): Chronic alcoholism: frequently overlooked cause of osteoporosis in men. *Am. J. Med.*, 80:393–397.

204. Stagni, N., de Bernard, B., Liut, G.F., Vittur, F., and Zanetti, M. (1980): Ca2 +-binding glycoprotein in avian bone induced by estrogen. *Connect. Tissue. Res.*, 7:121–125.

205. Stevenson, J.C., Abeyasekera, G., and Hillyard, C.J. (1982): Deficient calcitonin response to calcium infusion in postmenopausal osteoporosis. *Lancet*, i:693–695.

206. Stevenson, J.C., Abeyasekera, G., and Hillyard, C.J. (1983): Regulation of calcium-regulating hormones by exogenous sex steroids in early postmenopause. *Eur. J. Clin. Invest.*, 13:481–487.

207. Stevenson, J.C., Hillyard, C.J., MacIntyre, I., Cooper, H., Whitehead, M.I. (1979): A physiological role for calcitonin in protection of the maternal skeleton. *Lancet*, ii:767–770.

208. Stevenson, J.C., Meyers, C.H., Adjukiewicz, A.B. (1984): Racial differences in calcitonin and kalacalcin. *Calcif. Tissue. Int.*, 36:725–728.

209. Stevenson, J.C., White, M.C., Joplin, G.F., and MacIntyre, I. (1982): Osteoporosis and calcitonin deficiency. *Br. Med. J.*, 285:1010–1011.

210. Stevenson, S.L., Neer, R.M., Ridway, E.C., and Idibanski, A. (1986): Osteoporosis in Men with Hyperprolactinemic Hypogonadism. *Ann. Intern. Med.*, 104:777–782.

211. Stock, J.L., Coiderre, J.A., and Mallette, L.E. (1985): Effects of a short course of estrogen on mineral metabolism in postmenopausal women. *J. Clin. Endocrinol. Metab.*, 61:595–600.

212. Stryker, J.C. (1977): Use of hormones in women

over forty. *Clin. Obstet. Gynecol.*, 201:155–164.

213. Studd, J.W.W., Thom, M.H., and Paterson, M.E.L. (1979): The prevention and treatment of endometrial pathology in postmenopausal women receiving exogenous oestrogens. In: *Proceedings of the First International Congress on Hormones and Cancer*, edited by S. Iacobelli, et al. Raven Press, New York.

214. Szklo, M., Tonascia, J., and Gordis, L., et al. (1984): Estrogen use and myocardial infarction risk: a case control study. *Prev. Med.*, 13:510–516.

215. Taggart, H., Chestnut, C.H., III, Ivey, J.L., Baylink, D.J., Sisom, K., Huber, M.B., and Ross, B.A. (1982): Deficient calcitonin response to calcium stimulation in postmenopausal osteoporosis. *Lancet*, i:475–478.

216. Tiegs, R.D., Body, J.J., Wahner, H.W., Barta, J., Riggs, B.L., Heath, H., III. (1985): Calcitonin secretion in postmenopausal osteoporosis. *N. Engl. J. Med.*, 312:1097–1100.

217. Trotter, M., and Hixon, B.B. (1974): Sequential changes in weight, density and percentage weight of human skeletons from an early fetal period through old age. *Anat. Rec.*, 179:1–8.

218. Unger, A., Kay, A., and Griffin, A.J., et al. (1983): Disease activity and pregnancy associated with 2-glycoprotein in rheumatoid arthritis during pregnancy. *Brit. Med. J.*, 286:750–752.

219. Upton, G.V. (1982): The perimenopausal physiologic correlates and clinical management. *J. Reprod. Med.*, 27:1–28.

220. Vanderbroucke, J.P., Witteman, J.C.M., Valkenburg, H.A., Boersma, J.W., Cats, A., Festen, J.J.M., Hariman, A.P., Huber-Bruning, O., Rasker, J.J., and Weber, J. (1986): Noncontraceptive hormones and rheumatoid arthritis in perimenopausal and postmenopausal women. *J. Am. Med. Assoc.*, 255:1299–1303.

221. Vaishnav, R., Gallagher, J.A., Beresford, J.M., Poser, J., Russell, R.G.G. (1984): Direct effects of stanozolol and estrogens on human bone cell in culture. In: *Osteoporosis*, edited by C. Christiansen, et al., pp. 485–488. Aalborg Stiftsbogtrykkeri, Glostrup, Denmark.

222. Van Paassen, H.C., Poortman, J., Bogart-Creutzburg, I.H., Thijssen, J.H., Duursma, S.A. (1978): Oestrogen binding proteins in bone cytosol. *Calcif. Tissue. Res.*, 25:249–254.

223. van Paassen, H.C., Duursma, S.A., Roelofs, J.M., Sluys Veer, J.D., Andriesse, R., and Wigerinck, M.A.H.M. (1976): Biochemical parameters of bone metabolism in the pre-, peri-, and postmenopausal state. In: *Concensus on Menopausal Research*, edited by P.A. van Keep, R.B. Greenblat, and M. Albeaux-Fernet, p. 116. University Park Press, Baltimore.

224. Vermeulen, A., and Valdenek, L. (1978): Sex hormone concentrations in postmenopausal women: Relation to obesity, fat mass, age and years postmenopause. *Clin. Endocrinol.*, 9:59–66.

225. Wahl, P., Walden, C., and Knoff, R. (1983): Effect of estrogen/progestin potency on lipid/lipoprotein cholesterol. *N. Engl. J. Med.*, 308:862–867.

226. Wallace, R.B., Hoover, J., Barrett-Connor, E., et al. (1979): Altered plasma lipid and lipoprotein levels associated with oral contraceptive and oestrogen use. *Lancet*, 2:111–115.

227. Wallach, S., and Henneman, P.H. (1959): Prolonged estrogen therapy in postmenopausal women. *J. Am. Med. Assoc.*, 171:1637–1642.

228. Wallentin, L., and Larsson-Cohn, U. (1977): Metabolic and hormonal effects of postmenopausal oestrogen replacement treatment. II. Plasma lipids. *Acta Endocrinologica (KbH)*, 86:597–607.

229. Weaker, F.J., Herbert, D.C., and Sheridan, P.J. (1986): Do C-cells of the thyroid gland of the baboon contain estrogen receptors. *Acta Anat.*, 125:213–216.

230. Weinstein, R.S., and Gundberg, C.M. (1983): Serum osteocalcin reflects bone mineralization in osteopenic patients. *Clin. Res.*, 31:853A (abstr.).

231. Weiss, N.S., Szekely, D.R., Dallas, R., English, M.S., Abraham, I., and Schweid, A.I. (1979): Endometrial cancer in relation to patterns of menopausal estrogen use. *J. Am. Med. Assoc.*, 242:261–264.

232. Weiss, N.S., Ure, C.L., and Ballard, J.H. Decreased risk of fractures of the hip and lower forearm with postmenopausal use of estrogen. *N. Engl. J. Med.*, 303:1195–1198.

233. Whitehead, M.I., Lane, G., Morsman, J., Myers, C.H., Stevenson, J.C. (1984): Effect of castration on calcium regulating hormones. In: *Osteoporosis*, edited by C. Christiansen, et al., pp. 331–332. Aalborg, Stiftsbogtrykkeri, Glostrup, Denmark.

234. Whitehead, M.I., McQueen, J., and Beard, R.J. (1977): The effects of cyclical oestrogen therapy and sequential oestrogen/progestagen therapy on the endometrium of postmenopausal women. *Acta Obstet. Gynecol. Scand. (suppl.)*, 65:91–101.

235. Whitehead, M.I., McQueen, J., and King, R.J.B. (1979): Endometrial histology and biochemistry in climacteric women during oestrogen and oestrogen/progestogen therapy. *J. Roy. Soc. Med.*, 72(5):322–327.

236. Wilson, P.U.F., Garrison, R.J., and Castell, W.P. (1985): Postmenopausal estrogen use, cigarette smoking and cardiovascular morbidity in women over 50. *N. Engl. J. Med.*, 313:1038–1043.

237. Wingrave, S.J., and Kay, C.R. (1978): Reduction in incidence of rheumatoid arthritis associated with oral contraceptives. *Lancet*, i:569–571.

238. Yates, A.J.P., Gray, R.E.S., and Percival, R.C. Skeletal effects of stanozolol in osteoporosis. In: *Osteoporosis*, edited by C. Christiansen, et al., pp. 509–512. Aalborg Stiftsbogtrykkeri, Glostrup, Denmark.

239. Young, M.M., Jasani, C., Smith, D.A., and Nordin, B.E.C. (1968): Some effects of ethinyl oestradiol on calcium and phosphorous metabolism in osteoporosis. *Clin. Sci.*, 34:411–417.

240. Young, M.M., and Nordin, B.E.C. (1967): Effects of natural and artificial menopause on plasma and urinary calcium and phosphorous. *Lancet*, 2:118–120.

241. Ziel, H.K., and Finkle, W.K. (1975): Increased

risk of endometrial carcinoma among users of conjugated estrogens. *N. Engl. J. Med.*, 293:1167–1170.

242. Greenspan, S.L., Neer, R.M., Ridgway, E.C., and Klibanski, A. (1980): Osteoporosis in men with hyperprolactinemic hypogonadism. *Ann. Intern. Med.*, 104:777–782.

Osteoporosis: Etiology, Diagnosis, and Management, edited by B. Lawrence Riggs and L. Joseph Melton, III. Raven Press, New York © 1988.

13

Nutritional Factors In Bone Health

Robert P. Heaney

Creighton University, Omaha, Nebraska 68178

Osteoporosis is a condition of decreased bone mass and of increased bone fragility. Generally the two go together, and it is widely held that decreased mass is the factor principally responsible for the fragility. However, the two, while strongly associated, are not identical. Not all persons with reduced bone mass suffer clinically significant fractures, and some fractures generally considered to be osteoporotic (e.g., Colles') are often found in persons who have lost little or no bone mass. The fact that many persons with reduced mass do not fracture may be only because the fracture is a probabilistic occurrence, like a hurricane or an earthquake: not all persons suffer from such untoward events, even if they have the necessary preconditions, i.e., reduced bone mass on the one hand, or residence in an earthquake or hurricane zone, on the other. But it may also be that persons with reduced bone mass who do not fracture have a better quality of bone or suffer fewer falls. This distinction is important in discussing nutrition as a risk factor for osteoporosis, since virtually all that is known about the role of nutrition is in relation to the preservation and loss of bone mass. Essentially nothing is known about nutritional effects, if any, on bone quality or on propensity to fall. Thus bone mass, and not fracture, is the necessary focus of this chapter. For that reason, also, the discussion must necessarily be incomplete.

It may be helpful to note at the outset that, whereas it is relatively easy to be authoritative in dealing with a topic such as nutritional factors in anemia, where, for example, folate, B12, and iron all play clearly defined nutritional roles, it is not possible to bring the same degree of certitude to bear on the nutritional issues surrounding osteoporosis. At certain extremes of intake it seems clear that nutritional factors can cause osteoporosis, but it is not yet possible to be absolutely certain that nutritional abnormalities are important factors in all or even most patients with osteoporosis seen clinically. Further, competent scientists of many backgrounds disagree about the importance of nutrition. The evidence on both sides of this question has been extensively reviewed elsewhere (17,18). This chapter will not so much reconstitute this controversy as attempt to present a common-sense position that, if applied to a population at risk would at the very least be safe, in the sense that all reasonable nutritional steps will have been taken to prevent and/or treat the disorder.

Osteoporosis is like coronary artery disease, in that it is multifactorial. In both conditions nutritional factors are important. In both, experts disagree about their relative importance. In neither is it reasonable to expect that nutritional manipulations alone can solve the entirety of the problem. In both, the evidence supports a set of common-sense dietary steps that are probably of considerable value but which, at the very least, do little or no harm.

PRELIMINARY CONSIDERATIONS

Determinants of Bone Mass

Possession of a heavy bone mass is clearly known to be associated with reduced risk of osteoporotic fracture. Bone mass itself is determined by at least three broad groups of factors: genetic, mechanical, and endocrine/nutritional. All three interact and add to one another in any given individual (Fig.1). The bone mass one develops during growth is, like muscle mass, largely determined by genetic factors, and endocrine and nutritional factors are largely permissive. Mechanical loading can enhance or diminish this genetic impulse, but during growth it generally plays a less important role. However, as muturity is reached, mechanical loading becomes increasingly important: very simply peak bone mass must be used to be sustained. All persons lose bone with age after about age 35, probably to some degree because of decreased mechanical loading as persons advance from the rambunctiousness of childhood and adolescence to the relative gracefulness of maturity. Generally this loss of bone is in proportion to a corresponding loss of muscle (7), a fact that is often not recognized, but which underscores the lifelong importance of mechanical loading for the maintenance of musculoskeletal intergrity. And just as even the best possible nutrition cannot reverse or prevent muscle atrophy due to indolence and inactivity, so we should not expect nutritional therapy or prophylaxis to prevent or reverse bone loss due to the same factors.

The nutrients of most obvious importance in the context of bone health are, of course, calcium and phosphorus (as phosphate), since they comprise roughly 80 to 90% of the mineral content of bone. Also recognized as important, though of less clear significance in the context of osteoporosis, are trace elements such as manganese, copper, and zinc. These

are important for bone cell function, being necessary co-factors for collagen cross-linkage, mucopolysaccharide synthesis, alkaline phosphatase, and carbonic anhydrase (2,30). Skeletal deficiency states involving both the bulk phase minerals and one or more of the trace metals are well recognized in experimental animals, and in general the bony material in such deficiency states exhibits reduced mechanical strength. The extent to which any of these elements plays a significant role in human osteoporosis is still the subject of study.

Nutrition exerts two types of effects, one during growth when the supply of critical nutrients is inadequate to build the skeletal mass that is genetically programmed, and the other during maturity or later life, when intake is inadequate to meet extraskeletal demands for the bulk phase bone minerals. In both cases the organism straightforwardly optimizes its systems in favor of extraskeletal calcium homeostasis; skeletal integrity is given second priority. Indeed, an entirely adequate skeleton will be torn down in order to maintain extracellular fluid calcium ion concentration. The resulting skeletal condition is what we call osteoporosis, and several animal models of this type of osteoporosis have been recognized for many years (3,5,23,24). However, osteoporosis is an end-state condition rather than a specific disease with a unique cause, and it seems quite certain that there are other, non-nutritional mechanisms which can produce the same result. Thus, the finding that calcium deficiency causes osteoporosis in animals does not prove that osteoporosis in humans is caused by calcium deficiency. It shows only that it could be a cause; it shows what calcium deficiency will do to the skeleton; it does not define what level of intake constitutes calcium deficiency.

There are several important ways in which mechanical and nutritional factors interact. With the rise in use of labor-saving devices over the past 50 years there has been an inevitable decline in energy expenditure, and with it a corresponding decline in nutrient intake. This sets the scene for nutritional deficiency, since substances existing at low nutrient densities in

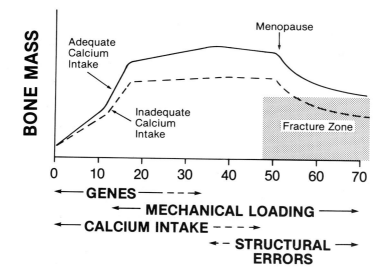

FIG. 1. Interaction of the principal determinants of bone mass at various stages throughout a woman's life. Peak skeletal mass is achieved at about age 35, after which age-related loss begins. This loss is temporarily accelerated at menopause as a result of estrogen loss. Genetic factors, as indicated, are most important early in life. Calcium intake is also believed to be of importance early, in terms of realizing the full genetic potential for bone mass. Its later importance is less certain. There is abundant evidence suggesting that it cannot reverse age-related loss or prevent the accelerated postmenopausal loss. However, acquired calcium dificiency may be a problem in many women after mid-life, and may aggravate age-related loss. This component of the total loss would, of course, be nutritionally related, and thus potentially preventable. Copyright © 1985, Robert P. Heaney, M.D., used with permission.

ordinary foodstuffs may no longer be consumed in adequate quantity when total food intake is reduced. Thus, from a single life-style change there arises both a decrease in the mechanical stimuli necessary to maintain the skeleton and a decrease in intake of certain nutrients which may thereby become nutritionally limiting and result in skeletal loss.

Another kind of interaction is perhaps seen in the osteoporosis found in young performance athletes, particularly women (9,27), and in anorectics (34). Generally their osteoporosis is attributed to estrogen deficiency, and while this doubtless plays an important role, it seems an unsatisfying explanation for the entirety of the problem. The performance athlete is typically very concerned about maintaining a low body weight, and hence voluntarily curbs intake, often ingesting a diet drawn from only a very narrow, and sometimes bizarre selection of foods. Reported studies make clear that the

average young women with this kind of problem, after making allowance for energy expended in running, ingests only about 800 to 1000 kCal/day for total metabolic and nutritional needs (9). Further, excessive perspiring during athletic activity is known to lead to loss of certain trace elements, notably zinc, and if not offset by adequate intake, creates a situation in which deficiency of some trace minerals can occur. Hence, it is not unlikely that multiple nutritional inadequacies play a role in this form of osteoporosis.

Heterogeneity of Skeletal Response

The probable heterogeneity of the osteoporotic syndrome is described elsewhere in the volume. But at a more fundamental level, bone itself is heterogeneous, at least in its tissue context if not in its intrinsic composition. Bone remodels to reshape itself to meet current uses and to replace damaged or otherwise inadequate material. But bone remodeling at the periosteal surface behaves differently from intracortical bone remodeling, and differently still from endosteal bone remodeling; similarly, trabecular bone is often said to behave differently from compact bone, though whether it is possible to lump all trabecular bone or all compact bone together, as if within type they were all the same, is questionable. Certainly trabecular bone in contact with red, hematopoietic marrow is exposed to quite a different local chemical environment than is trabecular bone exposed only to yellow, fatty marrow, and there is reason to believe that the two behave with corresponding differences. Further, since it is well-known that the proportion and distribution of red and yellow marrow change with age, it seems likely that one and the same bony region may well behave differently at different times in a person's life cycle.

We see this intrinsic heterogeneity reflected clinically in X-rays of patients with various disorders affecting the skeleton, for example, the subperiosteal resorption of hyperparathyroidism, the intracortical tunneling of high remodeling states (such as hyperthyroidism), the endosteal expansion of estrogen deficiency, and the metaphyseal rarefraction which is the first detectable sign of bone loss with immobilization or paralysis. We will note in what follows what appear to be counterpart differences in response to nutritional stress and therapy. It is important to make this point at the outset, since most clinical studies in live human beings sample the skeleton at only one, or at most two or three sites. However, probably no site adequately represents the others in all their diversity; thus it is easy to see how controversy can arise about the role or importance of virtually any factor that might be so studied.

CALCIUM

Requirements

The amount of calcium required to assure optimal nutrition, particularly after growth has been completed, is a subject of controversy.

National figures for Recommended Dietary Allowances (RDA's) range from a low of 400 to 500 mg/day for the World Health Organization for all adults to a high of 1000 mg/day for the U.S. for perimenopausal women. But many nutritionists and experts in the field of metabolic disease judge that these values, varying as they do over more than a two-fold range, are still wide of the mark, with positions ranging from an adult requirement as low as 200 mg/day to as high as 1500 mg/day. The 1984 NIH Consensus Conference on Osteoporosis (8) favored the high end of this range, and recommended an intake of 1000 mg/day for estrogen-replete perimenopausal women and 1500 mg/day for estrogen-deprived postmenopausal women. The basis for the NIH recommendation was not so much scientific proof as a calculated balancing of possible risks against possible benefits. Very simply, there was evidence supporting, though not conclusively establishing, the higher requirement values, and there was little or no evidence suggesting that such intakes, even if not helpful, would either produce much harm or result in much cost. Hence deciding in favor of the higher intake seemed the prudent thing to do. The evidence *pro* and *con* a high requirement has been reviewed elsewhere (17,18), and will only be summarized here.

All studies of calcium requirement based on metabolic balance methods indicate a high requirement in middle-aged women. Further, estrogen loss at menopause is associated with a deterioration in calcium balance performance, thus supporting the notion of an increased requirement after menopause. This deterioration consists of a combination of decreased intestinal absorptive efficiency and increased urinary excretion of calcium. The two, together, account for a negative balance shift of about 25 mg/day (21). Population-based studies give more equivocal results. Persons with high calcium intakes have been reported in some studies to show heavier skeletons than persons with low intakes, and sometimes the reported differences have been impressive and been associated with substantially lower fracture rates as well. At the other extreme, a few studies have shown no apparent difference in bone mass across substantial differences in current intake. Most studies show some correlation between current calcium intake and current bone mass, but generally the effect is relatively small.

Intervention studies show that calcium supplements can retard age-related bone loss in postmenopausal women for at least two years, but not at all bony sites. Thus several studies show virtually complete suppression of bone loss in various cortical sites such as the phalangeal bones and the metacarpals (1,25,33), but little or no effect on loss of bone from the metaphyseal bone of the distal radius (29,33)— *even in the same individuals.* Calcium supplements can retard the alveolar bone loss associated with tooth extraction and denture fitting (39,40), but not the osteoporosis of disuse associated with immobilization (15).

There are several possible reasons for this confusing picture. One explanation for this generally weak effect is the obvious fact that bone mass is more the result of integrated lifetime exposure to calcium than it is of current intake levels. Also, as mentioned earlier, bone is heterogeneous; it has slowly become clear that not all sites can be expected to respond in the same way. Further, also as suggested earlier, calcium intake is probably permissive, in the sense that calcium is required for, but does not itself cause, the skeleton to be of any given mass. That mass, instead, is determined by a combination of genetic and mechanical factors. As such, calcium is a threshold nutrient, relating to bone mass just as iron relates to hemoglobin mass. Below the threshold, intake is limiting, and one can expect to see a positive correlation between calcium intake and bone mass, just as below its threshold one expects to see a correlation between iron intake and hemoglobin mass. In neither case, however, does an intake above the threshold produce any further effect. The argument among nutritionists about calcium requirement centers on exactly this point. Some say that the range of commonly encountered intakes is above the threshold, and that is why one sees so little relation between calcium intake and bone mass in population studies. Others say that the usual intake

is below the threshold, and that is why one sees so much osteoporosis around the world.

What seems to be a useful middle ground between these positions can be expressed as follows: The threshold concept is valid and applicable to this problem, but the actual numerical value of the threshold differs from person to person over a wide range. Some have low thresholds, and others high. Thus whenever an inevitably mixed population is studied, the effect of variation in intake is diluted by the presence in the sample of persons whose intake, though different from that of others, is still above their particular threshold.

Factors Influencing Calcium Requirement

The reasons for this variation in intake threshold are many, and probably not all understood by any means. Genetic differences in the balance between end-organ responses to parathyroid hormone (and to $1,25(OH)_2D_3$) are one such. Thus U.S. blacks, known to have heavier bone mass from infancy onward (14), have recently been shown to have greater resistance to the bone resorptive effect of PTH (4). Thus, for any given circulating level of PTH, they make better use of dietary calcium and thereby tend to protect their skeletons. Other reasons include nutrient-nutrient and drug-nutrient interactions, and the effect of various comorbid conditions. Thus increased protein intake, by causing increased urine calcium without altering intestinal absorption, leads to decreased conservation of absorbed calcium. In effect this increases the calcium requirement (i.e., changes the threshold level for calcium as a nutrient). So, too, increased fiber intake decreases intestinal absorption (18). Increased sodium intake is known to lead to hypercalciuria and thus, as with protein, to increase the requirement for calcium.

The magnitude of these interactions is not known with certainty, but it appears that it can be substantial. Thus a doubling of protein intake has been shown in many different studies to lead to a 50% increase in urine calcium (19). By contrast a doubling of calcium intake produces only a 30 to 35% increase in urine calcium. Thus, surprising as it may seem, variations in protein intake have a greater effect on urine calcium than do variations in calcium intake itself. Sodium also can have a profound effect on urine calcium. The relation is complex and depends upon GFR, degree on hydration, and parathyroid status; but in general it can be said that an increase in urinary sodium carries with it an increase in urinary calcium (35).

Caffeine also increases urine calcium (19). Its effect is small, but not negligible, and when caffeine intake is high, the net effect is to increase calcium requirement substantially. Aluminum-containing antacids, by reducing phosphate absorption from the diet, lower plasma phosphate and thereby result in increased urinary calcium loss (38). Thus persons with chronic peptic ulcer disease and those with self-medicated indigestion, also may have elevated calcium requirements.

Additionally, other persons whose calcium intakes are below their respective thresholds may exhibit little effect from calcium intake variations because of other nutritional (or quasi-nutritional) factors that are, in effect, co-limiting with calcium. Vitamin D status is one such factor. Phosphatemia may well be another. The evidence suggesting that vitamin D insufficiency may be prevalent enough to explain the indifferent results often reported in population studies will be dealt with subsequently, as will the matter of phosphorus as a co-nutrient with calcium.

These interactions are described, not to make the point that excess protein, for example, is nutritionally bad, or to suggest that we should decrease our protein or caffeine intakes, but rather to explain why persons, particularly in different nations and with different standards of living and cultural practices, may well exhibit quite different calcium requirements.

Calcium Absorption and Vitamin D Status

Calcium absorptive efficiency has been noted by many investigators to decline with advancing age. An example is presented in Fig. 2, which shows the distribution of absorption values, adjusted to a mean calcium intake of 800 mg, in 273 healthy postmenopausal, estrogen-deprived women, at mean age 53.8 (20). In order just to meet obligatory extraintestinal losses, fractional absorption at this intake must be nearly 32%. Note, in Fig. 2, that 77% of the entire group absorbed less than this figure (the cross-hatched bars), and thus were of necessity in negative calcium balance.

While a decline in calcium absorption efficiency in mid-life might be thought to be a natural consequence of a declining need for calcium, exactly the opposite appears to be the case. PTH levels rise with age, and normally one would expect absorption to rise in parallel. The fact that it does not, that it declines instead, is thus something of a paradox. The reasons are inadequately understood, but they need exploring here, inasmuch as absorptive efficiency is crucial to the question of assuring adequate calcium nutrition.

At least four factors combine to explain the deterioration in absorptive efficiency. First is a decline with age in the circulating levels of $25(OH)D_3$, the precursor of the hormonally active form of vitamin D. This fall in $25(OH)D_3$ levels, which is probably due to a general decrease in average solar exposure as persons age, would not be expected to affect absorptive efficiency if D status were otherwise fully adequate. However, recent studies suggest that a large fraction of middle-aged and elderly adults have such marginal D levels that any fall inevitably results in a decline in absorptive efficiency. The crucial observation leading to this conclusion was the finding that administration of modest doses of $25(OH)D_3$ to apparently healthy adults would often raise circulating levels of $1,25(OH)_2D_3$, and that the degree of elevation of $1,25(OH)_2D_3$ produced was inversely proportional to the basal $25(OH)D_3$ level (12). Further, when $25(OH)D_3$ is administered, absorptive efficiency rises, alkaline phosphatase falls, and PTH levels drop as well. If the basal state of these persons had been one of vitamin D repletion, these changes would not have been expected to occur. These

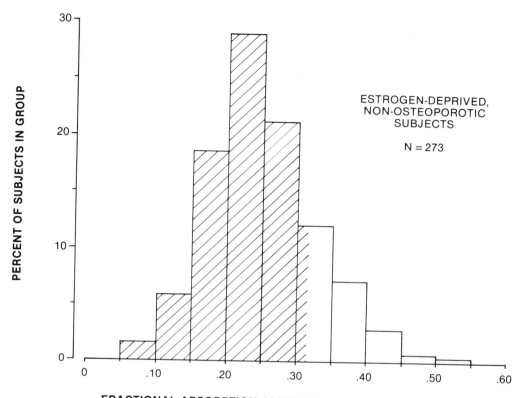

FIG. 2. Distribution of true fractional absorption of calcium in estrogen-deprived healthy, postmenopausal women. Absorption in each subject is adjusted to the mean intake of the group (0.80 g) in order to facilitate comparison (see 20). Copyright © 1985, Robert P. Heaney, M.D., used with permission.

findings therefore suggested that 25(OH)D$_3$ levels were limiting the amount of 1,25(OH)$_2$D$_3$ that the body could produce for any given level of circulating PTH. The point at which the effect disappears is equivalently the lower limit of normal values of 25(OH)D$_3$. Current estimates place that level at about 25-30 ng/ml in older individuals.

As a result of these findings it now appears that a distinction must be made between severe D deficiency, defined as 25(OH)D$_3$ levels generally below 5 ng/ml and associated with clinical and histologic osteomalacia, and less severe deficiency defined as 25(OH)D$_3$ levels in the range of 5 to 30 ng/ml, associated with calcium malabsorption, but not with histologic abnormality of bone (17,31). By this standard,

most elderly persons are to some degree vitamin D deficient.

The effect of the fall in 25(OH)D$_3$ levels with age is further compounded by two other age-related effects: a decline in perfusion of the endocrine kidney (expressed most familiarly as a fall in GFR) and, at least in some persons, a decline in the responsiveness of the renal 1-alpha-hydroxylase to circulating PTH. Both changes result in decreased production of 1,25(OH)$_2$D$_3$, and hence lead to impaired calcium absorption. Finally there is an increasing body of evidence indicating that there is, at least in some aging persons, and particularly in osteoporotics, some degree of resistance of the intestinal mucosa itself to the action of 1,25(OH)$_2$D$_3$ (13). As can be readily appreciated, these changes amount to an effective increase in the requirement for vitamin D with advancing age, a change which, ironically, is occurring at precisely a time in life when vitamin D status is deteriorating.

None of these changes is of an all-or-nothing character, and they all seem susceptible to being offset by assuring both adequate calcium intake and adequate D status (as reflected in a plasma $25(OH)D_3$ level at or above 25-30 ng/ml). It is not yet known how firm the boundary is between D sufficiency and insufficiency, or to what extent it should be considered to rise with age.

There is, understandably, a need to be concerned about vitamin D toxicity, particularly since it is possible for vitamin D-containing preparations to be obtained without perscription, and thus for persons to self-medicate and over-treat themselves. Further it is well-recognized that one of the features of vitamin D toxicity is excess bone resorption, surely an unwelcome development in a program intended to prevent osteoporosis. However, except for fueling in some few persons the tendency to overdo a good thing, emphasis on assuring adequate vitamin D status seems quite safe. $25(OH)D_3$ levels in young persons, or in populations living in sunny, southern latitudes, are generally in excess of 30 ng/ml, without the slightest evidence of vitamin D intoxication. By contrast, as has been noted earlier, $25(OH)D_3$ levels in older persons in northern latitudes are generally lower, often below 15 ng/ml. It would seem that whatever vitamin D intakes may be required to push those levels back up into the range 30 to 50 ng/ml would be quite safe. So long as $25(OH)D_3$ levels went no higher, the term "intoxication" would be quite inappropriate, and fear of such intoxication may cause us to err on the side of depriving our patients of a needed benefit.

PHOSPHORUS

Most investigation of human bone disease has focussed on the role of calcium. Nevertheless, as has been noted, other minerals are probably important as well, and may be limiting in certain situations. Phosphorus is an obvious example, since it is one of the bulk phase components of bone mineral, which normally contains about 2 mol of phosphate for every 3 mol of calcium (for a P:Ca molar ratio of 0.6). Clearly phosphate deficiency must limit the amount of bone mineral that can be deposited. Further, since hypophosphatemia is a strong stimulus to bone resorption (32), acquired phosphate deficiency could be predicted to lead to bone loss.

Deficiency of phosphate in the local internal environment also causes cellular malfunction. This is precisely what happens in the various osteomalacias, in which hypophosphatemia, though caused by many different mechanisms, is the ultimate reason for poor osteoblast function. This happens because of a combination of systemic hypophosphatemia and severe, local phosphorus depletion. The latter occurs because the mineralization of bone matrix inevitably withdraws minerals (Ca and P) from the extracellular fluid surrounding the osteoblast. Thus these cells are subjected chronically to low Ca and P concentrations. Presumably the osteoblast, as is known to be the case for muscle cells and other tissues, cannot function well in a low phosphorus environment (26). And while ambient concentrations of both calcium and phosphorus are reduced at actively mineralizing sites, the osteoblast, having its own internal supply of calcium, is probably more sensitive to the low P levels than it is to the low Ca levels. During growth in all mammals, the organism maintains osteoblast well-being by assuring an excess of phosphate, with the extracellular fluids containing phosphate in a molar ratio to calcium typically about 3 times higher than found in bone (i.e., 1.8 to 2.5). Thus, when bone matrix is mineralizing, ambient phosphate concentrations in the osteoblast's environment never fall below levels needed for optimal cell function. However, in the adult human, the levels of Ca and P in the ECF that we typically consider normal produce a P:Ca ratio as low as 0.65, very close to the ratio in bone, and thus any mineralization at all tends to subject the osteoblast to a low phosphate enviroment. This is particularly true for persons with plasma phosphate values at the low end of the ostensibly normal range. Because the plasma level elsewhere in the body remains relatively higher and thus the bone-forming site is continually supplied with mineral, the pathologic lesions of osteomalacia do not develop; but it is likely that the low ambient phosphate concentrations may limit the effectiveness of osteoblast function in many normal adults.

Control of ECF phosphate levels is loose and is relatively poorly understood. It is not entirely clear why adult human levels are as low as they are, though a fall in growth hormone secretion is surely one factor. Nevertheless, that ECF phosphate may be rate limiting with respect to optimal bone remodeling in the adult is suggested by work of Harris et al. (16), who showed in adult dogs that a regimen of phosphate supplements, sufficient to reproduce the normal alimentary phosphatemia several times a day, markedly stimulated bone remodeling, and more specifically, converted the endosteal surface (which is regularly dominated by resorption in adult dogs just as it is in adult humans) into a forming surface.

There is much confusion about the role of phosphate in adult nutrition, and questions have been raised as to whether there was not in fact cause for concern about the relatively high levels of phosphate present in the modern U.S. diet, and about the low Ca:P ratio characteristic of that diet (6). Some, even, have maintained that typical U.S. phosphate intakes contribute to the problem of osteoporosis (22). However, virtually all of the studies indicating a potentially harmful effect of excess phosphate have been performed in small or immature animals, in which basal ECF phosphate levels are normally high. Under such circumstances increased phosphate intakes produce even greater hyperphosphatemia, and may adversely effect calcium homeostasis by a variety of mechanisms that would not be operative at the substantially lower levels of ECF phosphate found in the adult human (e.g., direct physical chemical suppression of ECF (Ca^{2+}).

Further, two independent studies of the effect on calcium balance in adults of varing phosphate intakes over a wide range have both failed to show any hint of a deleterious effect (19,37). Additionally, many years' experience with the use of neutral phosphates in management of renal stone disease have also failed to suggest any harmful effect on bone.

Phosphate intake may be a matter of concern, however, not because of purported excess, but because of possible deficiency, as I have already suggested. With increased interest in maintaining adequate calcium intake, and with the likely use of calcium supplements, it could well develop that phosphate intake would become limiting in certain persons, especially elderly persons with low total nutrient intakes. When this is the case, any hoped-for beneficial effects of calcium supplements would be blunted or neutralized because there was not sufficient phosphate to sustain a positive shift in bone balance. Thus any regimen emphasizing medicinal calcium supplements needs to give adequate attention to the possibility of a need for additional phosphate as well.

TRACE MINERALS

It has been recognized for about fifty years that inadequate intake of certain minerals results in skeletal abnormalities, including deformities, reduced bone mass, and reduced bone strength. These minerals do not comprise a significant portion of the bulk mineral phase of bone, as do calcium and phosphorus, but they are instead components of metalloenzymes responsible for many cellular functions, including synthesis and breakdown of bone (2,30).

Manganese, for one, is a necessary co-factor for many enzymes involed in carbohydrate metabolism, and specifically for mucopolysaccharide synthesis. Deficiency is most apparent during growth, when chondrogenesis is reduced, bone matrix synthesis is impaired, and ash content and breaking strength of bone are reduced. It is not known what effects acquired manganese deficiency might have in the fully grown adult organism, though presumably new bone formation under manganese-deficient conditions in the adult would show the same intrinsic abnormalities then as during growth. Manganese is found in many different foods in the normal human diet and its requirement is believed to be in the range of 4 to 6 mg/day. Very little manganese is normally found in urine, and excretion is usually by the fecal route.

Copper is another trace mineral with many metabolic functions. One of importance in this context is its role in crosslinkage of collagen. Bone and tendon formed under conditions of copper deficiency are structurally weak, and animals grown on copper-deficient diets exhibit stunted growth. Like manganese, copper is normally excreted primarily through the feces.

Zinc deficiency results in stunted growth and inadequate collagen formation, among other problems. Zinc is a component of many enzymes, some of which (e.g., alkaline phosphatase, carbonic anhydrase) are linked with bone cell function. Zinc is an element widely believed to be marginal in the usual Western diet, and it is possible that many persons suffer from borderline zinc deficiencies. Zinc is excreted in urine and sweat as well as in the feces. (The latter is probably largely unabsorbed dietary zinc.)

Whether deficiencies of these minerals play any role in human osteoporosis, acquired in adult life, remains uncertain. As I have noted, dietary intake of performance athletes is often bizarre, and there is at least one well-publicized instance of a male athlete with multiple fractures and probable osteoporosis (at least some of whose fractures healed poorly), who confined himself to a very narrow range of foodstuffs, whose plasma manganese level was extremely low, and plasma copper moderately so, and who responded with bone healing and apparently increased bone density to a multivalent trace element cocktail containing manganese, copper, and zinc, among other substances (36). Zinc excretion is known to be enchanced by sweating, and it has been speculated that manganese may be lost in the same

way. Thus the combination of restricted dietary intake, strenuous exercise, and sweating may create a situation of trace mineral deficiency that may contribute to certain osteoporoses, specifically those found in performance athletes. But the problem may not be confined only to athletes. In one report plasma manganese levels were found to be significantly lower than normal in a group of osteoporotics. How widespread this finding may be is impossible to say, largely because most mainstream osteoporosis reasearch has not looked at these trace minerals.

PRACTICAL CONSIDERATIONS

It is a truism of nutrition that we don't know enough to take full control of our diets. Thus the best way to assure adequate nutrition is to consume a balanced diet derived from the widest possible variety of natural food sources. Hunter-gatherer tribes, able to maintain health by consuming a wide variety of seasonal foods, have been noted to develop nutritional deficiencies when they settle down to an agricultural economy and thereby reduce the range and variety of their food intake (11). Calcium intake seems no exception to this rule. Primitive humans, functioning at an otherwise unattractive stone-age level of existence, have been found to have calcium intakes in excess of 1500 mg/day, mostly from vegetable sources (10). It needs to be said that it is possible for more sophisticated, more civilized humans to do the same. While dairy products are a major source of calcium in the modern U.S. diet, they are not the only rich source by any means. Figure 3 displays the calcium content of a variety of human foods somewhat familiar to Western palates. Many of the richer, non-dairy sources are not in widespread use today, and it may be unrealistic to pretend that American eating practices are likely to change sufficiently to produce much of an increase in actual calcium intake despite the widespread availability of the element in natural sources. Nevertheless, it is important for health professionals to recognize that it is possible to construct high calcium

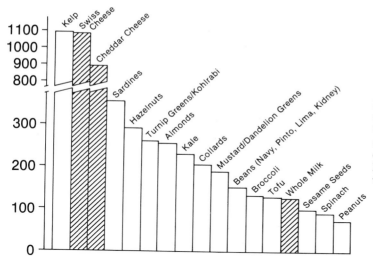

FIG. 3. Calcium contents of selected foods available to urbanized adults. Dairy products are highlighted for purposes of comparison. Copyright © 1985, Robert P. Heaney, M.D., used with permission.

diets from widely diverse sources. At least some of our patients can accept this information and use it to their profit.

Finally, it is important to be aware of the existance of many patients who may be at more than usual risk for calcium deficiency. Reference has been made to some of these patients in the foregoing, but it is useful to bring them together here.

1. *Postmenopausal, estrogen-deprived women.* As has been noted, after menopause women seem to use dietary calcium inefficiently, and, other things being equal, simply need more in their diets to maintain bone health.

2. *Women with diets high in protein, sodium, fiber, or caffeine.* As has been noted, these nutrients, to some degree important (or at least desirable) in their own right, alter the calcium requirement, each to varying degrees, but all in the same direction (upwards).

3. *Persons, especially women, ingesting aluminum-containing antacids.* Aluminum binds phosphate in the gut, lowers plasma phosphorus, and thereby raises urine calcium loss. Long-term treatment with these agents, generally for peptic disease or indigestion, may be an important contributor to the osteoporosis problem. Certainly, we

have recognized that gastrectomy is a contributing factor for many years (28), but it may well have been the long-term use of antacids, which inevitably precedes gastrectomy, that is the cause of the problem, rather than solely the malabsorption that may follow gastrectomy.

4. *Persons recovering from illness or immobility, particularly if prolonged.* In general, as has been noted above, we have about as much bone as we need for current mechanical loads. Bedrest for any reason leads to significant bone loss; sickness is certainly one such reason. Recovery from whatever may be the basic illness will leave a residue of unrepaired bone loss unless the diet contains a surplus of bone minerals. We have recognized a comparable need for increased intake of water-soluble vitamins and other critical nutrients during recovery from all kinds of catabolic episodes; a need for supplemental calcium, heretofore inadequately appreciated, is of this same sort.

5. *Persons who are inadvertently on low calcium diets.* Some diets, therapeutic or self-selected, are unwittingly deficient in calcium. A typical low-sodium diet, though intended as therapeutic, is one example. The diet of a typical alcoholic, clearly not therapeutic in intent, is another. Both tend

to be calcium-deficient, and both need to be supplemented by calcium.

CONCLUSION

It seems that the most practical suggestion that can be offered at this state of our understanding of these complex issues is to assure adequate calcium intake early in life. For many of our patients, it is, of course, too late to do that. But we can talk about their daughters, and about the importance of helping them change their dietary habits while there is still time for them to achieve their full skeletal potential. At the same time it remains important to assure adequate calcium intake even in the declining years, when the utilization of calcium in the diet deteriorates.

And finally, although its ultimate efficacy remains to be determined, it seems likely that special steps should be taken to assure adequate vitamin D status in both the middle-aged and the elderly. Since outside the sunbelt this cannot practically be achieved through solar exposure or usual dietary sources alone, it seems necessary that there be vitamin D fortification of the food chain, or routine vitamin D supplementation as a part of institutional or at least personal health maintenance regimens. The RDA for vitamin D in adults is currently about 200 IU/day (as contrasted with a figure of 400 during growth). While most elderly persons do not get even that much, it must be said that this figure is probably much too low. As has been noted, vitamin D requirements probably rise with age, rather than fall. It appears that total intakes on the order of 1000 IU/day may be required in the elderly for optimal balance in the Vitamin D-Ca-PTH control system. Toxicity need not be feared so long as serum 25(OH)D$_3$ levels do not exceed those found regularly in healthy young adults.

Addendum

It seems reasonably well established that a generous calcium intake contributes to enhanced bone mass during the phases of growth and consolidation of the skeleton and that extremely low levels of dietary calcium intake may cause bone loss after skeletal maturity. There is considerable controversy, however, about the calcium intake necessary to maintain bone mass in the adult. Since this chapter was received, there have been three longitudinal, densitometric studies measuring bone loss from the vertebrae that suggest a weaker effect of calcium intake than has been formerly believed. Using photon absorptiometry, Riis et al. (*N. Engl. J. Med.*, 316:173–177, 1987) found that a supplement of 1,500 mg of elemental calcium in women in the early postmenopause did not retard bone loss from the vertebrae or from the total skeleton significantly but did cause a moderate retardation of bone loss from the midradius. Using quantiative computed tomography, Ettinger et al. (*Ann. Intern, Med.*, 106:40–45, 1987) also found that 1,500 mg of elemental calcium supplement did not retard bone loss from the vertebrae in a similar group of women. However, treatment did reduce the minimal level of estrogen replacement required to retard bone loss, suggesting an estrogen-calcium interaction. Riggs et al. (*J. Clin. Invest.*, in press) studied rates of bone loss from the lumbar spine and midradius in women between the ages of 23 and 84 and found no effect of dietary calcium intake over the range of 260 to 2,035 mg/day, even after adjusting for contingent variables such as sex steroid levels and age. Thus, it seems clear that more studies are required to resolve this important issue. Until then, it seems reasonable to follow the recommendations of the recent NIH Conference on Osteoporosis that all adults consume a dietary calcium intake of at least 1,000 mg/day and that individuals judged to be at increased risk for osteoporosis should consume at least 1,500 mg/day (*Science* 235:833–834, 1987).

REFERENCES

1. Albanese, A.A., Edelson, A.H., Woodhull, M.L., Lorenze, E.J., Jr., Wein, E.H., and Orto, L.A. (1973): Effect of a calcium supplement on serum

cholesterol, calcium, phosphorus and bone density of "normal, healthy" elderly females. *Nutr. Rept. Int.*, 8:119–130.

2. Asling, C.W., and Hurley, L.S. (1963): The influence of trace elements on the skeleton. *Clin. Orthop.*, 27:213–264.

3. Bauer, W., Aub, J.C., and Albright, F. (1929): Studies of calcium and phosphorus metabolism. V. A study of the bone trabeculae as a readily available reserve supply of calcium. *J. Exp. Med.*, 49:145–161.

4. Bell, N.H., Green, A., Epstein, S., Oexmann, M.J., Shaw, S., and Shary, J. (1985): Evidence for alteration of the vitamin D-endocrine system in blacks. *J. Clin. Invest.*, 76:470–473.

5. Bodansky, M., and Duff, V.B. (1939): Regulation of the level of calcium in the serum during pregnancy. *J.A.M.A.*, 112:223–229.

6. Chinn, H.I. Effects of dietary factors on skeletal integrity in adults: calcium, phosphorus, vitamin D, and protein (1981): Prepared for Bureau of Foods, Food and Drug Administration, Department of Health and Human Services, Washington, D.C. FDA Contract No. 223-79-2275.

7. Cohn, S.H., Aloia, J.F., Vaswani, A.N. Zanzi, I., Vartsky, D., and Ellis, K.J. (1982): Age and sex related changes in bone mass measured by neutron activation. In : *Osteoporosis*. The Proceeding of an International Symposium held at the Jerusalem Osteoporosis Center in June 1981, edited by J. Menczel, G. C. Robin, M. Makin, and R. Steinberg, pp. 33–43. John Wiley & Sons, New York.

8. Consensus Conference, Osteoporosis (1984): *J.A.M.A.* 252:799–802.

9. Drinkwater, B.L., Nilson, K., Chesnut, C.H. III, Bremner, W.J., Shainholtz, S., and Southworth, M.B. (1984): Bone mineral content of amenorrheic and eumenorrheic athletes. *N. Eng. J. Med.*, 311:277–281.

10. Eaton, S.B., and Konner, M. (1985): Paleolithic nutrition. *N. Engl. J. Med.*, 312:283–289.

11. Fernandes-Costa, F.J., Marshall, J., Ritchie, C., van Tonder, S.V., Dunn, D.S., Jenkins, T., and Metz, J. (1984): Transition from a hunter-gatherer to a settled lifestyle in the !Kung San: effect on iron, folate, and vitamin B_{12} nutrition. *Am. J. Clin. Nutr.*, 40:1295–1303.

12. Francis, R.M., Peacock, M., Storer, J.H., Davies, A.E.J., Brown, W.B., and Nordin, B.E.C. (1983): Calcium malabsorption in the elderly: The effect of treatment with oral 25-hydroxyvitamin D_3. *Eur. J. Clin. Invest.*, 13:391–396.

13. Francis, R.M., Peacock, M., Taylor, G.A., Storer, J.H., and Nordin, B.E.C. (1984): Calcium malabsorption in elderly women with vertebral fractures: Evidence for resistance to the action of vitamin D metabolites on the bowel. *Clin. Sci.*, 66:103–107.

14. Garn, S.M. (1981): Stature, skeletal mass, and evolution. In: *Symposium of Nutrition and Evolution, Food, Man, Society*, edited by N. Kretchmer, pp. 97–106. Masson & Co., New York.

15. Hantman, D.A., Vogel, J.M., Donaldson, C.L., Friedman, R., Goldsmith, R.S., and Hulley, S.B. (1973): Attempts to prevent disuse osteoporosis by treatment with calcitonin, longitudinal compression and supplementary calcium and phosphate. *J. Clin. Endocrinol. Metab.*, 36:845–858.

16. Harris, W.H., Heaney, R.P., Davis, L.A., Weinberg, E.H., Coutts, R.D., and Schiller, A.L. (1976): Stimulation of bone formation *in vivo* by phosphate supplementation. *Calcif. Tissue Res.*, 22:85–98.

17. Heaney, R.P. (1986): Calcium, bone health, and osteoporosis. In: *Bone and Mineral Research, Annual 4*, edited by W.A. Peck. Elsevier Science Publishers, New York (in press).

18. Heaney, R.P., Gallagher, J.C., Johnston, C.C., Neer, R., Parfitt, A.M., and Whedon, G.D. (1982): Calcium nutrition and bone health in the elderly. *Am. J. Clin. Nutr.*, 36:986–1013.

19. Heaney, R.P., and Recker, R.R. (1982): Effects of nitrogen, phosphorus, and caffeine on calcium balance in women. *J. Lab. Clin. Med.*, 99:46–55.

20. Heaney, R.P., and Recker, R.R. (1987): Distribution of calcium absorption in middle-aged women. *Am. J. Clin. Nutr.*, (in press).

21. Heaney, R.P., Recker, R.R., and Saville, P.D. (1978): Menopausal changes in calcium balance performance. *J. Lab. Clin. Med.*, 92:953–963.

22. Jowsey, J. (1977): Osteoporosis: Dealing with a crippling bone disease of the elderly. *Geriatrics*, 32:41–50.

23. Jowsey, J., and Gershon-Cohen, J. (1964): Effect of dietary calcium levels on production and reversal of experimental osteoporosis in cats. *Proc. Soc. Exp. Biol. Med.*, 116:437–441.

24. Jowsey, J., and Raisz, L.G. (1968): Experimental osteoporosis and parathyroid activity. *Endocrinology*, 82:384–396.

25. Lee, C.J., Lawler, G.S., and Johnson, G.H. (1981): Effects of supplementation of the diets with calcium and calcium-rich foods on bone density of elderly females with osteoporosis. *Am. J. Clin. Nutr.*, 34:819–823.

26. Lotz, M., Zisman, E., and Bartter, F.C. (1968): Evidence for a phosphorus-depletion syndrome in man. *N. Engl. J. Med.*, 278:409–415.

27. Marcus, R., Cann, C., Madvig, P., Minkoff, J., Goddard, M., Bayer, M., Martin, M., Gaudiani, L., Haskell, W., and Genant, H. (1985): Menstrual function and bone mass in elite women distance runners. *Ann. Intern. Med.*, 102:158–163.

28. Melton, L.J., III, and Riggs, B.L. (1983): Epidemiology of age-related fractures. In : *The Osteoporotic Syndrome—Detection, Prevention, and Treatment*, edited by L.V. Avioli, pp. 45–72. Grune & Stratton, Inc., New York.

29. Nilas, L., Christiansen, C.C., and Rodbro, P. (1984): Calcium supplementation and postmenopausal bone loss. *Br. Med. J.*, 289:1103–1106.

30. Opsahl, W., Zeronian, H., Ellison, M., Lewis, D., Rucker, R.B., and Riggins, R.S. (1982): Role of copper in collagen cross-linking and its influence on selected mechanical properties of chick bone and tendon. *J. Nutr.*, 112:708–716.

31. Parfitt, A.M. (1983): Dietary risk factors for age-related bone loss and fractures. *Lancet*, 2:1181–1185.

32. Raisz, L.G. (1965): Bone resorption in tissue culture. Factors influencing the response to parathyroid hormone. *J. Clin. Invest.*, 44:103–116.

33. Recker, R.R., Saville, P.D., and Heaney, R.P. (1977): The effect of estrogens and calcium carbonate on bone loss in postmenopausal women. *Ann. Intern. Med.*, 87:649–655.

34. Rigotti, N.A., Nussbaum, S.R., Herzog, D.B., and Neer, R.M. (1984): Osteoporosis in women with anorexia nervosa. *N. Engl. J. Med.*, 311:1601–1606.

35. Robertson, W.G. (1976): Urinary excretion. In: *Calcium, Phosphate and Magnesium Metabolism*, edited by B.E.C. Nordin, pp. 113–161. Churchill Livingstone, Great Britain.

36. Saltman, P. (1985): Trace minerals in health and disease. In: *Frontiers in Longevity Research*, edited by R.J. Morin, pp. 162–182. Charles C Thomas, Springfield, Illinois.

37. Spencer, H., Kramer, L., Osis, D., and Norris, C. (1978): Effect of phosphorus on the absorption of calcium and on the calcium balance in man. *J. Nutr.*, 108:447–457.

38. Spencer, H., and Lender, M. (1979): Adverse effects on aluminum-containing antacid on mineral metabolism. *Gastroenterology*, 76:603–606.

39. Wical, K.E., and Swoope, C.C. (1974): Studies of residual ridge resorption Part II. The relationship of dietary calcium and phosphorus to residual ridge resorption. *J. Prosthet. Dent.*, 32:13–22.

40. Wical, K.E., and Brussee, P. (1979): Effects of a calcium and vitamin D supplement on alveolar ridge resorption in immediate denture patients. *J. Prosthet. Dent.*, 41:4–11.

Osteoporosis: Etiology, Diagnosis, and Management, edited by B. Lawrence Riggs and L. Joseph Melton, III. Raven Press, New York © 1988.

14

Hormonal Factors: PTH, Vitamin D, and Calcitonin

Richard Eastell, Hunter Heath III, Rajiv Kumar, and B. Lawrence Riggs

Division of Endocrinology, Metabolism, and Internal Medicine, Mayo Medical School, Mayo Clinic and Mayo Foundation, Rochester, Minnesota 55905

Parathyroid hormone, 1,25-dihydroxyvitamin D, and, possibly, calcitonin regulate calcium homeostasis in man. This chapter reviews the effect of aging on the plasma levels of these hormones and describes the role of these age-related changes in the pathogenesis of osteoporosis.

The classification of involutional osteoporosis proposed by Riggs and Melton (123,124) will be used here. Type I osteoporosis (postmenopausal osteoporosis) is most common in the age range 50 to 65 years and is manifested by vertebral fractures and Colles' fractures. The cause is probably different from that of age-related bone loss. Type II osteoporosis (senile osteoporosis) is common in the elderly and is manifested by fractures of the hip, pelvis, proximal humerus, and proximal tibia. It probably has the same cause as age-related bone loss.

PARATHYROID HORMONE

Parathyroid hormone, an 84-amino acid peptide is secreted by the parathyroid gland; the principal stimulus for secretion is a decrease in the plasma calcium concentration (45). The effect of parathyroid hormone (PTH) on the proximal renal tubule is to increase production of 1,25-dihydroxyvitamin D_3 [$1,25(OH)_2D_3$]

and to decrease phosphate reabsorption; the effect on the distal renal tubule is to increase calcium reabsorption (38). The long-term effect on bone is to increase bone remodeling (117). Thus, PTH plays a major role in regulating calcium homeostasis in man.

PTH is secreted mainly as the intact peptide, but in the liver and kidney it is cleaved, between amino acids 33 and 34 and between 36 and 37 (131), releasing biologically inactive mid-region and COOH-terminal fragments. The biologic half-life of the intact hormone is shorter than that of the COOH-terminal fragments, so the principal immunoreactive form of PTH (iPTH) in the plasma is heterogeneous COOH-terminal fragments (91). Because they are cleared by glomerular filtration, the accumulation of these fragments is particularly marked in renal impairment.

In radioimmunoassays for PTH, the antiserum may be directed against the COOH-terminal or mid-region sequences, the NH_2 terminus, or the intact hormone. Most of the assays used in the studies described below used antisera with mid-region specificity, although a few used antisera directed against the NH_2 terminus (42,54,89) or the intact hormone (54). It is difficult to interpret studies that find an increase in mid-region or COOH-terminal iPTH with age because creatinine clearance decreases with age, resulting in increased retention of PTH fragments.

Parathyroid function may be studied by measuring the biologic effect of PTH *in vivo*. PTH acts on the renal tubule to cause increased urinary excretion of cyclic AMP (cAMP) and decreased renal tubular reabsorption of phosphorus. cAMP in the urine originates either from the action of PTH on renal tubular cells (nephrogenous cAMP) or from filtration at the glomerulus. Thus, nephrogenous cAMP can be computed from (total urinary cAMP) minus (plasma cAMP) times (creatinine clearance) (17). Also, the theoretical renal phosphate threshold, TmP/GFR, may be estimated (147). PTH increases bone remodeling, and this results in increased serum levels of bone Gla protein (BGP) and increased urinary excretion of hydroxyproline.

Bioactive PTH may be measured by a cytochemical bioassay (23,59) or by a guanyl nucleotide-amplified renal adenylate cyclase assay (105). These recently introduced, laborious methods have not yet been widely applied to age-related changes in PTH.

Effect of Age on Parathyroid Function

Serum iPTH increases with age. Gallagher et al. (54) found an 80% increase in iPTH by "mid-region" assay and a 30% increase with an "intact" assay (Fig. 1) in women between the ages of 20 and 90 years. Similar findings (36,49,68,88,118,149) and even larger increases (13,111) have been reported.

Glomerular filtration rate (GFR) decreases with age. Increased iPTH values might result from retention of fragments that are inactive biologically but detected immunologically or from an increase in biologically active PTH or from both of these effects. Decreased renal function decreases plasma 1,25(OH)$_2$D$_3$ (see below), and this may stimulate PTH secretion indirectly via decreased plasma calcium or directly by an action on the parathyroid glands. PTH secretion is inhibited by 1,25(OH)$_2$D$_3$ *in vitro* (if incubated for > 2 hr [58,61]), and PTH gene transcription is inhibited by

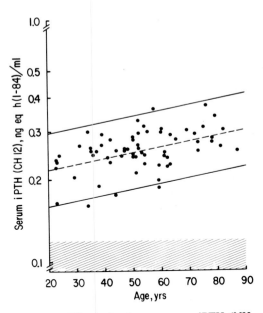

FIG. 1. Effect of aging on serum iPTH (NH$_2$ terminal antiserum) in 66 normal women. Hatched area represents limits of sensitivity of the assay. Lines show mean and 95% confidence limits. After Gallagher et al., ref. 54.

1,25(OH)$_2$D$_3$ both *in vitro* (21,126) and *in vivo* (130).

Four arguments support the idea that parathyroid function increases with age. First, radioimmunoassays using antisera directed against NH$_2$ terminal (42,54,89) or intact PTH determinants (54) show an increase in iPTH with age, although usually of smaller magnitude than found with COOH-terminal assays. Second, we have found an increase in bioactive PTH with age (M.S.Forero, R. Klein, R.A. Nissenson, K. Nelson, H. Heath III, C.D. Arnaud, and B.L. Riggs, unpublished data) as measured by the guanyl nucleotide-amplified renal adenylate cyclase assay of Nissenson et al. (105). Third, urinary cAMP excretion corrected for GFR increases by 30% between ages 20 and 90 years (36); nephrogenous cAMP doubles between these ages (68,88). Fourth, the TmP/GFR decreases with age by 30% between ages 20 and 90 years (13,68,88).

The increase in bioactive PTH probably results from a decrease in plasma ionized calcium (104,149). This decrease is not due to an increase in plasma phosphate because the latter actually decreases with age (49,149). More likely, it results from decreased intestinal absorption of calcium secondary to decreased plasma levels of $1,25(OH)_2D_3$ (see below).

Does the increase in serum PTH with age play a role in age-related bone loss and hence in type II osteoporosis? Primary hyperparathyroidism is associated with a decrease in bone mass to about 10% below that of age-matched controls, and this loss of bone is partially reversed by surgical removal of the adenoma (31,40,56,74,92). Osteopenia is most marked in postmenopausal women (113) and is associated with an increased risk of vertebral fractures (33). Conversely, hypoparathyroidism is associated with increased bone mass (65,128).

The bone loss associated with hyperparathyroidism is partly reversible and partly irreversible. Bone remodeling takes place at discrete foci known as bone remodeling units (BRU) (114). First, bone is resorbed by osteoclasts. Then, the resorption cavity is refilled by osteoblasts. In hyperparathyroidism, the number of BRU increases and bone mass decreases. If the disease is treated, the number of BRU decreases and bone mass increases—i.e., reversible bone loss. However, bone resorption can exceed new bone formation at each BRU (remodeling imbalance), causing bone to be lost irreversibly. Also, when trabecular plates are perforated there is no template for new bone formation and bone is lost irreversibly. The effect of these two mechanisms of irreversible bone loss is greater when bone remodeling increases, as with primary hyperparathyroidism and aging, and could explain why bone mass is only partially restored after parathyroidectomy for primary hyperparathyroidism.

There is good evidence that there is an age-related increase in bone turnover. Serum BGP and serum alkaline phosphatase activity may be considered to be markers of bone formation; urinary hydroxyproline is a marker of bone resorption. In some (36,43), but not all (22,96,115), studies, serum BGP increased with age, as did serum alkaline phosphatase activity (36,88). Urinary hydroxyproline excretion increases with age (36). Bone formation rate (BFR-v, %/year) increases in cortical bone (48) and trabecular bone (R. Eastell, P.D. Delmas, S.F. Hodgson, K.G. Mann, and B.L. Riggs, unpublished data), and the proportion of bone surface covered by osteoid increases with age (100), although these findings have not been confirmed by all workers (98,101). The increase in bone formation rate represents an increase in bone remodeling, because bone formation is coupled with bone resorption.

With increasing age, at each BRU there is a decrease in the amount of bone resorbed (44) and in the amount of bone formed (78). It is not known whether these two processes decrease by similar amounts, but it is likely that there is remodeling imbalance (114). If so, then an increase in the rate of bone remodeling would result in an increase in the rate of bone loss.

Parathyroid Function in Type I Osteoporosis

In about 10% of postmenopausal women with vertebral fractures there is an increase in serum iPTH (54,70, 118,141). This combination termed "type III osteoporosis" by Riggs et al. (119) is associated with low or normal serum ionized calcium and low-normal serum $1,25(OH)_2D_3$ levels; it may be due to an intrinsic defect in the enzyme 1α-hydroxylase in the kidney. These women have increased bone remodeling as determined by bone histomorphometry (70,141).

The levels of serum iPTH in type I osteoporosis usually are lower (Fig. 2) than those in age-matched controls (46,53,54,118). However, these findings were not confirmed by Bouillon et al. (16) who found no difference from controls or Fujita et al. (50) and Orimo and Shiraki (111) who found increases in serum iPTH.

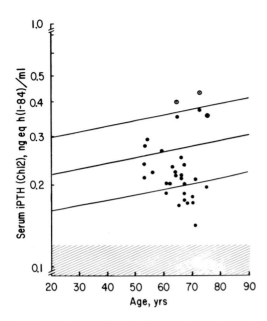

FIG. 2. Serum iPTH (NH_2 terminal antiserum) values in 31 women with type I osteoporosis and the normal mean and range shown in Fig. 1. Subgroup with high iPTH and low-normal plasma calcium and/or $1,25(OH)_2D_3$ reported by Riggs et al. (119). After Gallagher et al., ref. 54.

There is other evidence that PTH function is decreased in type I osteoporosis. Riggs et al. (121) reported decreased urinary excretion of cAMP, confirming an earlier observation by Lindsay and Sweeney (76). Gallagher et al. (54) reported increased TmP/GFR and plasma phosphate in patients with type I osteoporosis.

The above changes may be explained by an increase in bone resorption induced by the postmenopausal decrease in estrogen level (see Chapter 10, *this volume*). This increase would tend to increase plasma calcium and decrease plasma PTH. As a result, there would be an increase in TmP/GFR and a decrease in urinary cAMP.

VITAMIN D

The physiologically active form of the vitamin is $1,25(OH)_2D_3$ (18). Vitamin D is absorbed from the diet or is synthesized from precursors (provitamin D, previtamin D) in the epidermis in response to exposure of the skin to ultraviolet light (64). Vitamin D undergoes C-25 hydroxylation in the liver to 25-hydroxyvitamin D [25-(OH)-D]. The plasma concentration of 25-(OH)-D is a useful marker of vitamin D nutrition. This metabolite undergoes either C-1 or C-24 hydroxylation in the kidney to active $[1,25(OH)_2D_3]$ or inactive $[24,25-(OH)_2-D_3]$ forms of vitamin D (37).

The principal action of $1,25(OH)_2D_3$ is to increase intestinal calcium absorption (93). It also may act on bone to promote mineralization (90,137) and, at supraphysiologic levels, to stimulate bone resorption (86).

Plasma levels of 25-(OH)-D reflect vitamin D stores in the body. The levels are low in winter and high in summer, and they show a weak relationship to dietary vitamin D intake.

The plasma concentration of $1,25(OH)_2D_3$ is determined by its rate of production by renal 1α-hydroxylase activity and its rate of metabolic clearance (72). The activity of 1α-hydroxylase is increased by PTH, hypocalcemia and hypophosphatemia and decreased by $1,25-(OH)_2D_3$. Other factors are of lesser importance (37).

Effect of Age on Vitamin D Nutrition

Plasma levels of 25-(OH)-D decrease with age by more than 50 % (Fig. 3) (9,10,24, 28,53,55,62,79,82,110,127,145,148). There are several mechanisms that would decrease the plasma 25-(OH)-D level in elderly persons: 1) decreased dietary intake, 2) decreased vitamin D absorption, 3) decreased hepatic C25 hydroxylation, 4) increased metabolic clearance, 5) decreased epidermal vitamin D synthesis, and 6) decreased vitamin D-binding protein. We shall consider these mechanisms in turn.

1. Several groups have reported on the dietary consumption of vitamin D in the elderly (28,29,73). However, these studies did not include young controls. Elderly subjects commonly did not consume the Recommended Daily Allowance for vitamin D; however, this also may be true for younger subjects.

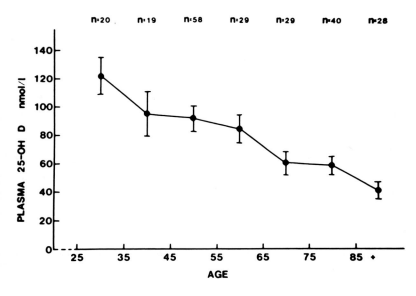
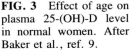

FIG. 3 Effect of age on plasma 25-(OH)-D level in normal women. After Baker et al., ref. 9.

2,3. The evidence on malabsorption of vitamin D in the elderly is conflicting. Barraguy et al. (10) administered ^{3}H-labeled vitamin D with a low-lipid meal to young (ages 30 to 58 years) and elderly (ages 68 to 98 years) subjects and found greater absorption by the young than by the elderly (13.2 % vs 7.6 % in 6 hr). Clemens et al. (27) gave 1.25 mg of vitamin D_2 in a single oral dose to young (ages 22 to 28 years) and elderly subjects (ages 57 to 88 years) and found similar increments in plasma 25-(OH)-D. Somerville et al. (135) gave low doses (12.5 μg/day) of vitamin D for 2 weeks then high doses (250 μg/day) to young (ages 24 to 48 years) and elderly (72 to 94 years) subjects and found similar increments in plasma 25-(OH)-D. One explanation for these apparently conflicting reports is that vitamin D absorption may be decreased in the elderly but the C25 hydroxylase activity may be increased as a result of the low levels of 25-(OH)-D and 1,25-$(OH)_2D_3$ in elderly subjects [see below for evidence on low 1,25$(OH)_2D_3$ levels in elderly; see Bell (11) for a review of C25 hydroxylase control by vitamin D metabolites].

4. The metabolic clearance rate of 25-(OH)-D has not been studied directly but the half-life of plasma 25-(OH)-D after administration of ^{3}H-labeled vitamin D was reported as 21 to 27 days (10) and did not increase with age. Clemens et al. (27) reported similar findings.

5. Plasma 25-(OH)-D increases in elderly subjects after exposure to ultraviolet light (30,133), and the response is similar to that in young subjects (34). MacLaughlin and Holick (85) reported a decrease in 7-dehydrocholesterol (provitamin D_3) content in skin biopsy specimens with aging. Furthermore, the conversion of provitamin D_3 to previtamin D_3 by ultraviolet light was decreased in skin from elderly subjects. Thus, vitamin D synthesis may be suboptimal in the elderly. Also, exposure to sunshine is often less in the elderly than in the young (9,62).

6. Changes in vitamin D-binding protein can cause profound changes in plasma 1,25-$(OH)_2D_3$ levels, such as the increase found in pregnancy or the decrease found in hepatic cirrhosis. However, vitamin D-binding protein concentrations do not change significantly with aging (49).

Thus, the plasma 25-(OH)-D level decreases with aging. The most important mechanisms are decreased sunshine exposure and decreased vitamin D absorption; mechanisms less well established include decreased dietary intake of vitamin D and decreased vitamin D production by the skin in response to ultraviolet light.

Effect of Age on Vitamin D Metabolism

Gallagher et al. (53) reported that plasma $1,25(OH)_2D_3$ levels decrease by 40% after age 65 years (Fig. 4). Decreases in plasma $1,25(OH)_2D_3$ with age also have been reported by others (27,32,49,87,144). However, three groups (26,39,84) were unable to find such a decrease. Plasma $1,25(OH)_2D_3$ concentration is affected by renal function and dietary calcium (53), and not all of the above papers reported these variables. Furthermore, the interassay variation of plasma $1,25(OH)_2D_3$ values under optimal conditions is about 15% (53,87) and so it may be difficult to detect small changes in $1,25(OH)_2D_3$ levels.

The most likely cause for the decrease in plasma $1,25(OH)_2D_3$ levels with aging is decreased renal 1α-hydroxylase activity. Tsai et al. (144) reported a smaller increment in plasma $1,25(OH)_2D_3$ concentration after 24-hr PTH infusion in elderly women than in young women. The increment in plasma $1,25(OH)_2D_3$ was inversely related to creatinine clearance. The increase in PTH with aging (see above) is

not sufficient to maintain plasma $1,25(OH)_2D_3$ in the elderly at the level found in young adults.

Intestinal calcium absorption decreases with age (Fig. 5), probably as a result of the decrease in plasma $1,25(OH)_2D_3$. This decrease is found by calcium balance studies (109), by jejunal perfusion studies (69), and by radiocalcium absorption tests (3,7,19,53). From age 20 years to age 80 years, the mean decrease in radiocalcium absorption is 40%.

Age-Related Bone Loss and Vitamin D Metabolites

In a study in Leeds, England, Baker et al. (8) found decreased levels of plasma 25-(OH)-D in patients with femoral neck fractures compared with age-matched controls. Half of the patients with fractures were house-bound and their dietary intake of vitamin D was less than that in controls. In Britain, few foods are fortified with vitamin D, and vitamin D deficiency is common in the house-bound. Patients with hip fracture in Finland (146), Israel (97), and the Netherlands (77) had low values of 25-(OH)-D with increased iPTH in the winter (after correction of the 25-(OH)-D values for low vitamin D-binding protein levels). In contrast, Lund et al. (83) reported normal levels of

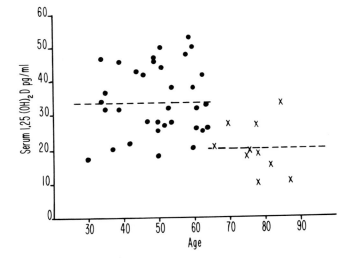

FIG. 4. Effect of age on plasma $1,25(OH)_2D_3$ levels in normal subjects under (●) and (x) over age 65 years. After Gallagher et al., ref. 53.

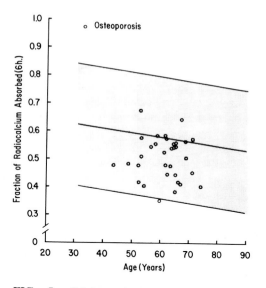

FIG. 5. Calcium absorption in 52 women with type I osteoporosis (o) and 95% confidence limits from 92 normal subjects. After Gallagher et al., ref. 53.

plasma 25-(OH)-D in Danish subjects with femoral neck fractures. In Denmark, food is supplemented with vitamin D and more than half of the elderly consume vitamin D supplements in the winter (82).

Bone histomorphometric findings in patients with femoral neck fracture in both England (1,2) and the United States (134) are consistent with, but not pathognomonic of, osteomalacia, i.e., increased proportion of bone surfaces covered by osteoid. This may have resulted from vitamin D deficiency because the proportion of osteoid surfaces with calcification fronts was decreased and the proportion of bone surfaces covered with osteoid was highest in late winter to spring, when plasma 25-(OH)-D was lowest (2).

A low concentration of vitamin D metabolites in plasma results in decreased calcium absorption. This would tend to cause a decrease in plasma calcium and thus secondary hyperparathyroidism, and this would cause decreased bone mass by the mechanisms described above. However, Tsai et al. (145) were unable to find any correlation between plasma

25-(OH)-D concentration and bone density in the radius or lumbar spine.

Vitamin D Metabolites and Type I Osteoporosis

Plasma 25-(OH)-D levels usually are normal in type I osteoporosis (53,108). However, increased mean plasma 25-(OH)-D levels have been described (79,136). In the report by Sorensen et al. (136), this was caused by previous therapy with vitamin D. Lore et al. (79,81) proposed that 25-hydroxylase activity may be increased in osteoporosis as a result of the low $1,25(OH)_2D_3$ levels found in osteoporosis. Bishop et al. (14) reported decreased mean levels of 25-(OH)-D. These reports did not always state whether cases and controls were matched for season (14,108). There are marked seasonal changes in plasma 25-(OH)-D, and failure to control for this vitiates the conclusions from such studies.

Plasma $1,25(OH)_2D_3$ levels reportedly are between 18% and 80% lower in patients with type I osteoporosis than in age-matched controls (Fig. 6) (4,53,81,84,111,121,136). In type I osteoporosis, no correlation was found between $1,25(OH)_2D_3$ and calcium absorption

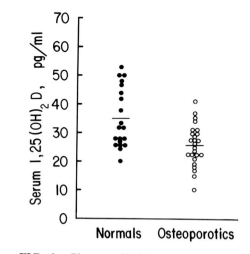

FIG. 6. Plasma $1,25(OH)_2D_3$ levels in 20 normal subjects (●) and 27 women with vertebral fracture (o). After Gallagher et al., ref. 53.

or between 1,25(OH)$_2$D$_3$ and dietary calcium (53), but 1,25(OH)$_2$D$_3$ was directly related to creatinine clearance (84). Nordin et al. (107,109) found no decrease in mean plasma 1,25(OH)$_2$D$_3$ level in type I osteoporosis. This negative finding may be related to the high interassay variation in the plasma 1,25(OH)$_2$D$_3$ assay, and the number of cases and controls described by Nordin (16 pairs) may not have been large enough to detect a significant difference. Also, the degree of decrease in plasma 1,25(OH)$_2$D$_3$ may be related to net bone resorption and hence to the severity of osteoporosis. Normal levels of 1,25(OH)$_2$D$_3$ were also reported in type I osteoporosis in three other studies (26,47,63).

Mean fractional calcium absorption is decreased by 20 to 30% in type I osteoporosis compared with age-matched controls (Fig. 5) (20,53,107,108,122,125). One group found no decrease (7).

Thus, plasma 1,25(OH)$_2$D$_3$ and intestinal calcium absorption probably decrease with age and may decrease further in type I osteoporosis.

Possible Mechanisms for Decrease in Intestinal Calcium Absorption in Type I Osteoporosis

Decreased calcium absorption could be caused by: (1) resistance of the intestine to the action of 1,25(OH)$_2$D$_3$; (2) intrinsic defect of 1α-hydroxylase activity; or (3) suppression of 1α-hydroxylase activity (in this model, increased net bone resorption due to estrogen deficiency would increase plasma calcium, suppress PTH, and thus suppress 1α-hydroxylase activity).

We favor mechanism 3 for the following reasons:

1. Treatment with "physiologic" doses of 1,25(OH)$_2$D$_3$ increases calcium absorption in type I osteoporosis to the same extent as in age-matched controls (51,53,125). This would support mechanisms 2 and 3 but not mechanism 1.

2. In type I osteoporosis, measures of parathyroid function (radioimmunoassay for PTH, reciprocal of plasma phosphate concentration) show a negative correlation with measures of bone resorption (bone histomorphometry, radiocalcium kinetics) as tested by canonical correlation analysis (120). Thus, increased bone resorption suppresses plasma PTH. Conversely, measures of parathyroid function show a positive correlation with measures of calcium absorption (fractional absorption of dietary calcium) by canonical correlation analysis. Thus, decreased plasma PTH results in decreased calcium absorption. This latter finding supports mechanism 3. According to mechanism 2, the primary defect in 1α-hydroxylase activity would result in decreased calcium absorption, decreased plasma calcium, and increased plasma PTH; mechanism 1 would also result in decreased calcium absorption and increased plasma PTH.

3. Slovik et al. (132) reported an increase in plasma 1,25(OH)$_2$D$_3$ after intravenous infusion of PTH in young subjects. This increase was smaller in elderly subjects with osteoporosis. Was this decreased response due to aging or to the mechanisms underlying osteoporosis? Tsai et al. (144) reported that the increase in 1,25(OH)$_2$D$_3$ in response to PTH infusion was not as great in older persons (Fig. 7A) and, by multiple regression analysis, showed that the age-related change was closely related to a decrease in creatinine clearance (Fig. 7B). Riggs et al. (121) and Sorensen et al. (136) reported normal increments in plasma 1,25(OH)$_2$D$_3$ after PTH stimulation in type I osteoporosis compared with age-matched controls. Thus, the effect of PTH on renal 1α-hydroxylase activity decreases with age, but this decrease is the same in type I osteoporosis as it is in age-matched controls. This would support mechanism 3 rather than 1 or 2.

4. To determine whether estrogen therapy would reverse the decreases in plasma 1,25(OH)$_2$D$_3$ and calcium absorption, Gal-

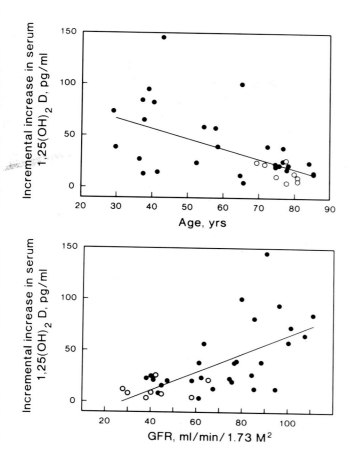

FIG. 7. Effect of age (A) and of creatinine clearance (B) on the incremental increase in serum $1,25(OH)_2D_3$ after 24-hr intravenous infusion of bovine PTH(1-34) in normal women (●) and women with hip fractures (o). After Tsai et al., ref. 144.

lagher et al. (52) administered conjugated estrogen for 6 months to 12 patients who had type I osteoporosis. They reported mean increases of 20 to 30% in plasma $1,25(OH)_2D_3$, fractional calcium absorption, and plasma iPTH. No changes were found in nine patients treated with placebo.

The above changes in vitamin D metabolites suggest that the primary defect in type I osteoporosis is estrogen deficiency and that the decrease in plasma $1,25(OH)_2D_3$ level is a consequence rather than a cause of type I osteoporosis.

CALCITONIN

Calcitonin is a 32 amino acid polypeptide secreted by the C cells of the thyroid in response to an increase in plasma calcium. Phar-

macologic doses of calcitonin (CT) decrease bone resorption and decrease reabsorption of phosphate and calcium in the renal tubule, but it is uncertain whether CT affects calcium homeostasis in adult humans (6).

CT is measured by radioimmunoassay. Most of the circulating immunoreactive CT (iCT) is present as molecules larger than monomeric CT and of questionable bioactivity. Body and Heath (15) devised an assay for monomeric CT that uses silica extraction (exCT). In this assay, 90% of either radioiodinated or unlabeled synthetic monomeric human CT was recovered. However, exCT levels were only 16% of iCT levels, and there was no correlation between basal levels of exCT and iCT. Thus, measurements of whole plasma iCT without prior extraction may not reflect levels of biologically active CT.

The CT secretion by the C cells of the thyroid may be tested by intravenous administration of calcium or pentagastrin. The dose of calcium given is in proportion to body weight because the increment in plasma calcium is dependent on the size of the calcium pool and the rate of movement of calcium out of this pool into bone, urine, and intestinal secretions.

Effects of Age on Calcitonin Secretion

There is disagreement about the effect of age on plasma CT concentrations and on the CT response to hypercalcemia. The disagreement may result partly from the difficulty in measuring monomeric CT and partly from the variable calcemic response to intravenous administration of calcium. Furthermore, the metabolic clearance rate of CT decreases with age (142), and this may explain why iCT levels reportedly peak later in elderly subjects (129).

Deftos et al. (35) reported a decrease in basal plasma iCT concentrations in men but not in women and a decrease in the response of iCT to hypercalcemia in both men and women. Morimoto et al. (103) found no change in basal iCT with age but a decrease in the response of iCT to hypercalcemia in men (women were not studied). Lore et al. (80) reported no effect of age on basal plasma iCT concentration; however, in a separate group of 30 women, the postmenopausal group had a lower plasma iCT than the premenopausal group. Body and Heath (15) reported that aging had no effect on either basal plasma iCT and exCT or on the response of iCT and exCT to hypercalcemia. A larger second study by the same group (142) confirmed these earlier findings. Anatomic studies of the thyroid gland have shown no decrease in C cell number with aging (71,112), and some have shown an increase (57).

Stevenson (138) proposed that a postmenopausal decrease in plasma CT causes osteoporosis. Also, because, at all ages, women have lower iCT and exCT levels than men, this may explain why women are at higher risk for osteoporosis. Estrogen replacement therapy decreases the rate of postmenopausal bone loss

(75,106,116) and causes an increase in midday plasma iCT (139). However, this latter finding was not confirmed by Hurley et al. (66) who measured both exCT and iCT (basal and calcium-stimulated) before and after ethynylestradiol therapy in 14 postmenopausal women and found no increase.

There is little evidence to suggest that a deficiency (such as after thyroidectomy) or an excess (such as with medullary thyroid carcinoma [MTC]) of CT has any effect on bone mass. Hurley et al. (67) reported *decreased* bone density of the lumbar spine in MTC and Emmertsen et al. (41) reported normal trabecular bone volume in iliac crest bone biopsy specimens taken from 14 patients with MTC. Melvin et al. (99) reported normal midradius bone mineral content in 18 patients with MTC. Conversely, Hurley et al. (67) found normal radius and lumbar spine bone densities in 21 patients after total thyroidectomy, whereas McDermott et al. (95) found decreased mid-radius and distal radius bone densities in 18 patients after total thyroidectomy. However, the latter group has now reported that the rate of bone loss is not increased in thyroidectomized persons (94). The basal level of iCT and the response of iCT to calcium infusion in patients with hip fracture are the same as in age-matched controls (12). Thus, because exCT does not decrease with aging, it is unlikely that plasma bioactive CT concentration decreases with aging. Even if there were a decrease, there is no consistent evidence that this would have a detrimental effect on bone mass.

Calcitonin Secretion in Type I Osteoporosis

Type I osteoporosis has been reported to be associated with low (102), normal (25), or slightly increased (143) plasma CT levels. Taggart et al. (140) and Zseli et al. (150) reported normal basal plasma iCT concentration but decreased iCT response to hypercalcemia. In another study, basal levels of exCT were higher in women with type I osteoporosis than in age-matched controls and responses of iCT and exCT to calcium infusions were normal

(143). As described above, there is no convincing evidence relating bone density to CT level.

CT therapy was effective in decreasing the rate of bone loss in patients with postmenopausal osteoporosis (5,60). This effect is pharmacologic rather than physiologic.

SUMMARY

We propose that the principal mechanism of age-related bone loss and type II osteoporosis is decreased $l\alpha$-hydroxylase activity. This decrease causes decreases in plasma $1,25(OH)_2D_3$ levels, calcium absorption, and plasma ionized calcium. In response to these changes, there is increased PTH secretion, which decreases plasma phosphate level and increases bone remodeling. The increased bone remodeling rate, in association with an imbalance of bone remodeling (due to impaired osteoblast activity), results in decreased bone mass. In elderly subjects living in countries with low ultraviolet light exposure, low plasma 25-(OH)-D levels may impair bone mineralization. CT probably plays no role in age-related bone loss.

Type I osteoporosis probably results from increased bone resorption due to factors interacting with estrogen deficiency. As a result, plasma calcium tends to increase and thus PTH secretion is suppressed. This increases plasma phosphate and decreases $1,25(OH)_2D_3$ and calcium absorption. CT probably plays no role in type I osteoporosis, although its concentration may change secondarily.

REFERENCES

1. Aaron, J.E., Gallagher, J.C., and Anderson, J. (1974): Frequency of osteomalacia and osteoporosis in fractures of the proximal femur. *Lancet*, 1:229–233.
2. Aaron, J.E., Gallagher, J.C., and Nordin, B.E.C. (1974): Seasonal variation of histological osteomalacia in femoral neck fractures. *Lancet*, 2:84–85.
3. Alevizaki, C.C., Ikkos, D.G., and Singhelakis, P. (1973): Progressive decrease of true intestinal calcium absorption with age in normal man. *J. Nucl. Med.*, 14:760–762.
4. Aloia, J.F., Cohn, S.H., Vaswani, A., Yeh, J.K.,

and Ellis, K. (1985): Risk factors for postmenopausal osteoporosis. *Am. J. Med.*, 78:95–100.
5. Aloia, J.F., Vaswani, A., Kapoor, A., Yeh, J.K., and Cohn, S.H. (1985): Treatment of osteoporosis with calcitonin, with and without growth hormone. *Metabolism*, 34:124–129.
6. Austin, L.A., and Heath, H., III (1981): Calcitonin: physiology and pathophysiology. *N. Engl. J. Med.*, 304:269–278.
7. Avioli, L.V., McDonald, J.E., and Lee, S.W. (1965): The influence of age on the intestinal absorption of ^{47}Ca in women and its relation to ^{47}Ca absorption in postmenopausal osteoporosis. *J. Clin. Invest.*, 44:1960–1967.
8. Baker, M.R., McDonnell, H., Peacock, M., and Nordin, B.E.C. (1979): Plasma 25-hydroxyvitamin D concentrations in patients with fractures of the femoral neck. *Br. Med. J.*, I:589–590.
9. Baker, M.R., Peacock, M., and Nordin, B.E.C. (1980): The decline in vitamin D status with age. *Age and Ageing*, 9:249–252.
10. Barraguy, J.M., France, M.W., Corless, D., Gupta, S.P., Switala, S., Boucher, B.J., and Cohen, R.D. (1978): Intestinal cholecalciferol absorption in the elderly and in younger adults. *Clin. Sci. Mol. Biol*, 55:213–220.
11. Bell, N.H. (1985): Vitamin D-endocrine system. *J. Clin. Invest.*, 76:1–6.
12. Beringer, T.R.O., Ardill, J., and Taggart, H.McA. (1986): Absence of evidence for a role of calcitonin in the etiology of femoral neck fracture. *Calcif. Tissue Int.*, 39:300–303.
13. Berlyne, G.M., Ben-Ari, J., Kushelevsky, A., Idelman, A., Galinsky, D., Hirsch, M., Shainkin, R., Yagil, R., and Zlotnik, M. (1975): The aetiology of senile osteoporosis: secondary hyperparathyroidism due to renal failure. *Quart. J. Med.*, 64:505–521.
14. Bishop, J.E., Norman, A.W., Coburn, J.W., Roberts, P.A., and Henry, H.L. (1980): Studies on the metabolism of calciferol. XVI. Determination of the concentration of 25-hydroxyvitamin D, 24,25-dihydroxyvitamin D and 1,25-dihydroxyvitamin D in a single two-milliliter plasma sample. *Min. Elect. Metab.*, 3:181–189.
15. Body, J.J., and Heath, H., III. (1983): Estimates of circulating monomeric calcitonin: physiological studies in normal and thyroidectomized man. *J. Clin. Endocrinol. Metab.*, 57:897–903.
16. Bouillon, R., Guerens, P., Dequecker, J., and De Moor, P. (1979): Parathyroid function in primary osteoporosis. *Clin. Sci.*, 57:167–171.
17. Broadus, A.E., Mahaffey, J.E., Martter, F.C., and Neer, R.M. (1977): Nephrogenous cyclic adenosine monophosphate as a parathyroid function test. *J. Clin. Invest.*, 60:771–783.
18. Brommage, R., and DeLuca, H.F. (1985): Evidence that $1,25$-dihydroxyvitamin D_3 is the physiologically active metabolite of vitamin D_3. *Endocrine Rev.*, 6:491–511.
19. Bullamore, J.R., Gallagher, J.C., Wilkinson, R., Nordin, B.E.C., and Marshall, D.H. (1970): Effect of age on calcium absorption. *Lancet*, 2:535–537.

20. Cannigia, A., Gennari, C., Bianchi, V., and Guideri, R. (1963): Intestinal absorption of ^{45}Ca in senile osteoporosis. *Acta Med. Scand.*, 173:613–617.

21. Cantley, L.K., Russell, J., Lettieri, D., and Sherwood, L.M. (1985): 1,25-Dihydroxyvitamin D$_3$ suppresses parathyroid hormone secretion from bovine parathyroid cells in tissue culture. *Endocrinology*, 117:2114–2119.

22. Catherwood, B.D., Marcus, R., Madvig, P., and Cheung, A.K. (1985): Determinants of bone gamma-carboxyglutamic acid-containing protein in plasma of healthy aging subjects. *Bone*, 6:9–13.

23. Chambers, D.J., Dunham, J., Zanelli, J.M., Parsons, J.A., Bitensky, L., and Chayen, J. (1978): A sensitive bioassay of parathyroid hormone in plasma. *Clin. Endocrinol. (Oxf.)*, 9:375–379.

24. Chapuy, M.-C., Durr, F., and Chapuy, P. (1983): Age-related changes in parathyroid hormone and 25-hydroxycholecalciferol levels. *J. Gerontol.*, 38:19–22.

25. Chesnut, C.H., III, Baylink, D.J., Sisom, K., Nelp, W.B., and Roos, B.A. (1980): Basal plasma immunoreactive calcitonin in postmenopausal osteoporosis. *Metabolism*, 29:559–562.

26. Christiansen, C., and Rodbro,P. (1984): Serum vitamin D metabolites in younger and elderly postmenopausal women. *Calcif. Tissue Int.*, 36:19–24.

27. Clemens, T.L., Zhon, X.-Y., Myles, M., Endres, D., and Lindsay, R. (1986): Serum vitamin D$_2$ and vitamin D$_3$ metabolite concentrations and absorption of vitamin D$_2$ in elderly subjects. *J. Clin. Endocrinol. Metab.*, 63:656–660.

28. Corless, D., Beer, M., Boncher, B.J., Gupta, S.P., and Cohen, R.D. (1975): Vitamin D status in long-stay geriatric patients. *Lancet*, 1:1404–1406.

29. Corless, D., Gupta, S.P., Sattar, D.A., Switala, S., and Boucher, B.J. (1979): Vitamin D status of residents of an old people's home and long-stay patients. *Gerontology*, 25:350–355.

30. Corless, D., Gupta, S.P., Switala, S., Barraguy, J.M., Boycher, B.J., Cohen, R.D., and Diffey, B.L. (1978): Response of plasma 25-hydroxyvitamin D to ultraviolet irradiation in long-stay geriatric patients. *Lancet*, 2:649–651.

31. Dalen, N., and Hjern, B. (1974): Bone mineral content in patients with primary hyperparathyroidism without radiological evidence of skeletal changes. *Acta Endocrinol. (Copenh.)*, 75:297–304.

32. Dandona, P., Menon, R.K., Shenoy, R., Houlder, S., Thomas, M., and Mallinson, W.J.W. (1986): Low 1,25-dihydroxyvitamin D, secondary hyperparathyroidism, and normal osteocalcin in elderly subjects. *J. Clin. Endocrinol. Metab.*, 63:459–462.

33. Dauphine, R.T., Riggs, B.L., and Scholz, D.A. (1975): Back pain and vertebral crush fractures: an unemphasized mode of presentation for primary hyperparathyroidism. *Ann. Intern. Med.*, 83:365–367.

34. Davie, M., and Lawson, D.E.M. (1980): Assessment of plasma 25-hydroxyvitamin D response to ultraviolet irradiation over a controlled area in young and elderly subjects. *Clin. Sci.*, 58:235–242.

35. Deftos, L.J., Weisman, M.H., Williams, G.W., Karpf, D.B., Frumar, A.M., Davidson, B.J., Par-

themore, J.G., and Judd, H.L. (1980): The influence of age and sex on plasma calcitonin in human beings. *N. Engl. J. Med.*, 302:1351–1353.

36. Delmas, P.D., Stenner, D., Wahner, H., Mann, K.G., and Riggs, B.L. (1983): Increase in serum bone γ-carboxyglutamic acid protein with aging in women. *J. Clin. Invest.*, 71:1316–1321.

37. DeLuca, H.F., and Schnoes, H.K. (1983): Vitamin D: recent advances. *Ann. Rev. Biochem.*, 52:411–439.

38. Dennis, V.W., Stead, W.W., and Myers, J.L. (1979): Renal handling of phosphate and calcium. *Ann. Rev. Physiol.*, 41:257–271.

39. Dokoh, S., Morita, R., Fukunaga, M., Yamamoto, I., and Torizuka, K. (1978): Competitive protein binding assay for 1,25-dihydroxyvitamin D in human plasma. *Endocrinol. Jpn.*, 25:431–436.

40. Eastell, R., Kennedy, N.S.J., Smith, M.A., Tothill, P., Edwards, C.R.W. (1986): Changes in total body calcium following surgery for primary hyperparathyroidism. *Bone*, 7:269–272.

41. Emmertson, K., Melsen, F., Mosekilde, L., Lund, B.I., Lund, B.J., Sorensen, O.H., Nielsen, H.E., Solling, H., and Hansen, H.H. (1981): Altered vitamin D metabolism and bone remodelling in patients with medullary thyroid carcinoma and hypercalcitoninemia. *Metab. Bone Dis. Rel. Res.*, 4:17–23.

42. Endres, D.B., Morgan, C.H., Garry, P.J., and Omdahl, J.L. (1986): Parathyroid function in a free-living elderly and young southwestern population. *J. Bone Min. Res.*, 1(S):342.

43. Epstein, S., Poser, J., McClintock, R., Johnston, C.C., Bryce, G., and Hui, S. (1984): Differences in serum bone gla protein with age and sex. *Lancet*, 1:307–310.

44. Eriksen, E.F., Mosekilde, L., and Melsen, F. (1985): Trabecular bone resorption depth decreases with age: differences between normal males and females. *Bone*, 6:113–123.

45. Fischer, J.A., Blum, J.W., Born, W., Dambacher, M.A., and Dempster, D.W. (1982): Regulation of parathyroid hormone secretion in vitro and in vivo. *Calcif. Tissue Int.*, 34:313–316.

46. Franchimont, P., and Heynen, G. (1976): Parathormone and calcitonin. In: *Radioimmunoassay in Various Medical and Osteoarticular Disorders*, pp. 101–107. J.B. Lippincott Co., Philadelphia.

47. Francis, R.M., Peacock, M., Taylor, G.A., Storer, J.H., and Nordin, B.E.C. (1984): Calcium absorption in elderly women with vertebral fractures: evidence for resistance to the action of vitamin D metabolites on the bowel. *Clin. Sci.*, 66:103–107.

48. Frost, H.M. (1969): Tetracycline-based histological analysis of bone remodelling. Editorial. *Calcif. Tissue Res.*, 3:211–237.

49. Fujisawa, Y., Kida, K., and Matsuda, H. (1984): Role of change in vitamin D metabolism with age in calcium and phosphorus metabolism in normal human subjects. *J. Clin. Endocrinol. Metab.*, 59:719–726.

50. Fujita, T., Orimo, H., Okano, K., Yoshikawa, M., Shimo, R., Inone, T., and Itami, Y. (1972): Radioimmunoassay of serum parathyroid hormone in

postmenopausal osteoporosis. *Endocrinol. Jpn.*, 19:571–577.

51. Gallagher, J.C., Jerpbak, C.M., Jee, W.S.S., Johnson, K.A., DeLuca, H.F., and Riggs, B.L. (1982): 1,25 Dihydroxyvitamin D_3: short- and long-term effects on bone and calcium metabolism in patients with postmenopausal osteoporosis. *Proc. Natl. Acad. Sci. USA*, 79:3325–3329.

52. Gallagher, J.C., Riggs, B.L., and DeLuca, H.F. (1980): Effect of estrogen on calcium absorption and serum vitamin D metabolites in postmenopausal osteoporosis. *J. Clin. Endocrinol. Metab.*, 51:1359–1364.

53. Gallagher, J.C., Riggs, B.L., Eisman, J., Hamstra, A., Arnaud, S.B., and DeLuca, H.F. (1979): Intestinal calcium absorption and serum vitamin D metabolites in normal subjects and osteoporotic patients. *J. Clin. Invest.*, 64:729–736.

54. Gallagher, J.C., Riggs, B.L., Jerpbak, C.M., and Arnaud, C.D. (1980): The effect of age on serum immunoreactive parathyroid hormone in normal and osteoporotic women. *J. Lab. Clin. Med.*, 95:373–385.

55. Garcia-Pascual, B., Peytremann, A., Courvoisier, B., and Lawson, D.E.M. (1976): A simplified competitive protein-binding assay for 25-hydroxy-calciferol. *Clin. Chim. Acta*, 68:99–105.

56. Genant, H.K., Heck, L.L., Lanzl, L.H., Rossman, K., Horst, J.V., and Paloyen, E. (1973): Primary hyperparathyroidism: a comprehensive study of clinical, biochemical and radiographic manifestations. *Radiology*, 109:513–524.

57. Gibson, W.G.H., Peng, T.-C., and Croker, B.P. (1982): Age-associated C-cell hyperplasia in the human thyroid. *Am. J. Pathol.*, 106:388–393.

58. Golden, P., Greenwalt, A., Martin, K., Bellorin-Font, E., Mazey, R., Klahr, S., and Slatopolsky, E. (1980): Lack of a direct effect of 1,25-dihydroxy-cholecalciferol on parathyroid hormone secretion by normal bovine parathyroid glands. *Endocrinology*, 107:602–607.

59. Goltzman, D., Henderson, B., and Loveridge, N. (1980): Cytochemical bioassay of parathyroid hormone: Characteristics of the assay and analysis of circulating hormone forms. *J. Clin. Invest.*, 65:1309–1317.

60. Gruber, H.E., Ivey, J.L., Baylink, D.J., Matthews, M., Nelp, W.B., Sisom, K., and Chesnut, C.H., III (1984): Long-term calcitonin therapy in postmenopausal osteoporosis. *Metabolism*, 33:295–303.

61. Gruson, M., Demignon, J., Del Pinto Montes, J., and Miravet, L. (1982): Comparative effects of some hydroxylated vitamin D metabolites on parathyrin secretion by dispersed rat parathyroid cells in vitro. *Steroids*, 40:275–285.

62. Guggenheim, K., Kravitz, M., Tal, R., and Kaufmann, N.A. (1979): Biochemical parameters of vitamin D nutrition in old people in Jerusalem. *Nutr. Metab.*, 23:172–178.

63. Haussler, M.R., Donaldson, C.A., Allegretto, E.A., Marion, S.L., Mangelsdorf, J., Kelly, M.A., and Pike, J.W. (1984): New actions of 1,25-dihydroxyvitamin D_3: possible clues to the pathogenesis of postmenopausal osteoporosis. In: *Copenhagen International Symposium on Osteoporosis*, edited by C. Christiansen, C.D. Arnau, B.E.C. Nordin, A.M. Parfitt, W.A. Peck, and B.L. Riggs, pp. 725–736, Aalborg Stiftsbogtrykkeri, Glostrup, Denmark.

64. Holick, M.F. (1985): The photobiology of vitamin D and its consequences for humans. *Ann. N. Y. Acad.*, 453:1–13.

65. Hossain, M., Smith, D.A., and Nordin, B.E.C. (1970): Parathyroid activity and postmenopausal osteoporosis. *Lancet*, 1:809–811.

66. Hurley, D.L., Tiegs, R.D., and Heath, H., III (1986): Does estrogen treatment in postmenopausal women affect calcitonin secretion? Abstract, *J. Bone Min. Res.*, 1(Suppl. 1):447.

67. Hurley, D.L., Tiegs, R.D., Wahner, H.W., and Heath, H., III (1986): Does prolonged calcitonin excess or deficiency affect bone mineral density in women? *J. Bone Min. Res.*, 1(Suppl. 1):240, (Abstr.)

68. Insogna, K.L., Lewis, A.M., Lipinski, B.A., Bryant, C., and Baran, D.T. (1981): Effect of age on serum immunoreactive parathyroid hormone and its biological effects. *J. Clin. Endocrinol. Metab.*, 53:1072–1075.

69. Ireland, P., and Fordtran, J.S. (1973): Effect of dietary calcium and age on jejunal calcium absorption in humans studied by intestinal perfusion. *J. Clin. Invest.*, 52:2672–2681.

70. Joly, R., Chapuy, M.C., Alexandre, C., and Meunier, P.J. (1980): Osteoporosis a' haut niveau de remodelage et fonction parathyroidienne. Confrontations histo-biologiques. *Pathol. Biol.*, 28:417–424.

71. Kendall, C.H., Cope, J., and McCluskey, E. (1985): C cell populations in thyroid: a postmortem study. *J. Pathol.*, 145:A83.

72. Kumar, R. (1984): Metabolism of 1,25-dihydroxy-vitamin D_3. *Physiol. Rev.*, 64:478–504.

73. Lawson, D.E.M., Paul, A.A., Black. A.E., Cole, T.J., Mandal, A.R., and Davie, M. (1979): Relative contributions of diet and sunlight to vitamin D state in the elderly. *Br. Med. J.*, 2:303–305.

74. Leppla, D.C., Snyder, W., and Pak, C.Y.C. (1982): Sequential changes in bone density before and after parathyroidectomy in primary hyperparathyroidism. *Invest. Radiol.*, 17:604–606.

75. Lindsay, R., Aitken, J.M., Anderson, J.B., Harte, D.M., MacDonald, E.B., and Clark, A.C. (1976): Long-term prevention of postmenopausal osteoporosis by oestrogen. *Lancet*, 1:1038–1040.

76. Lindsay, R., and Sweeney, A. (1978): Urinary cyclic-AMP in osteoporosis. *Scott. Med. J.*, 21:231–232, (Abstr.)

77. Lips, P., Bouillon, R., Jongen, M.J.M., van Ginkel, F.C., van der Vijgh, W.J.F., and Netelenbos, J.C. (1985): The effect of trauma on serum concentrations of vitamin D metabolites in patients with hip fracture. *Bone*, 6:63–67.

78. Lips, P., Courpron, P., and Meunier, P.J. (1978): Mean wall thickness of trabecular bone packets in the human iliac crest: changes with age. *Calcif. Tissue Res.*, 26:13–17.

79. Lore, F., Di Cairano, G., Signorini, A.M., and Caniggia, A. (1981): Serum levels of 25-hydroxy-vitamin D in postmenopausal osteoporosis. *Calcif. Tissue Int.*, 33:467–470.

80. Lore, F., Galli, M., Franci, B., and Martorelli, M.T. (1984): Calcitonin levels in normal subjects according to age and sex. *Biomed. Pharmacother.*, 38:261–263.

81. Lore, F., Nuti, R., Vattimo, A., and Caniggia, A. (1984): Vitamin D metabolites in postmenopausal osteoporosis. *Horm. Metab. Res.*, 16:58.

82. Lund, B., and Sorensen, O.H. (1979): Measurement of 25-hydroxyvitamin D in serum and its relation to sunshine, age and vitamin D. *Scand. J. Clin. Lab. Invest.*, 39:23–30.

83. Lund, B., Sorensen, O.H., and Christensen, A.B. (1975): 25-Hydroxycholecalciferol and fractures of the proximal femur. *Lancet*, 2:300–302.

84. Lund, B., Sorensen, O.H., Lund, B., and Agner, E. (1982): Serum 1,25-dihydroxyvitamin D in normal subjects and in patients with postmenopausal osteopenia. Influence of age, renal function and oestrogen therapy. *Horm. Metab. Res.*, 14:271–274.

85. MacLaughlin, J., and Holick, M.F. (1985): Aging decreases the capacity of human skin to produce vitamin D_3. *J. Clin. Invest.*, 76:1536–1538.

86. Maierhoffer, W.J., Gray, R.W., Cheung, H.S., and Lemann, J. (1983): Bone resorption stimulated by elevated serum 1,25-$(OH)_2$vitamin D concentrations in healthy men. *Kidney Int.*, 24:555–560.

87. Manolagas, S.C., Howard, J., Culler, F., Catherwood, B.D., and Deftos, L.J. (1982): Cytoreceptor assay for 1,25$(OH)_2$D: a simple, rapid and reliable test for clinical application. *Clin. Res.*, 30:527A, (Abstr.)

88. Marcus, R., Madvig, P., and Young, G. (1984): Age-related changes in parathyroid hormone and parathyroid hormone action in normal humans. *J. Clin. Endocrinol. Metab.*, 58:223–230.

89. Marcus, R., Minkoff, J., Young, G., Grant, B., and Segre, G.V. (1986): Age-related rise in parathyroid hormone: comparison of NH_2-terminal and mid-molecule assays. *J. Bone Min. Res.*, 1(Suppl):343.

90. Marie, P.J., Hott, M., and Garba, M.-T. (1985): Contrasting effects of 1,25-dihydroxyvitamin D_3 on bone matrix and mineral appositional rates in the mouse. *Metabolism*, 34:777–783.

91. Martin, K.J., Hruska, K.A., Freitag, J.J., Klahr, S., and Slatopolsky, E. (1979): The peripheral metabolism of parathyroid hormone. *N. Engl. J. Med.*, 301:1092–1098.

92. Martin, P., Bergman, P., Gillet, C., Fuss, M., Kinnaert, P., Corvilain, J., and van Geertruyden, J. (1986): Partially reversible osteopenia after surgery for primary hyperparathyroidism. *Arch. Intern. Med.*, 146:689–691.

93. Mayer, E., Kadowaki, S., Williams, G., and Norman, A.W. (1984): 1α,25-Dihydroxyvitamin D. In: *Vitamin D: Basic and Clinical Aspects*, edited by R. Kumar, pp. 259–302. Martinus Nijhoff Publishers, Hingham, Massachusetts.

94. McDermott, M.T., Hofeldt, F.D., and Kidd, G.S.

95. McDermott, M.T., Kidd, G.S., Blue, P., Crhaed, V., and Hofeldt, F.D. (1983): Reduced bone mineral content in totally thyroidectomized patients: possible effect of calcitonin deficiency. *J. Clin. Endocrinol. Metab.*, 56:936–939.

96. Melick. R.A., Farrugia, W., and Quelch, K.J. (1985): Plasma osteocalcin in man. *Aust. N. Z. J. Med.*, 15:410–416.

97. Meller, Y., Kestenbaum, R.S., Galinsky, D., and Shany, S. (1986): Seasonal variations in serum levels of vitamin D metabolism and parathormone in geriatric patients with fractures in southern Israel. *Isr. J. Med. Sci.*, 22:8–11.

98. Melsen, F., and Mosekilde, L. (1978): Tetracycline double-labeling of iliac trabecular bone in 41 normal adults. *Calcif. Tissue Res.*, 26:99–102.

99. Melvin, K.E.W., Tashjian, A.H., and Bordier, P. (1973): The metabolic significance of calcitonin-secreting thyroid carcinoma. In: *Clinical Aspects of Metabolic Bone Disease*, edited by B. Frame, A.M. Parfitt, and H. Duncan, pp. 193–201. Excerpta Medica, Amsterdam.

100. Merz, W.A., and Schenk, R.K. (1970): A quantitative histological study on bone formation in human cancellous bone. *Acta Anat.*, 76:1–15.

101. Meunier, P., Courpron, P., Edouard, C., Bernard, J., Bringuier, J., and Vignon, G. (1973): Physiological senile involution and pathological rarefaction of bone. Quantitative and comparative histological data. *Clin. Endocrinol. Metab.*, 2:239–256.

102. Milhaud, G., Benezech-Lefevre, M., and Moulchtar, M.S. (1978): Deficiency of calcitonin in age related osteoporosis. *Biomedicine*, 29:272–276.

103. Morimoto, S., Onishi, T., Okada, Y., Tanaka, K., Tsuji, M., and Kumahara, Y. (1979): Comparison of human calcitonin secretion after a 1-minute calcium infusion in young normal and in elderly subjects. *Endocrinol. Jpn.*, 2:207–211.

104. Morita, R., Yamamoto, I., Fukunaga, M., Dokoh, S., Konishi, J., Kousaka, T., Nakajima, K., Torizuka, K., Aso, T., and Motohashi, T. (1979): Changes in sex hormones and calcium regulating hormones with reference to bone mass associated with aging. *Endocrinol. Jpn.*, 26(Suppl):15–22.

105. Nissenson, R.A., Abbott, S.R., Teitelbaum, A.P., Clark, O.H., and Arnaud, C.D. (1981): Endogenous biologically active human parathyroid hormone: measurement by a guanyl nucleotide-amplified renal adenylate cyclase assay. *J. Clin. Endocrinol. Metab.*, 52:840–846.

106. Nordin, B.E.C., Horsman, A., Crilly, R.G., Marshall, D.H., and Simpson, M. (1980): Treatment of spinal osteoporosis in postmenopausal women. *Br. Med. J.*, 280:451–454.

107. Nordin, B.E.C., Peacock, M., Crilly, R.G., Francis, R.M., Speed, R., and Barkworth, S. (1981): Summation of risk factors in osteoporosis. In: *Osteoporosis: Recent Advances in Pathogenesis and Treatment*, edited by H.F. DeLuca, H.M. Frost, W.S.S. Jee, C. Johnston, Jr., and A.M. Parfitt, pp. 359–367. University Park Press, Baltimore.

108. Nordin, B.E.C., Peacock, M., Crilly, R.G., and

(1986): Calcitonin deficiency does not affect the rate of radial bone loss. *J. Bone Min. Res.*, 1:352.

Marshall, D.H. (1979): Calcium absorption and plasma 1,25(OH)₂D levels in postmenopausal osteoporosis. In: *Vitamin D, Basic Research and Its Clinical Application.* Proceedings of the Fourth Workshop on Vitamin D, Berlin, West Germany, February, 1979, edited by A.W. Norman, K. Schaeffer, D. Herrath, H.-G. Grigoleit, J.W. Coburn, H.F. DeLuca, E.B. Mawer, and T. Suda, pp. 99–106. Walter de Gruyter, Berlin.

109. Nordin, B.E.C., Wilkinson, R., Marshall, D.H., Gallagher, J.C., Williams, A., and Peacock, M. (1976): Calcium absorption in the elderly, *Calcif. Tissue Res.*, 21(Suppl):442–451.

110. Omdahl, J.L, Garry, P.J., Hunsaker, L.A., Hunt, W.C., and Goodwin, J.S. (1982): Nutritional status in a healthy elderly population: Vitamin D. *Am. J. Clin. Nutr.*, 36:1225–1233.

111. Orimo, H., and Shiraki, M. (1979): Role of calcium regulating hormones in the pathogenesis of senile osteoporosis. *Endocrinol. Jpn.*, 1:1–6.

112. O'Toole, K., Fenoglio-Preiser, C., and Pushparaj, N. (1985): Endocrine changes associated with the human aging process. III. Effect of age on the number of calcitonin immunoreactive cells in the thyroid gland. *Hum. Pathol.*, 16:991–1000.

113. Pak, C.Y.C., Steward, A., Kaplan, R., Bone, H., Nolz, C., and Browne, R. (1975): Photon absorptiometric analysis of bone density in primary hyperparathyroidism. *Lancet*, 2:7–8.

114. Parfitt, A.M. (1979): Quantum concept of bone remodeling and turnover: implications for the pathogenesis of osteoporosis. *Calcif. Tissue Int.*, 28:1–5.

115. Price, P.A., Parthemore, J.G., Deftos, L.J., and Nishimoto, S.K. (1980): New biochemical marker for bone metabolism: measurement by radioimmunoassay of bone gla protein in the plasma of normal subjects and patients with bone disease. *J. Clin. Invest.*, 66:878–883.

116. Recker, R.R., Saville, P.D., and Heaney, R.P. (1977): Effect of oestrogens and calcium carbonate on bone loss in postmenopausal women. *Ann. Intern. Med.*, 87:649–655.

117. Reeve, J., and Zanelli, J.M. (1986): Parathyroid hormone and bone. *Clin. Sci.*, 71:231–238.

118. Riggs, B.L., Arnaud, C.D., Jowsey, J., Goldsmith, R.S., and Kelly, P.J. (1973): Parathyroid function in primary osteoporosis. *J. Clin. Invest.*, 52:181–184.

119. Riggs, B.L., Gallagher, J.C., DeLuca, H.F., Edis, A.J., Lambert, P.W., and Arnaud, C.D. (1978): A syndrome of osteoporosis, increased serum immunoreactive parathyroid hormone, and inappropriately low serum 1,25-dihydroxyvitamin D. *Mayo Clin. Proc.*, 53:701–706.

120. Riggs, B.L., Gallagher, J.C., DeLuca, H.F., and Zinsmeister, A.R. (1982): Studies on the mechanism of impaired calcium absorption in postmenopausal osteoporosis. In: *Vitamin D.* Proceedings of the Fifth Workshop on Vitamin D, Williamsburg, Virginia, edited by A.W. Norman, K. Schaefer, D.-v. Herrath, and H.-G. Grigoleit, pp. 903–908, Walter de Gruyter, Berlin.

121. Riggs, B.L., Hamstra, A., and DeLuca, H.F. (1981): Assessment of 25-hydroxyvitamin D 1α-hydroxylase reserve in postmenopausal osteoporosis by administration of parathyroid extract. *J. Clin. Endocrinol. Metab.*, 53:833–835.

122. Riggs, B.L., Kelly, P.J., Kinney, V.R., Scholz, D.A., and Bianco, A.J. (1967): Calcium deficiency and osteoporosis. Observations in 166 patients and critical review of the literature. *J. Bone Joint Surg.* [Am.], 49:915–924.

123. Riggs, B.L., and Melton, J., III. (1983): Evidence for two distinct syndromes of involutional osteoporosis. Editorial. *Am. J. Med.*, 75:899–901.

124. Riggs, B.L., and Melton, L.J. III (1986): Medical Progress: Involutional osteoporosis. *N. Engl. J. Med.*, 314:1676–1686.

125. Riggs, B.L., and Nelson, K.I. (1985): Effect of long term treatment with calcitriol on calcium absorption and mineral metabolism in postmenopausal osteoporosis. *J. Clin. Endocrinol. Metab.*, 61:457–461.

126. Russell, J., Lettieri, D., and Sherwood, L.M. (1986): Suppression by 1,25(OH)₂D₃ of transcription of the pre-proparathyroid hormone gene. *Endocrinology*, 119:2864–2866.

127. Schmidt-Gayk, H., Goossen, J., Lendle, F., and Seidel, D. (1977): Serum 25-hydroxycholecalciferol in myocardial infarction. *Atherosclerosis*, 26:55–58.

128. Seeman, E., Wahner, H.W., Offord, K.P., Kumar, R., Johnson, W.J., and Riggs, B.L. (1982): Differential effects of endocrine dysfunction on the axial and appendicular skeleton. *J. Clin. Invest.*, 69:1302–1309.

129. Shamonki, I.M., Frumar, A.M., Tatanya, I.V., Meldrum, D.R., Davidson, B.H., Parthemore, J.G., Judd, H.L., and Deftos, L.J. (1980): Age-related changes in calcitonin secretion in females. *J. Clin. Endocrinol. Metab.*, 50:437–439.

130. Silver, J., Naveh-Many, T., Mayer, H., Schmelzer, H.J., and Popovtzer, M.M. (1986): Regulation by vitamin D metabolites of parathyroid hormone gene transcription in vivo in the rat. *J. Clin. Invest.*, 78:1296–1301.

131. Slatopolsky, E., Martin, K., Morrissey, J., and Hruska, K. (1982): Current concepts of the metabolism and radioimmunoassay of parathyroid hormone. *J. Lab. Clin. Med.*, 99:309–316.

132. Slovik, D.M., Adams, J.S., Neer, R.M., and Holick, M.F. (1981): Deficient production of 1,25-dihydroxyvitamin D in elderly osteoporotic patients. *N. Engl. J. Med.*, 305:372–374.

133. Snell, A.P., MacLennan, W.J., and Hamilton, J.C. (1978): Ultraviolet irradiation and 25-hydroxyvitamin D levels in sick old people. *Age and Ageing*, 7:225–228.

134. Sokoloff, L. (1978): Occult osteomalacia in American (USA) patients with fracture of the hip. *Am. J. Surg. Pathol.*, 2:21–30.

135. Somerville, P.J., Lien, J.W.K., and Kaye, M. (1977): The calcium and vitamin D status in an elderly female population and their response to administered supplemental vitamin D₃. *J. Gerontol.*, 32:659–663.

136. Sorensen, O.H., Lumholtz, B., Lund, B., Lund, B., Hjelmstrand, I.L., Mosekilde, L., Melsen, F.,

Bishop, J.E., and Norman, A.W. (1982): Acute effects of parathyroid hormone on vitamin D metabolism in patients with the bone loss of aging. *J. Clin. Endocrinol. Metab.*, 54:1258–1261.

137. Stern, P.H. (1980): The D vitamins and bone. *Pharmacol. Rev.*, 32:47–80.

138. Stevenson, J.C. (1982): Regulation of calcitonin and parathyroid hormone secretion by oestrogens. *Maturitas*, 4:1–7.

139. Stevenson, J.C., Abeyasekara, G., Hillyard, C.J., Phang, K.G., McIntyre, I., Campbell, S., Townsend, P.T., Young, O., and Whitehead, M.I. (1981): Calcitonin and the calcium-regulating hormones in postmenopausal women: effect of oestrogens. *Lancet*, 1:693–695.

140. Taggart, H., Chesnut, C.H., III, Ivey, J.L., Baylink, D.J., Sisom, K., Huber, M.B., and Roos, B.A. (1982): Deficient calcitonin response to calcium stimulation in postmenopausal osteoporosis? *Lancet*, 1:475–478.

141. Teitelbaum, S.L., Rosenberg, E.M., Richardson, C.A., and Avioli, L.V. (1976): Histological studies of bone from normocalcemic postmenopausal osteoporotic patients with increased circulating parathyroid hormone. *J. Clin. Endocrinol. Metab.*, 42:537–543.

142. Tiegs, R.D., Body, J.-J., Barta, J.M., and Heath, H., III (1986): Secretion and metabolism of monomeric human calcitonin: effects of age, sex, and thyroid damage. *J. Bone Min. Res.*, 1:339–349.

143. Tiegs, R.D., Body, J.-J., Wahner, H.W., Barta, J., Riggs, B.L., and Heath, H., III (1985): Calcitonin secretion in postmenopausal osteoporosis. *N. Engl. J. Med.*, 312:1097–1100.

144. Tsai, K.-S., Heath, H. III, Kumar, R., and Riggs, B.L. (1984): Impaired vitamin D metabolism with aging in women. Possible role in pathogenesis of senile osteoporosis. *J. Clin. Invest.*, 73:1668–1672.

145. Tsai, K.-S., Wahner, H.W., Offord, K.P., Melton, J. III, Kumar, R., and Riggs, B.L. (1987): Effect of aging on vitamin D stores and bone density in women. *Calcif. Tissue Int.*, 40:241–243.

146. Von Knorring, J., Slatis, P., Weber, T.H., and Helenius, T. (1982): Serum levels of 25-hydroxyvitamin D, 24,25-dihydroxyvitamin D and parathyroid hormone in patients with femoral neck fracture in southern Finland. *Clin. Endocrinol.*, 17:189–194.

147. Walton, R.J., and Bijvoet, D.L.M. (1975): Nomogram for derivation of renal threshold phosphate concentration. *Lancet*, 2:309–310.

148. Weisman, Y., Schen, R.J., Eisenberg, Z., Edelstein, S., and Harell, A. (1981): Inadequate status and impaired metabolism of vitamin D in the elderly. *Isr. J. Med. Sci.*, 17:19–21.

149. Wiske, P.S., Epstein, S., Bell, N.H., Queener, S.F., Edmondson, J., and Johnston, C.C. (1979): Increases in immunoreactive parathyroid hormone with age. *N. Engl. J. Med.*, 300:1419–1421.

150. Zseli, J., Szucs, J., Steczek, K., Szathmari, M., Kollin, E., Horvath, C., Gnoth, M., Hollo, I. (1985): Decreased calcitonin reserve in accelerated postmenopausal osteoporosis. *Horm. Metabol. Res.*, 17:696–697.

*Osteoporosis: Etiology, Diagnosis, and
Management*, edited by B. Lawrence Riggs and
L. Joseph Melton, III. Raven Press, New York
© 1988.

15

Drug Therapy of Osteoporosis: Calcium, Estrogen and Vitamin D

J. Chris Gallagher

Creighton University School of Medicine, Omaha, Nebraska 68131

There is controversy about the natural history of osteoporosis, some feel that it is a self-limiting disease (14) while others feel it is a progressive condition marked by periodic bouts of activity and remission (58). Because so little is known about the natural history of this disease, it is difficult to evaluate the efficacy of drugs in the treatment of osteoporosis unless long-term randomized and controlled double-blind studies have been performed that compare these agents with a placebo. Similar studies have been carried out in osteoporosis programs only in the last ten years, and then in a negligible amount of studies.

During the last 30 years the use of calcium supplements, estrogen or vitamin D, in the treatment of established osteoporosis has been a common practice amongst physicians worldwide. Few trials of these particular agents can satisfy the present criteria for drug efficacy in osteoporosis treatment, for the majority of studies preceded the mid-1970s when there were no control groups, or trials were too brief. For the above-mentioned reasons, it is difficult to do more than review studies that have been performed with these drugs, to attempt to understand their mechanism of action, and then to make a subjective assessment of their potential value in the treatment of osteoporosis.

Osteoporosis is a term that is used in different ways. For example, the loss of bone after the menopause in normal women is often referred to as postmenopausal osteoporosis, whereas others refer to it as age-related bone loss. The development of fractures in postmenopausal women also is often termed postmenopausal osteoporosis, whereas the development of fractures in elderly people over age 75 years is often referred to as senile osteoporosis. Recently the measurement of low bone density in individuals has been termed osteopenia or osteoporosis. For the purpose of this discussion on the treatment of osteoporosis the population includes patients with vertebral fractures, male and female, as well as unspecified patients.

CALCIUM THERAPY IN OSTEOPOROSIS

The role of calcium deficiency leading to osteoporosis was brought to attention by Nordin (43), who reviewed the studies linking calcium deficiency with osteoporosis in animals. Later, work by Jowsey and Raisz (28) found that osteoporosis did not occur in animals on a low calcium intake if the parathyroid glands were removed, thus, pointing to a central role for parathyroid hormone (PTH) in osteoporosis. Garn (22) and Solomon et al. (65), were unable to show a relationship between calcium intake and cortical bone mass. However, in a Yugoslav population Matkovic et al. (40) showed a higher bone mass in people from an area whose intake of calcium was high and lower bone mass in those from an area with habitual low calcium intake. Since then a number of prospective studies in postmenopausal women (27,42,50,59) have shown that supplementation with calcium has only a partial effect in preventing cortical bone loss and no effect in preventing trabecular bone loss (59). Calcium deficiency after the menopause may lead to more rapid bone loss (44), though these findings remain to be confirmed. The threshold level at which calcium deficiency leads to rapid bone loss, or the level at which calcium supplementation stops bone loss remains to be determined.

Effect of Calcium Supplements on Calcium Balance

Calcium supplements have been used in treatment of osteoporosis since the early 1950s. Yet, surprisingly, the amount of data is scarce; there are published results on only about 50 female patients and 9 male patients, and not all of these patients had vertebral fractures of the spine.

Some of the earlier studies tried to measure the efficacy of calcium by performing calcium balances on high calcium intakes. In 1959, Whedon et al. (70) reported the effects of calcium supplementation on calcium balance in 5 patients, one of whom was on cortisone. Calcium intakes varied from 400 to 2400 mg/day. In one patient calcium balance on a high calcium intake exceeded 600 mg/day and in another patient positive balance was 400 mg/day.

Surprisingly, urine calcium hardly changed although calcium intake had increased from 400 mg to 2400 mg/day. These results raise questions about the accuracy of calcium measurements performed at that time.

In 1961 Harrison et al. (25), carried out calcium balance studies on varying calcium intakes in 16 subjects, some of whom did not have fractures. Calcium intake was increased

on average from 7 to 40 mg/kg (420 to 2400 mg for a 132 lb patient). In balances performed immediately after transfer to a high calcium intake some osteoporotics developed more positive calcium balance than did normal subjects. In five of the osteoporotics who were restudied nine months later, calcium balance was positive in two, negative in two, and zero in one. Schwartz et al. (62), performed calcium balance studies on five males, three with fractures. They were initially balanced on a calcium intake of 1000 mg and then restudied on 3800 mg three to four months later. In one patient, urine calcium had increased by 80 mg and calcium balance by 590 mg. This patient was estimated to have gained 63 g of calcium during four months. If true, this would represent an unlikely increase of about 10% in total body calcium. Another patient was in 630 mg of positive calcium balance. Isotope studies of bone turnover showed that the calculated bone accretion rates declined by 50% over the long-term, and Schwartz noted that as bone turnover decreased the degree of positive balance decreased in parallel (63).

In a series of five acute calcium balances carried out at high calcium intakes, Lutwak and Whedon (38) used average values over 18 days to overcome the problem of variable transit time for stool calcium and improve the accuracy of the technique. In five patients measured on calcium intakes above 2 g/day, three of the five patients were in negative calcium balance at this intake. Three patients were followed on a high calcium intake for six months, and it was noted that calcium balance became more negative with time.

Many of these older studies on calcium balance probably suffered from significant analytic errors associated with high dietary calcium and incorrect fecal calcium measurements associated with variability in fecal excretion. Rose (60,61) demonstrated the fact that calcium balances on high calcium intakes had substantial errors. Using chromium sesquioxide as a new stool marker rather than carmine red, he showed that accurate correction of stool calcium was of such magnitude that it could change calcium balance from + 225 mg/day to zero! In four carefully studied patients, he could not demonstrate positive calcium balance in patients who had been on a calcium intake of 3 to 3.5 g/daily for four months, although calcium balance had been positive in the first 18 days (60).

Spencer et al. (67), studied three osteoporotic women over a prolonged period of time. They found less positive calcium balance than previously reported on higher calcium intakes, especially when patients were studied after one year, and they also described an intestinal absorptive defect of calcium in osteoporotics. These results were in contrast to the earlier studies by Harrison et al. (25) who showed an increase in calcium absorption in osteoporotics on a high calcium intake.

Calcium infusions administered daily for 12 days were used as a way of increasing calcium intake in seven patients (one female and six males aged 20 to 51 years) with osteoporosis (49). During the infusions calcium balance became positive and remained positive six months after the infusions were completed. Subsequently, histomorphometry performed on the iliac crest bone biopsies from these patients, six months after the infusions had been given, showed an increase in bone formation in three, and decreased resorption in four patients (29).

More recently, Nordin et al. (45) studied the short-term effect of calcium supplements on calcium balance in 12 osteoporotics using a daily balance technique and a better stool marker—polyethylene glycol. During the control period, the average calcium intake was 696 mg/day; three months later the balances were repeated on an average calcium intake of 1756 mg/day. Calcium balance improved from -40 to -13 mg/day; although this was not a statistically significant result, the changes appear to be realistic. Calcium kinetics showed a decrease in bone turnover, and this was confirmed by a significant decline in the hydroxyproline excretion. In another set of recent balance studies using chromium sesquioxide as the stool marker, 48 osteoporotic patients, 33 females, and 15 males, were first studied on a high calcium intake followed by a combination

of hormones or anabolic agents with calcium (68). Unfortunately, no control calcium balances were done on the patient's habitual intake before the study started. Patients were followed on the combination for periods varying from two to ten years with an average of 3.5 years follow-up. Most patients treated with estrogen or anabolic agents combined with calcium were found to be in positive calcium balance. At the end of the study after hormone therapy was discontinued a final balance study on the high calcium intake was carried out, and patients were found to be in negative calcium balance.

Effect of Calcium Supplements on Bone Histology

Besides calcium balances, there are more direct ways of looking at the effect of calcium on bone. A long-term study of the effect of calcium supplements on bone was carried out by Riggs et al. (55). They performed bone biopsies on 18 patients with osteoporosis, nine on 2 to 2.5 g calcium and nine on 1.5 to 2 g of calcium combined with vitamin D 50,000 U given twice weekly. In the first group, biopsies were performed before and after 3 to 4 months on calcium, and a signficant decrease in bone resorption was seen. In the second group, a decrease in bone resorption was again noted at four months but further biopsies done after one year showed not only a decrease in bone resorption but also a concomitant decline in bone formation. A significant decrease in serum immunoreactive parathyroid hormone was seen at four and 12 months, and it was suggested that this finding accounted for the significant decrease in bone turnover seen with long-term treatment.

Effect of Calcium Supplements on Vertebral Fracture

In two studies, data has been collected on the long-term effect of calcium on vertebral fractures. In 12 patients treated with calcium gluconate for an average of four years, no new vertebral fractures occurred during that time

(46); however, the authors point out that this group was carefully selected in that calcium was given only to those patients shown to have normal calcium absorption (usually most patients with spinal osteoporosis have low absorption of calcium, see vitamin D section). In the other study by Riggs, et al. (57), 27 patients received calcium carbonate, of 1.5 to 2.5 g/day, and 19 others were given in addition vitamin D (average 7,000 to 14,000 U/day). In the calcium and vitamin D-treated group there were 419 vertebral fractures per 1000 patient-years after approximately three years of treatment compared to 834 fractures/1000 patient-years in a similar group of women followed on no treatment for a period of two years. If the first year was excluded in the group treated with calcium, the average fracture rate for the second and third years only was 564/1000 patient-years. Neither of these treatment studies were randomized with a control group.

Effect of Calcium Supplements on Bone Density

There are virtually no studies of the effect of calcium on bone density in osteoporotics. In a study by Nordin et al. (45), the rate of bone loss on the metacarpal cortex decreased by 50% in the calcium group compared to that found in a parallel untreated group; however, the latter were followed only for an average of 1.4 years whereas the calcium group were followed for four years. Also, the calcium group were specially selected as noted above in that calcium absorption had to be normal. In a separate study comparing the effect of calcitonin with placebo on total body calcium in osteoporotics, the effect of calcitonin in patients with osteoporosis appeared to be dependent on the calcium intake (7). In this study both groups were supplemented to a total calcium intake of 1000 mg/day but those patients with the lowest calcium intake at baseline appeared to show a greater response to calcitonin, implying that the initial calcium intake may have modified the response to calcitonin. Apart from the results on metacarpal cortex and vertebral frac-

tures there is no other direct evidence that might support a case for calcium supplementation as the primary treatment for osteoporosis.

Conclusion

Unfortunately, only the most recent calcium balances in which a suitable stool marker was used are valid for interpretation. The earlier studies where calcium balance was reported to be positive at around 600 mg/day were probably erroneous due to analytical errors associated with a high calcium intake plus inadequate correction for delayed fecal excretion of calcium with suitable markers.

In the initial stage of treatment, calcium supplements probably inhibit bone resorption without affecting bone formation and thereby improve calcium balance, but positive bone balance lasts only a period of 3 to 6 months. Then, the subsequent decline in bone formation leads to reequilibration between resorption and formation at a reduced level of bone turnover. This will tend to reduce any imbalance between formation and resorption to minimum, leading to either zero or slightly negative calcium balance. It is possible that reduced secretion of PTH and $1,25(OH)_2D_3$ are partly responsible for lower bone turnover. Important questions for future research with calcium should focus on whether a reduction in bone activators such as PTH and vitamin D are important for bone health, *vis à vis* the repair of microfractures through the remodeling process. It is not at all clear what the calcium requirement figure is for osteoporotics. There is a need for long-term studies of the effects of calcium supplements in osteoporotics. Until that work is completed, it is suggested that the calcium intake be set at 1000 to 1500 mg/day. There is as yet no clear evidence to show that calcium is absorbed any differently from food or calcium supplements. About 25% of osteoporotics have lactase deficiency and self select a low calcium intake because of milk intolerance (41). In this group one can use calcium carbonate (40% elemental calcium), calcium lactate (9% elemental), calcium gluconate

(10% elemental), or calcium phosphate (30% elemental) to supplement the diet.

EFFECT OF ESTROGENS IN OSTEOPOROSIS

The evidence linking estrogen deficiency to bone loss is much stronger than that for calcium. Women who undergo an early menopause have reduced bone density later on in life (52), and women with gonadal deficiency such as Turner's syndrome develop osteoporosis earlier than expected (4). Women who develop estrogen deficiency from excessive athletic activity or hyperprolactinemia also show signs of osteoporosis determined from bone density studies (15). Estrogen therapy effectively stops postmenopausal bone loss (27,34,50), which is in marked contrast to the effects of calcium. Whether women with osteoporosis have more marked estrogen deficiency is controversial. Two studies have shown lower estrogen activity (12,17) while another study showed no differences between osteoporotic and controls (13). It has been suggested (47) that lower estrogen levels in osteoporosis are due to decreased production of androstenedione from the adrenals which is the main precursor of estrogen in postmenopausal women. Significantly lower levels of androstenedione have been found in osteoporotics less than age 60 but not in those older than 60 years (12,47). These findings infer that reduced production of androstenedione may be important in the pathogenesis of those with early onset of the disease recently termed type I osteoporosis.

The same introductory comments in the section on calcium can be applied to the use of estrogens in the treatment of osteoporosis. No controlled trials comparing estrogen with placebo have ever been conducted in patients with established osteoporosis.

Effect of Estrogens on Calcium Balance

After his original observations establishing a link between estrogen deficiency and osteoporosis, Albright carried out long-term studies of the effect of estrogen on calcium balance (1). Measurements on estrogen showed that calcium absorption increased, urine calcium decreased, and calcium balance became positive. These findings were confirmed by others over the next few years. Lafferty et al. (31) showed that calcium balance improved in three out of four osteoporotics treated with estrogen but calcium balance became less positive with time and even negative after treatment lasting one year. The kinetic studies of bone turnover showed a decrease in bone resorption with no change in bone formation during the first few weeks. After long-term treatment, however, kinetic measurements showed a decline in bone formation indicating that a marked reduction in bone turnover occurred on estrogen. It became clear that the decrease in bone resorption accounted for the fall in urine calcium despite the increase in intestinal absorption. Presumably, in the early phase of estrogen treatment absorbed calcium is taken up by bone before bone formation declines. With long-term treatment there is less need for absorbed calcium and there may be a decrease in absorption. Lafferty suggested that the decline in bone formation that occurred on estrogens was the explanation for the relative ineffectiveness of long-term estrogen therapy since it only arrested the progress of the disease rather than curing it by increasing bone density. In this respect, the changes on estrogen are similar to those seen with calcium supplementation. Similar findings were reported by Gordan and Eisenberg (23), who showed that long term therapy with estrogen caused a decrease in both bone formation and resorption. Recently, more precise calcium balance studies utilizing a stool marker were carried out in 13 patients by Marshall et al. (39,47); they demonstrated an improvement in calcium balance from -106 to -32 mg/day after 3 to 4 month treatment with estrogen. Unlike some earlier studies, calcium absorption did not increase significantly after estrogen therapy, however, in his group calcium absorption was normal before treatment. Two other studies have demonstrated a rise in radiocalcium absorption in osteoporotics treated with estrogen and in both groups calcium absorption was low before treatment (8,19). This increase in calcium absorption has been attributed to significant increases in serum levels of PTH and 1,25 $(OH)_2D_3$ (19). There is only one study of the effect of estrogen combined with calcium in the treatment of osteoporotics (68). Calcium balances were performed after six months on estrogen and calcium and generally showed positive calcium balance. When estrogen was discontinued, calcium balance became negative even though the patients remained on a high calcium intake. An example of the estrogen effect on calcium balance is shown in Fig. 1.

Effect of Estrogen on Bone Histology

Estrogen effect on bone has been measured directly in bone biopsies using histomorphometry. In 30 women, Riggs et al. (53) showed a decrease in bone surfaces involved in resorption and no change in formation surfaces after 3 to 4 months of treatment. After long-term treatment (2 to 3 years), however, a significant decline occurred in bone formation as well as bone resorption (54). These findings are in close agreement with the kinetic studies by Lafferty et al. (31) described above. Serum PTH increased significantly in patients on estrogens, yet bone turnover did not increase although there was a trend for resorption activity to be higher on the long term biopsies.

Effect of Estrogen on Height and Vertebral Fractures

A number of studies have looked at the effect of estrogen on the spine. Indirectly, this was first done by Henneman and Wallach (26), who evaluated the change in height of 22 patients who had been started on estrogen 4 to 20 years earlier by Albright. Height loss stopped immediately in ten patients, within two years in six patients, within three years in one patient, and continued in the remaining five patients. Whether height loss is a good indirect estimate of vertebral collapse has been disputed by some (69). Gordan et al. (24) ran-

domized 220 osteoporotic patients to treatment with either estrogen or anabolic drugs but did not have a control group. The fracture rate was 40/1000 patient-years on anabolic drugs, 25/1000 on 0.6 mg conjugated estrogens, and 3/1000 patient-years on 1.25 mg conjugated estrogens. The average follow-up for the estrogen group was ten years but less than two years for the anabolic-treated group. In another nonrandomized study, 15 osteoporotics treated with 25 μg daily of ethinylestradiol for an average period of two years, had a vertebral fracture rate identical to that of 32 untreated patients followed for an average for 1.3 years (46). In contrast, a recent retrospective survey of vertebral fracture rates in osteoporotics treated with different drugs showed that the vertebral fracture rate on a combination of estrogens and calcium (220/1000 patient years) was only half that of patients given calcium supplements alone (564/1000 patient years) and one quarter that of an untreated group (57).

Effect of Estrogen on Bone Density

There have been no studies of the estrogen effect on trabecular bone, and only one study on cortical bone (46) in established cases of osteoporosis. In 13 osteoporotics treated with estrogen, no decrease in metacarpal cortical thickness was seen, while a parallel control group showed significant declines in metacarpal cortical thickness.

Conclusion

The results tell us more about the mechanism of action of estrogens on bone than about their efficacy in established osteoporosis. Like calcium supplements, estrogen treatment over a period of several months reduces bone resorption and leads to a temporary increase in calcium balance that is offset later by a decline in bone formation. Unlike calcium, estrogen increases serum parathyroid hormone and 1,25-dihydroxyvitamin D, but whether this difference in response from that seen with calcium is important for the bone remodeling process remains unclear. The most convincing data so far comes from the studies by Riggs et al. (57), where vertebral fracture rates were much lower on estrogen and calcium than on calcium alone.

TREATMENT OF OSTEOPOROSIS WITH VITAMIN D ANALOGUES

A significant proportion of patients with osteoporosis have malabsorption of calcium (8,17,19) measured by either radiocalcium or calcium balance techniques. A number of groups have demonstrated reduced serum levels of 1,25-dihydroxyvitamin D and it is likely that this finding accounts mainly for the reduced calcium absorption in most patients (2,5,9,18,32,35). Some patients may have a primary defect in the gut itself since a small number of patients have low calcium absorption with high levels of 1,25-dihydroxyvitamin D (16,18). We have never seen a patient fail to

increase calcium absorption after oral administration of synthetic 1,25-dihydroxyvitamin D3; thus, the defect in calcium absorption is subtle. For the majority of patients with low calcium absorption it is suggested that the pathogenesis is as follows:

increased bone resorption → slight elevation of serum calcium → reduced PHT secretion → reduced 1,25-dihydroxyvitamin production → reduced calcium absorption (56).

Osteoporotics on a low calcium diet fail to adapt by increasing calcium absorption (18), thereby aggravating calcium deficiency. Logically one should normalize calcium absorption in those with malabsorption by using a vitamin D compound, and avoid using any therapy that might switch off production of PTH and 1,25-dihydroxyvitamin D thereby reducing calcium absorption.

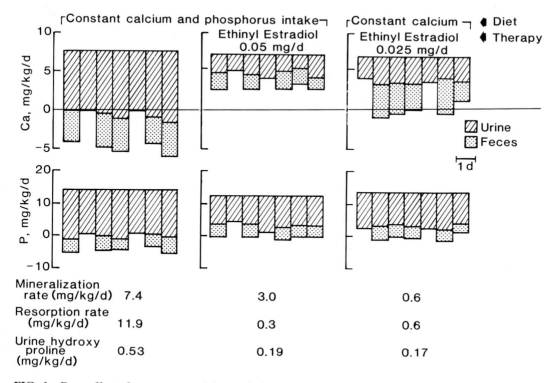

FIG. 1 Dose effect of estrogen on calcium and phosphorus balance and bone turnover. Calcium and phosphorus intake are plotted from the top of the figure. Balance is positive if values lie above zeroline and negative if they lie below. Note the increase in calcium absorption, the decrease in urine calcium, and decline in bone mineralization and resorption rates.

Use of Vitamin D₂

Vitamin D_2 was one of the first of the vitamin D compounds used in the treatment of osteoporosis. Gallagher et al. (18), showed that osteoporotics with impaired calcium absorption had a variable response to vitamin D_2. In some patients calcium absorption responded to 1000 U daily but many required 10,000 or 20,000 U daily, and several did not show any increase in absorption until the dose reached a level of 40,000 U daily. Later it was suggested that the low absorptive response in this group was due to resistance at the gut level to the circulating form of vitamin D (16); non-responders to the low dose were usually over age 70 years; whereas responders were younger than 70 years. The results of calcium balances on different doses of vitamin D_2 in these same patients have recently been summarized (45). In seven patients given 10,000 U daily, calcium balance on a calcium intake of 728 mg/d improved from -132 to -48 mg/day. In eight patients treated with 20,000 U daily and eight patients treated with 40,000 U daily, there was no real change in calcium balance; however, in the latter groups the mean calcium intake was 554 mg and 448 mg/day, respectively. That may have been too low for patients to have the chance to develop positive calcium balance. Anderson used 9,000 U vitamin D to treat four patients with osteoporosis, and three showed a definite improvement in calcium balance (3). Buring treated 23 patients for one year with vitamin D_2, 35,000 U daily, and a calcium supplement, but no effect on bone mass could be demonstrated (6).

Use of 1αOHD₃

In a study reported first by Sorensen (66) and later by Lund (37), 22 Danish osteoporotic patients were treated with 1 μg/day of 1αOHD₃ for five years. Spine density increased by 1% at 2 years, and by 5% at the end of 5 years treatment. In the same patients, radial density at the 2 cm and 8 cm sites increased significantly by 3 months, continued to increase for 24 months and gradually returned to baseline by the end of 5 years; the study was uncontrolled. Lindholm et al. (33) treated 25 Swedish osteoporotics for two years with 1 μg of 1αOHD₃ and a calcium supplement. Clinical symptoms improved, and an increase in radial density was seen. In a study of the effect of 1αOHD₃ in osteoporotic patients in England, calcium balances were performed before and after either 1 or 2 μg of 1αOHD₃ (11,39), (see Fig. 2). Calcium absorption improved in all patients given 2 μg/day but not in those given 1 μg. Although calcium balance increased in the group given the larger dose, it still remained negative. When estrogen was combined with 1αOHD₃, calcium balance became more positive in seven of the nine patients on the 2 μg dose, and positive in four of the seven patients on 1μg of 1αOHD₃. Shiraki et al. carried out a large controlled multi-treatment study in Japanese osteoporotic patients (64). A control group of 23 patients were compared to 11 patients given 1 μg daily of 1αOHD₃, and nine patients on 0.5 μg of 1αOHD₃. After two years of treatment, radial density had decreased by 13% in the control group whereas the group on a low dose showed a gain of 7% in radial density and the group; on a high dose showed an increase of 11% in radial density. After stopping treatment with 1αOHD₃ rapid bone loss occurred within a few months. In a single group study, Krolner et al. (30), treated 21 Danish ostseoporotic women with 0.5 to 1.0 μg of 1αOHD₃ and showed an increase of 5.5% in lumbar spine density after two years.

Use of 1,25 Dihydroxyvitamin D₃

Cannigia et al. (10), treated osteoporotic patients in Italy with 1 μg/day of $1,25\text{-}(OH)_2D_3$ only if they had impaired calcium absorption and followed them for 3 years. Calcium absorption was normalized in all patients, and bone mineral density measured at the mid-radius site increased by about 6% over 3 years.

In two recent studies utilizing calcium balance techniques, osteoporotic patients in the

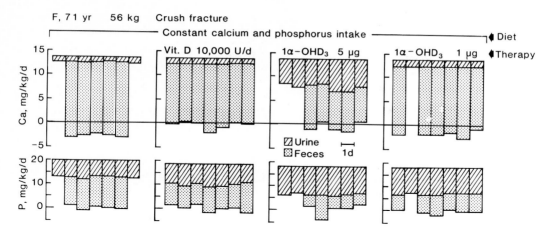

FIG. 2 Effect of vitamin D_2 or $1\alpha OHD_3$ on calcium and phosphorus balance. Calcium and phosphorus intake are plotted from the top of the figure. Balance is positive if it lies above the zeroline and negative if below. This diagram compares the effect of vitamin D_2 10,000 U (250 μg) daily, 5 μg, and 1 μg of $1\alpha OHD_3$ on calcium and phosphorous absorption and balance. Daily administration of 5 μg of $1\alpha OHD_3$ was more potent than 1 μg of $1\alpha OHD_3$ which was more potent than vitamin D_2 10,000 U on calcium absorption. An optimal dose for normalizing absorption would probably be 2 μg $1\alpha OHD_3$ since urine calcium excretion was too high on 5 μg of $1\alpha OHD_3$.

USA were randomized to either placebo or $1,25(OH)_2D_3$ and followed for a period of one to two years. In one study (20), there was a significant improvement in calcium balance, which changed from negative (-55 mg/day) to positive ($+5$ mg/day) during the first 6 months. At the end of two years calcium balance became negative (-25 mg/day) although it was still improved compared to baseline. In the second study (51), no significant difference was seen between the treatment or placebo groups at the end of one year since both groups showed an improvement in calcium balance. In this study it was thought that the change in calcium balance in the control group was due to an increase in calcium intake during the final balance period. Lund et al. (36) randomly assigned 27 Danish patients to treatment with either estrogen alone or estrogen plus 0.5 μg of $1,25$-dihydroxyvitamin D_3 for a period of two years. Patients on combined therapy showed an increase of 0.7% in radial density, whereas the group on estrogen alone had a decrease of 1% by the end of one year. Nordin (48) compared the effects of calcium alone with a combination of 0.25 μg of $1,25(OH)_2D_3$ and a calcium sup-

plement. The group on calcium alone had a decrease of 3.3%/year in radial density measured at the distal site and the group on calcium and $1,25$-dihydroxyvitamin D had a decrease of 1.6% per year. When an anabolic hormone was combined with calcium and $1,25$-dihydroxyvitamin D_3 there was an increase of 25% in radial density. Shiraki et al. (64) treated 22 patients with 0.5 μg of $1,25$-$(OH)_2D_3$ and compared the results to those in 35 controls. The patients on placebo had a decrease of 12% in radial density over two years, while the group on $1,25(OH)_2D_3$ showed no significant bone loss.

Effect of 1,25 Dihydroxyvitamin D_3 on Fracture Rates

Two studies have compared the effect of calcitriol and placebo on vertebral fracture rates over a one year period (20,51). In one center, vertebral fracture rates were reduced by 75% at the end of 1 year, and in the other center, vertebral fracture rates were reduced by 50% at the end of 1 year. In both centers, all patients were crossed over from placebo to calcitriol at the end of the first year, and vertebral fractures in years 2 and 3 in both centers were 50% lower than the first year. However, since there were no corresponding placebo groups for years 2 and 3, the significance of these long-term results is not clear.

Since calcitriol increases calcium absorption in osteoporotic patients, the question remains whether or not calcium supplements are as effective as calcitriol. Gallagher and Recker (21), compared the effect of high-dose calcitriol with that of calcium supplements in 10 osteoporotic patients. Patients were treated with 2 µg of 1,25-dihydroxyvitamin D_3 daily for a period of 6 months and placed on a calcium intake of 500 mg/day. Bone biopsies were performed before treatment and after 6 months. After the second biopsy was completed, patients were crossed over to calcium supplements (1.5 g/day) and underwent a third bone biopsy after 4 to 6 months on calcium. On average there was a doubling in the bone formation rate and in the double tetracycline-labelling of bone after high dose 1,25-dihydroxyvitamin D_3 therapy, whereas the reverse occurred in the same patients treated with calcium supplements. Thus, bone remodeling was increased by calcitriol and depressed by calcium supplements. Patients treated with lower doses of calcitriol, 0.5 µg/day, do not appear to show a decrease in bone formation rate or tetracycline labelling, although one might expect a decrease in bone turnover if the effect of calcitriol were simply to increase calcium absorption.

Despite the fact that all studies with vitamin D analogues have not been placebo-controlled, the results of the administration of calcitriol and its analogues on calcium balance, bone density, and vertebral fracture rates are similar, and suggest that this group of compounds have efficacy in the treatment of osteoporotic patients. The most likely explanation for the effect of these agents is their ability to increase calcium absorption and improve calcium balance. Such an effect should result in an increase in bone density if bone turnover is normal. The fact that bone formation rates do not decrease on long-term treatment with low doses of calcitriol suggests also that calcitriol stimulates bone turnover directly, in contrast to the effect of calcium supplements which is to increase calcium absorption and decrease bone turnover after several months. Although this mechanism for calcium may be an advantage in patients with high-turnover osteoporosis or in those with an inadequate dietary calcium intake, it may be undesirable for patients with low-turnover osteoporosis. However, because of the lack of controlled studies in patients treated with calcium, these arguments remain hypothetical. It is still not clear whether calcitriol is more beneficial than calcium in patients with low-turnover osteoporosis, and further studies are needed with both agents in order to establish relative efficacy in the treatment of osteoporosis. Because of the potency of newer analogues of vitamin D on calcium absorption, further data are needed with respect to the incidence of hypercalcemia and hypercalcuria and long-term safety of these compounds on renal function. Newer analogues of vitamin D that have a greater effect on bone than gut would be desirable and efforts to synthesize these compounds are presently underway.

ACKNOWLEDGMENTS

This work was supported in part by grant AM-29792 from the National Institutes of Health.

REFERENCES

1. Albright, F. (1947): The effect of hormones on osteogenesis in man. *Horm. Res.,* 1:293–353.
2. Aloia, J.F., Cohn, S.H., Vaswani, A., Yeh, J.K., Yuen, K., and Ellis, K. (1985): Risk factors for postmenopausal osteoporosis. *Am. J. Med.,* 78:95–100.
3. Anderson, I.A. (1950): Postmenopausal osteoporosis, clinical manifestations, and the treatment with oestrogens. *Quart. J. Med.,* 19:67–96.
4. Beals, R.K. (1973): Nosologic and genetic aspects of scoliosis. *Clin. Orthop.,* 93:23–32.
5. Bishop, J.E., Norman, A.W., Coburn, J.W., Roberts, P.A., and Henry, H.L. (1980): Studies in the metabolism of calcified 16. Determination of the

concentration of 25-hydroxyvitamin D 24-25 dihydroxyvitamin and 1,25 dihydroxyvitamin D in a single 2 milliliter plasma sample. *Miner Electrolyte Metab.,* 3:181–189.

6. Buring, K., Hulth, G., Nilsson, B.E., Westlin, N.E., and Wiklund, P.E. (1974): Treatment of osteoporosis with vitamin D. *Acta. Med. Scand.,* 195:471–472.

7. Burnell, J.M., Baylink, D.J., Chesnut, C.H., and Teubner, E.J. (1986): The role of skeletal calcium deficiency in postmenopausal osteoporosis. *Calcif. Tissue. Int.,* 38:187–192.

8. Caniggia, A., Gennari, C., Bianchi, V., and Guideri, R. (1963): Intestinal absorption of Ca in senile osteoporosis. *Acta. Med. Scand.,* 173:613.

9. Caniggia, A., Nuti, R., Lorie, F., and Vattimo, A. (1984): The hormonal form of vitamin D in the pathophysiology and therapy of postmenopausal osteoporosis. *J. Endocrinol. Invest.,* 7:373–378.

10. Caniggia, A., Nuti, R., Lorie, F., and Vattimo, A. (1985): 1,25 (OH) 2 vitamin D3 in the long-term treatment of postmenopausal osteoporosis. In: *Vitamin D. A Chemical, Biochemical and Clinical Update,* edited by A.W. Norman, K. Schaefer, H. -. G. Grigoleit, and D.V. Herrath, pp. 986–995. Walter de Gruyter & Co., Berlin-New York.

11. Crilly, R.G., Marshall, D.H., Horsman, A., and Nordin, B.E.C. (1980): 1 alpha hydroxy D3 with and without oestrogen in the treatment of osteoporosis. In: *Osteoporosis: Recent Advances in Pathogenesis and Treatment,* edited by H.F. DeLuca, H.M. Frost, W.S.S. Jee, and C.C. Johnston. University Park Press, Baltimore.

12. Crilly, R.G., Francis, R.M., and Nordin, B.E.C. (1981): Steroid hormones, ageing and bone. *Clin. Endocrinol. Metab.,* 19:115–139.

13. Davidson, B.J., Riggs, B.L., Wahner, H.W., and Judd, H.L. (1983): Endogenous cortisol and sex steroids in patients with osteoporotic spinal fractures. *Obstet. Gynecol.,* 61:275–8.

14. Dent, C.E. (1955): Idiopathic osteoporosis. *Proc. R. Soc. Med.,* 48:574.

15. Drinkwater, B.L., Nilson, K., Chesnut, C.H., Bremner, W.J., Shainholtz, S., and Southworth, M.B. (1984): Bone mineral content of amenorrheic and eumenorrheic athletes. *N. Engl. J. Med.,* 311:277–81.

16. Francis, R.M., Peacock, M., Taylor, G.A., Storer, J.H., and Nordin, B.E.C. (1984): Calcium malabsorption in elderly women with vertebral fractures: Evidence for resistance to the action of vitamin D metabolites on the bowel. *Clin. Sci.,* 66:103–107.

17. Gallagher, J.C., Aaron, J., Horsman, A., Marshall, D.H., Wilkinson, R., and Nordin, B.E.C. (1973): The crush fracture syndrome in postmenopausal women. *Clin. Endocrinol. Metab.,* 2:293–315.

18. Gallagher, J.C., Riggs, B.L., Eisman, J., Hamstra, A., Arnaud, S.B., and DeLuca, H.F. (1979): Intestinal calcium absorption and serum vitamin D metabolites in normal subjects and osteoporotic patients. *J. Clin. Invest.,* 64:729–736.

19. Gallagher, J.C., Riggs, B.L., and DeLuca, H.F. (1980): Effect of estrogen on calcium absorption and serum vitamin D metabolites in postmenopausal osteoporosis. *J. Clin. Endocrinol. Metab.,* 51:1359–1364.

20. Gallagher, J.C., Jerpbak, C.M., Jee, W.S.S., Johnson, K.A., DeLuca, H.F., and Riggs, B.L. (1982): 1,25-Dihydroxyvitamin D3: Short- and long-term effects on bone and calcium metabolism in patients with postmenopausal osteoporosis. *Proc. Natl. Acad. Sci.,* 79:3325–3329.

21. Gallagher, J.C., and Recker, R.R. (1985): A comparison of the effects of calcitriol or calcium supplements. In: *Vitamin D, A Chemical, Biochemical and Clinical Update,* edited by A.W. Norman, K. Schaefer, H. -. G. Grigoleit, and D.V. Herrath, pp. 971–975. Walter de Gruyter & Co., Berlin-New York.

22. Garn, S.M. (1970): *The Earlier Gain and Later Loss of Cortical Bone in Nutritional Perspective.* Charles C Thomas, Springfield.

23. Gordan, G.S. and Eisenberg, E. (1963): The effect of estrogens, androgens and corticoids on skeletal kinetics in man. *Proc. Roy. Soc. Med.,* 56:1027–1029.

24. Gordan, G.S., Picchi, J., and Roof, B.S. (1973): Antifracture efficacy of long-term estrogens for osteoporosis. *Trans. Assoc. Am. Phys.,* 86:326–332.

25. Harrison, M., Fraser, R., and Mullan, B. (1961): Calcium metabolism in osteoporosis. *Lancet,* 1:1015–1019.

26. Henneman, P.H., and Wallach, S. (1957): The use of androgens and estrogens and their metabolic effects. *Arch. Intern. Med.,* 100:715–723.

27. Horsman, A., Gallagher, J.C., Simpson, M., and Nordin, B.E.C. (1977): Prospective trial of oestrogen and calcium in postmenopausal women. *Br. Med. J.,* 2:789–92.

28. Jowsey, J., and Raisz, L.G. (1968): Experimental osteoporosis and parathyroid activity. *Endocrinology,* 82:384.

29. Jowsey, J., Hoye, R.C., Pak, C.Y.C., and Bartter, F. (1969): The treatment of osteoporosis with calcium infusions*. *Am. J. Med.,* 47:17–22.

30. Krolner, B., Nielsen, S.P., Lund, B., Lund, B.J., Sorensen, O.H., and Jacobsen, S. (1980): Lumbar spine bone mineral content in post-menopausal osteoporosis. *Calcif. Tissue. Int.,* 31S:77A.

31. Lafferty, F.W., Spencer, G.E., and Pearson, O.H. (1964): Effects of androgens, estrogens and high calcium intakes on bone formation and resorption in osteoporosis*. *Am. J. Med.,* 36:514–528.

32. Lawoyin, S., Zerwekh, J.E., Glass, K., and Pak, C.Y.C. (1980): Ability of 25-hydroxyvitamin D3 therapy to augment serum 1,25- and 24, 25-dihydroxyvitamin D in postmenopausal osteoporosis. *J. Clin. Endocrinol. Metab.,* 50:593–596.

33. Lindholm, T.S., Nilsson, O.S., Kyhle, B.R., Elmstedt, E., Lindholm, T.C., and Eriksson, S.A. (1981): Failures and complications in treatment of osteoporotic patients treated with 1 di-hydroxyvitamin D3 supplemented by calcium. In: *Osteoporosis,* edited by C. Christiansen, C.D. Arnaud, B.E.C. Nordin, A.M. Parfitt, W.A. Peck, and B.L. Riggs, pp. 351–357. Aalborg Stiftsbogtrykkeri, Glostrup, Denmark.

34. Lindsay, R., Aitken, J.M., Anderson, J.B., Hart,

D.M., MacDonald, E.B., and Clarke, A.C. (1976): Long term prevention of postmenopausal osteoporosis by oestrogen. *Lancet,* I:1038–1040.

35. Lund, B., Sorensen, O.H., Lund, B., and Agner, E. (1982): Serum 1,25-dihydroxyvitamin D in normal subjects and in patients with postmenopausal osteopenia. Influence of age, renal function and oestrogen therapy. *Horm. Metab. Res.,* 14:271–274.

36. Lund, B., Holm, P., Egsmose, C., Sorensen, H., Friis, T., and Delling, G. (1984): A controlled double-blind study comparing the effect of estrogen with estrogen and 1,25-dihydroxyvitamin D3 in postmenopausal osteoporosis. In: *Osteoporosis,* edited by C. Christiansen, C.D. Arnaud, B.E.C. Nordin, and A.M. Parfitt, W.A. Peck, and B.L. Riggs, pp. 763–676. Aalborg Stiftsbogtrykkeri, Glostrup, Denmark.

37. Lund, B., Sorensen, O.H., Andersen, R.B., Lund, B., Mosekilde, L., Egsmose, C., Storm, T.L., and Nielsen, S.P. (1985): Long-term treatment of senile osteopenia with 1 di-hydroxycholecalciferol. In: *Vitamin D. A Chemical, Biochemical and Clinical Update,* edited by A.W. Norman, K. Schaefer, H.-G. Grigoleit, and D.V. Herrath, pp. 1039–1040. Walter de Gruyter & Co., Berlin–New York.

38. Lutwak, L., and Whedon, G.D. (1963): Osteoporosis. *Drug Metab,*:1–39.

39. Marshall, D.H., Gallagher, J.C., Guha, P., Hanes, F., Oldfield, W., and Nordin, B.E.C. (1977): The effect of 1 alpha-hydroxycholecalciferol and hormone therapy on the calcium balance of post-menopausal osteoporosis. *Calcif. Tissue. Res.,* 225:78–84.

40. Matkovic, V., Kostial, K., Simonovic, I., Buzina, R., Brodarec, A., and Nordin, B.E.C. (1979): Bone status and fracture rates in two regions of Yugoslavia. *Am. J. Clin. Nutr.,* 32:540–9.

41. Newcomer, A.D., Hodgson, S.F., McGill, D.B., and Thomas, P.J. (1978): Lactase Deficiency: Prevalence in Osteoporosis. *Ann. Intern. Med.,* 89:218–220.

42. Nilas, L., Christiansen, C., and Rodbro, P. (1984): Calcium supplementation and post-menopausal bone loss. *Br. Med. J.,* 289:1103–6.

43. Nordin, B.E.C. (1960): Osteoporosis, osteomalacia and calcium deficiency. *Clin. Orthop.,* 17:253.

44. Nordin, B.E.C., Horsman, A., and Gallagher, J.C. (1974): The effect of vitamin D on bone loss in spinal osteoporosis. *Symp. Bone Mineral Determinations,* 1:59.

45. Nordin, B.E.C., Horsman, A., and Marshall, D.H. (1979): Calcium requirement and calcium therapy. *Clin. Orthop.,* 140:216–239.

46. Nordin, B.E.C., Horsman, A., Crilly, R.G., Marshall, D.H., and Simpson, M. (1980): Treatment of spinal osteoporosis in postmenopausal women. *Br. Med. J.,* 280:451–454.

47. Nordin, B.E.C., Peacock, M., Aaron, J., Crilly, R.G., Heyburn, P.J., Horsman, A., and Marshall, D. (1980): Osteoporosis and osteomalacia. *Clin. Endocrinol. Metab.,* 9:1.

48. Nordin, B.E.C., Chatterton, B.E., Walker, C.J., Steurer, T.A., Horowitz, M., and Need, A.G. (1985): The effect of calcium, hormones and Ro-
caltrol therapy on forearm bone loss in normal and osteoporotic postmenopausal women. In: *Vitamin D. A Chemical, Biochemical and Clinical Update,* edited by A.W. Norman, K. Schaefer, H.-G. Grigoleit, and D.V. Herrath, Walter de Gruyter & Co., Berlin–New York.

49. Pak, C.Y.C., Zisman, E., Evens, R., Jowsey, J., Delea, C.S., and Bartter, F.C. (1969): The treatment of osteoporosis with calcium infusions. *Am. J. Med.,* 47:7–16.

50. Recker, R.R., Saville, P.D., and Heaney, R.P. (1977): Effect of estrogens and calcium carbonate on bone loss in postmenopausal women. *Ann. Intern Med.,* 87:649–55.

51. Recker, R.R., Gallagher, J.C., and Heaney, R.P. (1984): The metabolic effects of treatment with calcitriol in patients with postmenopausal osteoporosis. *Clin. Res.,* 32(2):406A.

52. Richelson, L.S., Whaner, H.W., Melton, L.J., and Riggs, B.L. (1984): Relative contributions of aging and estrogen deficiency to postmenopausal bone loss. *N. Engl. J. Med.,* 311:1273–1275.

53. Riggs, B.L., Jowsey, J., Kelly, P.J., Jones, J.D., and Maher, F.T. (1969): Effect of sex hormones on bone in primary osteoporosis. *J. Clin. Invest.,* 48:1065–1072.

54. Riggs, B.L., Jowsey, J. Goldsmith, R.S., Kelly, P.J., Hoffman, D.L., and Arnaud, C.D. (1972): Short- and long-term effects of estrogen and synthetic anabolic hormone in postmenopausal osteoporosis. *J. Clin. Invest.,* 51:1659–1663.

55. Riggs, B.L., Jowsey, J., Kelly, P.J., Hoffman, D.L., and Arnaud, C.D. (1974): Effects of oral therapy with calcium and vitamin D in primary osteoporosis. *J. Clin. Endocrinol. Metab.,* 42:1139–1144.

56. Riggs, B.L., Gallagher, J.C., DeLuca, H.F., and Zinmeister, A.,R. (1981): Studies on the mechanism of impaired calcium absorption in postmenopausal osteoporosis. In: *Vitamin D. Clinical, Biochemical and Clinical Endocrinology of Calcium Metabolism,* edited by A.W. Norman, K. Schaefer, H.-.G. Grigoleit, and D.V. Herrath, pp. 903–908. Walter de Gruyter & Co., Berlin–New York.

57. Riggs, B.L., Seeman, E., Hodgson, S.F., Taves, D.R., and O'Fallon, W.M. (1982): Effect of the fluoride/calcium regimen on vertebral fracture occurrence in postmenopausal osteoporosis: comparison with conventional therapy. *N. Engl. J. Med.,* 306:446–50.

58. Riggs, B.L., and Melton, L.J. (1986): Involutional osteoporosis. *N. Engl. J. Med.,* 314:1676–1686.

59. Riis, B., Thomsen, K., and Christiansen, C. (1987): Does calcium supplementation prevent postmenopausal bone loss? *New Engl. J. Med.,* 316:173–177.

60. Rose, G.A. (1964): The study of the treatment of osteoporosis with fluoride therapy and high calcium intake. *Postgrad. Med. J.,* 40:158–163.

61. Rose, G.A. (1967): A critique of modern methods of diagnosis and treatment of osteoporosis. *Clin. Orthop.,* 55:17–41.

62. Schwartz, E., Panariello, V.A., and Saela, J. (1965): Radioactive calcium kinetics during high

calcium intake in osteoporosis*. *J. Clin. Invest.*, 44:1547–1560.

63. Schwartz, E., Chokas, W.V., and Panariello, V.A. (1964): Metabolic balance studies of high calcium intake in osteoporosis. *Am. J. Med.*, 36:233–249.

64. Shiraki, M., Orimo, H., Ito, H., Akiguchi, I., Nakao, J., and Takahashi, R. (1985): Long-term treatment of postmenopausal osteoporosis with active vitamin D3, 1-alpha-hydroxycholecalciferol (1-OHD3) and 1,24 dihydroxycholecalciferol (1,24(OH)2D3). *Endocrinol. Jpn.*, 32:305–315.

65. Solomon, L. (1968): Osteoporosis and fracture of the femoral neck in the South African Bantu. *J. Bone Joint Surg.*, 50:2.

66. Sorensen, O.H., Andersen, R.B., Christensen, M.S., Friis, T., Hjorth, L., Jorgensen, F.S., Lund, B., and Melsen, F. (1977): Treatment of senile osteoporosis with 1 di-hydroxyvitamin D3. *Clin. Endocrinol.*, 7:169S–175S.

67. Spencer, H., Jacob, M., Lewin, I., and Samachson, J. (1964): Absorption of calcium in osteoporosis. *Am. J. Med.*, 37:223–234.

68. Thallasinos, N.C., Gutteridge, D.H., Joplin, G.F., and Fraser, T.R. (1982): Calcium balances in osteoporotic patients on long-term oral calcium therapy with and without sex hormones. *Clin. Sci.*, 62:221.

69. Urist, M.R., Gurvey, M.S., and Fareed, D.O. (1970): Long-term observations on aged women with pathological osteoporosis. In: *Osteoporosis*, edited by U.S. Barzel, p. 3., Grune & Stratton, New York.

70. Whedon, G.D. (1959): Effects of high calcium intakes on bones, blood and soft tissue; relationship of calcium intake to balance in osteoporosis. *Fed. Proc.*, 18:1112–1118.

Osteoporosis: Etiology, Diagnosis, and Management, edited by B. Lawrence Riggs and L. Joseph Melton, III. Raven Press, New York © 1988.

16

Drug Therapy: Calcitonin, Bisphosphonates, Anabolic Steroids, and hPTH (1–34)

Charles H. Chesnut III

Osteoporosis Research Center, University of Washington School of Medicine, Seattle, Washington 98195

GENERAL ASPECTS OF THERAPY (10,12)

Osteoporosis is defined as a reduction in bone mass per unit volume (skeletal osteopenia) to a level leading to fracture, particularly of the spine, distal radius, and proximal femur. Treatment of such osteoporosis of whatever cause (corticosteroid-induced, postmenopausal, etc.) may be divided into symptomatic therapy and therapy for the underlying disease (skeletal osteopenia). Symptomatic therapy is usually related to previously occurring skeletal fractures and involves analgesia, short-term limitation of activity, back bracing if appropriate, and time. Therapy for skeletal osteopenia, on the other hand, may require specific agents [such as calcitonin, bisphosphonates, anabolic steroids, and possibly the 1–34 fragment of parathyroid hormone (PTH)] administered intermittently or continually for extended periods. This chapter will deal with the latter form of therapy; it is imperative that the patient, and practitioner, realize that such treatment of underlying skeletal osteopenia is not directed primarily towards symptom relief, although if further fractures are prevented, the symptoms of the disease will obviously be reduced.

As previously noted, the principal, although not the sole, determinant of skeletal fracture in the osteoporotic patient is the amount of bone mass present. This observation may be used in the formulation of a therapeutic program based primarily upon modification or stabilization of bone mass. To understand such a therapeutic program, some knowledge of the concepts of bone remodeling is necessary. Bone is constantly turning over, or remodeling, in response to calcium requirements, mechanical stress, etc.; as noted in Fig. 1B the initial event is an increase in bone resorption, as mediated by the osteoclast. An increase in bone formation, as mediated by the osteoblast, generally follows. The processes of bone resorption and bone formation are normally and perhaps homeostatically "coupled"; an increase or decrease in bone resorption will produce a corresponding increase or decrease in bone formation, such that the net change in bone mass is zero. In many cases of osteoporosis, particularly of the postmenopausal variety, bone resorption is thought to be increased over normal resorption levels, without a corresponding increase in bone formation, leading to a net loss in bone mass (Fig. 1C); bone remodeling is "negatively uncoupled". In other cases of osteoporosis, particularly corticosteroid-

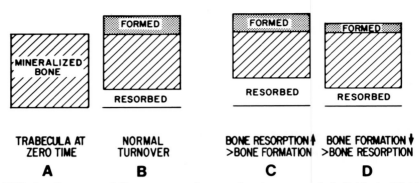

FIG. 1.   Bone remodeling sequences in normal and osteoporotic individuals (10,12).

induced, a primary decrease in bone formation may occur, also resulting in a reduction in bone mass (Fig. 1D).

If inadequate skeletal mass is a principal determinant of increased fracture risk in osteoporotic patients, the goal of treatment should be either preventive or restorative, depending upon the patient's bone mass and fracture history. For example, in an aging woman with a relatively normal bone mass and no previous fractures, the goal of therapy should be the prevention of an osteopenic state sufficient to increase the risk of fracture. Attaining this goal involves slowing of the bone loss that normally occurs with aging and estrogen-depletion. On the other hand, in a woman with a low bone mass and a history of previous fracture, treatment should be directed toward restoration of bone mass to a level at which fracture risk is substantially reduced. Attainment of this goal will involve a slowing of bone mass loss as well as replacement of bone previously lost.

In terms of bone remodeling (Fig. 1), prevention of bone mass loss and/or restoration of bone previously lost may be accomplished by decreasing bone resorption, increasing bone formation, or both. To prevent osteopenia, a decrease in bone resorption may suffice, provided that bone formation is maintained at a normal level. Bone mass restoration, however, ideally requires an increase in bone formation as well as a decrease in bone resorption; an increase in bone resorption with a greater increase in bone formation, or a decrease in bone resorption with a lesser decrease in bone for-

mation, will also result in the desired net positive bone mass change. In other words, such therapeutic maneuvers attempt to "positively uncouple" the normal coupling mechanisms of bone remodeling.

Calcitonin, Bisphosphonate, Anabolic Steroid, and hPTH (1-34) Therapy (8,11)

Several therapeutic agents slow the loss of bone mass, probably by primarily decreasing bone resorption. Such agents include oral calcium (dietary or supplemental), estrogen, calcitonin, bisphosphonates, and congeners of vitamin D, and may be termed "anti-bone resorbers." These agents may, with the possible exception of calcitonin, bisphosphonates, and congeners of vitamin D (that may also restore bone mass previously lost), be of primarily prophylactic value, i.e., they prevent significant bone loss. While, as noted previously, it is theoretically possible that an anti-bone resorbing agent could increase bone mass due to an "uncoupling" of normal skeletal coupling mechanisms (resulting in a decrease in bone resorption without a corresponding decrease in bone formation), such an increase may be both transient and of questionable clincial benefit, due to an anticipated reinstitution of normal coupling phenomena.

As shown in Fig. 2, use of an anti-bone resorbing agent prior to loss of bone mass below a hypothetical fracture threshold would be reasonable; bone mass would remain above the fracture threshold, presumably sufficient to

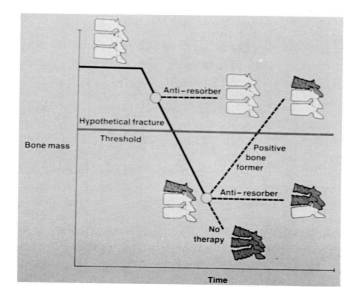

FIG. 2. Therapy of osteoporosis based upon an effect on bone mass; darker vertebrae represent vertebral compression fractures (10,11,12).

prevent fractures. However, the benefit of these anti-bone resorbing agents, with again the exception of calcitonin and vitamin D congeners, as the sole therapy in the individual with preexisting osteoporotic fractures (and with therefore low bone mass by definition) is as yet unproven; again, as shown in Fig. 2, the use of such a therapeutic agent alone, without restoration of previously lost bone mass, would presumably allow further fractures. The individual would remain at risk for further fracture due to inadequate bone mass.

On the other hand, some agents appear capable of restoring bone mass previously lost, and possibly of preventing further fractures. Sodium fluoride, the anabolic steroids, and potentially the 1–34 fragment of parathyroid hormone would be classified as such "positive bone formers." As noted in Fig. 2, the positive bone formers, either alone or in combination with anti-bone resorbing agents, would theoretically increase bone mass above the hypothetical fracture threshold and thereby decrease the incidence of subsequent fracture.

CALCITONIN

Calcitonin is a 32 amino acid polypeptide hormone derived in mammals from C cells of the thyroid gland, and from the ultimobranchial glands of lower species. Human, salmon, porcine, and eel calcitonin preparations are currently available for therapeutic administration; the activity of the different calcitonins are expressed in MRC (Medical Research Council) units or IU (International Units), with salmon calcitonin the most potent of all currently available preparations.

Calcitonin is a potent inhibitor acutely of osteoclast activity, and subsequently of bone resorption (which is reflected in a lowering of serum calcium); it probably functions physiologically to protect against hypercalcemia by preventing calcium release from bone. No direct effect of calcitonin on bone formation has been definitively elucidated. As a physiologic and pharmacologic inhibitor of bone resorption, calcitonin therefore possesses an obvious therapeutic rationale for usage in osteoporosis. A number of other observations also support its potential efficacy in postmenopausal osteoporosis, including those of decreasing calcitonin levels with advancing age and lower calcitonin levels in women compared to men (14), and a possible deficiency in calcitonin reserve (response of calcitonin to calcium infusion) in postmenopausal osteoporotic females compared to age matched normal females (35).

Such a calcitonin deficiency would presumably result in increased bone resorption and increased bone wasting. In general, the age, gender, and postulated osteoporosis–specific changes in calcitonin secretion are consistent with a role for calcitonin in the development of decreased bone mass; however, the recent finding of Tiegs et al. (38) concerning monomeric calcitonin raise significant questions regarding the role of calcitonin deficiency in the etiology of postmenopausal osteoporosis.

Early studies did not confirm such a therapeutic rationale, but these limited clinical trials with porcine (13,20) and synthetic salmon calcitonin (21,40) were either uncontrolled, of short duration, or utilized a comparatively small number of subjects. More recent studies however have utilized more stringent study design criteria, and have demonstrated a more promising role for calcitonin in the treatment of osteoporosis. Agrawal et al. (1) noted a significant increase in total body calcium (total bone mass) as determined by the total body calcium-neutron activation analysis (TBC-NAA) procedure in a subgroup of osteoporotic males. In addition, in a two-year controlled study Gruber et al. (18) demonstrated (Fig. 3) a transient, but significant, increase in total bone mass (as measured by TBC-NAA) through 18 months in 24 postmenopausal osteoporotic (spinal compression fractures) females; subjects received synthetic salmon calcitonin in a daily dosage of 100 MRC units, plus supplemental calcium, and vitamin D. A decrease in bone resorption was documented on iliac crest bone biopsy at study conclusion (26 months). The slight increase in total bone mass (+2%, +14.5 g of TBC, Fig. 3) through 18 months may have been due to a transient "uncoupling" of bone resorption and formation, but at the concluding bone biopsy bone apposition rate was decreased. Also, in this study total bone mass may have been decreasing at 18 months; this finding, in combination with other observed serum and urine changes, suggested a developing resistance to the drug's action, possibly due to reinstitution of normal coupling mechanisms, or perhaps more likely, to a down regulation of receptor sites (i.e., a persistent saturation of calcitonin receptor sites on osteoclasts) consequent to a continuous daily administration of 100 MRC units of calcitonin. Such a possible "plateau" effect may indicate a decrease in drug effectiveness associated with continuous and prolonged therapy, and is also observed with calcitonin treatment of Paget's disease.

A possible analgesic effect of calcitonin, particularly in patients with metastatic bone disease, has been described (17); whether such analgesia, hypothetically mediated by ß-endorphins, would occur in osteoporotic subjects treated with calcitonin is conjectural at best.

Safety is an outstanding characteristic of calcitonin administration; it is perhaps the safest of currently available therapies for osteoporosis. Transient facial flushing and nausea, rare vomiting and diarrhea, and mild inflammation or itching at the site of injection (as noted below, the drug is administered intramuscularly or subcutaneously) are comparatively rare side-effects, and should not necessitate drug discontinuation.

Synthetic salmon calcitonin is currently approved by the Food and Drug Administration as the drug Calcimar for treatment of the postmenopausal osteoporotic patient; human and eel calcitonin are utilized in Europe or Japan but are not approved for usage in the United States. The USV Rorer Pharmaceutical Company of Fort Washington, Pennsylvania, is the pharmaceutical vendor; the cost is approximately $15.00/vial, with each vial containing 2 cc or 200 MRC units. The recommended dosage is 100 MRC units daily by either intramuscular or subcutaneous injection (as a polypeptide the drug is inactivated by gastric secretions if administered orally); it should be given with adequate calcium (at least 1000 mg of elemental calcium daily) and possibly vitamin D (a multivitamin daily with 400 IU of D_2 is sufficient). A recent editorial (31) advises the administration of 2000 mg of elemental calcium 8 to 10 h following calcitonin administration, to block calcitonin's hypocalcemic effect and subsequent parathyroid hormone secretion; such therapy, however, remains of hypothetical value at present.

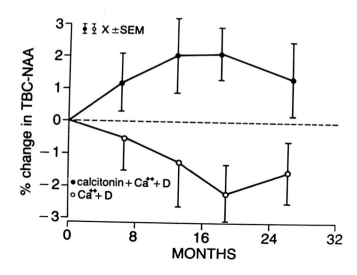

FIG. 3. Percent change in TBC–NAA (total body calcium-neutron activation analysis) in 24-treated (●) and 21 control (0) patients (11).

Calcitonin, therefore, would appear to be primarily an antiresorbing agent, and would have potential value in preventing bone loss prior to such loss occurring. It would, however, also appear to be of value in the osteoporotic patient with fractures and a reduced bone mass, as in addition to slowing bone mass loss over a period of at least two years it significantly increased bone mass through 18 months (Fig. 3), possibly by a transient "uncoupling of coupling". Presumably calcitonin therapy is of limited long-term (greater than 18 months) value in replacing bone previously lost; it should, however, be noted that in the osteoporotic patient possibly greater benefit could be achieved with a lesser calcitonin dosage administered intermittently. Perhaps 50 MRC units of synthetic salmon calcitonin administered every second or third day would be of greater therapeutic efficacy than 100 MRC units administered continuously, although clinical trials would be necessary to prove such efficacy. In addition, utilization of calcitonin in combination with other therapeutic agents known to stimulate bone formation (such as sodium fluoride or anabolic steroids) may provide a greater therapeutic effect in the osteoporotic subject. Further clinical trials are definitely indicated to assess the possibly beneficial effects of intermittent and/or combination therapy in osteoporotic patients; in this regard a previous study (26) does suggest a positive effect of oral phosphate (that transiently stimulates bone remodeling and possibly bone formation) "pulsed" intermittently in combination with parenterally administered synthetic salmon calcitonin, also administered intermittently. However, the combination of calcitonin alternating with human growth hormone was not found to be of benefit (3).

While calcitonin does appear to be of value in the patient with osteoporosis and fractures, its greatest potential may lie in the prevention of this disease. Ideally, to be utilized prophylactically a therapeutic modality should be of proven therapeutic efficacy, should be safe, and should possess an acceptable route of administration and an acceptable cost. In terms of these requirements calcitonin would be a quite reasonable therapeutic agent: it does slow bone mass loss, and is uniquely safe compared to the majority of other osteoporosis therapies. Expense, however, must be reduced, and an alternative mode of administration to the current parenteral route must be developed. In terms of the latter requirement, administration of the drug nasally by intranasal spray would be acceptable; such routes of administration are under evaluation (25,28).

BISPHOSPHONATES

The bisphosphonates (also known as diphosphonates) are analogues of endogenous pyrophosphate, possessing P-C-P bonds, that are resistant to enzymatic hydrolysis and possess a high-binding affinity for hydroxyapatite crystal. The therapeutic rationale for their usage in a variety of metabolic bone diseases (including Paget's disease, hypercalcemia of malignancy, heterotopic ossification, and postmenopausal osteoporosis) is basically an inhibition of bone remodeling, particularly bone resorption, by a variety of mechanisms, including inhibition of growth and dissolution of hydroxyapatite crystal (*in vitro*) (30), and possibly an interference with osteoclast function and/or attachment to bone surfaces. Three bisphosphonates, ethane-1-hydroxy-1, 1-diphosphonate (EHDP), 3-amino-1-hydroxy-propylidine-1-diphosphonate (APD), and dichloromethylene diphosphonate (CI_2MDP, clodronate), are, or have been, utilized in clinical practice, or in research studies.

While therapeutic efficacy has been demonstrated for the bisphosphonates in those diseases with increased bone remodeling and bone resorption, (such as Paget's disease), few studies are available confirming such efficacy in osteoporosis. Heaney et al. (19) observed a decrease in both bone resorption and bone accretion, as assessed by calcium balance and radiocalcium kinetic studies, in a group of postmenopausal osteoporotic females treated with EHDP in a dosage of 20 mg/kg/day for 12 months; however, while a decrease in bone mineralization (accretion) was noted, the authors postulated that a lesser dosage of EHDP could conceivably reduce bone accretion less than bone resorption and that such "positive uncoupling" of the components of bone remodeling could, if persistent, lead to positive calcium balance and a beneficial effect upon bone mass. Therein lies a basic hypothesis for bisphosphonate usage in osteoporosis: that the decrease in bone remodeling known to occur with these agents will involve a greater reduction in bone resorption than in bone formation, that such actions on remodeling will be persistent, and that such a preferential and potentially beneficial effect will vary according to dosage, duration of administration, and type of bisphosphonate utilized.

A recent double-blind controlled study (11) from our laboratory tested such a hypothesis; the bisphosphonate clodronate was administered intermittently through approximately 11 months to 24 of 46 postmenopausal osteoporotic females. As noted in Fig. 4 a substantial increase in total bone mass as assessed by the TBC-NAA technique was noted when clodronate was administered in an intermittent dosage of 1200 to 1600 mgm daily (on drug for 1 month, off drug for 3 months, on drug for 3 months, etc.). As a potent inhibitor of bone resorption (documented in this study by a significant decrease in total urinary hydroxyproline, a marker for bone remodeling and specifically bone resorption), the expected efficiency of clodronate would be primarily in slowing bone mass loss. However, as noted in Fig. 4, the observed 6% increase in total bone mass suggests a continuous uncoupling of bone resorption and bone formation, persisting for months after medication discontinuation, with suppression of bone resorption but continuation of bone formation, and net accrual of bone mass. Whether other bisphosphonates (EHDP, APD) share in this apparent beneficial effect on osteoporotic bone is unproven; the Heaney et al. study (19) notwithstanding, definitive studies of these bisphosphonates in osteoporosis have not been performed, although 2 large clinical trials assessing EHDP efficacy are underway.

The bisphosphonates, orally administered, are generally well-tolerated with occasional, generally mild, nausea and diarrhea the rare side-effect in Paget's patients treated with EHDP and clodronate; a transient elevation in body temperature has been noted in similar patients treated with APD (39). Serum phosphorous is frequently elevated, and parathyroid hormone occasionally elevated, the latter particularly with clodronate administration (24). Significant hematologic effects of clodronate have not been confirmed.

A more worrisome potential complication of bisphosphonate therapy is a mineralization defect leading to osteomalacia and possible increased risk of fracture; such a complication

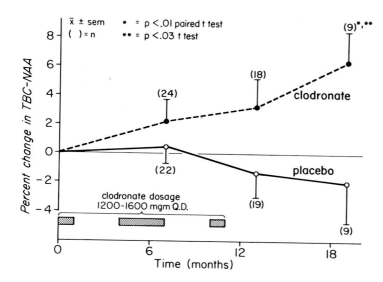

FIG. 4. Percent change in TBC–NAA in 24 treated (●) and 22 control (0) patients; treated patients received clodronate daily, 1200 to 1600 mg, intermittently over 11 months (on drug 1 month, off 3 months, on 3 months, off 3 months, and on 1 month) (11).

appears to be associated with EHDP (6) rather than with clodronate or APD, and with high (10 to 20 mg/kg/day) persistent (greater than 6 months) EHDP dosage, although lower dosages (5mg/kg/day) have also been incriminated (5).

The bisphosphonates are experimental therapeutic agents for osteoporosis, and are not currently approved by the Food and Drug Administration as treatment for this disease (EHDP is approved for the treatment of Paget's disease under the trade name Didronel). The precise dosage and administration (continuous vs intermittent dosing) schedule remains unproven; in ongoing studies with EHDP a dosage of 400 mg daily, 2 weeks of every 3 months, in sequential combination with oral phosphate, is utilized. The current cost of EHDP (Didronel) is $60.00 per 100 tablets (200 mg tablet); Norwich Eaton Pharmaceuticals, Inc., of Norwich, New York, is the supplier.

While the bisphosphonates must be viewed as potentially effective in the overall treatment of osteoporosis, their principle value (as anti-bone resorbers) may be in prophylaxis. Such a statement assumes future prophylactic studies confirming their therapeutic efficacy and long term safety; their oral route of administration, and their relative inexpensiveness, are definite assets for a potential prophylactic agent. As

noted previously, appropriate synergistic combination programs (i.e., bisphosphonates as anti-bone resorbers plus sodium fluoride as a positive bone former) also deserve further study.

ANABOLIC STEROIDS

The anabolic steroids, synthetic derivatives of the androgen testosterone, were developed in an attempt to dissociate the anabolic effects of testosterone from its masculinizing effects. As early as 1947, Reifenstein and Albright suggested a beneficial effect of methyltestosterone in osteoporosis as defined by calcium balance techniques (29); subsequent studies (32) with anabolic steroids noted an effect similar to those of estrogens with a decrease in bone resorption as the primary skeletal effect. In general, until relatively recently the role of these agents in the treatment of osteoporosis was, at best, uncertain; three studies of the effects of anabolic steroids performed during the past eight years have, however, demonstrated decidedly positive results.

In two of these studies (2,7) treatment with the anabolic steroid methandrostenolone produced a signficant increase in total bone mass as determined by the TBC-NAA technique. In a third study (9) the anabolic steroid stanozolol, when combined with a daily 1000 mg calcium intake, substantially improved total bone mass status in 21 postmenopausal osteoporotic women during 29 months of study participation (Fig. 5). Also, the lack of new spinal compression fractures in the stanozolol-treated patients suggested an improvement in spinal structural integrity.

In addition, data from this latter study suggested possible mechanisms of action of stanozolol, and probably of other anabolic steroids, in postmenopausal osteoporosis: a primary renal effect resulting in a decrease in urinary calcium, with a subsequent rise in serum calcium and a counterregulatory decrease in serum parathyroid hormone. Presumably such a decrease results in a decrease in bone resorption. In addition, a direct stimulation of bone formation, as assessed by iliac-crest bone-biopsy techniques, was noted. Such an effect on bone formation was unsuspected; subsequent *in vitro* (4) and *in vivo* (15) studies (the latter demonstrating an increase in skeletal alkaline phosphatase, a marker for bone formation) following stanozolol therapy have, however, confirmed such a stimulatory effect. Hence stanozolol and, presumably, other anabolic steroids function as positive bone formers in the treatment of postmenopausal osteoporosis.

The anabolic steroids, orally administered, are generally well-tolerated from a gastrointestinal standpoint, but have significant systemic side-effects (8). As 17-methylated heterocyclic steroids these agents can be expected to produce liver function test abnormalities, including occasional (and reversible) elevations of serum bilirubin, alkaline phosphatase, and other liver enzymes. In addition, sodium retention and masculinizing effects (an increase in facial hair, acne, hoarseness) have been noted in some individuals receiving anabolic steroids. Also, when administered continuously at high dosage (two to three times that recommended for osteoporosis) for extended periods, anabolic steroids have been associated with hepatomas and peliosis hepatis (blood filled hepatic cysts). Lastly, and perhaps most worrisome, an effect of anabolic steroids on serum lipids has been noted, with a reduction in high density lipoproteins and an elevation in low density lipoproteins (34); such lipoprotein changes are of at least theoretical concern because of the possible effect of these alterations on the rate of atherogenesis.

As noted, the majority of the anabolic steroids currently available are administered orally (stanozolol: Winstrol, oxandrolone: Anavar) or intramuscularly (nandrolone: Dura-

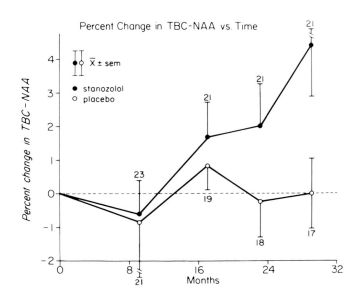

FIG. 5. Percent change in TBC–NAA in 23-treated (●) and 21 control (0) patients (9).

bolin). The dosage of stanozolol utilized in previous osteoporosis studies (9) was 2 mg by mouth three times a day, three out of every four weeks; 100 stanozolol tablets are $30.85. Winthrop-Breon Laboratories of New York, New York, is the purveyor of stanozolol. Such dosage and cost considerations are of generally academic interest as the Food and Drug Administration has recently withdrawn approval for the usage of these drugs in osteoporosis, most likely due to their side effects.

As medications with positive (increasing bone formation) and negative (significant side-effects) attributes, where do the anabolic steroids fit into the osteoporosis therapeutic armamenterium? In the elderly osteoporotic female with compression fractures and low bone mass who is not responding to other medications, the anabolic steroids such as stanozolol may be of value, either alone or in combination with anti-resorbing agents such as calcitonin or diphosphonates. The risk-benefit ratio (future hypothetical atherogenic potential vs possible fracture prevention) is acceptably low. These agents would, however, be contraindicated for long-term prophylactic usage, particularly in the premenopausal female. It should also be kept in mind that the anabolic steroids are not FDA-approved for osteoporosis treatment.

hPTH (1-34)

PTH is an 84 amino acid polypeptide hormone, with multiple direct and indirect effects upon the skeleton: while its primary skeletal effect may be an increase in bone resorption secondary to osteoclast stimulation, it is also known to increase bone formation and trabecular bone mass in humans and animals (36), and to produce osteosclerosis in patients with primary and secondary hyperparathyroidism (16,22). This it appears that the resorptive effects of parathyroid hormone on bone can be separated from its formative effects (37). In addition, the biologically active amino-terminal portion of human parathyroid hormone (hPTH 1-34) has been synthesized, and found to increase bone turnover and trabecular bone vol-

ume on iliac crest bone biopsies from osteoporotic patients. A therapeutic rationale appears to exist for the usage of this specific parathyroid hormone fragment as an anabolic positive bone former.

Data regarding the efficacy, and mechanism of action, of synthetic hPTH (1-34) dervies from two clinical studies: Reeve et al. (27) observed a substantial increase in iliac trabecular bone volume, rate of new bone formation, and radiocalcium accretion (as determined by radiocalcium kinetics) in a limited number (9 to 21) of osteoporotic subjects treated daily over a 6 to 24 month period with 100 μg of subcutaneously-administered hPTH (1-34). Calcium balance, calcium absorption, and cortical bone density (as determined primarily by radial single photon absorptiometry techniques) did not, however, change. The authors concluded that the failure to increase dietary calcium absorption may have limited a possible increase in cortical bone mass, and, perhaps disconcertingly, that the observed increase in trabecular bone may have been at the expense of cortical bone (since the balance studies showed no net retention of either calcium or phosphate). Slovik et al. (33) studied the effects of short-term (3 to 4 weeks) subcutaneous administration of hPTH (1-34) at a dosage of 450 or 750 U/day in six osteoporotic subjects; in patients receiving 450 U calcium absorption increased, calcium and phosphate balance improved but a minimal increase in radiocalcium accretion was observed. In subjects receiving the higher dosage an increase in urinary calcium, no improvement in calcium absorption, and a negative calcium balance occurred; such occurrences were felt to either lead to, or to be the result of, net bone breakdown in the high dosage group. It was concluded that low dosages of hPTH (1-34) may promote bone formation, but that higher dosages would result in a deleterious increase in bone resorption; the authors further speculated that the long-term usefulness of hPTH (1-34) in osteoporosis could be limited by its failure to *consistently* increase calcium absorption, calcium balance, and calcium accretion.

The safety of hPTH (1–34) appears reasonable; transient mild hypercalcemia, and a mild (but again transient) itching and redness at the site of injection, are the two side-effects observed to date. As the drug remains primarily an experimental therapeutic agent and research tool, and is not currently approved for treatment of osteoporosis by the Food and Drug Administration. Limited information is available on its dosage (other than as noted previously) and expense. The primary provider of hPTH (1–34) is the USV Rorer Pharmaceutical Company, Fort Washington, Pennsylvania.

The future usage of PTH, and specifically hPTH (1–34), in the treatment of osteoporosis remains unclear at this time; among its negative attributes are its less than desirable necessity of parenteral injection, an apparent negative effect on cortical bone mass, a possibly narrow therapeutic window (with excessive dosage resulting in adverse skeletal effects), and an overall lack of definitive efficacy data. It appears unlikely that hPTH (1–34) will achieve a major role as a single therapy for the prevention or treatment of postmenopausal osteoporosis. However, it is quite possible that this hormone fragment could be utilized in a combination therapeutic program; its positive attributes of stimulation of bone formation (in appropriate dosage) and overall bone turnover could make it an attractive treatment modality when used intermittently in combination with an agent inhibiting bone resorption.

It should also be noted that a bovine PTH (1–34) is available; such a preparation would presumably have little application for osteoporosis therapy as it produces neutralizing antibodies after several weeks of injections in humans (23).

MONITORING THE RESPONSE TO THERAPY (8)

Therapy in osteoporosis implies prevention or reversal of bone wasting; many practitioners and patients assume that such therapy will decrease pain. In general, with the possible exception of calcitonin, the previously discussed therapeutic agents will have no direct effect on pain (although, as noted previously, these agents may indirectly decrease pain if fractures are prevented). Pain, and/or subjective improvement in the patient's sense of well-being, cannot be used in establishing the presence or absence of a therapeutic response; other techniques must be employed as a measure of response to treatment. Among these techniques are the various methods for bone mass quantitation, such as dual photon absorptiometry and computerized axial tomography (CT), that are currently available in many medical centers.

For many practicing physicians, however, radiography may be the sole method available for monitoring therapy. Successful treatment of osteoporosis ultimately includes the prevention of new fractures, and the absence of new radiographic fractures is an important indication of a positive response to treatment. The occurrence of a new fracture during the second year of therapy or thereafter should indicate a lack of therapeutic response; it is generally accepted however that a fracture occurring within the first 6 to 12 months of therapy does not always indicate a treatment failure. Factors contributing to the occurrence of a fracture, such as microfractures of individual bony trabeculae, may occur some time (perhaps even months) before the actual fracture; a predisposition to fracture may therefore exist before the initiation of therapy, and it may be impossible for any currently available therapy to reverse this predisposition within a relatively short period.

The monitoring of therapeutic response implies an ability to determine how long a specific medication should be continued, i.e., the duration of therapy. Such data are not currently available with the medications discussed in this chapter, as studies with these agents have only extended through 24 to 30 months. Presumably, the absence of new fractures and/or the improvement or stabilization of bone mass would indicate a continuation of therapy, although the ultimate duration of treatment will depend on other factors such as expense, cost of administration, and side-effects.

Usage of Calcitonin, Bisphosphonates, Anabolic Steroids, and hPTH in other than Postmenopausal Osteoporosis

The previous discussions regarding calcitonin, the bisphosphonates, the anabolic steroids, and hPTH have primarily pertained to the usage of these medications in postmenopausal osteoporosis; there is limited definitive information regarding their efficacy in other osteoporotic conditions, including steroid-induced osteopenia, the bone-wasting associated with rheumatoid arthritis and immobilization, etc. Presumably these agents would have value in such conditions, but dosage, dosing schedules, and efficacy must await controlled clinical trials. Also, their usage in osteoporotic males is empirical at present; while anabolic steroids might appear suited for usage in the male osteoporotic patient, their potential for side effects, even in the male, must be considered.

CONCLUSIONS

Osteoporosis, particularly postmenopausal osteoporosis, is a common, morbid, and extremely expensive disease, particularly of the elderly. The therapeutic agents discussed in this chapter offer some expectation of reducing this incidence and expense. It must, however, be remembered that individual patient responses to these various medications will obviously vary; since osteoporosis is a heterogeneous disease, therapeutic responses would also presumably be heterogeneous. Nevertheless, the average response of bone mass to these therapeutic perturbations would indicate potential value for the prevention of osteoporosis (calcitonin and bisphosphonates), and for the treatment of osteoporosis after the disease occurred (the anabolic steroids and possibly the human fragment of parathyroid hormone). In the future there will undoubtedly be further utilization of these individual agents in combination therapies, and as part of sequential therapeutic programs.

REFERENCES

1. Agrawal, R., Wallach, S., Cohn, S., Tessier, M., Verch R., Hussain, M., and Zanzi, I. (1981): Calcitonin treatment of osteoporosis. In: *Calcitonin 1980. Chemistry, Physiology, Pharmacology, and Clinical Aspects,* edited by A. Pecile, pp. 237–246, Excerpta Medica, Amsterdam.
2. Aloia, J.F., Kapoor, A., Vaswani, A., and Cohn, S.H. (1981): Changes in body composition following therapy of osteoporosis with methandrostenolone. *Metabolism,* 30:1076–1079.
3. Aloia, J.F., Vaswani, A., Kapoor, A., Yeh, J.K., and Cohn, S.H. (1985): Treatment of osteoporosis with calcitonin, with and without growth hormone. *Metabolism,* 34:124–129.
4. Beresford, J.N., Gallagher, J.A., Poser, J., Gowen, M., Couch, M., Yates, A.J.P., Kanis, J.A., and Russell, R.G.G. (1983): Effects of the anabolic steroid, stanozolol, on human bone cells *in vitro*. In: XVII European Symposium on Calcified Tissues, abstr. 97.
5. Boyce, B.F., Fogelman, I., Ralston, S., Smith, L., Johnston, E., and Boyle, I.T. (1984): Focal osteomalacia due to low-dose diphosphonate therapy in Paget's disease. *Lancet,* 1:821–824.
6. Canfield, R., Rosner, W., Skinner, J., McWhorter, J., Resnick, L., Feldman, F., Kammermans, S., Ryan, K., Kunigonis, M., and Bohne, W. (1977): Diphosphonate therapy of Paget's disease of bone. *J. Clin. Endocrinol. Metab,* 44:96–106.
7. Chesnut, C.H., Nelp, W.B., Baylink, D.J., and Denney, J.D. (1977): Effect of methandrostenolone on postmenopausal bone wasting as assessed by changes in total bone mineral mass. *Metabolism,* 26:24–56.
8. Chesnut, C.H., and Baylink, D.J. (1983): The role of anabolic steroids in the treatment of osteoporosis. *Geriat. Med. Today,* 2:21–29.
9. Chesnut, C.H., Ivey, J.L., Gruber, H.E., Matthews, M., Nelp, W.B., Sisom, K., and Baylink, D.J. (1983): Stanozolol in postmenopausal osteoporosis: therapeutic efficacy and possible mechanisms of action. *Metabolism,* 32:571–580.
10. Chesnut, C.H. (1984): Treatment of postmenopausal osteoporosis. *Comprehen. Ther.,* 10(7):41–47.
11. Chesnut, C.H. (1984): Synthetic salmon calcitonin, diphosphonates, and anabolic steroids in the treatment of postmenopausal osteoporosis. In: *Osteoporosis. Proceedings of the Copenhagen International Symposium on Osteoporosis,* edited by C. Christiansen, C.D. Arnaud, B.E.C. Nordin, A.M. Parfitt, W.A. Peck, and B.L. Riggs, pp. 549–555, Aalborg Stiftsbogtrykkeri, Glostrup, Copenhagen.
12. Chesnut, C.H. (1984): An appraisal of the role of estrogens in the treatment of postmenopausal osteoporosis. *J. Am. Geriat. Soc.,* 32:604–608.

13. Cohn, S.H., Dombrowski, C.S., Hauser, W., Klopper, J., and Atkins, H.L. (1971): Effects of porcine calcitonin on calcium metabolism in osteoporosis. *J. Clin. Endocrinol.*, 33:719–728.

14. Deftos, L.J., Weisman, J.H., Williams, G.W., Karpf, D.B., Frumar, A.M., Davidson, B.J., Parthmore, J.G., and Judd, H.L. (1980): Influence of age and sex on plasma calcitonin in human beings. *N. Engl. J. Med.*, 302:1351–1353.

15. Farley, J.R., Chesnut, C.H., and Baylink, D.J. (1981): Improved method for quantitative determination in serum of alkaline phosphatase of skeletal origin. *Clin. Chem.*, 27:2002–2007.

16. Genant, H.K., Baron, J.M., Paloyan, E., and Jowsey, J. (1975): Osteosclerosis in primary hyperparathyroidism. *Am. J. Med.*, 59:104–113.

17. Gennari, C. (1981): Calcitonin and bone metastasis of cancer. In: *Calcitonin 1980. Chemistry, Physiology, Pharmacology, and Clinical Aspects,* edited by A. Pecile, pp. 277–287. Excerpta Medica, Amsterdam.

18. Gruber, H.E., Ivey, J.L., Baylink, D.J., Matthews, M., Nelp, W.B., Sisom, K., and Chesnut, C.H. (1984): Long-term calcitonin therapy in postmenopausal osteoporosis. *Metabolism,* 33:295–303.

19. Heaney, R.P., and Saville, P.D. (1976): Etidronate disodium in postmenopausal osteoporosis. *Clin. Pharmacol. Ther.*, 20:593–604.

20. Jowsey, J., Riggs, B.L., Goldsmith, R.S., Kelly, P.J., and Arnaud, C.D. (1971): Effects of prolonged administration of porcine calcitonin in postmenopausal osteoporosis. *J. Clin. Endocrinol.*, 33:752–758.

21. Jowsey, J., Riggs, B.L., Kelly, P.J., and Hoffman, D.L. (1978): Calcium and salmon calcitonin in treatment of osteoporosis. *J. Clin. Endocrinol. Metab.*, 47:633–639.

22. Lalli, A.F., and Lapides, J. (1965): Osteosclerosis occurring in renal disease. *Am. J. Roentagen,* 93:924–926.

23. Melick, R.A., Gill, J.R., Berson, S.A., Yalow, R.S., Bartter, F.C., Potts, J.T., and Aurbach, G.D. (1967): Antibodies and clinical resistance to parathyroid hormone. *N. Engl. J. Med.*, 276:144–147.

24. Meunier, P.J., Chapuy, M.C., Alexandre, C., Bressot, C., Edouard, C., Vignon, E., Mathieu, L., and Trechel, V. (1979): Effects of disodium dichloromethylene diphosphonate (Cl₂MDP) on Paget's disease of bone. *Lancet,* 2:489–492.

25. Pontiroli, A.E. Alberetto, M., and Pozza, G. (1985): Intranasal calcitonin and plasma calcium concentrations in normal subjects. *Br. Med. J.*, 290:1390–1391.

26. Rasmussen, H., Bordier, P., Auquier, L., Eisinger, J.B., Kuntz, D., Caulin, F., Argemi, B., Gueris, J., and Julien, A. (1980): Effect of combined therapy with phosphate and calcitonin on bone volume in osteoporosis. *Metab. Bone Dis. Relat. Res.*, 2:107–111.

27. Reeve, J., Meunier, P.J., Parsons, J.A., Bernat, M., Bijvoet, O.L.M., Courpron, P., Edouard, C., Klenerman, L., Neer, R.M., Renier, J.C., Slovik, D., Vismans, F.J.F.E., and Potts, J.T. (1980): Anabolic effect of human parathyroid fragment on trabecular bone in involutional osteoporosis: a multicentre trial. *Br. Med. J.*, 280:1340–1344.

28. Reginster, J.V., Albert, A., and Franchimont, P. (1985): Salmon calcitonin nasal spray in Paget's disease of bone: preliminary results in five patients. *Calcif. Tissue. Int.*, 37:577–580.

29. Reifenstein, E.C., and Albright, F. (1947): The metabolic effects of steroid hormones in osteoporosis. *J. Clin. Invest.*, 26:24–56.

30. Reitsma, P.H., Teitelbaum, S.L., Bijvoet, O.L.M., and Kahn, A.J. (1982): Differential action of the bisphosphonates (3-amino-1-hydroxypropylidene)-1, 1-bisphosphonate (APD) and disodium dichloromethylidene bisphosphonate (Cl₂MDP) on rat macrophage-mediated bone resorption in vitro. *J. Clin. Invest.*, 70:927–933.

31. Rico, H. (1985): The use of calcitonin as osteolytic drug. *Calcif. Tissue. Int.*, 37:105–106.

32. Riggs, B.L., Jowsey, J., Goldsmith, R.S., Kelly, P.J., Hoffman, D.L., and Arnaud, C.D. (1972): Short- and long-term effects of estrogen and synthetic anabolic hormone in postmenopausal osteoporosis. *J. Clin. Invest.*, 51:1659–1663.

33. Slovik, D.M., Neer, R.M., and Potts, J.T. (1981): Short-term effects of synthetic human parathyroid hormone—(1–34) administration on bone mineral metabolism in osteoporotic patients. *J. Clin. Invest.*, 68:1261–1271.

34. Taggart, H.A., Applebaum-Bowden, D., Haffner, S., Warnick, G.R., Cheung, M.D., Albers, J.J., Chesnut, C.H., and Hazzard, W.R. (1982): Reduction in high density lipoproteins by anabolic steroid (stanozolol) therapy for postmenopausal osteoporosis. *Metabolism,* 3:1147–1152.

35. Taggart, H.M., Chesnut, C.H., Ivey, J.L., Baylink, D.J., Sisom, K., Huber, M.B., and Roos, B.A. (1982): Deficient calcitonin response to calcium stimulation in postmenopausal osteoporosis. *Lancet,* 1:475–477.

36. Tam, C.S., Bayley, A., Cross, E.G., Murray, T.M., and Harrison, J.E. (1982): Increased bone apposition in primary hyperparathyroidism: measurements based on short interval tetracycline labeling of bone. *Metabolism,* 31:759–765.

37. Tam, C.S., Heersche, J.N.M., Murray, T.M., and Parsons, J.A. (1982): Parathyroid hormone stimulates the bone apposition rate independently of its resorptive action: differential effects of intermittent and continuous administration. *Endocrinology,* 110:506–512.

38. Tiegs, R.D., Body, J.J., Wahner, H.W., Barta, J., Riggs, B.L., and Heath, H. (1985): Calcitonin secretion in postmenopausal osteoporosis. *N. Engl. J. Med.*, 312:1097–1100.

39. van Breukelen, F.J.M., Bijvoet, O.L.M., and Van Oosterom A.T. (1979): Inhibition of osteolytic bone lesions by (3-amino-1-hydroxypropylidene)-1, 1-biphosphonate (A.P.D.). *Lancet,* 1:803–805.

40. Wallach, S., Cohn, S.H., Atkins, H.L., Ellis, K.J., Kohberger, R., Aloia, J.F., and Zanai, I. (1977): Effect of salmon calcitonin on skeletal mass in osteoporosis. *Curr. Ther. Res.*, 22:556–571.

Osteoporosis: Etiology, Diagnosis, and Management, edited by B. Lawrence Riggs and L. Joseph Melton, III. Raven Press, New York © 1988.

17

Treatment of Osteoporosis with Sodium Fluoride

Erik F. Eriksen, Stephen F. Hodgson, and B. Lawrence Riggs

Division of Endocrinology, Metabolism, and Internal Medicine, Mayo Medical School, Mayo Clinic and Mayo Foundation, Rochester, Minnesota 55905

The severe decrease in bone mass seen in osteoporosis is caused by an imbalance between bone resorption and bone formation during the bone remodeling process (discussed in Chapter 2, *this volume*). Bone remodeling proceeds at discrete foci in cortical and trabecular bone called "bone remodeling units." It is initiated by osteoclasts that resorb bone to form tunnels in cortical bone and lacunae on the surface of trabecular bone. The bone removed during the resorption phase (normal duration, 3 to 5 weeks) (19) is then replaced by bone newly formed by osteoblasts during the formation phase (normal duration, 3 to 5 months) (18). The end result of this remodeling cycle is the creation of new bone structural units (Haversian systems in cortical bone, and new osteonal packets or walls in trabecular bone), thus repairing microdamage and securing the mechanical integrity of bone.

The ideal therapeutic agent for osteoporosis should increase bone mass to a level above the fracture threshold (Fig. 1). Theoretically, this can be accomplished by either inhibition of bone resorption or sustained stimulation of bone formation in excess of the bone resorptive activity.

The effects of estrogens, calcitonin, and calcium on bone mass are mainly due to inhibition of bone resorption. No direct effects on bone formation have been demonstrated so far (64). These agents may protect against further bone loss from perforative resorption of trabecular plates (61) and thicken existing trabeculae. The decrease in resorptive activity, however, leads to a decrease in bone formation because there is tight coupling between resorption and formation at each bone remodeling unit (24). Small transient increases in bone mass may occur in the first few months after initiation of treatment when the resorption phase is depressed while the formation phase in bone remodeling units that were initiated prior to therapy is being completed. After approximately 6 months, however, bone formation also decreases and no further increase in bone mass occurs (24,60). Newer approaches, e.g., treatment regimens involving selective manipulation of separate bone cell populations (ADFR) or formation-stimulating regimens using parathyroid hormone (PTH) 1–34, and vitamin D (25,84), seek to overcome the problems of decreased bone formation fragments by cyclic administration of inhibitors of bone resorption and stimulators of bone formation (see Chapter, 2, *this volume*). At present, however, these newer approaches have to be considered experimental. Moreover, most of the regimens reported so far use expensive peptides that have to be administered parenterally. Of these regi-

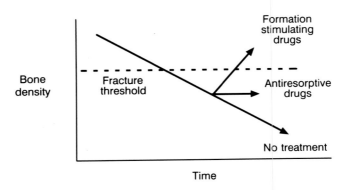

FIG. 1. Model for the effect of treatment on bone loss. As bone loss ensues, bone mineral density (BMD) falls below the fracture threshold and fractures begin to occur. If the patient receives no treatment or ineffectual treatment, there is continued bone loss, and as bone density levels become progressively lower, there is an increased number of fractures. If an antiresorptive drug is given, bone mass is maintained. Because BMD remains below the fracture threshold, the patient will remain at risk for fractures, albeit at a lower rate because further bone loss is prevented. A formation-stimulating drug, however, will substantially increase bone mass to above the fracture threshold, thereby preventing further fractures. From *Cecil Textbook of Medicine,* 18th Edition, with permission from W. B. Saunders Company, Philadelphia, Pennsylvania.

mens, only fluoride therapy has been widely evaluated. Moreover, fluoride is inexpensive, can be administered orally and has a well documented positive effect on bone mass in humans.

FLUORIDE AND THE SKELETON

Fluorine is one of the most avid of the bone-seeking elements. Absorption of fluoride is efficient (more than 90% after an oral dose) (16,50). Fifty percent of the absorbed dose is rapidly deposited in the skeleton, and most of the remainder is excreted in the urine. Fluoride levels measured in bone are proportional to dietary intake over a wide range (49). No homeostatic regulation of fluoride levels has been demonstrated in man (91). Serum and bone fluoride concentrations are in equilibrium, which means that fasting serum and urine fluoride levels provide reliable indices of previous fluoride intake (91).

The fluoride content of foods is low; the daily dietary intake of fluoride is only about 0.3 to 0.5 mg (40). Fluoridated drinking water provides an additional intake of 1 mg/day. An intake of 1 to 2 mg/day decreases the incidence

of dental caries in children but has no demonstrable effect on bone structure. It has been argued, however, that fluorine is an essential trace element and is responsible for growth and maintenance of bone and teeth (54).

The clinical manifestations of higher fluoride intake depend on dosage. A fluoride intake of 2 to 4 mg/day (achieved by drinking water that contains fluoride at 2 to 4 ppm (as may occur in some aquafers in the western United States) produces mottling of the enamel of erupting teeth (37). At 8 mg/day there is a 10% incidence of radiographically apparent osteosclerosis. Intakes of 20 to 80 mg/day (as may occur in inhabitants of the Punjab region of India and workers exposed to cryolite [Na_6AlF_3]) may produce crippling fluorosis after 10 to 20 years. This disease is characterized by dense bones, exostoses, neurologic complications due to bony overgrowth, osteoarthritis, and ligamentous calcification; however, there often is a remarkable increase in bone mass (Fig. 2), even in the absence of symptomatic fluorosis (74,83).

Three stages of fluoride effects on skeletal structure have been observed (41): (1) bone fluoridation (i.e., increased bone fluoride content without detectable changes in bone struc-

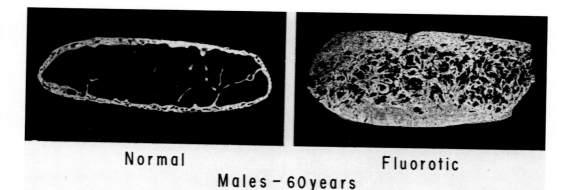

FIG. 2. Comparison of microradiographs of transverse section of ribs in a 60-year-old normal man and one from the Punjab area of India with endemic fluorosis. From *Bone and Mineral Research Annual 2* (1984) with permission from Elsevier, New York.

ture), occurring at bone fluoride contents less than 2,500 ppm; (2) bone mottling (comparable to mottling of enamel), occurring at levels between 2,500 and 5,000 ppm; and (3) bone fluorosis (gross and radiographic abnormalities), occurring at fluoride levels exceeding 5,000 ppm. Fluoride-induced bone mottling is caused by a direct effect on osteoblasts, leading to the production of an abnormal bone matrix (that calcifies abnormally or inadequately) and microscopically abnormal osteocytes. Unstained sections of mottled osteons have a brownish discoloration. Histologically, signs of acclerated bone remodeling with production of abnormal, nonlamellar bone (so-called woven bone) are present. In the cortex the outer zone of laminar bone is replaced by Haversian systems, and increased porosity due to increased numbers of resorptive canals may be seen. This may induce a compensatory addition of new periosteal woven bone. Coarsened and thickened trabeculae may give a radiographic appearance of dense trabeculation, and the abundance of nonlamellar, woven bone may produce a "pseudopagetoid" picture. At very high skeletal fluoride levels the bone assumes an osteomalacic appearance with wide osteoid seams and poorly mineralized bone (Fig. 3).

Of these various skeletal effects of fluoride, only osteosclerosis increases bone strength.

The other changes, architectural disorganization of the trabecular network, osteopenia, and impaired mineralization, will decrease bone strength and increase the risk of fracture. Therefore, fluoride must be administered under careful control to maximize the osteosclerotic component and minimize the other undesirable effects.

Mechanism of Action of Fluoride

Effects on Bone Resorption

Some evidence suggests that fluoride may affect bone resorption. *In vitro*, fluoride decreases the solubility of bone mineral (17), and fluoride pretreatment decreases the bone resorption induced by parathyroid hormone (28). Baylink et al. (5,6) reported increased resorptive activity in endosteal areas of bone formed prior to initiation of fluoride therapy. Whether these phenomena can be ascribed to direct cellular effects of fluoride on the skeleton or to secondary hyperparathyroidism is still unknown. The long-term effects of fluoride on bone resorption seem to be different. In osteoporotics treated with fluoride for 2 to 5 years, a decrease in bone resorptive activity has been demonstrated by calcium kinetic and histomorphometric methods (11,20).

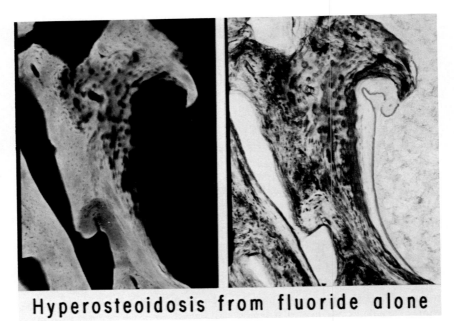

Hyperosteoidosis from fluoride alone

FIG. 3. One-hundred micron section of bone from a patient receiving fluoride alone. Left panel shows microradiograph. New bone formed during fluoride therapy is recognized by area of low mineral density with irregular mineralization (woven bone). Right panel shows transillumination of section displaying thick osteoid seams.

Fluorine substitutes isomorphically for hydroxyl in the crystal lattice of the apatite in bone, forming fluorohydroxyapatite (17). This substitution increases bone crystallinity and decreases solubility and chemical reactivity of bone crystals leading to a more stable mineral system. Changes in apatite crystallinity could explain the inhibition of bone resorption seen after fluoride treatment. Whether fluoride also acts via direct effects on osteoclasts is unknown. High levels of fluoride liberated from fluoride-containing bone during the resorptive process, however, might inhibit osteoclastic activity and explain the discrepancy between the acute and chronic therapeutic effects (17).

Effects on Bone Formation

Both indirect and direct cellular mechanisms have been suggested as explanations for the observed increase in bone formation during chronic fluoride administration. Bone cells are responsive to changes in electrical currents in their environment (22). Bone crystals may act as transducers for mechanical stress, generating piezo-electric currents in bone that may affect osteoblast activity (3). The increased rigidity of crystalline fluorohydroxyapatite might enhance these piezoelectric currents. This could explain the more pronounced effect of fluoride on the weight-bearing axial skeleton (vertebral column and *os ilium*) than on non-weight-bearing bones such as the radius. Farley et al. (21) demonstrated direct effects of fluoride on osteoblast-like cells *in vitro:* at concentrations of fluoride in the media comparable to therapeutic levels in humans, there was increased proliferation and differentiation of bone cells.

A positive balance between resorption and formation, demonstrated by calcium balance and calcium-kinetic analysis of bone turnover, has been found after 2 to 4 years of fluoride treatment. The positive balance is attributable to a decrease in resorption rate with a concomitant increase in bone formation rate (11).

Historical Background

Prompted by studies showing lower prevalence of osteoporosis in areas with moderately high fluoride levels in the drinking water (9,51), Rich et al. started to treat osteoporotic patients with fluoride (66,67) on the rationale that induction of subclinical fluorosis would strengthen the skeleton without causing other problems. They found that such treatment increased calcium retention. Several studies were conducted to test fluoride treatment of primary osteoporosis (Table 1). However, in a histologic study in 1967, Baylink and Bernstein (6) demonstrated that the increased formation was followed by an increase in resorption, excessive osteoid formation, and poor mineralization of newly formed bone. These adverse findings led to a waning of interest in the use of fluoride for the treatment of osteoporosis.

Subsequent studies at the Mayo Clinic in the 1970s, however, showed that the initial unfavorable results could be controlled by three factors: 1) duration of treatment before evaluation; 2) use of calcium supplements; and 3) dosage of sodium fluoride administered (45). Rich et al. (66,67) demonstrated that there was little effect on calcium retention in the initial months after start of fluoride therapy. This led to the premature conclusion that there was limited benefit. But after 12 to 18 months of treatment, increases in bone mass were detected (44). Moreover, optimization of fluoride dosage (44) and the use of calcium supplements (35,44) led to improved results and a decrease in histopathologic changes in bone. Resolution of the initial problems with fluoride therapy has led to its extensive use in osteoporosis during the last decade.

Although sodium fluoride therapy for osteoporotic patients has been authorized by regulatory bodies in several European countries, it has not been approved for clinical use in the United States. The Food and Drug Administration approval awaits the outcome of two ongoing large, controlled studies (at the Mayo Clinic and at the Henry Ford Hospital). Until then, sodium fluoride use in American patients with osteoporosis should be restricted to clinical investigation.

Treatment Regimens

Dosage of Sodium Fluoride

In previous studies the dosages ranged from 18 to 200 mg/day (2.2 mg of sodium fluoride is equivalent to 1 mg of fluoride ion). Jowsey et al. (44) (Fig. 4) demonstrated that the extent of bone formation surfaces in iliac crest bone biopsy samples increased in proportion to fluoride dosage, over the range of 30 to 90 mg/day ($r = 0.72$; $p < 0.005$). Dosages of sodium fluoride below 50 mg/day stimulated bone formation inconsistently, whereas dosages above 80 mg/day induced formation of abnormal, woven bone and increased the incidence of side effects (44). Thus, the therapeutic window is narrow. The extent of resorptive surface correlated inversely ($r = -0.78$; $p < 0.005$) with the dosage of calcium (300 to 1,500 mg/day) received by the subjects. On the basis of these results, we recommend a sodium fluoride dosage of 60 mg/day and a daily supplement of 1,500 mg of calcium. Fluoride dosage should then be adjusted on the basis of serum fluoride values: the optimal therapeutic range is 5 to 15 μM at 24 hr after the last sodium fluoride dose (87).

Calcium and Vitamin D Supplements

Studies performed in the late 1960s and early 1970s strongly suggested that the excessive osteoid formation and incomplete mineralization of new bone seen after fluoride therapy could be diminished by giving vitamin D and calcium supplements (44,45). As assessed by macroradiography of serial bone biopsy samples, normal fully mineralized lamellar bone (formed during combined fluoride, calcium, and vitamin D therapy) was found to be superimposed on poorly mineralized bone with an abnormal, mosaic appearance (formed during therapy with fluoride alone) (45). These find-

TABLE 1. *Results of fluoride treatment of osteoporosis*

Investigators date of study	Patients studied, no.	NaF, mg/day	Supplementary therapy		Duration of therapy (month)	Major findings
			Calcium	Vitamin D[a]		
Rich and Ensinck, 1961 (66)	6	50	No	No	3–4	Ca retention in all
Rich et al., 1964 (67)	4	100–200	No	No	1–18	3 responded; mean Ca retention, + 138 mg/day
Cohen and Rubini, 1965 (13)	3	75–150	No	No	4	No change in 1; Ca retention in 2
Rose, 1965 (75)	4	100	No	No	8–10	Minimal improvement in external Ca balance in 1; no significant change in 3
Bernstein and Cohen, 1967 (8)	20	50–150	No	No	2–24	Mean change in Ca balance, + 27 mg/day
Baylink and Bernstein, 1967 (6)	20	15–200	No	No	5–15	Biopsies in 15 patients showed increased bone formation and resorption; new bone was poorly mineralized and osteoid tissue was excessive
Lukert et al., 1967 (53)	7	50–100	No	No	1	Labile Ca pool decreased; no change in other ^{45}Ca parameters or Ca balance
Jowsey et al., 1968 (45)	3	25–90	Some did	Some did	7–24	Biopsies showed increased bone formation; excessive osteoid tissue and incomplete mineralization of new bone diminished by vitamin D and Ca supplements
Jowsey and Kelly, 1968 (42)	3	25	Yes	Yes	30	Biopsies showed increased bone formation and decreased bone resorption
Spencer et al., 1969 (85)	1	25	No	No	1–2	No change in Ca absorption or external Ca balance
Merz et al., 1970 (55)	16	50—75	No	No	Varying intervals	Bone volume markedly increased on iliac biopsies
Schenk et al., 1970 (77)	16	25	No	No	1–22	Bone formation and osteoid tissue markedly increased
Thiébaud et al., 1970 (88)	13	70–150	No	No	4–10	Histologic evidence of fluorosis on bone biopsies; no change in urinary hydroxyproline excretion
Jowsey et al., 1972 (44)	11	80–90	Yes	Yes	12–18	Certain doses of NaF, vitamin D, and Ca stimulated formation of histologically normal new bone
Ryckwaert et al., 1972 (76)	14	50–80	No	No	12–31	Trabecular volume in iliac bone increased in half of the patients at 1 year and in 10 of 11 after 2 years
Haas et al., 1973 (30)	11	100	No	No	12–24	Bone formation increased as assessed by radiocalcium kinetics and bone biopsy
Inkovaara et al., 1975 (38)	237	50	No	No	6	Aged persons who had prophylactic fluoride therapy had more fractures than controls
Chlud, 1977 (12)	40	50–100	No	No	12	By clinical and radiographic criteria 2/3 of patients with involutional osteoporosis responded

TABLE 1. (*continued*)

Investigators date of study	Patients studied, no.	NaF, mg/day	Supplementary therapy		Duration of therapy (month)	Major findings
			Calcium	Vitamin D[a]		
Hauswaldt et al., 1977 (36)	14	60–80	No	No	> 48	Increases in trabecular volume in iliac bone in 8
Parsons et al., 1977 (62)	15	40	Yes	Yes	48	Increases in bone mass and radio-calcium accretion with positive Ca balance in most
Vokrouhlická et al., 1977 (89)	12	30–50	No	Yes	12–24	Of 2 who had bone biopsy, only 1 responded
Baud et al., 1978 (4)	57	60	Some did	Some did	> 12	On iliac biopsy, those receiving Ca and vitamin D had lowest frequency of mottling and highest degree of mineralization and crystallinity
Dambacher et al., 1978 (14)	56	50–100	No	No	36	Radiographic vertebral density increased but appendicular cortical bone decreased
Franke, 1978 (23)	43	20–80	No	No	12–72	About 3/4 benefitted clinically
Hansson and Roos, 1976 (31)	9	50	Yes	Yes	18–24	Significant increase in spinal bone density in 5
Olah et al., 1978 (58)	14	50–100	No	Yes	< 52	Biopsy showed increase in bone mass; vitamin D did not prevent mineralization defect
Reutter and Olah, 1978 (65)	27	80–120	No	No	36	Increase in iliac trabecular bone mass and suggestion of decreased fracture rate
Ringe et al., 1978 (73)	23	65	No	No	25	Increased iliac trabecular bone mass but bone mass of radius decreased by densitometry
Vose et al., 1978 (90)	45[b]	50	Yes	No	48	Subjects receiving NaF had increase in density of phalanx and fewer hip fractures
Riggs et al., 1980 (71)	36	40–65	Yes	Some did	48–72	1/3 had increased spinal bone mass on radiographs and decreased fracture incidence
Briancon and Meunier, 1981 (10)	74	50	Yes	Yes	24	Most had histologic evidence of increased bone formation and trabecular bone volume; only 8 had mineralization impairment
Harrison et al., 1981 (33)	16	50	Yes	Yes	36	Response assessed by neutron activation analysis of torso variable (− 10.5% to + 21%); subgroup that also received estrogen had best response
Aloia et al., 1982 (1)	18	45	Yes	No	21	Patients also received estrogen; significant increase in total body Ca with time
Riggs et al., 1982 (72)	61	40–60	Yes	Some did	48–72	Decrease in vertebral fracture rate compared with controls; effects of estrogen and fluoride were additive
Kuntz et al., 1984 (47)	19	50	No	Some did	12–58	In fluoride-treated group, trabecular bone volume increased but metacarpal indices and Ca content of hand unchanged; 25-OH-D supplementation did not prevent mineralization defect

TABLE 1. (*continued*)

Investigators date of study	Patients studied, no.	NaF, mg/day	Supplementary therapy		Duration of therapy (month)	Major findings
			Calcium	Vitamin D[a]		
Lane et al. 1984 (48)	10	40–70	Yes	Yes	23–64	Fracture rate down from 1.25 per patient-year to 0.33 after 18 months of therapy
Charles et al., 1985 (11)	20	40–60	Yes	Yes	12–24	Positive Ca balance achieved; vitamin D supplementation increased Ca absorption
Eriksen et al., 1985 (20)	24	40–60	Yes	Yes	60	Positive trabecular bone balance and significant increase in trabecular bone volume achieved; vitamin D and Ca supplementation did not prevent mineralization deficit in 21
Power and Gay 1986 (63)	24	40–60	Yes	Yes	5–7	Fracture incidence decreased only in 8 with radiologic signs of fluorosis

[a]Pharmacologic dosage.

[b]In this clinical trial in elderly inmates of a home for the mentally retarded, controls received placebo, oxymetholone, or phosphate treatment.

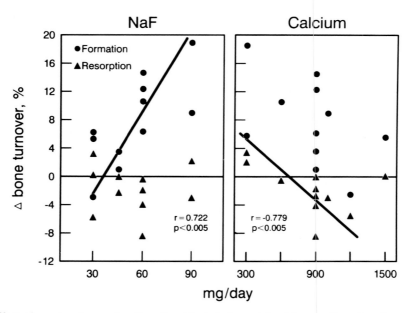

FIG. 4. Effect of varying doses of sodium fluoride and elemental calcium on bone forming and resorbing surfaces as assessed by microradiography of iliac crest biopsies. Incremental change in bone surfaces assessed by comparing baseline and one-year bone biopsy samples. Note that stimulation of bone-forming surfaces was dose related. Dosages of less than 45 mg of sodium fluoride daily failed to produce a uniform stimulation, whereas dosages of 90 mg daily produced bone of abnormal structure. Bone-resorbing surfaces were inversely related to the dosage of supplemental elementary calcium. Data redrawn from Jowsey et al. (1972) as redrawn by Riggs. From *Bone and Mineral Research Annual 2* (1984) with permission from Elsevier, New York.

ings were corroborated subsequently by Baud et al. (4). Calcium supplementation also decreases bone resorptive activity by as yet unknown mechanisms (35,44,52) (Fig. 4). It had been proposed that the increase in bone resorption after therapy with fluoride alone may be caused by secondary hyperparathyroidism induced by an accelerated demand for calcium as a result of accelerated bone formation (5). However, direct effects of fluoride on osteoclasts also may play a role.

The fluoride-induced mineralization defect and the beneficial effects of calcium and vitamin D supplementation have to be related to the duration of therapy. In the early studies (4,45) that found beneficial effects of calcium and vitamin D supplementation, treatment periods were less than 2 years. Briancon and Meunier (10) found that only 8 of 74 patients had mineralization defects when studied histologically after 2 to 3 years of treatment. By contrast, in histologic studies after 4 to 5 years of treatment, most patients had mineralization defects despite calcium and vitamin D administration. After 52 and 60 months of therapy, respectively, Olah et al. (58) and Eriksen et al. (20) demonstrated a pronounced mineralization defect in the majority of patients treated with sodium fluoride, calcium, and vitamin D.

In the Eriksen et al. study, a new technique was used that provides a three-dimensional reconstruction of the total remodeling sequence; there was no significant change in final resorption depth between pre- and posttreatment biopsy samples. However, the resorption rate was 50% lower in the posttreatment biopsy samples. Thus, the treatment regimen removed the activity of resorptive cells, but the final result of bone resorption, i.e., the final depth of the lacuna, was unchanged. The bone formation period was prolonged from 302 days to 1,020 days in the posttreatment biopsies. The mineralization lag time (an index describing the time from initiation of bone matrix synthesis to mineralization of the matrix), normally about 20 days, was prolonged to 108 days in the posttreatment biopsies, which indicates the presence of a mineralization defect. Moreover, a decrease in osteoblastic matrix synthesis

could be demonstrated. Despite the inhibition of bone formation, however, a positive balance between resorption and formation and an increase in trabecular bone volume were demonstrated.

The cause of the fluoride-induced mineralization defect is unknown. The severity of the mineralization defect seems to increase with increased dose. At 60 mg of sodium fluoride per day, tetracycline labels in bone were sharp and uniform but at 90 mg/day the newly formed bone failed to fix tetracycline label (44).

The mechanism by which fluoride inhibits bone mineralization and calcium ameliorates this abnormality have not been established. The $Ca \times PO_4$ product in serum is unchanged during fluoride therapy, and serum levels of 25-hydroxyvitamin D are normal. Fluoride does not seem to be a crystal poison either; on the contrary, it enhances crystal growth (17). After they incorporate, fluoride apatite crystals are larger (there is increased thickness, but the length is the same). This structural change in bone crystals might affect their binding to organic matrix constituents (17). Johnson (41) hypothesized that the osteoid tissue formed during fluoride therapy does not calcify normally. Furthermore, fluoride increases the bone matrix content of dermatan sulfate, a mineralization inhibitor (86). Using subcutaneous implanted endochondreal bone in rats, Eanes and Reddi (17) found delayed uptake of ^{45}Ca in fluoride-treated animals. On the basis of histologic and biochemical data, they concluded that the mineralization defect was caused by retarded matrix development, leading to a decreased number of matrix sites for crystal nucleation.

The rationale for the use of vitamin D is to increase intestinal calcium absorption and thus increase bone mineralization. Indeed, a recent study of calcium kinetics has demonstrated an increased intestinal absorption of calcium after treatment with calcium, fluoride, and vitamin D for 2 years (11).

The studies on side effects after vitamin D supplementation are still conflicting. In a group of 163 patients with a mean observation time of 2.8 years (total, 460 patient-years), Hasling et al. (34) did not find one case of persistent or symptomatic hypercalcemia. Urinary excretion of calcium was unchanged, and no case of kidney stones developed. During the treatment period, the mean serum calcium for the entire group decreased, in agreement with the findings of Parsons et al. (62). However, other studies have found more hypercalcemia and hypercalciuria in patients treated with vitamin D plus calcium, compared with patients treated with calcium alone (71). Kuntz et al. (47) could not demonstrate that addition of 25-hydroxyvitamin D_3 decreased the extent of the fluoride-induced mineralization defect. Moreover, a Mayo Clinic study was unable to demonstrate any further decrease in fracture incidence when vitamin D was added to a fluoride treatment regimen (71). Therefore, it is questionable whether addition of vitamin D to the regimen is beneficial.

Intermittent or Continuous Treatment

In an attempt to decrease the mineralization defect and the frequency of side-effects, various types of cyclic fluoride regimens have been suggested. Pulse doses of fluoride over a period of weeks or months theoretically should increase osteoblast number without significantly increasing bone resorptive activity. After a certain period of time (e.g., 1 formative period) a new pulse could be given. This regimen might decrease the risk of fluoride-induced mineralization defects and the incidence of side-effects because fluoride levels in serum would be increased only for short periods. Thus, as a result of maximal effects on mitogenesis and increased mineralization of bone matrix, one might expect reversals of the negative bone balance in osteoporotics to be even more pronounced than those found with continuous-treatment regimens.

AVAILABLE FORMS OF SODIUM FLUORIDE

In the United States, sodium fluoride is only available in low-potency (2 to 5 mg) tablets.

Combination with calcium carbonate has been shown to decrease the irritant effect of fluoride on the gastric mucosa. The beneficial effect has been attributed to calcium carbonate serving as an antacid. Due to increased fluoride absorption in the presence of increased calcium ion in the intestine, concomitant administration of calcium and fluoride requires that fluoride dosage be increased by approximately 25% to achieve the same net fluoride absorption (43).

Slow-release capsules have also been introduced in order to minimize gastrointestinal side effects. In a recent study, Pak et al. (59) found a substantial reduction in side-effects. In 101 patients treated over a median period of 2 years, the incidence of gastrointestinal symptoms was 6% and the incidence of lower extremity of pain was 8%. However, this form is not yet available for use in the United States.

Side-Effects

Symptomatic skeletal fluorosis has not occurred after fluoride treatment for up to 6 years. The doses of fluoride administered therapeutically to osteoporotic patients, however, have been within the lower range of the dosage that Hodge (37) estimated would lead to skeletal fluorosis after 10 years of ingestion. But side-effects have occurred in 30% to 50% of treated patients in several large series. The two main types, periarticular and gastrointestinal side-effects, affected a mean of 34.6 and 20.5% of treated patients, respectively (Table 2).

A lower extremity pain syndrome, consisting of periarticular or foot pain and occasionally tenderness around the large joints, has been described. These symptoms always disappear within several weeks after discontinuation of treatment. They may recur again (in half of the patients) after therapy is reinstituted at a lower fluoride dosage. The underlying mechanism is still subject to speculation. Scintigraphic findings suggest the possibility of a chemical periostitis at sites of skeletal pain (81). In Mayo Clinic patients, no evidence of chemical synovitis or synovial effusions was found (57,71). A recent study (78) demonstrated that radiographs taken within 2 weeks

TABLE 2. *Incidence of side-effects of fluoride therapy for osteoporosis*

Authors	Incidence[a]	
	Gastrointestinal	Periarticular
Ryckwaert et al. (76)	3/14	—
Chlud (12)	6/40	5/40
Baud et al. (4)	14/57	—
Dambacher et al. (14)	—	33/56
Franke (23)	—	15/43
Reutter and Olah (65)	2/27	12/27
Ringe et al. (73)	2/23	11/23
Briancon and Meunier (10)	16/74	24/74
Harrison et al. (33)	1/16	3/16
Riggs et al. (71)	14/61	10/61
Aloia et al. (1)	3/18	—
Hasling et al. (34)	40/163	61/163
Total	101/493 (20.5%)	174/503 (34.6%)

[a]Expressed as number of subjects with symtoms/number of patients studied. These are listed only if the report had a specific comment on presence or absence of symptoms.

after onset of articular symptoms invariably were negative. However, when new radiographs were taken 4 weeks after onset of symptoms, changes suggestive of healing stress fractures could be demonstrated at sites displaying increased uptake on bone scans. O'Duffy et al. (57) performed ^{99m}Tc hydroxymethylene diphosphonate scintigraphy in 11 osteoporotic women in whom periarticular pain developed and in 12 nonsymptomatic osteoporotics on fluoride and calcium. The women with periarticular pain showed an increased number of foci of abnormal uptake, and in five of them radiography revealed stress fractures. The authors concluded that the periarticular pain resulted from intense regional bone turnover which may be complicated by stress microfractures (Fig. 5).

Schnitzler (78,79) reported that lower extremity stress fractures occurred in all of eight patients who had acute lower extremity pain syndrome while they were on fluoride treatment. Schulz et al. (80) found new periosteal and endosteal bone growth in 67% of fluoride-treated osteoporotics with periarticular pain although they failed to detect stress fractures. The incidence of the lower extremity pain syndrome increases with increased serum fluoride levels (87). Although it has been suggested

that very large increases in serum alkaline phosphatase might herald increased occurrence of pain syndromes (7,46), another group was unable to demonstrate any correlation between alkaline phosphatase responses over the first two years of fluoride therapy and the incidence of skeletal pain (34).

Gastrointestinal symptoms are mainly due to irritation of the gastric mucosa. This irritation produces epigastric pain, nausea, vomiting, and, occasionally, iron-deficiency anemia due to gastrointestinal bleeding from superficial mucosal ulceration. A few cases of ulceration and hematemesis have been reported (34). These side-effects are thought to be elicited by a direct irritating effect of fluoride ion on the gastric mucosa or by the formation of hydrofluoric acid. The frequency of gastric side-effects can be reduced by concomitant administration of calcium carbonate with the sodium fluoride or by administration of the fluoride with meals.

Other side-effects occur more rarely; occasionally there is loss of hair or growth of small bone spurs. Even more unusual are toxic effects such as optic neuritis (26), peripheral neuritis (23,71), degenerative diseases of the central nervous system (71), and the presence of giant cells in bone marrow (15). These isolated occurrences may be coincidences. Hasling et al. (34) reported small but significant decreases in serum levels of coagulation factors in the absence of liver dysfunction. No adverse effects on thyroid or renal function could be demonstrated.

It was found that 40% of side-effects occurred during the first year, 14% during the second year, and 12% during the third and final year of the study. Thus, the accumulation of fluoride in the skeleton does not appear to increase the incidence of side effects. Over a 5-year period, only 5% to 10% of patients had to discontinue treatment because of side-effects.

Chronic renal failure and osteomalacia are contraindications to fluoride therapy. Because the kidney is the main route of fluoride excretion, renal failure may lead to toxic accumulation of fluoride. In azotemic patients treated

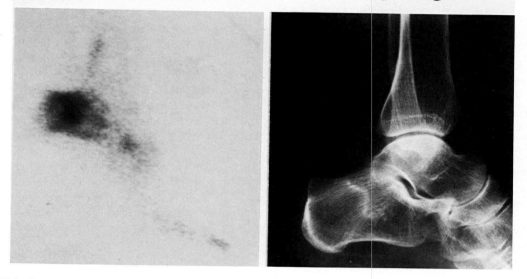

FIG. 5. Findings in a 62-year-old woman treated with 75 mg of sodium fluoride daily for 18 months. Patient developed acute pain in the heel. Isotope scintigram showed localized uptake, and a radiograph of the foot taken four weeks after onset of pain showed a typical stress fracture. From Eastell et al. in *Clinics in Obstetrics and Gynecology* with permission from W.B. Saunders Company, Philadelphia, Pennsylvania.

with fluoride, severe fluorosis with bilateral hip fractures has been reported (27). Osteomalacia may be aggravated by fluoride-induced inhibition of mineralization. Previous hip fracture may constitute a relative contraindication.

EFFECTS ON BONE MASS

Effects on Trabecular and Cortical Bone

Studies on iliac crest bone have demonstrated that fluoride therapy substantially increases trabecular bone of the axial skeleton, at times into the normal range (14,31,62,71). Dual-photon absorptiometric studies have demonstrated increases of 1% per month in bone mineral content of the spine after 18 to 24 months of therapy (31).

These dramatic effects on trabecular bone are not accompanied by increases in the predominantly cortical bone of the appendicular skeleton. On the contrary, fluoride therapy may decrease cortical bone mass. Bone remodeling in cortical bone increases during fluoride treatment (88) but the positive balance achieved in trabecular bone does not occur. Resorption and formation seem to be in relative balance, but the increased bone turnover leads to increased porosity of cortical bone. Bang et al. (2) reported an increase in trabecular bone in 43 men who had industrial fluorosis, but this increase was accompanied by a 2.5-fold increase in cortical bone porosity. Single-photon absorptiometric studies by Ringe et al. (73), Dambacher et al. (14), and Riggs (69) showed a significant decrease in bone mineral density in the radius. Dambacher et al. (14) found significant decreases in metacarpal and diaphyseal cortex thickness in fluoride-treated patients, but Lane et al. (48) were unable to demonstrate any changes in clinical thickness in iliac crest bone biopsy specimens after fluoride therapy.

These differences in responses of cortical and trabecular bone to fluoride therapy raise a question as to whether the bone is redistributed from the cortex, e.g., from the hip to the vertebrae. This could lead to an increased incidence of hip fractures in fluoride-treated patients. Indeed, in a randomized series of elderly patients treated with either placebo or sodium fluoride (50 mg/day) for 6 months, the fluoride-treated group had a significantly higher incidence of hip fractures (38). Gutteridge et al. (29) reported that 5 of 16 patients undergoing treatment with sodium fluoride, calcium, and vitamin D had a total of 11 femoral fractures over an observation period of 4 years; no fractures occurred in a control group observed for 3 years. However, these findings were contradicted by a recent multicenter study (70) on the occurrence of hip fractures in which 418 fluoride-treated osteoporotics observed for more than 1,000 patient years were compared with 120 osteoporotics who had been followed prospectively for 3 years prior to initiation of fluoride therapy. No significant difference could be demonstrated between the incidences of hip fractures in the two groups (1.6 and 1.8%, respectively). The expected incidence of hip fracture in nonosteoporotic women of the same age in the general community was found to be 0.5%. Thus, untreated osteoporotics were at greater risk for hip fractures but fluoride treatment did not appear to add to this risk. Power and Gay (63) also found no relationship between hip fracture and fluoride treatment. Finally, in a recent study in Finland, Simonen and Laitinen (82) found that fluoridation of drinking water in one community (1 mg/liter) led to a significantly lower incidence of hip fractures compared with communities with only trace amounts of fluoride in the water.

Because of the seriousness of hip fractures, the question of increased risk for hip fracture in fluoride-treated patients is a key issue in assessing the risks and benefits of sodium fluoride treatment. Prospective studies evaluating changes in bone mineral density of the hip and fracture risk are currently under way.

Antifracture Efficacy

Fluoride-containing bone has increased crystallinity and decreased elasticity (92). Therefore, increased bone mass may not necessarily signify decreased fracture risk. Studies in experimental animals have shown variable effects of fluoride on bone strength; both increased strength (68) and decreased bone strength (92) have been reported.

There have been a few studies of the occurrence of vertebral fractures in osteoporotic patients during fluoride therapy. In a three-year randomized study of patients with multiple myeloma, Harley et al. (32) found similar incidences of vertebral fracture in the placebo group and in the two groups receiving sodium fluoride, 25 or 200 mg/day. Briancon and Meunier (10) reported new vertebral fractures in 9 of 26 patients on sodium fluoride, calcium, and vitamin D compared with 11 of 16 in a previously reported series of patients treated with a homeopathic dose of calcitonin. Riggs et al. (72) reported the occurrence of new vertebral fractures in patients undergoing five different treatment regimens who were chosen according to identical entry criteria and then followed prospectively for up to 4 years; the groups were comparable in age and number of vertebral fractures at entry. Compared with no treatment, treatment with calcium decreased the fracture rate to 50% while treatment with calcium + fluoride or calcium + estrogen decreased the fracture rate to 25%. Treatment with all three agents (calcium, fluoride, and estogen) decreased the fracture rate to 10% of the rate seen in untreated osteoporotics (Fig. 6).

The even more profound effect of fluoride together with estrogen and calcium can be ascribed to the synergistic stimulatory effects of fluoride on bone formation and the inhibitory effects of estrogen on bone resorption. Addition of vitamin D to the therapeutic regimens containing fluoride either failed to decrease the fracture rate further or decreased it only marginally.

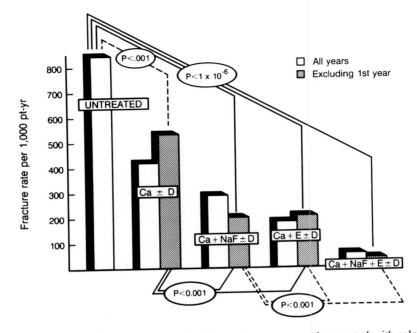

FIG. 6.   Rates of vertebral fracture in groups of patients who are untreated or treated with calcium supplements, calcium supplements plus sodium fluoride, calcium supplements plus estrogen, or calcium supplements plus sodium fluoride plus estrogen. Some of the patients also received pharmacologic doses of vitamin D. Analysis of covariants, however, failed to show a difference between those receiving vitamin D and those that were not. Data are given both for all years of treatment or excluding the first year of treatment, as sodium fluoride requires at least one year to increase bone mass. Data are from Riggs et al. (1982) with permission from the Massachusetts Medical Society.

In a group of 10 osteoporotics, Lane et al. (48) found a reduction in fracture rate from 1.25/patient year before treatment to 0.33/patient year after 18 months of treatment. Thereafter, no further fractures occurred. Over a mean follow-up period of 55 months, the mean fracture rate was only 0.11/patient year.

Power and Gay (63) recently reported that fracture incidence decreased only in the 8 of 24 fluoride-treatment patients in whom radiographic fluorosis developed; moreover, these 8 patients were younger and closer to menopause than the 16 patients without radiographic fluorosis.

DIFFERENCES IN INDIVIDUAL RESPONSIVENESS

Several recent studies indicate that responsiveness of bone to fluoride shows profound variability among individuals. Riggs et al. (72) found that 15 of 27 patients with postmenopausal osteoporosis had a radiographically apparent increase in trabecular bone mass (i.e., increased trabecular thickening). New vertebral fractures occurred only 1/6th as frequently in these patients as in the remainder. Briancon and Meunier (10) found that trabecular bone volume doubled for their group of 28 patients as a whole but there was a subgroup of 7 of these patients in whom there was no increase in trabecular bone volume. They speculated that patients with very low bone volumes had the highest risk of being nonresponders.

Lane et al. (48) found no correlation between initial osteoid characteristics and response to treatment. However, relative increases in trabecular bone volume and trabecular width correlated inversely with initial trabecular volume and width. This indicates that, contrary to the hypothesis of Meunier et al. (56), patients with low bone mass respond better than patients with high bone mass.

Eriksen et al. (20) reported that 4 of 24 patients on a regimen of fluoride, calcium, and vitamin D_2 had no increase in trabecular bone volume over a 5-year treatment period. In a study using serial determination of alkaline phosphatase levels in patients, Ivey et al. (39) found that 42% had an excellent response, with a quick and persistent increase in alkaline phosphatase activity; 32% had an intermediate response with a slow, gradual increase within the normal range; and 21% did not respond or responded only minimally. Thus, about 25% of patients undergoing treatment with fluoride fail to have an adequate therapeutic response. However, at present, no criterion on which selection of responders can be based has been devised.

The cause or causes of the individual variability in response to fluoride is not well understood. The amount of bone present prior to initiation of treatment is not a major factor. In the Mayo Clinic study, no differences between responders and nonresponders could be demonstrated in terms of severity of osteoporosis or number of vertebral fractures (72). The bioavailability of fluoride also was not a determinant of responsiveness in that study because responders and nonresponders received similar mean cumulative doses of sodium fluoride and had similar mean serum fluoride concentrations during therapy.

It has been claimed that poor response in serum alkaline phosphatase activity might identify the patients with poor response in therapy (7), but in other studies no difference was demonstrated (34). Preliminary data from our ongoing fluoride study indicate that patient compliance may be an important determinant of nonresponsiveness.

ROLE OF FLUORIDE IN THE TREATMENT OF OSTEOPOROSIS

The mitogenic effects of fluoride make it a useful agent for the treatment of osteoporotic patients with low bone turnover in whom the main objective of treatment is to increase bone turnover in order to induce formation of new trabecular structures. In patients with high bone turnover, the mitogenic effect probably will be less important, but the patient might still benefit from the creation of the positive balance between resorption and formation that has been demonstrated in patients on fluoride therapy. High bone turnover increases the risk of performative resorption and thus the risk for disintegration of the trabecular network (see Chapter 2, *this volume*). Therefore, further increase in bone turnover due to ingestion of fluoride might have deleterious effects on trabecular architecture. These effects have not been demonstrated in practice.

Further clinical trials on the effects of fluoride in combination with antiresorptive agents such as estrogen, calcitonin, and diphosphonates should be performed. Estrogen seems to enhance the antifracture efficacy of fluoride (72), but in patients with low turnover this agent probably would be of little value. Calcitonin also might potentiate the positive effects of fluoride by virtue of its inhibitory action on osteoclasts. Certain diphosphonate analogs in higher doses create mineralization defects. Therefore, one might hesitate to use these agents in combination with fluorides. Whether these theoretical objections have any bearing in clinical practice remains to be established.

REFERENCES

1. Aloia, J.F., Zanzi, I., Vaswani, A., Ellis, K., and Cohn, S.H. (1982): Combination therapy for osteoporosis with estrogen, fluoride, and calcium. *J. Am. Geriatr. Soc.,* 30:13–17.
2. Bang, S., Baud, C.A., Boivin, G., Demeurisse, C., Gössi, M., Tochon-Danguy, H.J., and Very, J.M. (1978): Morphometric and biophysical study of bone tissue in industrial fluorosis. In: *Fluoride and Bone,* edited by B. Courvoisier, A. Donath, and C.A. Baud, pp. 168–175. Hans Huber Publishers, Bern, Switzerland.
3. Bassett, C.A.L. (1968): Biologic significance of piezoelectricity. *Calcif. Tissue Res.,* 1:252–272.
4. Baud, C.A., Lagier, R., Bang, S., Boivin, G., Gössi, M., and Tochon-Danguy, H.J. (1978): Treatment of osteoporosis with NaF, calcium or/and phosphorus, and vitamin D: histological, morphometric and biophysical study of the bone tissue. In: *Fluoride and Bone,* edited by B. Courvoisier, A. Donath, and C.A. Baud, pp. 290–292. Hans Huber Publishers, Bern, Switzerland.

5. Baylink, D., Wergedal, J., Stauffer, M., and Rich, C. (1970): Effects of fluoride on bone formation, mineralization, and resorption in the rat. In: *Fluoride and Medicine*, edited by T.L. Vischer, pp. 37–69. Hans Huber Publishers, Bern, Switzerland.

6. Baylink, D.J., and Bernstein, D.S. (1967): The effects of fluoride therapy on metabolic bone disease: a histologic study. *Clin. Orthop.*, 55:51–85.

7. Baylink, D.J., Duane, P.B., Farley, S.M., and Farley, J.R. (1983): Monofluorophosphate physiology: the effects of fluoride on bone. *Caries Res.*, 17 (Suppl. 1):56–76.

8. Bernstein, D.S., and Cohen, P. (1967): Use of sodium fluoride in the treatment of osteoporosis. *J. Clin. Endocrinol. Metab.*, 27:197–210.

9. Bernstein, D.S., Sadowsky, N., Hegsted, D.M., Guri, C.D., and Stare, F.J. (1966): Prevalence of osteoporosis in high- and low-fluoride areas in North Dakota. *J.A.M.A.*, 198:499–504.

10. Briancon, D., and Meunier, P.J. (July 1981): Treatment of osteoporosis with fluoride, calcium, and vitamin D. *Orthop. Clin. North Am.*, 12:629–648.

11. Charles, P., Mosekilde, L., and Taagehøj Jensen, F. (1985): The effects of sodium fluoride, calcium phosphate, and vitamin D_2 for one to two years on calcium and phosphorus metabolism in postmenopausal women with spinal crush fracture osteoporosis. *Bone*, 6:201–206.

12. Chlud, K. (1977): Zur Behandlung der Osteoporose mit einem protrahiert wirksamen Natrium-Fluorid-Präparat. *Z. Rheumatol.*, 36:126–139.

13. Cohen, M.B. and Rubini, M.E. (1965): The treatment of osteoporosis with sodium fluoride. *Clin. Orthop.*, 40:147–152.

14. Dambacher, M.A., Lauffenburger, Th., Lämmle, B., and Haas, H.G. (1978): Long term effects of sodium fluoride in osteoporosis. In: *Fluoride and Bone*, edited by B. Courvoisier, A. Donath, and C.A. Baud, pp. 238–241. Hans Huber Publishers, Bern, Switzerland.

15. Duffey, P.H., Tretbar, H.C., and Jarkowski, T.L. (1971): Giant cells in bone marrows of patients on high-dose fluoride treatment. *Ann. Intern. Med.*, 75:745–747.

16. Dustin, J.-P. (1970): Monitoring of fluoride dosage during treatment of bone disease. In: *Fluoride in Medicine*, edited by T.L. Vischer, pp. 178–189. Hans Huber Publishers, Bern, Switzerland.

17. Eanes, E.D., and Reddi, A.H. (1979): The effect of fluoride on bone mineral apatite. *Metab. Bone Dis. Rel. Res.*, 2:3–10.

18. Eriksen, E.F., Gundersen, H.J., Melsen, F., and Mosekilde, L. (1984): Reconstruction of the formative site in iliac trabecular bone in 20 normal individuals employing a kinetic model for matrix and mineral apposition. *Metab. Bone Dis. Rel. Res.*, 5:243–252.

19. Erikson, E.F., Melsen, F., and Mosekilde, L. (1984): Reconstruction of the resorptive site in iliac trabecular bone: a kinetic model for bone resorption in 20 normal individuals. *Metab. Bone Dis. Rel. Res.*, 5:235–242.

20. Eriksen, E.F., Mosekilde, L., and Melsen, F. (1985): Effect of sodium fluoride, calcium, phosphate, and vitamin D_2 on trabecular bone balance and remodeling in osteoporotics. *Bone*, 6:381–389.

21. Farley, J.R., Wergedal, J.E., and Baylink, D.J. (1983): Fluoride directly stimulates proliferation and alkaline phosphatase activity of bone-forming cells. *Science*, 222:330–332.

22. Fitzsimmons, R., Farley, J.R., Adey, R.A., and Baylink, D.J. (1986): Evidence that action of electric field (EF) exposure to increased bone cell proliferation in vitro is selective for alkaline phosphatase (ALP) rich cells and dependent on mitogenic activity release. *J. Bone Mineral Res.*, S1, (Abstr.) 157.

23. Franke, J. (1978): Our experience in the treatment of osteoporosis with relatively low sodium-fluoride doses. In: *Fluoride and Bone*, edited by B. Courvoisier, A. Donath, and C.A. Baud, pp. 256—262. Hans Huber Publishers, Bern, Switzerland.

24. Frost, H.M. (1969): Tetracycline-based histological analysis of bone remodeling (editorial). *Calcif. Tissue Res.*, 3:211–237.

25. Frost, H.M. (1979): Treatment of osteoporoses by manipulation of coherent bone cell populations. *Clin. Orthop.*, 143:227–244.

26. Geall, M.G., and Beilin, L.J. (1964): Sodium fluoride and optic neuritis. *Br. Med. J.*, 2:355–356.

27. Gerster, J.C., Charhon, S.A., Jaeger, P., Boivin, G., Briancon, D., Rostan, A., Baud, C.A., and Meunier, P.J. (1983): Bilateral fractures of femoral neck in patients with moderate renal failure receiving fluoride for spinal osteoporosis. *Br. Med. J.*, 287:723–725.

28. Goldhaber, P. (1967): The inhibition of bone resorption in tissue culture by nontoxic concentrations of sodium fluoride. *Isr. J. Med. Sci.*, 3:617–626.

29. Gutteridge, D.H., Price, R.I., Nicholson, G.C., Kent, G.N., Retallack, R.W., Devlin, R.D., Worth, G.K., Glancy, J.J., Michell, P., and Gruber, H. (1984): Fluoride in osteoporotic vertebral fractures—trabecular increase, vertebral protection, femoral fractures. In: *Osteoporosis*, edited by C. Christiansen, C.D., Arnaud, B.E.C. Nordin, A.M. Parfitt, W.A. Peck, and B.L. Riggs, Jr., pp. 705–707. Aalborg Stiftsbogtrykkeri, Glostrup, Denmark.

30. Haas, H.G., Lauffenburger, Th., Guncaga, J., Lentner, Ch., Olah, A.J., and Dambacher, M.A. (1973): Bone turnover in osteoporosis, studied with sodium fluoride (abstract). *Eur. J. Clin. Invest.*, 3:235.

31. Hansson, T., and Roos, B. (1976): Osteoporoses: effect of combined therapy with sodium fluoride, calcium, and vitamin D on the lumbar spine in osteoporosis. *Am. J. Roentgenol.*, 126:1294–1296.

32. Harley, J.B. (Chairman), Schilling, A., and Glidewell, O. (Acute Leukemia Group B and Eastern Cooperative Oncology Group) (1972): Ineffectiveness of fluoride therapy in multiple myeloma. *N. Engl. J. Med.*, 286:1283–1288.

33. Harrison, J.E., McNeill, K.G., Sturtridge, W.C., Bayley, T.A., Murray, T.M., Williams, C., Tam, C., and Fornasier, V. (1981): Three-year changes in bone mineral mass of postmenopausal osteoporotic patients based on neutron activation analysis of the central third of the skeleton. *J. Clin. Endocrinol. Metab.*, 52:751–758.

34. Hasling, C., Nielsen, H.E., Melsen, F., and Mose-

kilde, L. (1987): The safety of osteoporosis treatment with sodium fluoride, calcium phosphate and vitamin D. *Miner. Electrolyte Metab.* (in press).

35. Hauck, H.M., Steenbock, H., and Parsons, H.T. (1933): The effect of the level of calcium intake on the calcification of bones and teeth during fluorine toxicosis. *Am. J. Physiol.*, 103:489–493.

36. Hauswaldt, Ch., Fuchs, Ch., Hesch, R.-D., Köbberling, J., and Unger, K.-O. (1977): Histomorphometrische Untersuchungen und Beckenkamm-Biopsien bei Fluorid-Langzeittherapie der Osteoporose. *Dtsch. Med. Wochenschr.*, 102:1177–1180.

37. Hodge, H.C. (1960): Notes on the effects of fluoride deposition on body tissues. *Arch. Industrial Health*, 21:350–352.

38. Inkovaara, J., Heikinheimo, R., Jarvinen, K., Kasurinen, U., Hanhijarvi, H., and Iisalo, E. (1975): Prophylactic fluoride treatment and aged bones. *Br. Med. J.*, 3:73–74.

39. Ivey, J.L., Farley, J.R., and Baylink, D.J. (1981): Alkaline phosphatase response in sodium fluoride-treated osteoporotics. *Clin. Res.*, 29:95. (abstr.)

40. Jenkins, G.N. (1967): Fluoride. *World Rev. Nutr. Diet.*, 7:138–203.

41. Johnson, L.C. (1965): Histogenesis and mechanisms in the development of osteofluorosis. In: *Fluorine Chemistry*, edited by J.H. Simons, Vol. 4, pp. 424–441. Academic Press, New York.

42. Jowsey, J., and Kelly, P.J. (1968): Effect of fluoride treatment in a patient with osteoporosis. *Mayo Clin. Proc.*, 43:435–443.

43. Jowsey, J., and Riggs, B.L. (1978): Effect of concurrent calcium ingestion on intestinal absorption of fluoride. *Metabolism*, 27:971–974.

44. Jowsey, J., Riggs, B.L., Kelly, P.J., and Hoffman, D.L. (1972): Effect of combined therapy with sodium fluoride, vitamin D and calcium in osteoporosis. *Am. J. Med.*, 53:43–49.

45. Jowsey, J., Schenk, R.K., and Reutter, F.W. (1968): Some results of the effect of fluoride on bone tissue in osteoporosis. *J. Clin. Endocrinol. Metab.*, 28:869–874.

46. Kanis, J.A., and Meunier, P.J. (1984): Should we use fluoride to treat osteoporosis?: a review. *Quart. J. Med.*, 53:145–164.

47. Kuntz, D., Marie, P., Naveau, B., Maziere, B., Tubiana, M., and Ryckewaert, A. (1984): Extended treatment of primary osteoporosis by sodium fluoride combined with 25 hydroxycholecalciferol. *Clin. Rheumatol.*, 3:145–153.

48. Lane, J.M., Healey, J.H., Schwartz, E., Vigorita, V.J., Schneider, R., Einhorn, T.A., Suda, M., and Robbins, W.C. (October 1984): Treatment of osteoporosis with sodium fluoride and calcium: effects on vertebral fracture incidence and bone histomorphometry. *Orthop. Clin. North Am.*, 15:729–745.

49. Largent, E.J. (1954): Metabolism of inorganic fluorides. In: *Fluoridation as a Public Health Measure*, edited by J.H. Shaw, pp. 49–78. American Association for the Advancement of Science, Washington, D.C.

50. Leone, N.C. (1960): The effects of the absorption of fluoride. I. Outline and summary. *Arch. Industrial Health*, 21:324–325.

51. Leone, N.C., Stevenson, C.A., Hilbish, T.F., and Sosman, M.C. (1955): A roentgenologic study of a human population exposed to high-fluoride domestic water: a ten-year study. *Am. J. Roentgenol.*, 74:874–885.

52. Lindemann, G. (1965): Experimental chronic fluorosis in young rats receiving supplementary doses of vitamin D. *Acta Odontol. Scand.*, 23:575–592.

53. Lukert, B.P., Bolinger, R.E., and Meek, J.C. (1967): Acute effect of fluoride on ^{45}calcium dynamics in osteoporosis. *J. Clin. Endocrinol. Metab.*, 27:828–835.

54. Mertz, W. (1981): The essential trace elements. *Science*, 213:1332–1338.

55. Merz, W.A., Schenk, R.K., and Reutter, F.W. (1970): Paradoxical effects of vitamin D in fluoride-treated senile osteoporosis. *Calcif. Tissue Res.*, 4 Suppl:49–50.

56. Meunier, P.J., Sellami, S., Briançon, D., and Edouard, C. (1981): Histological heterogeneity of apparently idiopathic osteoporosis. In: *Osteoporosis: Recent Advances in Pathogenesis and Treatment*, edited by H.F. DeLuca, H.M. Frost, W.S.S. Jee, C.C. Johnston, Jr., and A.M. Parfitt, pp. 293–301. University Park Press, Baltimore.

57. O'Duffy, J.D., Wahner, H.W., O'Fallon, W.M., Johnson, K.A., Muhs, J.M., Beabout, J.W., Hodgson, S.F., and Riggs, B.L. (1986): Mechanism of acute lower extremity pain syndrome in fluoride-treated osteoporotic patients. *Am. J. Med.*, 80:561–566.

58. Olah, A.J., Reutter, F.W., and Dambacher, M.A. (1978): Effects of combined therapy with sodium fluoride and high doses of Vitamin D in osteoporosis. A histomorphometric study in the iliac crest. In: *Fluoride and Bone*, edited by B. Courvoisier, A. Donath, and C.A. Baud, pp. 242–248. Hans Huber Publishers, Bern, Switzerland.

59. Pak, C.Y.C., Sakhaee, K., Gallagher, C., Pariel, C., Peterson, R., Zerwekh, J.E., Lemke, M., Britton, F., and Adams, B. (1987): Attainment of therapeutic fluoride levels in serum without major side effects using a slow release preparation of sodium fluoride in postmenopausal osteoporosis. *Bone Miner. Res.* (in press).

60. Parfitt, A.M. (1980): Morphologic basis of bone mineral measurements: transient and steady state effects of treatment in osteoporosis (editorial). *Min. Electrolyte Metab.*, 4:273–287.

61. Parfitt, A.M. (1984): Age-related structural changes in trabecular and cortical bone: cellular mechanisms and biomechanical consequences. *Calcif. Tissue Int.*, 3(Suppl.) 1:123–128.

62. Parsons, V., Mitchell, C.J., Reeve, J., and Hesp, R. (1977): The use of sodium fluoride, vitamin D and calcium supplements in the treatment of patients with axial osteoporosis. *Calcif. Tissue Res. [Suppl.]*, 22:236–240.

63. Power, G.R.I., and Gay, J.D.L. (1986): Sodium fluoride in the treatment of osteoporosis. *Clin. Invest. Med.*, 9:41–43.

64. Raisz, L.G., and Kream, B.E. (1983): Regulation of bone formation. Part 2. *N. Engl. J. Med.*, 309:83–89.

65. Reutter, F.W., and Olah, A.J. (1978): Bone biopsy findings and clinical observations in longterm treatment of osteoporosis with sodium fluoride and vitamin D₃. In: *Fluoride and Bone*, edited by B. Courvoisier, A. Donath, and C.A. Baud, pp. 249–255. Hans Huber Publishers, Bern, Switzerland.

66. Rich, C., and Ensinck, J. (1961): Effect of sodium fluoride on calcium metabolism of human beings. *Nature*, 191:184–185.

67. Rich, C., Ensinck, J., and Ivanovich, P. (1964): The effects of sodium fluoride on calcium metabolism of subjects with metabolic bone diseases. *J. Clin. Invest.*, 43:545–556.

68. Rich, C., and Feist, E. (1970): The action of fluoride on bone. In: *Fluoride in Medicine*, edited by T.L. Vischer, pp. 70–87. Hans Huber Publishers, Bern, Switzerland.

69. Riggs, B.L. (1984): Treatment of osteoporosis with sodium fluoride: an appraisal. *Bone Mineral Res.*, 2:366–393.

70. Riggs, B.L., Baylink, D.J., Kleerekoper, M., Lane, J.M., Melton, L.J., III, and Meunier, P.J. (1987): Incidence of hip fractures in osteoporotic women treated with sodium fluoride (submitted for publication).

71. Riggs, B.L., Hodgson, S.F., Hoffman, D.L., Kelly, P.J., Johnson, K.A., and Taves, D. (1980): Treatment of primary osteoporosis with fluoride and calcium: clinical tolerance and fracture occurrence. *J.A.M.A.*, 243:446–449.

72. Riggs, B.L., Seeman, E., Hodgson, S.F., Taves, D.R., and O'Fallon, W.M. (1982): Effect of the fluoride/calcium regimen on vertebral fracture occurrence in postmenopausal osteoporosis: comparison with conventional therapy. *N. Engl. J. Med.*, 306:446–450.

73. Ringe, J.D., Kruse, H.P., and Kuhlencordt, F. (1978): Long term treatment of primary osteoporosis by sodium fluoride. In: *Fluoride and Bone*, edited by B. Courvoisier, A. Donath, and C.A. Baud, pp. 228–232. Hans Huber Publishers, Bern, Switzerland.

74. Roholm, K. (1937): *Fluorine Intoxication: a Clinical-Hygienic Study; With a Review of the Literature and Some Experimental Investigations*, H.K. Lewis and Company, London.

75. Rose, G.A. (1965): A study of the treatment of osteoporosis with fluoride therapy and high calcium intake. *Proc. R. Soc. Med.*, 58:436–440.

76. Ryckwaert, A., Kuntz, D., Teyssedou, J.-P., Tun Chot, S., Bordier, Ph., and Hioco, D. (1972): Étude histologique de l'os chez des sujets ostéoporotiques en traitement prolongé par le fluorure de sodium. *Rev. Rhum. Mal. Osteoartic.*, 39:627–634.

77. Schenk, R.K., Merz, W.A., and Reutter, F.W. (1970): Fluoride in osteoporosis: quantitative histological studies on bone structure and bone remodelling in serial biopsies of the iliac crest. In: *Fluoride in Medicine*, edited by T.L. Vischer, pp. 153–168. Hans Huber Publishers, Bern, Switzerland.

78. Schnitzler, C.M. (1984): Stress-fractures in fluoride therapy for osteoporosis. In: *Osteoporosis*, edited by C. Christiansen, C.D. Arnaud, B.E.C. Nordin, A.M. Parfitt, W.A. Peck, and B.L. Riggs, Jr., pp.

629–634, Aalborg Stiftsbogtrykkeri, Glostrup, Denmark.

79. Schnitzler, C.M., and Solomon, L. (1986): Histomorphometric analysis of a calcaneal stress fracture: a possible complication of fluoride therapy for osteoporosis. *Bone*, 7:193–198.

80. Schulz, E.E., Engstrom, H., Sauser, D.D., and Baylink, D.J. (1986): Osteoporosis: radiographic detection of fluoride-induced extra-axial bone formation. *Radiology*, 159:457–462.

81. Schulz, E.E., Libanati, C.R., Farley, S.M., Kirk, G.A., and Baylink, D.J. (1984): Skeletal scintigraphic changes in osteoporosis treated with sodium fluoride: concise communication. *J. Nucl. Med.*, 25:651–655.

82. Simonen, O., and Laitinen, O. (1985): Does fluoridation of drinking-water prevent bone fragility and osteoporosis? *Lancet*, 2:432–434.

83. Singh, A., Jolly, S.S., Bansal, B.C., and Mathur, C.C. (1963): Endemic fluorosis: epidemiological, clinical and biochemical study of chronic fluorine intoxication in Punjab (India). *Medicine (Baltimore)*, 42:229–246.

84. Slovik, D.M., Daly, M.A., Doppelt, J.H., Potts, J.T., Jr., Rosenthal, D.J., and Neer, R.M. (1986): Increases in vertebral body density of postmenopausal osteoporotics after alternating treatment with bPTH (1–34) fragment and 1,25(OH)₂D₃: an interim report. *XIth International Conference on Calcium Regulating Hormones and Bone Metabolism*, Abstr. 14, Nice, France.

85. Spencer, H., Lewin, I., Fowler, J., and Samachson, J. (1969): Effect of sodium fluoride on calcium absorption and balances in man. *Am. J. Clin. Nutr.*, 22:381–390.

86. Susheela, A.K., and Jha, M. (1983): Cellular and histochemical characteristics of osteoid formed in experimental fluoride poisoning. *Toxicol. Lett.*, 16:35–40.

87. Taves, D.R. (1970): New approach to the treatment of bone disease with fluoride. *Fed. Proc.*, 29:1185–1187.

88. Thiébaud, M., Zender, R., Courvoisier, B., Baud, C.A., and Jacot, C. (1970): The action of fluoride on diffuse bone atrophies. In: *Fluoride in Medicine*, edited by T.L. Vischer, pp. 136–142. Hans Huber Publishers, Bern, Switzerland.

89. Vokrouhlická, O., Hrba, J., Horn, V., and Palovsky, V. (1977): Treatment of osteoporosis with large doses of sodium fluoride. *Rev. Czech. Med.*, 23:104–108.

90. Vose, G.P., Keele, D.K., Milner, A.M., Rawley, R., Roach, T.L., and Sprinkle, E.E., III (1978): Effect of sodium fluoride, inorganic phosphate, and oxymetholone therapies in osteoporosis: a six-year progress report. *J. Gerontol.*, 33:204–212.

91. Waterhouse, C., Taves, D., and Munzer, A. (1980): Serum inorganic fluoride: changes related to previous fluoride intake, renal function and bone resorption. *Clin. Sci.*, 58:145–152.

92. Wolinsky, I., Simkin, A., and Guggenheim, K. (1972): Effects of fluoride on metabolism and mechanical properties of rat bone. *Am. J. Physiol.*, 223:46–50.

Osteoporosis: Etiology, Diagnosis, and Management, edited by B. Lawrence Riggs and L. Joseph Melton, III. Raven Press, New York © 1988.

18

Orthopaedic Consequences of Osteoporosis

Joseph M. Lane, Charles N. Cornell, and John H. Healey

Metabolic Bone Disease Section, The Hospital for Special Surgery, Division Orthopaedic Surgery, Memorial Sloan-Kettering Cancer Center, New York, New York 10021

END RESULT OF OSTEOPOROSIS

Loss of Structural Integrity, Fractures, and Consequent Deformity

Osteoporosis is a problem of epidemic proportions in the United States (see Chapter 5, *this volume.*) The magnitude of this disorder has recently been evaluated by Holbrook, Grazier, Kelsey and Stauffer, in their study, "The Frequency of Occurrence, Impact and Cost of Selected Musculoskeletal Conditions in the United States" (30). This extensive evaluation of musculoskeletal disorders clearly demonstrates that the incidence of osteoporosis increases dramatically with age and that women are more frequently affected than men. Other investigators have reached similar conclusions (33,38,62,71). In a study of a group in Michigan, more than half the women age 45 and older showed evidence of osteoporosis as defined by osteopenia on spinal x-rays. Osteoporosis was demonstrated in nine out of ten women after age 75, and was associated with wedge fractures of vertebrae in one out of every five women. It is believed that 70% of all fractures occurring in women older than 45 are related to osteoporosis (44,57), and it has been estimated that osteoporosis accounts for more than $6 billion in economic costs annually (30).

The primary fractures most often seen by orthopaedists in patients with osteoporosis are vertebral fractures, hip fractures, and forearm (Colles') fractures (Fig. 1). Although spinal fractures lead to deformity and Colles' fractures produce dysfunction, hip fractures severely affect the ultimate quality of life and challenge survival (30,32). One patient in twenty past the age of 65 currently occupying a hospital bed is recovering from a hip fracture. In the best of hands, 40% of patients sustaining a hip fracture will not survive two years following this injury. Of the patients originating from a nursing home, 70% will not survive one year (4,29,30,35,39). Only one-third of patients following a hip fracture will return to a life-style and level of independence comparable to that prior to the injury.

Appropriate treatment of skeletal injuries secondary to osteoporosis requires an understanding of the effect of osteoporosis on: (1) bone's material and structural properties, (2) the mechanisms of fracture, and (3) the mode of fracture healing. Following these topics, the management of spine, hip, Colles' and pelvic fractures will be discussed.

BONE BIOMECHANICS

The skeleton serves as a mineral reserve, hemopoetic repository, and structural support.

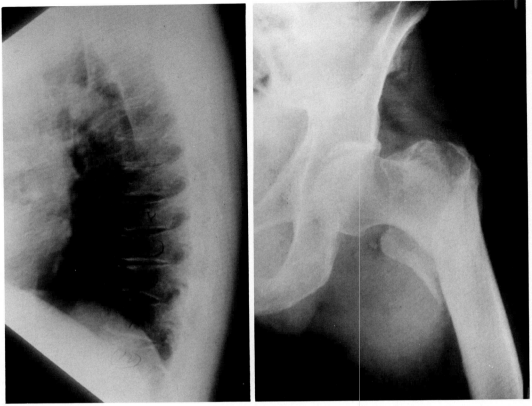

A   **B**

FIG. 1.   Radiographs illustrating typical osteopenic fractures. **A:** Lateral radiograph of thoracic spine demonstrating wedge fractures of T9, T10, and T12. **B:** AP radiograph of an intertrochanteric fracture of left hip.

The structural elements have important biomechanical properties (see Chapter 4, *this volume*). Bone is a composite material consisting of type 1 collagen (tensile strength) and hydroxyapatite mineral (compressive strength) (10). It is anisotropic in structure and consistency (46). Histologic and microradiographic analyses have shown that bone has well-defined areas of nonmineralized osteoid, partially mineralized osteoid, and fully mineralized osteoid. Nonmineralized osteoid usually constitutes 1 to 2% of the total bone volume. Although all mature bone is essentially lamellar, the cortex is relatively compact, with a high volume to surface ratio. Interspaced within the cortex are Haversian canals with a central blood vessel. Circumferential rings are applied around the vessel to form each osteon. *Cutting cones* of osteoclasts can be seen removing old cortical bone to be replaced or remodeled with a new osteonal system.

Trabecular bone is also largely lamellar, but it has a high surface to volume ratio. Rather than remodeling by *tunneling resorption* within the trabeculae, there is remodeling upon the surface. Osteoclasts initially carve out Howship's lacunae. Within these lacunae, osteoblastic bone formation occurs secondarily.

The material properties of bone are governed by the microdensity of the material. Carter and co-workers (10) demonstrated that in a homogenous material, the compressive strength of bone is proportional to the square of the density. When not homogenous, however, the ma-

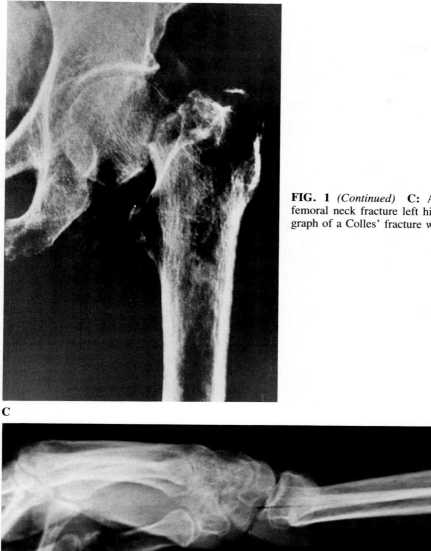

FIG. 1 *(Continued)* **C:** AP radiograph of a femoral neck fracture left hip. **D:** Lateral radiograph of a Colles' fracture with dorsal tilt.

C

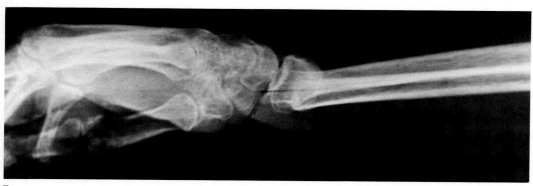

D

terial's weakest point is the area of least density, and failure or fractures occur at such sites (Fig. 2). The area between the two cortical end plates of the ilium, for example, contains trabecular bone of low density. The central third of the medullary canal frequently has the lowest density of trabeculae and is the site where failure occurs during compressive and shear testing. This emphasizes the importance of the structural distribution of the bone mass.

Bone geometry determines bone strength (34,61). The tensile strength of a solid rod is the same as that of a tube with the same cross-sectional area of material. However, the tube

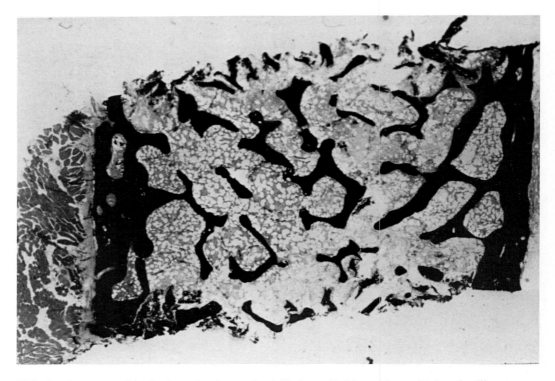

FIG. 2.   Low power histologic study of an undecalcified transilial bone biopsy. Trabeculae illustrate connectivity to cortex at endosteal area. There is minimal connectivity in the midportion of the medullary canal and this area has weakest structural strength to shear loads.

has a greater moment of inertia and is significantly stronger than the rod when withstanding bending or torsion stresses (see Fig. 3, Chapter 4, *this volume*). Consequently, the farther the material is distributed away from the center of the object, the stronger is the structural strength of that material in torsion and bending (67). An example of this principle is seen in the femoral diaphysis of an aging individual. As one grows older, the outer periosteal diameter increases, as does the inner endosteal diameter. This shifts the bone mass further from the epicenter of the bone. Theoretically, these changes in bone geometry have the potential to maximize skeletal strength for any given amount of bone mass and could partially compensate for the decreased bone mass that accompanies aging (43). For instance, a 10% increase in the diameter of a long bone can compensate for a 30% decrease in bone mass.

In reality (7,42), increases in the diameter of long bones rarely exceed 2% of the original diameter. Furthermore, although this process has been demonstrated to occur in males (21,49), there are data which suggest that the female skeleton does not widen with aging. In addition, certain parts of the skeleton, such as the femoral neck, are deficient in periosteum and cannot compensate for loss of endosteal bone mass. These observations partially explain the predilection for fracture of the femoral neck in elderly females.

Careful dissection of the tibia demonstrates another principle of structural distribution and material properties. The anterior and posterior aspects of the diaphysis are, respectively, under the greatest tensile and compressive stresses due to the bowing of the tibia and the greater strength of muscles in the posterior compartment of the leg. The medial and lateral aspects of the tibia are in a more neutral plane and sustain significantly less tensile and compressive loads. Analysis of the tibial cortices shows that the osteonal count is greatest in the medial and lateral aspects of the diaphysis in the neutral plane, and lowest in the area of anterior diaphysis under the greatest tension. Symmetric stressing of the tibia in animals has clearly demonstrated the inhibition of osteonal remodeling and the development of bone apposition on the outer diameters of the anterior and posterior tibial cortex (73). Immobilization of the tibia and calcium deficiency lead to an increase in osteonal remodeling in the unstressed medial and lateral tibia.

Two concepts can be generated from these studies: modeling and remodeling (Fig. 3). In modeling, general appositional growth occurs on the surface of the loaded bone at the greatest distance from the epicenter of the bone. It does not follow Frost's (21) metabolic bone unit concept of resorption followed by formation, but instead manifests direct formation without resorption. Modeling is illustrated clinically by periosteal bone formation in stressed bones. It is also seen following aseptic necrosis, in which the dead trabeculae provide a lattice upon which new appositional bone growth occurs. Lastly, it is clearly illustrated in the external fracture callus, where bone formation occurs without preliminary bone resorption.

Conversely, remodeling involves an initial process of removing bone from within. This is illustrated by the cutting cone oteoclastic resorption of cortical bone or Howship's lacunar indentations into trabecular bone. In both instances, the bone is temporarily weakened during the remodeling process before it is partially restrengthened by new bone formation. Furthermore, the initial mineralization is incomplete so that the new metabolic bone unit is significantly decreased in compressive strength compared to the preexisting highly mineralized bone. Lastly, the production of porosities and subsequent reossification during the remodeling process results in a multicomponent bone rather than a single unit of reinforced collagen. This remodeled bone differs from reinforced concrete which is produced in its entirety at one time. It more resembles the process of boring holes into preexisting concrete and producing microfractures and weakness. Plugging up the holes with new concrete will never reproduce its original strength. Thus, osteonal and remodeled bone is initially significantly weaker than the cortical bone it replaced.

According to Wolff's Law (72), form follows function. The skeleton, and particularly

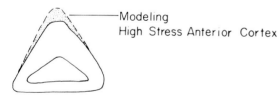

Modeling
High Stress Anterior Cortex

Remodeling
Low Stress Medial/Lateral Cortex

FIG. 3. Modeling represents appositional bone deposition on periphery of structure. Remodeling is turnover within original dimensions of structure. Modeling occurs on most loaded regions; remodeling occurs on least loaded areas of bone.

the osteoblasts and osteoclasts, does respond to structural demands. A clear distinction must be made between modeling and remodeling in this regard, however. Immobilization will lead to bone resorption, particularly in the unstressed areas. The body recognizes skeletal stress, perhaps by a piezoelectric feedback, and will only remodel the least stressed bone. There is a possibility that the physiologic signal of exercise may be reproduced through such bioelectricity. Studies from Brighton (65) and others have indicated that capacitive coupling can prevent loss of bone from disuse osteoporosis. Whether bioelectricity can mimic the signal from exercise and can actually lead to augmentation of bone mass is uncertain. Although augmented production of bone can occur in the young, there is little to indicate that people past the age of 45 can markedly increase their bone mass unless they are starting from a state of major deprivation.

Stringent exercise, on the other hand, will lead to modeling of the skeletal area that is repetitively stressed. In the younger age group, studies by Jacobson (31) and co-workers have demonstrated that when comparing tennis players to high performance swimmers and typical college co-eds, the swimmers and co-eds had comparable bone mass while the tennis players with a high level of "*impact loading*" had significantly greater trabecular bone within the spine. Stress loading against gravity of an impact nature leads to augmented bone mass. Exercise has also been shown to be partially protective even in patients with anorexia nervosa (51). In this patient population as compared to normal individuals, the authors demonstrated a significant diminution in bone mass in those anorectic individuals who did not exercise. However, in the anorexic individuals who carried out a general exercise program regularly, bone mass was not statistically different from controls. Consequently, exercise can partially protect bone mass from loss even in short periods of nutritional deprivation.

Exercise, therefore, can maintain bone mass by inducing modeling and augmented bone formation in impact loaded bones in an effort to increase the structural strength of the loaded areas. Conservative levels of exercise will retain bone mass but not lead to appositional bone growth. Investigators have analyzed the postmenopausal population and demonstrated that a reasonable level of exercise such as walking five miles a week, dancing, and limited forceful activity can decrease the traditional postmenopausal loss of bone from 2% per year to less than 0.5% (9) per year. Other studies have noted that exercise can also limit the tendency for remodeling of stressed bones and thereby prevent loss of bone strength.

Normal metabolic circumstances avoid rapid bone turnover or production of excess osteoid and protect bone's mechanical structure. Enhanced remodeling runs the risk of producing microweaknesses. Patients with hyperparathyroidism, hyperthyroidism, and even Paget's disease, with its enhanced bone mass, all have hypermetabolic remodeling states and are noted for their high incidence of stress fractures. Efforts to strengthen bone by promoting the remodeling process are less likely to succeed than those that augment bone by direct modeling. The implications of modeling and remodeling are clear in terms of osteoporosis. Bone which has undergone significant remodeling and porosity has markedly weakened microstructure.

Conversely, modeled bone maintains an intact microstructure without faults or stress risers, while augmenting lamellar bone mass by appositional growth.

Mechanism of Fracture

Bone consists of both cortical and trabecular bone, and there are different structural roles for each of these two types. Areas in which large impact stresses are applied from many directions do best with the trabecular bone pattern. Cortical bone's primary function is protection against torque and bending loads. Cortical bone forms slowly and its dimensions have been developed in response to a long history of specific recurring stresses. The vertebral body consists of a cortical outer shell and a large trabecular interior bone volume. Hayes and co-workers (10) have shown that removing the cortex lessens the mechanical strength of the vertebral body during compressive testing only by 7%. Consequently, 93% of the compressive strength of the vertebral body is maintained by the trabecular bone. This has similarly been noted in the subchondral area of the femur and the proximal tibia. The femoral neck has little trabecular bone and depends upon cortical bone for its integrity. It fails mainly in torque and bending modes for which trabecular bone has little protective role.

Those areas of the skeleton rich in trabecular bone sustain the first ravages of osteoporosis due to the high surface to volume ratio. The metaphyses of the distal radius and proximal humerus, and the vertebral bodies lose trabecular bone early after menopause, and these are the sites of early postmenopausal fractures. Cortical bone is slower in dissolution due to its low surface to volume ratio. Its loss occurs later during so-called "senile osteoporosis" and results in cortical bone fractures in areas such as the hip (27).

These fractures occur either from repetitive microinjury with propagation of the fracture line (fatigue failure) or from acute trauma (27). Bone is a viscoelastic substance in which load may deform the bone but, once the load is removed, the bone will regain its original shape (Fig. 4). Once the point of elasticity has been surpassed, however, permanent plastic deformation will occur. At that point, remodeling or modeling of the bone will occur in an effort to regain structural strength. If this process is deficient, microfractures may coalesce, leading to a weakened cortex and subsequent fracture following mild trauma. The classical example of this process is the stress fracture. These fractures are most frequently seen in the rib, pubic ramus, tibia and femoral neck.

Acute trauma can be superimposed on these microfractures. As a consequence, it is uncertain what initiates hip fractures. Many observers contend that over 50% of hip fractures result from torque-induced failure of the femoral neck cortex and that the fracture is completely sustained before the patient strikes the floor. The majority of spinal trabecular fractures, on the other hand, certainly represent repetitive

injuries with microcollapse leading to ultimate deformity. Most patients are unaware of a specific event leading to each vertebral fracture.

Unfortunately, noninvasive measures of bone density only report gross mass per unit volume. Bone is not homogenous and that volume contains areas of decreased density with microstructural imperfections. Despite this limitation, Melton (44) at the Mayo Clinic has shown that the femoral hip fracture rate clearly depends upon gross bone mass. He found 4/1,000 hip fractures per year in patients with femoral bone mass of $< 1.0 \ g/cm^2$ as identified on the dual beam absorptiometry instrumentation. A 50% decrease in mass was associated with a fourfold increase in hip fracture incidence. Thus, a gross loss of bone mass increases fracture rate in an exponential manner, and the hip fracture incidence is related to the bone density squared. This clinical evidence corroborates laboratory tests where bone strength is also related to the square of the bone density (10).

Load distribution may accentuate fracture risk, however. Healey (26) has shown that 58% of patients with idiopathic osteoporosis develop scoliosis. Conversely, 76% of patients with adult idiopathic kyphoscoliosis will have osteoporosis (Fig. 5). Furthermore, patients with unstable idiopathic scoliosis ($> 30°$ curves) have a spinal bone density 2 SD below the age-adjusted mean. The kyphoscoliosis shifts body weight, increasing the load upon the anterior vertebral body trabecular bone. This stress concentration, in turn, accentuates the fracture risk of selected vertebrae. The major sites of fracture occurrence are (1) the apex of the kyphus, (2) the transition between the thoracic and the lumbar vertebral bodies, and (3) the apex of the lumbar scoliotic curve. Kyphoscoliosis, then, is a clear risk and contributes to the specific site of fractures.

Fracture Healing

Fracture healing classically utilizes endochondral bone repair (27,36,58). Six clear stages have been identified. These include the following: (1) stage of impact, (2) stage of in-

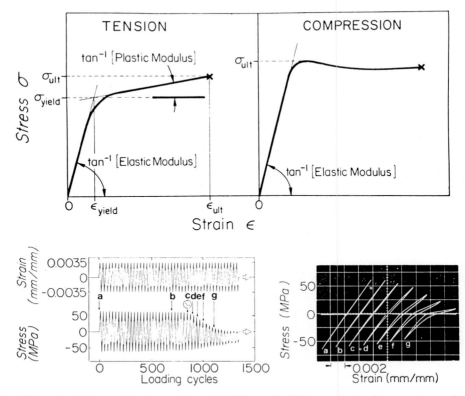

FIG. 4. Biomechanical considerations of material failure. **A:** Either under tension or compression loads material undergoes a reversible elastic deformation followed by plastic unreversible deformation until failure (x) as demonstrated by stress/strain plots. **B:** Under cyclic loading, failure occurs each cycle into the plastic region of the stress/strain curve. (From Carter D.R., and Spenbler, D.M. (1978): Mechanical properties and composition of cortical bone. *Clin. Orthop.*, 135:192–217, with permission.)

duction, (3) stage of inflammation, (4) stage of soft callus, (5) stage of hard callus, and (6) stage of remodeling/modeling. The stage of impact occurs from the moment of initiation of injury to the dissipation of energy. This leads to both soft tissue and bony trauma. It is followed by the stage of induction in which a series of inductive factors such as kinins, electronegativity, low pH, and low oxygen tension all initiate the process of tissue repair. Specific agents, e.g., bone morphogenic protein, may be important to induce and modulate repair. The stage of inflammation follows, during which time there is bone resorption of the necrotic osseous tissue, the initiation and development of vasoformative elements, and the ingrowth of primitive mesenchymal tissue. The stage of soft callus is the conversion of primitive mesenchymal tissue into soft chondroid el-

ement. The stage of hard callus involves the calcification of the cartilage bars, deposition of fiber bone upon the cartilage bars and, ultimately, its conversion into lamellar bone. The last stage of remodeling and modeling reorganizes the microscopic and anatomical structure of the bone, restoring maximal strength to the bone.

Osteoporosis seriously compromises the latter two stages of hard callus and remodeling (36). The synthesis of bone and its mineralization is keenly dependent upon calcium supplied either from diet or calcium reserves in bone. Osteoporotic patients have a low calcium pool, with inadequate dietary calcium and a poor structural calcium bank. Callus mineralization is thus slowed. The stage of remodeling and modeling is further prolonged because of the competition for calcium with the rest of the

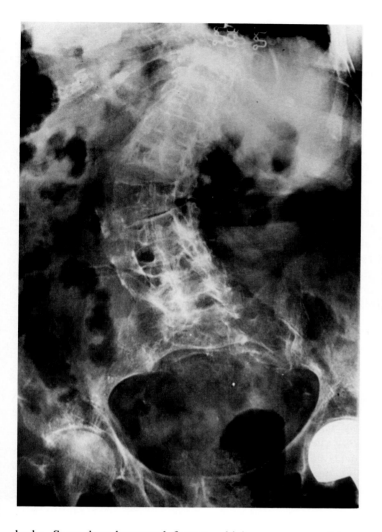

FIG. 5. AP radiograph of lumbar scoliosis in a patient who has previously had a hemiarthroplastic replacement for a right hip fracture. The left lumbar scoliosis demonstrates a lateral spondylolethesis at L3–L4 in an osteopenic skeleton.

body. Secondary hormonal factors which are already active to maintain calcium homeostasis at the expense of the osteoporotic skeleton may also seriously compromise fracture healing. Consequently, while the first stages through the soft callus stage may proceed without interference in osteoporosis, the mineralization and the ultimate remodeling of the callus are prolonged (19). Hip fractures in the elderly remain positive by bone scan well into the third year, and union cannot be fully ascertained until that period of time. Healing can be stimulated by physiological levels of vitamin D, nutritional levels of calcium adequate for that individual (1500 mg elemental calcium/day), normal nitrogen balance (adequate calorie intake) and

appropriate exercise stimulation (63). Exercise aligns collagen in bone deposition, particularly during the stage of remodeling and modeling. However, osteoporotic individuals are rarely supported with appropriate calcium and vitamin therapy following a fracture. Studies at The Hospital for Special Surgery have demonstrated a 10% systemic bone loss in the unaffected skeleton following long bone fractures even in the face of "adequate" calcium intake.

Management of Fractures

The impact of skeletal loss becomes most vividly apparent as the skeleton begins to fail in its ability to withstand required loads. When this occurs, osteoporosis becomes a disease state which alters the quality of life and challenges survival. The severe economic consequences of this disorder also begin to emerge.

A reasonable return of function following fracture in elderly patients can only be achieved by early, definitive stabilization of the injured extremities. Immobilization of the patient as a whole rather than definitive operative treatment places the patient at risk of pulmonary decompensation, venoembolic disease, decubitus formation, and further musculoskeletal deterioration from which recovery becomes unlikely. In recent years, the treatment of osteoporotic fractures has improved considerably as a result of improvements in the design of internal fixation devices and understanding of the biology and mechanics of fracture healing in osteoporotic bone.

At The New York Hospital Cornell Medical Center and The Hospital for Special Surgery, an osteoporosis center has been developed which has attracted a large referral population with osteoporosis and skeletal failure. Because of this, a considerable experience with treatment of fractures in the elderly has been gained. Based upon this experience, the following principles have been conceived and have guided the formulation of our treatment protocols:

1. Elderly patients are best served by rapid, definitive fracture care aimed at early restoration of mobility and function. In most cases, these patients are healthiest on the day of injury and are in the best shape for surgery at that time. Nevertheless, many concurrent illnesses are often present and should be thoroughly evaluated prior to surgery. Survival is often benefited by judicious medical tune-up which is used to treat reversible medical decompensations that may have caused or resulted from the injury (35). Similarly, surgical procedures should be kept simple to minimize operative time, blood loss, and physiologic stress upon these patients.
2. The aim of intervention should be to achieve stable fracture fixation that allows early return of function. For the lower extremity, this implies early weight-bearing. Although anatomic restoration is important for intraarticular fractures, metaphyseal and diaphyseal fractures are probably best managed by efforts to achieve stability rather than anatomic reduction.
3. The primary mode of failure of internal fixation results from bone failure rather than implant failure. The strength of bone is directly related to its mineral density (10). Osteoporotic bone, therefore, lacks the strength to hold plates and screws securely. Furthermore, comminution is generally more extensive in osteoporotic fractures. Internal fixation devices should be chosen which allow compaction of fracture fragments into stable patterns that minimize stresses at bone-impact interfaces. Furthermore, implants should be chosen which minimize stress shielding to avoid further skeletal decompensation as a result of intervention. For these reasons, sliding nail-plate devices and intramedullary devices which are load-sharing and allow settling into stable patterns are ideal.

The remainder of this chapter will review the current treatment of Colles', hip, vertebral and pelvic fractures, which constitute the most common skeletal injuries in osteoporotic patients. A summary of the treatment protocols used by the authors will also be presented.

HIP FRACTURES

Hip fractures present a major risk for permanent morbidity and mortality in patients with osteoporosis. The incidence of hip fractures increases with longevity; approximately 32% of women and 17% of men by the age of ninety will have sustained a hip fracture (22,44). It is disturbing that the age- and sex-adjusted hip fracture rates have increased significantly since World War II. Hip fracture rates may have been affected by several factors. Studies from Finland have indicated that populations on fluoridated water (one part per million) have one-third the fracture rate patients on nonfluoridated water as corrected per decade (59). Patients in high calcium intake areas in Yugoslavia (41) have been shown to have one-third to one-fourth the fracture rate of patients from areas with low indigenous calcium in their diet. The latter dietary calcium intake is comparable to the average American intake.

Sodium fluoride has been utilized successfully to decrease vertebral fractures, but its effect on hip fracture is uncertain (37,50). Augmented fracture rates have been suggested for a group of patients in Australia under treatment with sodium fluoride (1 mg/kg/day) in a preliminary study reported to the American Society for Bone and Mineral Research. However a large collaborative study by Riggs and others (50) has suggested that, in fact, the hip fracture rate is not increased. Long-term studies of patients on fluoride therapy at The Hospital for Special Surgery have suggested a 50% decreased rate of fractures after two years of fluoride treatment (37).

The two predominant types of hip fracture are the subcapital femoral neck and intertrochanteric hip fractures (Fig. 6). Each fracture presents different requirements for fixation and a different set of complications (see below). Subcapital fractures are associated with a high risk of nonunion and/or aseptic necrosis of the femoral head. Intertrochanteric fractures have a low risk of nonunion but can lead to malalignment, including retroversion and varus deformities with cut-out of the internal fixation. These fractures all require open reduction and internal fixation or hemiarthroplasty (Fig. 7). A study at New York Hospital (57) demonstrated that of 77 patients, one-third had evidence of hyperosteoidosis (more than 5% trabecular osteoid). Although 40% had marked trabecular bone loss, all patients over 50 had decreased bone mass compared to young individuals. Twenty-five percent had increased metabolic turnover indices, including high osteoclast count. In this study, bone histomorphometry appeared to be a good predictor of outcome following treatment for femoral neck fracture. Patients who had trabecular bone volume that was within 60% of normal had 85 to 90% suc-

cessful union, while patients who had severe trabecular bone loss (< 60% of normal) had less than a 33% union rate in women, and a 50% union rate in men. These authors concluded that significant metabolic bone disease, particularly osteoporosis, leads to a high rate of unsuccessful union following femoral neck fractures. Intertrochanteric fractures have not been comparably studied.

Femoral Neck Fractures

Femoral neck fractures remain as one of the unsolved problems in orthopedics today. They are problematic because of a high incidence of nonunion and avascular necrosis that occurs in spite of adequate treatment. Closed reduction and pin or screw fixation using a variety of implants is consistently associated with a 14% incidence of nonunion, and a 15% incidence of avascular necrosis and symptomatic segmental collapse. Arnold has demonstrated that these complications can be minimized by accurate reduction and fixation but, in his reported series, patients with severe osteopenia had a higher incidence of failure secondary to loss of bony fixation (2,3). Using iliac crest biopsy data, Arnold (3) and Sceleppi (57) have shown that in spite of accurate reduction and pinning, patients with trabecular bone volumes less than 15% of normal have a significantly higher risk of poor results. These findings are corroborated in studies from other institutions. Although these studies are based upon fractures fixed by closed reduction and Knowles pinning, no significant difference has been consistently reported using other devices such as sliding nail plate implants (6,11,14,20).

The treatment options for femoral neck fractures are reduction and internal fixation versus hemiarthroplasty (Fig. 7). The dilemma in treatment arises from incomplete knowledge of when to choose either method. Clearly, if one performed only arthroplasty procedures, the complications associated with these fractures would not appear.

Hemiarthroplasty, however, is associated with its own complications and is clearly not a panacea for this injury (53,60). The major dis-

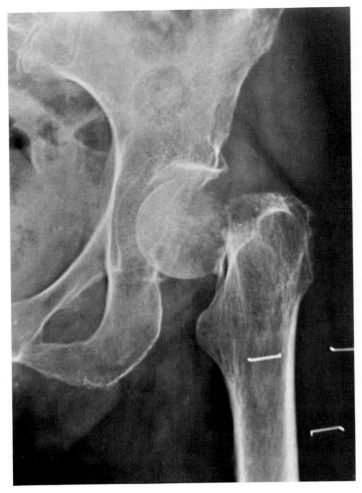

FIG. 6. **A:** AP radiograph of an intracapsular fracture of the femoral neck.

A

advantage of hemiarthroplasty is its inability to provide hip function equal to that of an intact hip joint. Long-term complications of dislocation, loosening and breakage of implants and late infection occur with regular frequency following arthroplasty and are avoided by closed reduction and internal fixation. In addition, it has been traditionally reported that hemiarthroplasty is associated with a higher perioperative morbidity, although in our most recent series, postoperative morbidity was nearly equal to that of closed reduction and pinning. In addition, as experience with the technique of arthroplasty has improved and as newer, more durable and functional designs have been introduced, the results of primary treatment with hemiarthroplasty have improved. As a result, the indications for primary hemiarthroplasty in our hands have expanded.

Our current protocol for treatment of displaced femoral neck fractures relies upon closed reduction and internal fixation using Knowles pins or compression screws as the primary form of treatment. In our most recent, comprehensive review of 251 patients who underwent closed reduction and Knowles pinning for femoral neck fractures between 1979 and 1981, 80% of patients with Garden III or IV fractures in whom good reductions were obtained, had good to excellent results at six

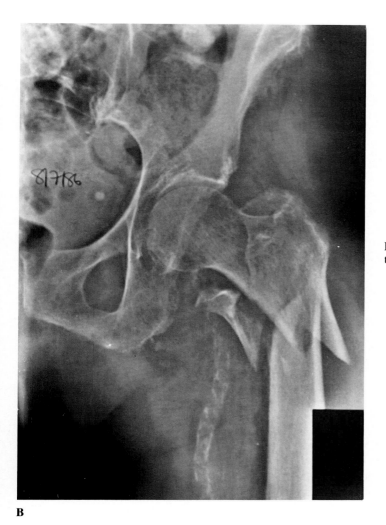

FIG. 6 *(Continued)* **B:** An intertrochanteric hip fracture.

B

months (3). The review reemphasized that good results are achieved only if reduction is adequate. Primary hemiarthroplasty using a cemented bipolar prosthesis is selected for patients who are physiologically 70 years of age (i.e., life expectancy is five years) and who are active household or community ambulators. Nonambulatory patients are not treated primarily by hemiarthroplasty unless the fracture is a pathologic one due to metastatic disease. Patients with severe demineralizing bone disease are also selected for hemiarthroplasty, as are patients with neurologic disorders who require immediate ambulation and who cannot comply with partial weight-bearing physical therapy

protocols. Hemiarthroplasty is also chosen if stable reduction cannot be obtained at surgery. In a recent review of 120 cemented bipolar hemiarthroplasties performed for displaced femoral neck fracture at The New York Hospital, the early postoperative mortality was 4%, with a 5% six-month mortality. The survival rate at six months was not improved by treating the acute fracture by closed reduction and pinning followed by delayed hemiarthroplasty if the primary Knowles pinning failed. One early and two late dislocations occurred and one patient required repeat surgery because of a disengagement of the prosthetic head from the bipolar bearing. At five-year follow-up,

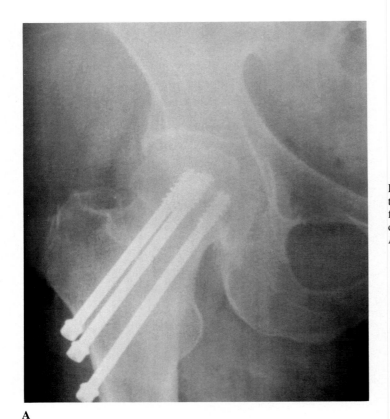

FIG. 7. Treatment of hip fractures. **A:** AP radiograph of a femoral neck hip fracture reduced and stabilized with three Asnis pins.

A

only two hips demonstrated radiographic loosening, one of which required revision as well. These encouraging results have prompted us to be more aggressive in use of primary hemiarthroplasty in the treatment of displaced femoral neck fractures in patients older than 70 years (5).

Intertrochanteric Fractures

Intertrochanteric fractures also primarily affect elderly women with metabolic bone disease. These fractures have received less attention and notoriety than femoral neck fractures because nonunion and avascular necrosis are uncommon. However, the incidence of malunion with resulting varus, shortening and external rotation deformity is significant and can be disabling. Traditional treatment of intertrochanteric fractures utilized fixed nail/side plate devices such as the Jewett Nail. Because of

poor bone quality, these devices were beset with problems of high rates of loss of fixation and pin penetration into the hip joint (45,54). A fixed nail plate device is a load-bearing device. It does not allow impaction of the fracture into a stable position and, therefore, requires stable reduction of the fracture fragments to be successful. In the absence of stable reduction, high loads are generated at the interface between the trabecular bone of the femoral head and the nail. This inevitably predisposes to loss of fixation when metabolic bone disease is significant. As such, fixed nail plate devices violate our principles of design of internal fixation devices for osteoporotic fracture. The medial displacement osteotomy was conceived to rectify this situation by creating bony stability, but the osteotomy, itself, is technically demanding and results in a shortened limb with weakened abductor power (18,54). In addition, failure of fixation follow-

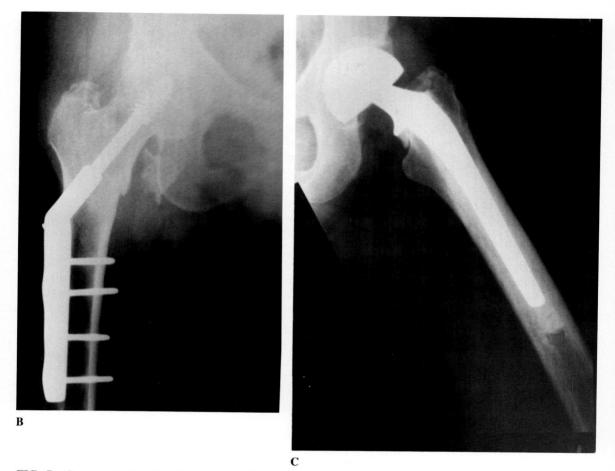

B

C

FIG. 7. *(Continued)* **B:** AP radiograph of a femoral intertrochanteric hip fracture reduced and stabilized with a Richards hip compression screw. **C:** AP radiograph of a femoral neck hip fracture corrected with a bipolar hemiarthroplasty.

ing medial displacement osteotomy is reported to vary from 10 to 30% (16,48). Sliding hip screws represent an improvement over fixed nail plate devices in that they allow controlled impaction of the fracture until a stable fracture is achieved. Thus, the device has load-sharing properties that reduce the stresses between implant and bone (Fig. 7B).

Significantly improved results are achieved with such devices (14,49). Nonetheless, in spite of these improvements in design, a significant incidence of malunion and loss of fixation still occurs. Medial displacement osteotomy does not appear to significantly improve results when a sliding nail plate device is used.

Intramedullary condylocephalic nails provide the advantages of intramedullary fixation with less intraoperative blood loss and fewer wound infections. However, they achieve results similar to the sliding nail plate, while providing a whole new set of complications (12,47,52). For a four-year period extending from 1979 through 1983, Ender's nails were used primarily at The New York Hospital and The Hospital for Special Surgery Fracture Service for treatment of stable and unstable intertrochanteric fractures. Although operative time and surgical blood loss were less, the complication rates related to nail penetration, back out and loss of fixation were such that we have since reverted to anatomic reduction and internal fixation using sliding nail plate devices. We continue to use this method as our treatment of choice for stable and unstable intertrochanteric fractures.

The key to success in using sliding nail plate devices is attention to detail and a thorough understanding of the principles of design. To achieve optimal purchase, the screw must be placed in the center of the femoral head and must engage subchondral bone. New screw designs with extra large thread intended to improve ''the bite'' in soft bone have been introduced (Richards) and, when necessary, methyl methacrylate can be used to provide adjunctive fixation (8).

In addition, the amount of impaction by the fracture should be anticipated. Grossly unstable fractures are best treated with short barrels which allow maximal slide. It is not uncommon for the screw to slide completely down a long barrel side plate converting the device into a fixed device with resultant loss of fixation (Fig. 8).

SPINAL COMPRESSION FRACTURES

Spinal compression fractures are ubiquitous in patients with severe osteopenia. Urist (68) reports that 96% of patients in a typical population with osteopenia have collapse fractures of the spine. The distribution of fractures is clearly related to the structural alignment of the spine, with the majority occurring at the apex of the thoracic kyphus, the transitional zone of the thoracolumbar spine and at the apex of a lumbar scoliotic curve. The occurrence of fractures in the dorsal spine results in an accentuation of the thoracic kyphosis. This gives rise to the so-called ''Dowagher's hump''. Fractures are somewhat less frequent in the lumbar spine. Lumbar back pain is common, however, and most often results from increased lordotic posturing necessary to compensate for the increased thoracic kyphosis.

Most fractures are unrecognized at the time of onset and are often found in the course of a routine examination. Acute fractures may be quite painful, however, leading to disability for up to six weeks. Acute compression fractures (1) in osteopenic patients typically result from minor trauma of everyday activities such as stooping, standing from a sitting position, or a minor fall. Patients who suffer spinal compression fractures generally pass through two stages: the acute fracture stage and, secondly, through the state of postural back pain. Pain usually develops very quickly and can be quite severe and associated with paraspinal muscle spasm. As a result of this, the patient often may poorly localize the pain; therefore, the entire spine should be evaluated. In patients with multiple previous fractures, bone scans are often more helpful than plain films in delineating the acutely fractured level. The clinical course is marked by acute, severe back pain and occasionally an ileus.

The acute treatment consists of conservative bed rest, hot packs, muscle relaxants and physical activity as soon as possible (1,66). Orthotics should only be utilized to mobilize the patient. Once the patient is ambulatory, the orthotics should be removed because they lead to a stress bypass and discourage bone retention within the spine. Long-term treatment should consist of an exercise program to maintain strength and flexibility (see Chapter 19, *this volume*). Thoracic extension exercises strengthen the upper back muscles supporting the thoracic spine. Abdominal strengthening exercises help to support the lumbar spine. Secondary arthritis associated with malalignment may lead to areas that require specific exercises. Severe secondary scoliosis may require a custom-fitted orthotic.

Major surgical indications following spinal fractures relate mainly to acute spinal canal impingement. Fortunately, neurologic compromise resulting from spinal instability or canal compromise is exceedingly rare. Three percent of patients at The Hospital for Special Surgery develop sensory level and neuromuscular evidence of cord compression. CT scan, MRI, and myelograms may be necessary in any patients with persistent day and night pain and neurological findings. These fractures may re-

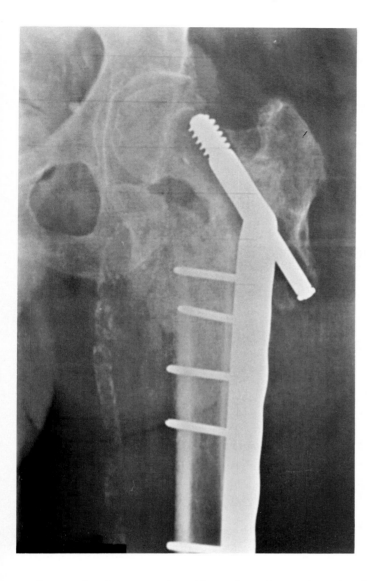

FIG. 8. AP radiograph of an unstable intertrochanteric fracture stabilized with a Richards Screw. The fracture has impacted fully converting the sliding nail plate device into a fixed device with subsequent cut-out of the femoral head.

quire anterior decompression akin to the technique utilized for tuberculosis (28). The incorporation of the bone grafts, usually from the iliac crest may take prolonged periods of time. Therefore, these patients require protection in a (prenyl) brace starting four vertebral bodies above the level of fusion for a period as long as nine months.

A dilemma facing the physician is the diagnosis and appropriate treatment for the patient presenting with a previously unrecognized compression fracture of the thoracic or lumbar spine. An algorithm has been created at The Hospital for Special Surgery which has been useful in guiding the workup of these patients to the correct diagnosis (see Fig. 9). Initially, the question to be raised is whether a sufficiently high degree of trauma (such as falling down a flight of stairs or other significant injury) was present to account for the fracture. Lifting a window or tripping on the carpeting are insufficient trauma in this regard. In the face of major trauma, the orthopaedist must decide whether the fracture is stable (treated

ALGORITHM FOR WORK-UP OF OSTEOPENIA

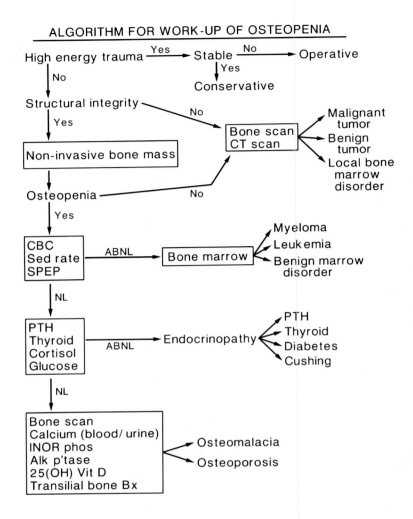

FIG. 9. An algorithm for work-up of osteopenia (see text).

conservatively) or unstable (requiring operative intervention and stabilization with instrumentation). In the absence of major trauma, it is critical to determine whether in fact there is structural continuity of the fractured vertebral body. If X-rays do not show any evidence of clear structural deficiency, the degree of generalized osteopenia should be determined. Noninvasive techniques including quantitative CT scan (24), and dual beam absorptiometry (69,70) appear to be very efficacious. Further studies of the vertebral body, including a bone scan and CT scan, are warranted if structural deficiencies are identified. These studies may reveal meta-

static or primary malignant tumors. The nontumorous diseases that could lead to localized structural insufficiency include Paget's disease and hemangioma of bone.

In the face of generalized osteopenia, the differential diagnosis centers on bone marrow abnormality, endocrinopathy, osteoporosis or osteomalacia. An abnormal sedimentation rate, CBC or serum protein electrophoresis suggest a bone marrow disorder, and diagnosis of myeloma, leukemia or other hematological disorder should be considered. If hematological screening studies are negative, blood studies should be done to measure thyroid function, parathyroid function, estrogen and endogenous steroid levels and glucose. Elevations in 24-hr urine collection of hydroxyproline (derived from bone collagen turnover) should be found in high turnover conditions produced by hormonal imbalances. If endocrinopathy studies are negative, the differential diagnosis of osteopenia rests between osteoporosis and osteomalacia. Alkaline phosphatase, calcium, phosphorous and vitamin D levels may be helpful. However, the ultimate diagnosis may require a transilial bone biopsy to differentiate osteomalacia and osteoporosis. Unfortunately, osteoid mineralization defects are commonly missed by noninvasive investigation. At The Hospital for Special Surgery, 25% of patients presenting with compression fractures to the orthopaedic service had endocrinopathies; 2% had marrow abnormalities; and 30% demonstrated abnormal hyperosteoidosis on their bone biopsy. The remainder had pure osteoporosis or a combination of osteoporosis plus one of the above mentioned disorders.

COLLES' FRACTURE

Fractures of the distal radius are indigenous in the population of postmenopausal patients. Abraham Colles' description (15) of 170 years ago can hardly be improved upon today. Although it was classically held that significant deformity of the distal radius can be associated with relatively normal function, it is now clear that the multitude of complications that arise from this injury can be avoided by accurate reduction which restores the normal relationship of the distal radioulnar joint, followed by early mobilization of the hand and upper extremity.

Closed reduction and casting under local or regional anesthesia is the treatment of choice for most Colles' fractures. In the absence of severe dorsal comminution or extensive intraarticular involvement, this method leads to accurate reduction, rapid healing, and early return of function. The key to a stable reduction is achieving a ''hooked'' reduction of the volar cortex that provides a hinge to maintain dis-

traction force on the intact dorsal periosteum. An adequate reduction implies no radial shortening and at least a neutral angulation of the distal radial articular surface in the anteroposterior plane (Fig. 10). Without this complete reduction, the fracture complex remains unstable and can readily settle in plaster. Reduced fractures then require two weeks of above elbow immobilization, followed by four weeks of below elbow immobilization. The major complications of this form of treatment occur secondary to overly constrictive dressings, that results in swelling of fingers and late stiffness, and attempts to hold unstable fractures in an exaggerated position of palmar flexion, that results in carpal tunnel compression, wrist and finger stiffness and possibly a high incidence of reflex sympathetic dystrophy (23). Sarmiento (55, 56) has recently advocated a functional cast brace method of treatment that allows early hand function in an attempt to avoid these complications, but recent reports suggest that results are not significantly different from conventional casting (64).

Clancy has recently reported a very favorable experience with Kirschner wire fixation of Colles' fracture that allows use of closed reduction and casting in more unstable fracture patterns (13). Unstable, severely comminuted fractures of the distal radius are best treated by distraction devices, either pins in plaster or external fixation (17, 25). These methods allow early hand and elbow motion if properly applied but can result in fairly significant wrist stiffness. We, therefore, advocate no more than six weeks of treatment by this method. After this immobilization, the arm is placed in a cast or removable splints for additional time if the fracture is not sufficiently healed. Grossly displaced intraarticular factures are probably best dealt with by open reduction of the distal radial articular surface and bone grafting of metaphyseal comminution combined with either external or internal fixation.

In all cases, prompt reduction and stabilization of these fractures under adequate anesthesia and avoidance of constrictive dressings or exaggerated positions are the most important

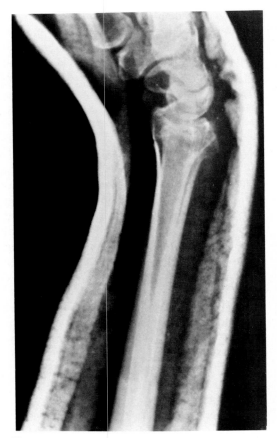

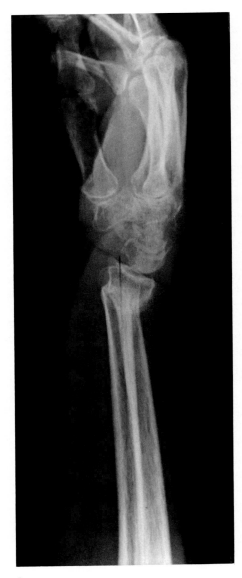

A

FIG. 10. **A:** Lateral radiograph of a Colles' fracture with dorsal displacement. **B:** Lateral radiograph after the fracture has been reduced. A stable reduction was achieved. Stability is gained by exact reduction of the volar cortex seen in this case.

elements of successful outcome. The method of treatment chosen must allow adequate motion of the fingers and upper extremity and should be followed by vigorous, supervised physical therapy until maximum function is restored.

PELVIC FRACTURES

Pelvic fractures, particularly about the pubic rami, occur frequently in the osteoporotic population. They may be more frequent in those individuals with underlying hyperosteoidosis.

Therapy is predominantly directed toward resolving the symptoms rather than restoring skeletal continuity. Healing always occurs even with conservative management. Mobilization using a walker initially, followed by crutches may be sufficient. Pain should be the guide for weight-bearing, and no operative intervention is warranted.

SUMMARY

We have discussed the biomechanical and biomaterial properties of bone and emphasized the microenvironment. The microdensity of bone tissues determines the resistance to compressive forces. The structural orientation of bone critically determines its ability to withstand torsion and bending forces. Highly remodeled bone is brittle and fractures easily due to the multiple reversal planes within the bony plates. Conversely, augmentation of bone on the periphery by modeling leads to increased material microstrength and structural macrostrength. Consequently, appositional modeling augments while remodeling diminishes bone strength.

Hip fractures, spinal fractures, Colles' fractures and pelvic fractures have been discussed in terms of their pathophysiology and treatment. An algorithm has been presented for the differential diagnosis of patients presenting with a recently discovered spinal compression fracture.

The hallmark of osteoporosis treatment is its prevention. Reasonable nutrition, including appropriate calcium and vitamin D, preservation of proper hormonal balance (estrogen supplementation), coupled with appropriate exercise is the essence of preventing the development of osteoporosis, particularly in the high risk individual (40). Truly osteoporotic individuals require more than repair of their fractures. Appropriate reestablishment of exercise and nutrition in these individuals may lead to protection of the remaining bone mass and enhance fracture healing. Specific therapeutic modalities for the treatment of osteoporosis including sodium fluoride, estrogen/progesterone, calcitonin and bone remodeling programs have been discussed in greater detail elsewhere in this volume.

ACKNOWLEDGMENT

This manuscript was supported in part by The National Institutes of Health (2P 30 CA 29502).

REFERENCES

1. Aitken, M. (1984): Management of osteoporosis. In: *Osteoporosis in Clinical Practice,* edited by M. Aitken. John Wright and Sons, Ltd., Bristol.
2. Arnold, W.D., Lyden, J.P., and Minkoff, J. (1974): Treatment of intracapsular fractures of the femoral neck. *J. Bone Joint Surg.,* 56-A:254–262.
3. Arnold, W.D. (1984): The effect of early weight-bearing on the stability of femoral neck fractures treated with Knowles pins. *J. Bone Joint Surg.,* 66-A:847–852.
4. Avioli, L.V. (1981): Postmenopausal osteoporosis: Prevention versus cure. *Fed. Proc.* 40:2418–2422.
5. Bochner, R., Lyden, J.P., and Burstein, A.H. (1987): Follow-up of bipolar hemiarthroplasties performed for femoral neck fracture. Twenty-first Meeting of American Academy of Orthopedic Surgeons, San Francisco, January, 1987.
6. Baker, G.I., and Barrick, E.F. (1978): Follow-up notes on articles previously published in the Journal: Deyerle treatment of femoral neck fractures. *J. Bone Joint Surg.,* 60-A:269–271.
7. Barr, D. (1985): Doctoral Thesis. University of West Virginia.
8. Bartucci, E.J., Gonzalez, M.H., Cooperman, D.R., Freedberg, H.I., Barmada, R., and Laros, G.S. (1985): The effect of adjunctive methylmethacrylate on failures of fixation and function in patients with intertrochanteric fractures and osteoporosis. *J. Bone Joint Surg.,* 67-A:1094–1107.
9. Cann, C.E., Genant, H.K., Ettinger, B., and Gordan, G.S. (1980): Spinal mineral loss in oophorectomized women: Determination by quantitative computed tomography. *J.A.M.A.,* 244:2056–2059.
10. Carter, D.R., and Hayes, W.C. (1977): The compressive behavior of bone as a two-phase porous structure. *J. Bone Joint Surg.,* 59-A:954–962.
11. Cassebaum, W.H., and Parkes, J.C. (1973): Treatment of displaced intracapsular fractures of the hip utilizing the Richards screw. *J. Bone Joint Surg.,* 55-A:1309. (Abstr.)
12. Chapman, M.W., Bowman, W.E., Csongradi, J.J., and Day, L.J. Trafton, P.G., and Bovill, E.G., Jr. (1981): The use of Ender's pins on extracapsular fractures of the hip. *J. Bone Joint Surg.,* 63-A:14–28.
13. Clancy, G.J. (1986): Percutaneous Kirschner wire fixation of Colles' fractures. *J. Bone Joint Surg.,* 67-A:1008–1014.

14. Clawson, D.K. (1964): Intracapsular fractures of the femur treated by the sliding screw plate fixation method. *J. Trauma*, 4:753–756.

15. Colles, A. (1814): On the fracture of the carpal extremity of the radius. *Edinb. Med. Surg. J.*, 10:182–186.

16. Conrad, J.J. (1971): Medial displacement fixation of unstable intertrochanteric fractures of the hip. *Bull. Hosp. Joint Dis.*, 32:54–62.

17. Cooney, W.P., III (1980): External mini-fixations: Clinical applications and techniques. In: *Continuing Educational Course on External Fixation*, edited by R.M. Johnston, pp. 155–171. Year Book Medical Publishers, Chicago.

18. Dimon, J.H., III, and Hughston, J.C. (1967): Unstable intertrochanteric fractures of the hip. *J. Bone Joint Surg.*, 49-A:440–450.

19. Einhorn, T.A., Bonnarens, F., and Burstein, A.H. (1986): The contributions of dietary protein and mineral to the healing of experimental fractures. A biomechanical study. *J. Bone Joint Surg.*, 68-A:1389–1395.

20. Fielding, J.W. (1980): The telescoping Pugh nail in the surgical management of the displaced intracapsular fracture of the femoral neck. *Clin. Orthop.*, 152:123–130.

21. Frost, H.M. (1969): Tetracycline-based histological analysis of bone remodeling. *Calcif. Tissue Res.*, 3:211–237.

22. Gallagher, J.C., Melton, L.J., Riggs, B.L., and Bergstralh, E (1980): Epidemiology of fractures of the proximal femur in Rochester, Minnesota. *Clin. Orthop.*, 150:163–171.

23. Gelberman, R.H., Szabo, R.M., and Mortensen, W.W. (1984): Carpal tunnel pressures and wrist position in patients with Colles' fractures. *J. Trauma*, 24:747–749.

24. Genant, H.K., Cann, C.E., Ettinger, B., and Gordan, G.S. (1984): Quantitative computed tomography of vertebral spongiosa: A sensitive method for detecting early bone loss after oophorectomy. *Ann. Intern. Med.*, 97:699–705.

25. Green, D.P. (1975): Pins and plaster treatment of comminuted fractures of the distal end of the radius. *J. Bone Joint Surg.*, 57-A:304–310.

26. Healey, J.H., and Lane, J.M. (1985): Structural scoliosis in osteoporotic women. *Clin. Orthop.*, 195:216–223.

27. Heppenstall, B.R. (1980): Fracture healing. In: *Fracture Treatment and Healing*, edited by R.B. Hepenstall, pp. 35–64. W.B. Saunders Company, Philadelphia.

28. Hodgson, A.R., and Stock, F.E. (1960): Anterior spine fusion for the treatment of tuberculosis of the spine: The operative findings and results of treatment in the first one-hundred cases. *J. Bone Joint Surg.*, 42-A:295–310.

29. Holbrook, T.L., Grazier, K.L., Kelsey, J.L., and Stauffer, R.N. (1984): *Human and Economic Impact of Injuries and Crippling Disorders of the Musculoskeletal System*. American Academy of Orthopaedic Surgeons, Chicago.

30. Holbrook, T.L., Grazier, K., Kelsey, J.L., and Stauffer, R.N. (1984): Specific musculoskeletal conditions. In: *The Frequency of Occurrence, Impact and Cost of Selected Musculoskeletal Conditions in the United States*. pp. 24–72. American Academy of Orthopaedic Surgeons, Chicago.

31. Jacobson, P.C., Beaver, W., Grubb, S.A., Taft, T.N., and Talmage, R.V. (1984): Bone density in women: College athletes and older athletic women. *J. Orthop Res.*, 2:328–332.

32. Jensen, G.F., Christiansen, C., Boesen, J., Hegedus, V., and Transbol, I. (1982): Epidemiology of postmenopausal spinal and long bone fractures. *Clin. Orthop.*, 166:75–81.

33. Johnston, C.C., Jr., Norton, J.A., Jr., Khairi, R.A., and Longcope, C. (1979): Age-related bone loss. In: *Osteoporosis II*, edited by U.S. Barzel, pp. 91–100. Grune and Stratton, New York.

34. Jowsey, J. (1977): Bone morphology: Bone structure. In: *Metabolic Diseases of Bone*, edited by C.B. Sledge, pp. 41–47. W.B. Saunders Company, Philadelphia.

35. Kenzora, J.E., McCarthy, R.E., Lowell, J.D., and Sledge, C.G. (1984): Hip fracture mortality: Relation to age, treatment, preoperative illness, time of surgery, and complications. *Clin. Orthop.*, 186:45–56.

36. Lane, J.M. (1980): Metabolic bone disease and fracture healing. In: *Fracture Treatment and Healing*, edited by R.B. Heppenstall, pp. 946–962. W.B. Saunders Company, Philadelphia.

37. Lane, J.M., Healey, J.H., Schwartz, E., Vigorita, V.J., Schneider, R., Einhorn, T.A., Suda, M., and Robbins, W.C. (1984): Treatment of osteoporosis with sodium fluoride and calcium: Effects of vertebral fracture incidence and bone histomorphometry. *Orthop. Clin. North Am.*, 15:729–745.

38. Lane, J.M., Vigorita, V.J., and Falls, M. (1984): Osteoporosis: Current diagnosis and treatment. *Geritarics*, 39:40–47.

39. Lane, J.M., and Vigorita, V.J. (1985): Osteoporosis. *Univ. Pennsylvania Orthop. J.*, 1:22.

40. Lane, J.M. (1985): Osteoporosis as a preventable nutritional disease. *J. Clin. Med. Nutr.*, Apr:23.

41. Matković, V., Kostial, K., and Šimonović, I., Buzina, R., Brodarec, A., and Nordin, B.E.C. (1979): Bone status and fracture rates in two regions of Yugoslavia. *Am. J. Clin. Nutr.*, 32:540–549.

42. Martin, B.R., Pickett, J.C., and Zinaich, S. (1980): Studies of skeletal remodeling in aging men. *Clin. Orthop.*, 149:268–282.

43. Martin, R.B., and Atkinson, P.J. (1977): Age and sex-related changes in the structure and strength of the human femoral shaft. *J. Biomech.*, 10:223–231.

44. Melton, L.J., III, and Riggs, B.L. (1983): Epidemiology of age-related fractures. In: *The Oteoporotic Syndrome: Detection, Prevention, and Treatment*, edited by L.V. Avioli, pp. 45–72. Grune and Stratton, New York.

45. Møller, B.N., Lucht, U., Grymer, F., and Bartholdy, N.J. (1984): Instability of trochanteric hip fractures following internal fixation. *Acta Orthop. Scand.*, 55:517–520.

46. Moss, M.L. (1980): The design of bones. In: *Scientific Foundations of Orthopaedics and Trauma-*

tology, edited by R. Owen, J. Goodfellow, and P. Bullough, pp. 59–66. W.B. Saunders Company, Philadelphia.

47. Olerud, S. Stark, A., and Gillstrom, P. (1980): Malrotation following Ender nailing. *Clin. Orthop.*, 147:139–142.

48. Rao, J.P., Banzon, M.T., Weiss, A.B., and Rayhack, J. (1983): Treatment of unstable intertrochanteric fractures with anatomic reduction and compression hip screw fixation. *Clin. Orthop.*, 175:65–71.

49. Riggs, B.L., and Melton, L.J., III (1983): Evidence for two distinct syndromes of involutional osteoporosis. *Am. J. Med.*, 75:899–901.

50. Riggs, B.L., Seeman, E., Hodgson, S.F., Taves, D.R., and O'Fallon, W.M. (1982): Effect of the fluoride/calcium regimen on vertebral fracture occurrence in postmenopausal osteoporosis: Comparison with conventional therapy. *N. Engl. J. Med.*, 306:446–450.

51. Rigotti, N.A., Nussbaum, S.R., Herzog, D.B., and Neer, R.M. (1984): Osteoporosis in women with anorexia nervosa. *N. Engl. J. Med.*, 311:1601–1606.

52. Russin, L.A., and Sonni, A. (1980): Treatment of intertrochanteric and subtrochanteric fractures with Enders' intramedullary rods. *Clin. Orthop.*, 148:203–212.

53. Salvati, E.A., Artz, T., Aglietti, P., and Asnis, S.E. (1974): Endoprostheses in the treatment of femoral neck fractures. *Orthop. Clin. North Am.*, 5:757–777.

54. Sarmiento, A. (1963): Intertrochanteric fractures of the femur. *J. Bone Joint Surg.*, 45-A:706–722.

55. Sarmiento, A., Pratt, G.W., Berry, N.C., and Sinclair, W.F. (1975): Colles' fractures: Functional bracing in supination. *J. Bone Joint Surg.*, 57-A:311–317.

56. Sarmiento, A., Zagorski, J.B., and Sinclair, W.F. (1980): Functional bracing of Colles' fractures: A prospective study of immobilization in supination vs. pronation. *Clin. Orthop.*, 146:175–183.

57. Scileppi, K.P., Stulberg, B., Vigorita, V.J., Lane, J.M., Vossburgh, R., Bullough, P.G., and Arnold, W.D. (1981): Bone histomorphometry in femoral neck fractures. *Surg. Forum*, 32:543–545.

58. Sevitt, S. (1980): Healing of fractures in man. Chapter 32. In: *Scientific Foundations and Orthopaedics and Traumatology*, edited by R. Owen, J. Goodfellow, and P. Bullough, pp. 258–273. W.B. Saunders Company, Philadelphia.

59. Simonen, O., and Laitinen, O. (1985): Does fluoridation of drinking-water prevent bone fragility and osteoporosis? *Lancet*, 2:432–434.

60. Smith, D.M., Oliver, C.H., Ryder, C.T., and Stinchfield, F.E. (1975): Complications of Austin Moore arthroplasty: Their incidence and relationship to potential predisposing factors. *J. Bone Joint Surg.*, 57-A:31–33.

61. Smith, R.W., Jr., and Walker, R.R. (1964): Femoral expansion in aging women: Implications for osteoporosis and fractures. *Science*, 145:156–157.

62. Spencer, H. (1982): Osteoporosis: Goals of therapy. *Hosp. Prac.*, 17:131–148.

63. Steier, A., Gegalia, I., Schwartz, A., Rodan, A. (1967): Effect of vitamin D_2 and fluoride on experimental bone fracture healing in rats. *J. Dent. Res.*, 46:675–680.

64. Stewart, H.D., Innes, A.R., and Burke, F.D. (1984): Functional cast bracing for Colles' fractures: A comparison between cast-bracing and conventional plaster casts. *J. Bone Joint Surg.*, 66-B:749–753.

65. Tadduni, G.T., and Brighton, C.T. (1985): The treatment of disuse osteoporosis in the rat with a capacitively coupled electrical signal. *Orthop. Trans.*, 9:227–228. (Abstr.)

66. Tobis, J.S. (1970): Physical medicine for the osteoporotic patient. In: *Osteoporosis*, edited by U.S. Barzel, pp. 133–139. Grune and Stratton, New York.

67. Trotter, M., and Peterson, R.R. (1967): Transverse diameter of the femur: On roentgenograms and on bones. *Clin. Orthop.*, 52:233–239.

68. Urist, M.R., Gurvey, M.S., and Fareed, D.O. (1970): Long-term observations on aged women with pathological osteoporosis. In: *Osteoporosis*, edited by U.S. Barzel, pp. 3–37. Grune and Stratton, New York.

69. Wahner, H.W., Dunn, W.L., and Riggs, B.L. (1983): Noninvasive bone mineral measurements. *Sem. Nucl. Med.*, 13:282–289.

70. Wahner, H.W., Dunn, W.L., and Riggs, B.L. (1984): Assessment of bone mineral. Part 2. *J. Nucl. Med.*, 25:1241–1253.

71. Wallach, S. (1978): Management of osteoporosis. *Hosp. Prac.*, 13(Dec.):91–98.

72. Wolff, J. (1892): *Das Gesetz der Transformation de Enochen*. Hirschwald, Berlin.

73. Wright, T.M., and Hayes, W.C. (1980): Mechanics of fracture and fracture propagation. Chapter 31. In: *Scientific Foundations of Orthopaedics and Traumatology*, edited by R. Owen, J. Goodfellow, and P. Bullough, pp. 252–258. W.B. Saunders Company, Philadelphia.

Osteoporosis: Etiology, Diagnosis, and Management, edited by B. Lawrence Riggs and L. Joseph Melton, III. Raven Press, New York © 1988.

19

Exercise and Physical Therapy

Mehrsheed Sinaki

Department of Physical Medicine and Rehabilitation, Mayo Clinic and Mayo Foundation; Mayo Medical School, Rochester, Minnesota 55905

To fulfill its function as mechanical support for the body, bone must be able to withstand the stresses of daily living (Chapter 4, *this volume*). It follows that physical activity should influence skeletal integrity—inactivity may be conducive to age-related bone loss, while exercise could confer prophylactic benefit. Activity must also be considered in the management of patients with symptomatic osteoporosis. This chapter reviews the effect of physical activity on bone mass and summarizes current knowledge of physical therapeutic measures for osteoporosis, especially spinal osteoporosis with vertebral fracture.

IMMOBILIZATION AND BONE LOSS

Bone is exposed to constantly changing patterns of loading and adapts to these changes through alterations in bone mass and skeletal geometry (28). The concept that a bone develops the structure most suited to resist the forces acting upon it is often credited to Wolff, who in 1892 postulated that when a bone is bent under a mechanical load, it modifies its structure by bony apposition in the concavity and by resorption in the convexity (89). The influence of this principle, known as Wolff's law, on bone modeling and remodeling is covered in Chapter 18 (*this volume*). Since Wolff's time, studies

have shown that bone is affected positively by activity (40) and that mechanical stress and strain on bones as a result of muscle tension and pressure help prevent bone loss (1,29,85). Conversely, bone is influenced negatively by reduction of its load-carrying role by fracture fixation implants and prosthetic joint replacements (12,55,80,81), while inactivity and the absence of pressure transmitted to bone or the absence of tension applied to bone by muscle or both (89) are thought to produce disuse osteoporosis.

Immobilization and weightlessness clearly result in accelerated bone loss (10). Stevenson in 1952 (75) studied 85 patients who were immobilized for various diseases and found bedridden patients to have radiographic reductions in bone density that he attributed to disturbances in calcium metabolism. More recently, Krølner and Toft examined 34 adults hospitalized for low back pain who required therapeutic bed rest; the bone mineral content in the lumbar spine decreased about 0.9% per week as assessed with dual photon absorptiometry (42). An even greater rate of trabecular bone loss occurred among adolescent girls at bed rest after operation for scoliosis (30), and in patients with spinal cord injuries (51). Early increases in bone turnover have generally been noted throughout the skeleton in quadriplegia

(56), although bone loss from the lower extremities may predominate (87). After the loss of 30% or more of trabecular bone volume, however, a new steady state is reached and bone mass is then maintained (32,51). Nonetheless, fracture risk may be increased in such patients (17,87).

Similar metabolic effects have been reported in healthy individuals at complete bed rest. Deitrick et al. (20) found that calcium loss increased for about five to six weeks in normal healthy persons in bed with plaster fixation of the lower extremities and then maintained a consistently high level until function was resumed. Concomitant with this phenomenon was an associated nitrogen loss, an indication that both calcium and protein were being lost more rapidly than under normal conditions. Muscle strength deteriorated during the period of immobilization, but no change was seen in the skeleton using the insensitive technique of serial radiographs on two subjects (20). In another study, in which three healthy men were restricted to complete bed rest for 30 to 36 weeks, there were marked elevations in urinary calcium, phosphorus, and hydroxyproline levels associated with loss of approximately a third of bone mass from the central os calcis (22). These data suggest that bed rest can lead to excessive bone loss and to clinically important osteoporosis.

Significant bone loss was also found among astronauts on early flights, although the amount of loss did not correlate well with the duration of time in space (49). Subsequent studies on the Apollo flights confirmed the loss of bone mineral from the os calcis in some but not all crew members, but the previous observation of substantial bone loss from the distal forearm was not replicated (83). Data from the Skylab program also identified bone loss as an important potential problem for prolonged space flight. The levels of loss observed after 59 and 84 days were thought to be of no clinical concern, but the negative calcium balance was estimated at about four g per month; the risk of fracture could be high if such losses persist during longer flights (63). Although there is some evidence that exercise and load bearing in space can reduce bone loss, the possibly adverse influences of very long or repetitive flights have not been well-quantified (64) and there are indications that bone mass lost in space is not completely recouped upon return to earth (79).

The determinants of disuse osteoporosis are less clear. It seems that weight-bearing and physical activity both act as mechanical stimuli for bone growth and remodeling (45), although various groups have argued for the predominance of one or the other. The value of weight-bearing in preserving bone mass was emphasized by Whedon and Shorr (86); in several studies they described, patients lost calcium while they were confined to bed, and this loss did not subside until they were ambulatory. Direct standing for two or more hr per day has reversed the changes in mineral metabolism induced by bed rest (10,36) but supine exercises performed rigorously for as long as four hours daily seem ineffective (62,66).

Wyse and Pattee (90), on the other hand, postulated that the "stresses and strains" on bone result primarily from muscular contractions rather than weight-bearing. Using a tilt table, they evaluated the direct effect of weight-bearing through the lower extremities in patients with paraplegia. Such weight-bearing did not affect calcium, phosphorus, or nitrogen metabolism in these patients, and the disuse osteoporosis associated with paraplegia did not respond to weight-bearing (90). In 1961, Abramson and Delagi (3) reviewed the literature and reexamined Abramson's earlier (2) hypothesis regarding the necessity of weight-bearing for the prevention of disuse osteoporosis. They also concluded that weight-bearing is much less effective than muscle contraction in limiting bone loss and suggested that muscle action is the most effective stress on bone for maintaining bone mass.

Although there is evidence to support the concept that the absence of pressure forces on the skeleton is primarily responsible for disuse osteopenia, possibly by altering piezoelectric forces within the bone (9), the exact mechanism whereby bone mineral is lost is uncertain (31,76). Biochemical studies in paraplegia reveal that rates of bone formation and bone resorption are both increased during the early stages but that it is the disproportionate increase in bone resorption which appears to be the basic pathologic effect (14). This probably results from increased remodeling activation, along with a remodeling imbalance, e.g., more bone is resorbed than is formed in each cycle (Chapter 2 *this volume*). In severe cases, extensive resorption is seen in all three bone envelopes—endosteal, Haversian and periosteal (38). The bone resorption leads to hypercalcemia, increased urinary calcium, phosphorus, and hydroxyproline and to negative calcium and phosphorus balance (76), while increased urinary nitrogen is probably due to the muscle atrophy that accompanies disuse (1). These changes result in depressed serum iPTH levels, lowered plasma $1,25(OH)_2D_3$ and diminished intestinal calcium absorption (76).

Attempts to reverse these effects with diet or drugs have not been very successful. Freeman (27) investigated the use of vitamin D for prevention or reduction of the loss of calcium in patients with spinal cord injuries. Liberal doses of vitamin D in more than 25 patients failed to alter the excretion of calcium, and no change was noted when administration of vitamin D was discontinued. More recent attempts with vitamin D, calcitonin, or diphosphonates have achieved little more by way of preventing bone loss in patients at bed rest (60,67), but calcitonin (53) and diphosphonates (52) have shown some sparing effect in paraplegia.

Although mechanical forces must be present to maintain bone mass, it is difficult to extrapolate data from the extremes of space flight and immobilization to bone loss during aging. While the effect of inactivity on bones has been recognized for years (20,42), the potential effect of inactivity on postmenopausal osteoporosis has been emphasized only recently (92). Thus, decreased physical activity with aging—nearly half of elderly individuals are sedentary compared with less than a fifth of young adults (13)—may lead to a reduction in muscle mass (16) because the less that muscle contraction is used, the less muscle bulk is maintained. This tenet was expressed by Ayre

(8) and Eccles (25), who believed that contraction through the whole range of joint motion was important. Moreover, a substantial and increasing proportion of people are disabled as they grow older (46), and this has a negative influence on activity as well.

Further, muscle mass and bone mass are directly related. Doyle et al. (23) compared the ash weight of the third lumbar vertebral body with the weight of the left psoas muscle from 46 routine autopsy cases and found a significant correlation. They proposed that the weight of a muscle reflects the force that it exerts on the bones to which it is attached and that muscle weight is an important determinant of bone mass. This position is supported by similar observations in vivo of a positive correlation between bone mineral density of the lumbar spine and strength of the extensor muscles of the back (70). Likewise, associations between bone mass and exercise history or fitness are reported by some (11,15,61) but not all workers (39,91,93).

Consequently, the parallel decline in muscle mass and bone mass with age, at least in men (78), probably is more than coincidence (26), and inactivity may account for some of the bone loss previously associated with aging *per se* (6). It may be possible to increase muscle mass and fitness through exercise, however, even in elderly individuals (7,74). Thus, there is some hope that bone mass can also be increased or at least the rate of loss slowed (see below).

PHYSICAL ACTIVITY AND BONE GAIN

While physical inactivity has been implicated in bone loss, exercise has been suggested as one of the determinants of bone gain. The effects of exercise are most dramatically illustrated in studies of athletes. Jones et al. (40) studied roentgenograms of the humeri in a group of 84 professional tennis players and found pronounced bone hypertrophy on the playing side. The cortical thickness on the playing side was 34.9% more in men and 28.4% more in women than that on the contralateral side. Similarly, bone density measured with single photon absorptiometry was greater in the dominant arm of adolescent baseball players (84) and in the favored leg among a diverse group of athletes (57). However, benefit is confined to exercised limbs. While Huddleston et al. (34) confirmed the excess bone mass in the playing arm of experienced senior tennis players compared with the contralateral arm and the greater mass of the playing arm compared with the dominant arm of normal elderly men, the nonplaying arm of the tennis players was no different from the nondominant arm of the other men.

Although very intensive physical activity can augment bone mass over a fairly short period of time (50), no improvement was seen with a less severe regimen (19), and long-term athletic activity is probably more important. Nilsson et al. (58) compared the bone mineral content of 24 male weight lifters and 21 professional ballet dancers (8 men and 13 women) with that of age-matched healthy controls. Bone mineral content in the proximal tibia and fibula, measured with photon absorptiometry, was higher in both dancers and weight lifters. Increased width of these bones was found predominantly in the dancers, even though they were shorter and weighed less than their controls. These data suggest that physical activity, when started early in life, results in high bone mineral content and increased dimensions of the bones of the lower limbs. This supposition is borne out in studies of older distance runners, who have increased axial and appendicular bone mass (5,19,44). A high reservoir of bone mass at midlife may delay the clinical manifestations of involutional osteoporosis in later life. Although attention has recently been drawn to potential adverse consequences of prolonged exertion, as observed in female marathon runners who became amenorrheic (24), this should not be interpreted as a denial of the value of exercise in maintaining skeletal integrity.

Limited experimental evidence supports the hypothesis that physical activity may also slow involutional bone loss. Aloia et al. (4) evaluated the effect of exercise on the prevention of involutional bone loss in 18 postmenopausal women. One group of subjects exercised three times a week for about one hr, while the others continued with their usual daily activities. Total and regional bone mass were measured before and after one year of exercise. Bone mineral content of the radius did not change significantly in either group, but total body calcium increased in the exercise group and decreased in the sedentary group. In contrast, an increase in bone mineral content of the radius was seen in a small group of nursing home residents who exercised 30 min a day three times a week (71) and after two or three years of individualized aerobic exercise among a group of middle-aged women (72). Bone loss in the radius was less and the moment of inertia greater among postmenopausal women engaged in a program of aerobic dancing (88). In each of these studies, nonexercising controls generally continued to lose bone. Krølner et al. (43) found no effect of exercise on bone mineral content of the forearm among 31 women ages 50 to 73 years with previous Colles' fractures. However, after eight months of exercise, one hr twice weekly, bone mineral content of the lumbar spine had increased by 3.5% in the exercise group but had decreased 2.7% among the unexercised controls. The authors suggested that the discrepancy between forearm and spine might be due to a differential exercise response in trabecular and cortical bone and concluded that exercise can inhibit or reverse involutional bone loss from the lumbar vertebrae in normal women (43). However, none of these investigations randomized the exercise intervention and the outcome was not assessed in a blinded manner. Thus, the benefit of moderate exercise of the sort that older individuals might undertake has not been firmly established (18).

PHYSICAL MANAGEMENT OF OSTEOPOROSIS

Symptoms of Osteoporosis

Osteoporosis is asymptomatic until fractures occur. While limb fractures are usually evident clinically, some vertebral fractures, particularly the wedge fractures associated with type II (senile) osteoporosis, may not bring the patient to a physician's attention. Limb fractures aside, the osteoporotic patient who seeks medical care is usually one in whom the reduction of bone mass is so advanced that vertebral compression fractures are identifiable roentgenographically. Such fractures occur most frequently in the lower thoracic and upper lumbar areas, but the midthoracic and lower lumbar vertebrae are also often affected (66). Cervical and upper thoracic vertebrae are rarely, if ever, involved.

Vertebral fractures are often manifested by the appearance of pain at the involved level of the spine. In patients with symptomatic osteoporosis, back pain is usually a major complaint and can be acute or chronic. The pain may develop gradually or occur suddenly when a patient falls, lifts a heavy object, or performs some other activity. Indeed, acute pain that occurs in the absence of a previously known fracture should strongly suggest a vertebral compression fracture, especially in a patient in whom osteoporosis has previously been diagnosed. Sometimes a minor fall or even an affectionate hug may lead to fracture of a vertebra or rib. Some vertebral fractures may not be apparent on roentgenograms for up to four weeks after the injury (59), but roentgenographic or other evidence (Chapter 7, *this volume*) is necessary for a firm diagnosis of fracture.

Involutional bone loss contributes to the susceptibility of bones to fracture in elderly persons (35,65). While patients can have severe spinal osteoporosis without experiencing vertebral fractures, this is improbable unless routine activities such as lifting and bending are avoided. Certainly, their susceptibility is much greater than that of women without the disease, and it is essentially only a matter of time before exposure to even mild trauma will cause vertebral compression. Fortunately, compression rather than displacement of vertebral bones is the rule. Treatment of compression fractures must focus on relief of pain and prevention of further fractures. The fractures will heal in time, although the resulting bone deformity will remain.

Acute Pain

Acute back pain is usually due to a recent vertebral fracture. It can be diminished by bed rest for up to one to two weeks (on a hard mattress with a soft covering such as synthetic sheepskin or a two-inch foam pad), although prolonged bed rest can aggravate bone loss. The patient should be in the supine position with a thin pillow under the head and a pillow of regular thickness under the knees to avoid undue strain on the spine. Some patients may have less pain if they lie on the side rather than on the back. This position should be allowed, and a small pillow should be used to fill the hollow of the flank, if present. With this latter position, the patient usually feels more comfortable with hips and knees somewhat flexed. Placing a small pillow between the knees decreases the strain on the lower back caused by adduction at the hip. Proper positioning of the patient and correct use of pillows are crucial factors in the effectiveness of bed rest. The patient may need complete bed rest, be permitted a bedpan, or have bathroom privileges, depending on the intensity of the pain and the discomfort encountered when the upright posture is assumed.

Moderate heat (47) and a gentle massage (41) of the paraspinal muscles will help decrease pain resulting from spasms. Application of heat for 20 to 30 min with an infrared lamp is usually recommended. The distance between the lamp and the area that is to be treated should be about 18 to 24 in. This type of heat application is inexpensive and easy to use. Massage should be done exclusively with gentle stroking because deep massage and heavy pressure may exacerbate the pain.

In addition to physical therapy, mild analgesics may be used when needed to relieve pain. One should be hesitant about using strong analgesics and resort to them only in the most refractory cases, and then only for brief periods. Constipation can be especially distressing to a patient with persistent back pain. Steps should be taken to avoid this problem; if present, it should be treated.

If acute pain persists despite a trial of bed rest, one should consider prescribing a back support for the patient to wear during ambulatory activities. Back supports can be obtained off the shelf or by mail order. However, for small-framed women less than five feet tall, they should probably be custom-fitted. A properly fitted back support is appreciated more than any other treatment measure by most patients. Full-support, rigid polypropylene braces, or bivalved body jackets (Fig. 1), are preferred and usually give the best relief (68). Unfortunately, some patients, usually elderly persons, do not tolerate rigid back braces. These braces are obviously confining, and some of the jackets may weigh as much as four pounds. In these instances, a semirigid (48) thoracolumbar support with shoulder straps is a

good alternative (Fig. 2). The shoulder straps help remind patients with kyphotic posture to avoid stooping. Rigid back braces, which are usually better tolerated by young patients, provide stronger support (48).

Chronic Pain

Chronic pain may be due to vertebral fractures *per se* or may result from kyphotic or scoliotic changes in the spine, with inappropriate stretching of ligaments. In patients with severe kyphosis, pressure of the lower part of the rib cage over the pelvic rim causes significant loin pain and tenderness (82). Therefore, this type of chronic pain needs to be treated primarily with measures that improve posture. These include proper back extension exercises and use of a back support.

Improving the muscular support of the spine by proper strengthening exercises should be

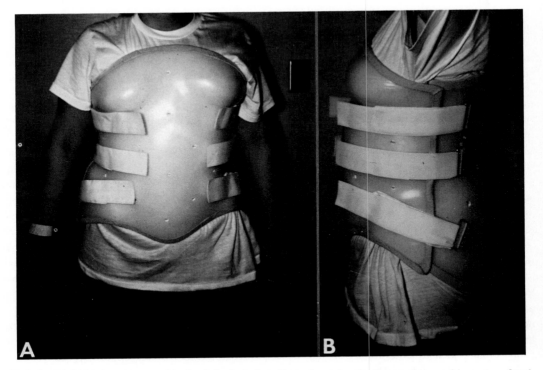

FIG. 1   Rigid back support, or bivalved, body jacket. Brace is made of polypropylene and is custom fitted. **A:** Anterior view. **B:** Lateral view. From Sinaki, ref. 68. By permission of Mayo Foundation.

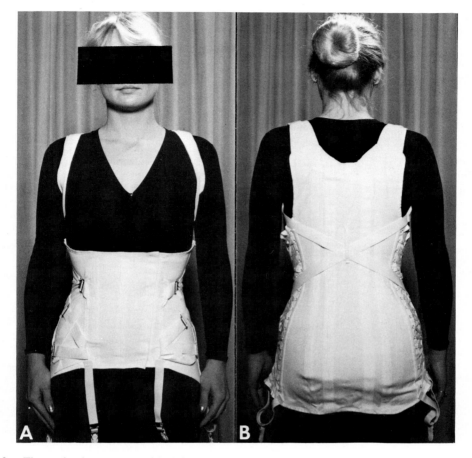

FIG. 2. Thoracolumbar support with rigid or semirigid stays applied on each side of spine. Addition of shoulder straps would further decrease kyphotic posture or remind patient to avoid severe stooping. Proper padding can be added to shoulder straps to decrease pressure over bony prominences. **A:** Anterior view. **B:** Posterior view.

tried whenever possible. Extension exercises are recommended (Fig. 3), along with exercises to reduce lumbar lordosis (Fig. 4). Many persons with back pain, osteoporotic or otherwise, may not realize that weak abdominal muscles also add to their problem. Thus, back extension exercises should be complemented by isometric abdominal muscle strengthening exercises. These improve the muscular support of the spine, but they should be done in a way that does not cause undue ligamentous strain (Figs. 5 and 6). The patient should lie supine while placing the hands under the ischial tuberosities to decrease pelvic tilt, and elevate both

lower extremities 10° to 15° with the knees fully extended (Fig. 7). The degree of lumbar flexion with this exercise does not seem to exceed the degree of lumbar flexion assumed in a usual sitting posture. The exercise program should be individualized for each patient according to the severity of bone loss and the patient's ability, ranging from back extension exercises while prone for some to pectoral stretching and back extension while sitting for others.

Flexion exercises (Fig. 8) are not recommended because they can increase the vertical compression forces on the vertebral body, in-

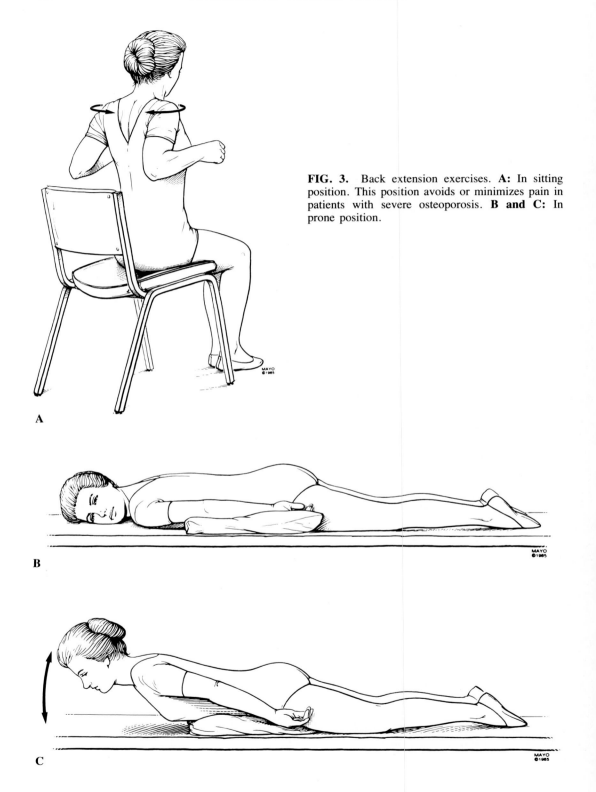

FIG. 3. Back extension exercises. **A:** In sitting position. This position avoids or minimizes pain in patients with severe osteoporosis. **B and C:** In prone position.

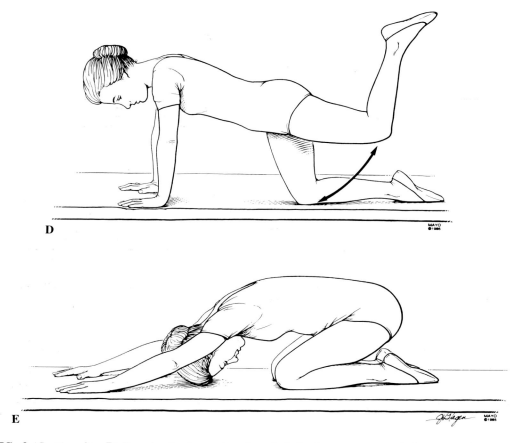

D

E

FIG. 3 *(Continued).* **D:** Exercise for improving strength in lumbar extensors and gluteus maximus muscles. **E:** In cat-stretch position. **A, C,** and **D,** redrawn from Sinaki, ref. 68. By permission of Mayo Foundation.

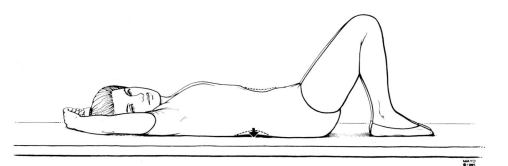

FIG. 4. Exercise to decrease lumbar lordosis with isometric contraction of lumbar flexors. By permission of the Mayo Foundation.

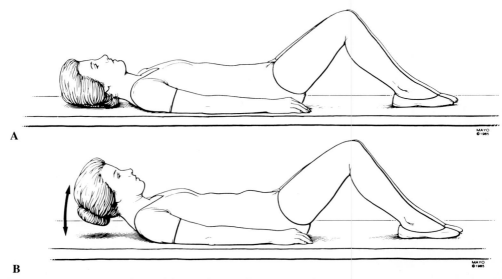

FIG. 5. A and **B:** Technique of isometric exercise to strengthen abdominal muscles. **B,** redrawn from Sinaki, ref. 68. By permission of Mayo Foundation.

crease the possibility of occurrence of anterior wedge fractures, and further increase the kyphosis. In a study by Sinaki and Mikkelsen (69), 59 women with postmenopausal spinal osteoporosis and back pain had been instructed in a treatment program that included back strengthening extension exercises in 25, back strengthening flexion exercises in 9, and combined extension and flexion exercises in 19; no therapeutic exercises were prescribed in 6. Their ages ranged from 49 to 60 years (mean, 56 years). Follow-up ranged from 1 to 6 years (the mean for the groups was 1.4 to 2 years). All the patients had spinal roentgenographic studies before treatment and at follow-up examinations, at which time any further wedging and compression were recorded. Additional vertebral fractures, by group, occurred as follows: extension group, 16%; flexion group, 89%; extension and flexion group, 53%; and no exercise group, 67%. In comparison with the extension group, the occurrence of wedging or compression fractures was significantly higher in the flexion group and in the extension and flexion group. The authors concluded that significantly more vertebral compression fractures occur in patients with postmenopausal

spinal osteoporosis who follow a back strengthening exercise program that involves flexion of the spine than in those who perform extension exercises. Therefore, extension or isometric exercises seem to be more appropriate for patients with postmenopausal osteoporosis.

Back supports are used in an attempt to support and correct posture as much as possible (Figs. 2, 9, 10, 11, and 12). Semirigid or rigid back supports are used, depending on the severity of the spinal osteoporosis and the patient's tolerance. Back supports can correct posture by: (1) reminding the patient to avoid strenuous bending during daily physical activities; (2) preventing the patient from increasing the kyphotic posture, which would increase the compression forces on the spine; (3) providing symptomatic relief of pain as an adjunct to physical therapeutic measures; and (4) decreasing the contributory role of weak abdominal muscles to the kyphotic posture.

The efficiency of lumbar supports was studied by Morris et al. (54), who found that lumbar braces increase the intraabdominal pressure of the wearer at rest by compressing the abdomen and turning the abdomen into a semirigid

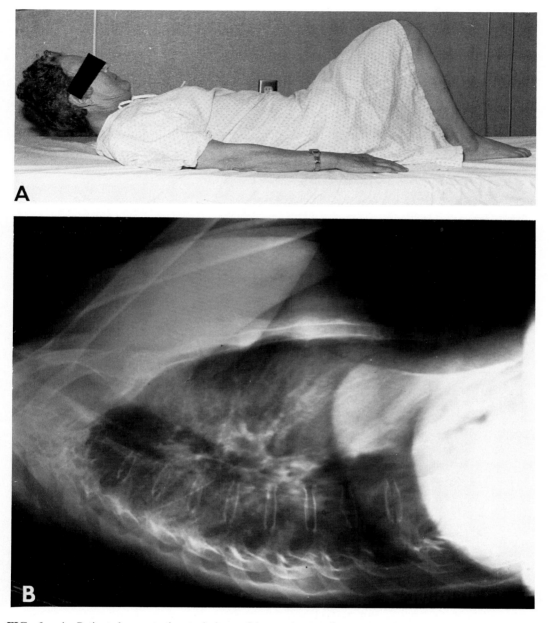

FIG. 6.   A: Patient demonstrating technique of isometric exercise to strengthen abdominal muscles. **B:** Roentgenogram of spine during performance of exercise. Dorsal kyphosis was not increased.

cylinder. This pressure within the abdominal cavity is believed to influence the load on the spine by supporting the trunk anteriorly. When such a support is worn, the weight of the upper half of the body rests both on the vertebral col-

umn and on the semirigid cylinder. In very overweight patients, the amount of compression must be increased to provide the same support. According to the law of Laplace, the tension in the wall of a container necessary to

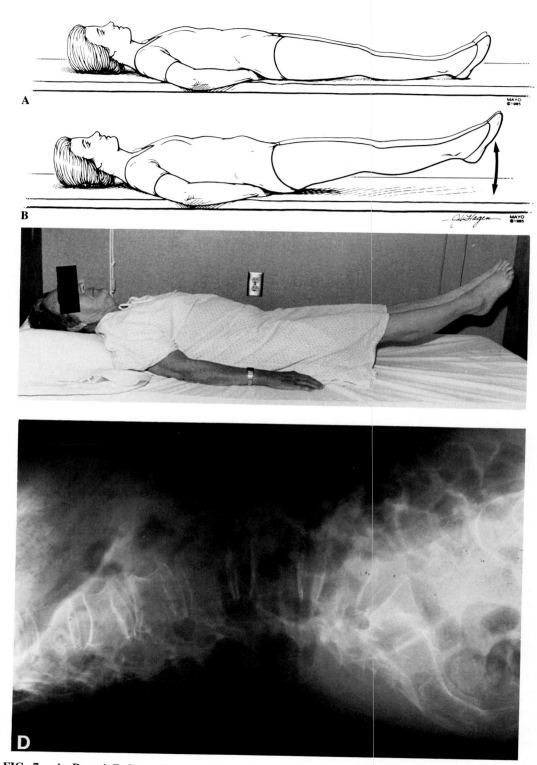

FIG. 7. A, B, and **C:** Isometric exercise to strengthen abdominal muscles. **D:** Roentgenogram of spine during performance of exercise. Lumbar flexion was not increased. **B,** redrawn from Sinaki, ref. 68. By permission of Mayo Foundation.

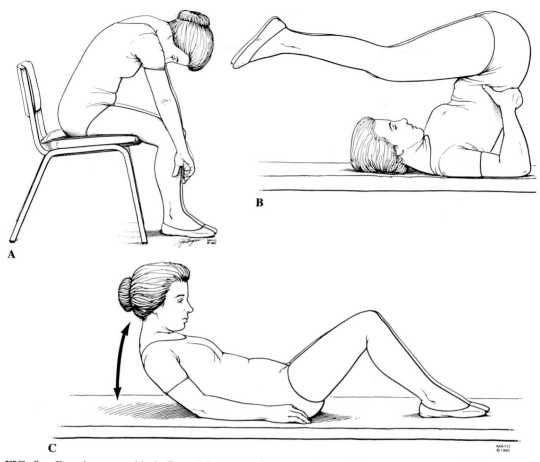

FIG. 8. Exercises to avoid. **A, B,** and **C:** Spinal flexion exercises which are *not* recommended for patients with spinal osteoporosis. **A,** redrawn from Sinaki, ref. 68. By permission of Mayo Foundation.

contain a given pressure on the contents is inversely proportional to the curvature of the wall and directly proportional to the radius of curvature at any point (77). Thus, the tension in the wall of a container required to exert a particular pressure must be greater if the radius of the curvature is greater. To provide an overweight patient with a sufficient amount of intraabdominal pressure to support the lumbar spine, one must increase the tightness of the support. Since this would be very uncomfortable for the overweight patient, the improper bending and stooping postures that expose the spine to undue strain can be eliminated through rigid bracing, which does not have any abdom-

inal contact but prevents the patient from bending by two-point contact at sternum and pubis (Fig. 13).

The purpose of supporting the spine is to permit ambulation while allowing rest for the painful area of the back. Supports used for pain sometimes have to be applied for a prolonged period, in which case atrophy of the back muscles may result. Physiotherapy is necessary in order to prevent this atrophy. The program should include exercises that strengthen the trunk muscles and provide muscular stability. Good results can be obtained by training patients to perform isometric exercises while they are wearing their back supports.

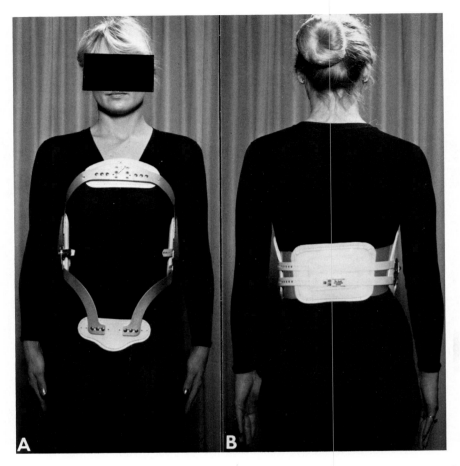

FIG. 9. Jewett brace—used to prevent lumbar and thoracic flexion when patient has acute pain due to recent compression fracture of spine. Proper fitting requires proper contact at base of sternum and over pubic bone. **A:** Anterior view. **B:** Posterior view.

Severe Kyphotic Posture

Complications of vertebral fracture other than pain also need to be considered. Chest deformities disturb relationships between the insertions and origins of respiratory muscles and may tend to flatten the diaphragm. This may lead to easy fatigability, related either to the kyphotic posture with undue ligamentous stretch or to a reduction in vital capacity as the result of the abnormal posture. Treatment of such restrictive disorders includes attempts to loosen contractures of the involved muscles and stiffened joints, improve chest expansion, and rectify the anatomic alterations as much as possible (33). Stretching exercises of the pectoral muscles and other respiratory muscles, such as the intercostals, are important. Deep-breathing exercises combined with pectoral stretching and thoracic spine extension are recommended (Fig. 14). Many of these exercises can even be accomplished when the patient is fitted with a back support, which is sometimes necessary to reduce the pain. Indeed, some patients may be unable to follow the exercise program without back support for the pain. In patients experiencing intercostal pain, attempts

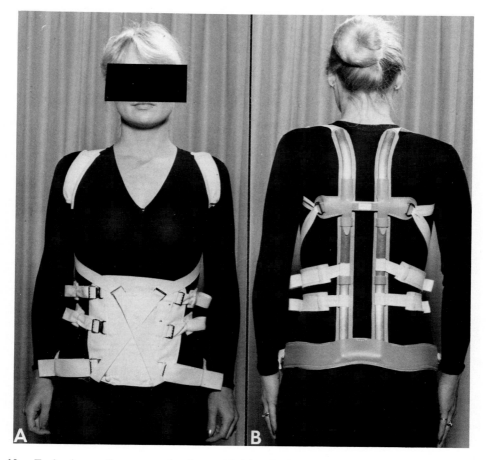

FIG. 10. Taylor brace. Some extension is provided but flexion of spine is not eliminated. **A:** Anterior view. **B:** Posterior view.

should be made to control the kyphosis and ligamentous strain of the thoracic spine by the application of a semirigid thoracolumbar support with shoulder straps (Fig. 15). In patients with multiple compression fractures, severe kyphosis, and pain, application of a molded polypropylene body jacket (Fig. 1) may be feasible. In these patients, the sudden development of spinal pain with exertional activities indicates the need for a spinal roentgenograph.

Patients should also be instructed to avoid stooping during daily activities (73). The patient's desk and chair may need to be adjusted and a thin pillow placed against the backrest of the chair for better support of the lower back.

A hard mattress with plywood applied over the box spring will improve spinal support during sleep and prevent aggravation of the kyphotic posture, which could occur with a soft, sinking mattress. Patients should also try to avoid sleeping on their sides in stooped postures. Synthetic sheepskin over the mattress provides a soft contact over the spinous processes and decreases the possibility of developing pressure sores.

Assistive Devices

The drastic event in osteoporosis is fracture. As noted in previous chapters, osteoporosis is

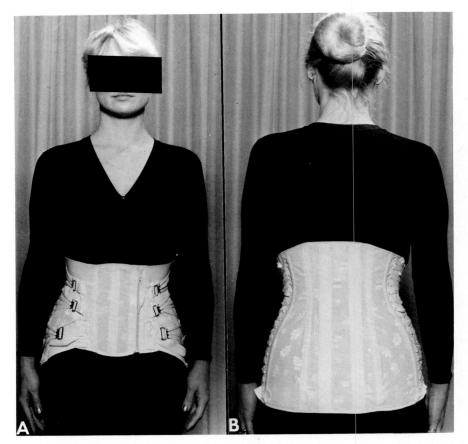

FIG. 11. Lumbosacral support for increasing intraabdominal pressure and improving muscular support of lower back. It mainly supports lower thoracic and lumbosacral spine. Stays may be rigid or semirigid. **A:** Anterior view. **B:** Posterior view.

generally a necessary but not sufficient cause of age-related limb fractures. These are generally associated with a specific episode of trauma, usually a fall. In elderly persons, the prevalence of failing vision, muscle weakness, incoordination, and faulty posture is increased, and falls occur frequently. The use of assistive devices (canes or walkers) is of utmost importance to improve a patient's safety of gait.

Gait-assistive devices include the usual cane, supportive canes with a broader base of support and prongs, walkers, and wheeled

walkers (Fig. 16). If the patient has primarily unilateral low-back pain referred to the buttock and hip areas, the use of a cane in the hand opposite to the painful side is helpful in decreasing the pain related to weight-bearing (21). Canes also increase the base of support, which in itself improves the patient's balance. Walkers, if wheeled, eliminate the strain (although mild) on the osteoporotic spine that would otherwise result from lifting the walker. Walkers are more supportive than canes and are used for limited ambulatory activities.

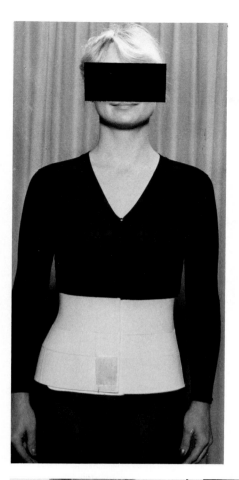

FIG. 12 Elastic lumbosacral support, anterior view, which does not immobilize the spine. Extreme flexion and extreme extension are restricted, whereas lateral bending and rotation are unaffected. It supports primarily by increasing intraabdominal pressure and transforming abdominal cavity into semirigid cylinder capable of transmitting stresses through abdomen rather than through spine.

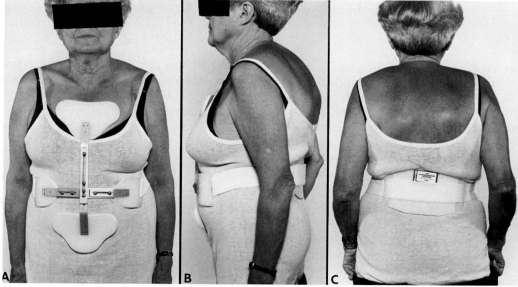

FIG. 13. Patient with osteoporosis of spine and compression fractures was unable to tolerate increased intraabdominal pressure with use of abdominal back support because of hiatal hernia. Patient was fitted with Jewett brace satisfactorily. **A:** Anterior view. **B:** Lateral view. **C:** posterior view.

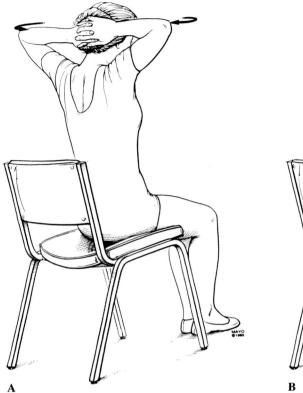
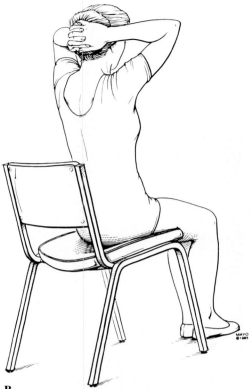

A   **B**

FIG. 14.   A and **B:** Deep-breathing exercise combined with pectoral stretching and back extension exercise. Patient sits on a chair, locks her hands behind her head, and inhales deeply while she gently extends her elbows backward. While exhaling, she returns to the starting position. This is repeated 10 to 15 times. **A,** redrawn from Sinaki, ref. 68. By permission of Mayo Foundation.

PREVENTIVE MEASURES

In spinal osteoporosis, prevention of further bone loss and vertebral compression fractures (the most common disabling deformity of osteoporosis) is an important goal. Because the morbid event is fracture, the most important criterion for successful treatment of established osteoporosis is reduction of the fracture rate. The fractures lead to dorsal kyphosis ("dowager's hump"), a progressive decrease in height, and, often, acutely painful and disabling fractures in the dorsal and lumbar regions. Therefore, preventive measures are necessary. Patients should be instructed to avoid bending and heavy lifting. Jarring of the spine can be decreased with the proper use of shoes with rubber heels. Use of a cane provides better balance, reduces the possibility of falls, and decreases the low-back pain resulting from weight-bearing. Early instruction on the principles of proper posture may decrease the rate of worsening of the kyphosis. In order to avoid straining flexion of the spine, patients should avoid heavy lifting and carry any weights close to the spine. Patients should also be instructed in pectoralis stretching, deep breathing, and back extension exercises to help avoid or decrease stooping.

When pursuing recreational activities, patients should practice the same caution as they do with therapeutic exercises. Not all types of exercise are appropriate for these patients because of the fragility of their vertebrae. Exer-

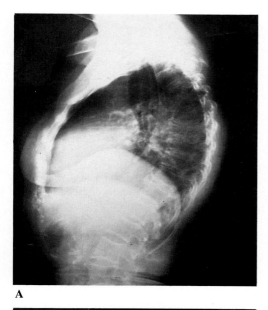

A

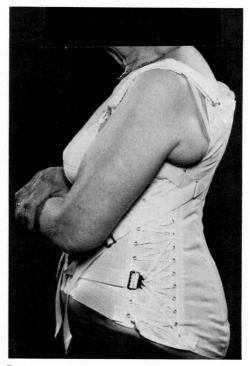

B

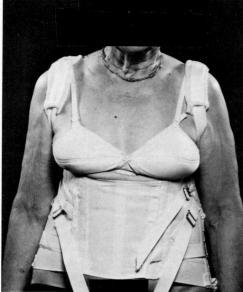

C

FIG. 15. Patient with osteoporosis and compression fractures. **A:** Roentgenogram of thoracic spine, lateral view, shows osteoporosis and compression fractures of several midthoracic and lower thoracic vertebral bodies. Lateral (**B**) and anterior (**C**) photographs show patient fitted with semirigid thoracolumbar support with shoulder straps to decrease kyphotic posture. Stays are semirigid; if replaced with rigid stays, support is transformed into rigid back support.

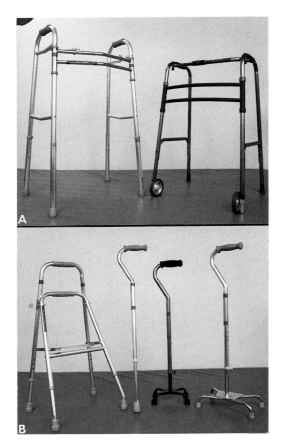

FIG. 16. Gait-assistive devices for patients with osteoporosis. **A:** Walker (left) and wheeled walker (right). **B:** (from left), Walkane, cane, and two types of broad-base canes, for stability.

cises that place flexion forces on the vertebrae, whether or not accompanied by extension strengthening exercises, tend to cause an increased number of vertebral fractures. Unfortunately, some activities that seem harmless are anything but benign. Golfing, a favorite among elderly persons, can be harmful because the players tend to stoop. Bowling involves similar risks. However, patients who enjoy these sports and who would feel a psychologic loss in giving them up should be advised to wear an adequate back support to prevent stooping. Preferably, patients with spinal osteoporosis should participate in recreational activities such as swimming, which do not predispose the back to strain. Swimming is ineffective for improving bone mineral density of the spine but is an important exercise for fitness (37). Walking is better, but bicycling is also acceptable if

the patient has a proper posture and avoids bending positions (sits up straight). If an exercise program is to be prescribed for patients with spinal osteoporosis, however, a cautious approach is recommended.

REFERENCES

1. Abramson, A.S. (1948): Atrophy of disuse: a definition. *Arch. Phys. Med.*, 29:562–570.
2. Abramson, A.S. (1948): Bone disturbances in injuries to the spinal cord and cauda equina (paraplegia): their prevention by ambulation. *J. Bone Joint Surg.*, 30-A:982–987.
3. Abramson, A.S., and Delagi, E.F. (1961): Influence of weight-bearing and muscle contraction on disuse osteoporosis. *Arch. Phys. Med. Rehabil.*, 42:147–151.
4. Aloia, J.F., Cohn, S.H., Ostuni, J.A., Cane, R., and Ellis, K. (1978): Prevention of involutional bone loss by exercise. *Ann. Intern. Med.*, 89:356–358.

5. Aloia, J.F., Stanton, H., Cohn, S.H., Babu, T., Abesamis, C., Kalici, N., and Ellis, K. (1978): Skeletal mass and body composition in marathon runners. *Metabolism*, 27:1793–1796.

6. Aloia, J.F. (1981): Exercise and skeletal health. *J. Am. Geriatr. Soc.*, 29:104–107.

7. Aniansson, A., Ljungberg, P., Rundgren, Å., and Wetterqvist, H. (1984): Effect of a training programme for pensioners on condition and muscular strength. *Arch. Gerontol. Geriatr.*, 3:229–241.

8. Ayre, W.B. (1945): Disuse atrophy of skeletal muscle. *Can. Med. Assoc. J.*, 53:352–355.

9. Bassett, C.A.L. (1968): Biologic significance of piezoelectricity. *Calcif. Tissue Res.*, 1:252–272.

10. Birge, S.J., and Whedon, G.D. (1968): *Hypodynamics and Hypogravics; The Physiology of Inactivity and Weightlessness*, edited by M. McCally, p. 213. Academic Press, New York.

11. Black-Sandler, R., LaPorte, R.E., Sashin, D., Kuller, L.H., Sternglass, E., Cauley, J.A., and Link, M.M. (1982): Determinants of bone mass in menopause. *Prev. Med.*, 11:269–280.

12. Brown, I.W., and Ring, P.A. (1985): Osteolytic changes in the upper femoral shaft following porous-coated hip replacement. *J. Bone Joint Surg.*, 67-B:218–221.

13. Casperson, C.J., Christenson, G.M., and Pollard, R.A. (1986): Status of the 1990 physical fitness and exercise objectives—evidence from NHIS 1985. *Public Health Rep.*, 101:587–592.

14. Chantraine, A., Nusgens, B., and Lapiere, Ch.M. (1986): Bone remodeling during the development of osteoporosis in paraplegia. *Calcif. Tissue Int.*, 38:323–327.

15. Chow, R.K., Harrison, J.E., Brown, C.F., and Hajek, V. (1986): Physical fitness effect on bone mass in postmenopausal women. *Arch. Phys. Med. Rehabil.*, 67:231–234.

16. Cohn, S.H., Vartsky, D., Yasumura, S., Sawitsky, A., Zanzi, I., Vaswani, A., and Ellis, K.J. (1980): Compartmental body composition based on total-body nitrogen, potassium, and calcium. *Am. J. Physiol.*, 239:E524–E530.

17. Comarr, A.E., Hutchinson, R.H., and Bors, E. (1962): Extremity fractures of patients with spinal cord injuries. *Am. J. Surg.*, 103:732–738.

18. Cummings, S.R., Kelsey, J.L., Nevitt, M.C., and O'Dowd, K.J. (1985): Epidemiology of osteoporosis and osteoporotic fractures. *Epidemiologic Rev.*, 7:178–208.

19. Dalén, N., and Olsson, K.E. (1974): Bone mineral content and physical activity. *Acta Orthop. Scand.*, 45:170–174.

20. Deitrick, J.E., Whedon, G.D., and Shorr, E. (1948): Effects of immobilization upon various metabolic and physiologic functions of normal men. *Am. J. Med.*, 4:3–36.

21. Denham, R.A. (1959): Hip mechanics. *J. Bone Joint Surg.*, 41-B:550–557.

22. Donaldson, C.L., Hulley, S.B., Vogel, J.M., Hattner, R.S., Bayers, J.H., and McMillan, D.E. (1970): Effect of prolonged bed rest on bone mineral. *Metabolism*, 19:1071–1084.

23. Doyle, F., Brown, J., and Lachance, C. (1970): Relation between bone mass and muscle weight. *Lancet*, 1:391–393.

24. Drinkwater, B.L., Nilson, K., Chesnut, C.H., III, Bremner, W.J., Shainholtz, S., and Southworth, M.B. (1984): Bone mineral content of amenorrheic and eumenorrheic athletes. *N. Engl. J. Med.*, 311:277–281.

25. Eccles, J.C. (1941): Disuse atrophy of skeletal muscle. *Med. J. Aust.*, 2:160–164.

26. Ellis, K.J., and Cohn, S.H. (1975): Correlation between skeletal calcium mass and muscle mass in man. *J. Applied Physiol.*, 38:455–460.

27. Freeman, L.W. (1949): The metabolism of calcium in patients with spinal cord injuries. *Ann. Surg.*, 129:177–184.

28. Frost, H.M. (1983): A determinant of bone architecture: The minimum effective strain. *Clin. Orthop.*, 175:286–292.

29. Gillespie, J.A. (1954): The nature of the bone changes associated with nerve injuries and disuse. *J. Bone Joint Surg.*, 36-B:464–473.

30. Hansson, T.H., Roos, B.O., and Nachemson, A. (1975): Development of osteopenia in the fourth lumbar vertebra during prolonged bed rest after operation for scoliosis. *Acta Orthop. Scand.*, 46:621–630.

31. Hattner, R.S., and McMillan, D.E. (1968): Influence of weightlessness upon the skeleton: a review. *Aerospace Med.*, 39:849–855.

32. Heaney, R.P. (1962): Radiocalcium metabolism in disuse osteoporosis in man. *Am. J. Med.*, 33:188–200.

33. Helmholz, H.F., Jr., and Stonnington, H.H. (1982): Rehabilitation for respiratory dysfunction. In: *Krusen's Handbook of Physical Medicine and Rehabilitation*, edited by F.J. Kottke, G.K. Stillwell, and J.F. Lehmann, Third Edition, pp. 771–786. W.B. Saunders Company, Philadelphia.

34. Huddleston, A.L., Rockwell, D., Kulund, D.N., and Harrison, R.B. (1980): Bone mass in lifetime tennis athletes. *J.A.M.A.*, 244:1107–1109.

35. Iskrant, A.P., and Smith, R.W., Jr. (1969): Osteoporosis in women 45 years and over related to subsequent fractures. *Public Health Rep.*, 84:33–38.

36. Issekutz, B., Jr., Blizzard, J.J., Birkhead, N.C., and Rodahl, K. (1966): Effect of prolonged bed rest on urinary calcium output. *J. Appl. Physiol.*, 21:1013–1020.

37. Jacobson, P.C., Beaver, W., Grubb, S.A., Taft, T.N., and Talmage, R.V. (1984): Bone density in women: college athletes and older athletic women. *J. Orthop. Res.*, 2:328–332.

38. Jenkins, D.P., and Cochran, T.H. (1969): Osteoporosis: The dramatic effect of disuse of an extremity. *Clin. Orthop.*, 64:128–134.

39. Johnell, O., and Nilsson, B.E. (1984): Life-style and bone mineral mass in perimenopausal women. *Calcif. Tissue Int.*, 36:354–356.

40. Jones, H.H., Priest, J.D., Hayes, W.C., Tichenor, C.C., and Nagel, D.A. (1977): Humeral hypertrophy in response to exercise. *J. Bone Joint Surg.*, 59-A:204–208.

41. Knapp, M.E. (1982): Massage. In: *Krusen's Handbook of Physical Medicine and Rehabilitation*, edited

by F.J. Kottke, G.K. Stillwell, and J.F. Lehmann, Third Edition, pp. 386–388. W.B. Saunders Company, Philadelphia.

42. Krølner, B., and Toft, B. (1983): Vertebral bone loss: An unheeded side effect of therapeutic bed rest. *Clin. Sci.*, 64:537–540.

43. Krølner, B., Toft, B., Pors Nielsen, S., and Tondevold, E. (1983): Physical exercise as prophylaxis against involutional vertebral bone loss: A controlled trial. *Clin. Sci.*, 64:541–546.

44. Lane, N.E., Bloch, D.A., Jones, H.H., Marshall, W.H., Jr., Wood, P.D., and Fries, J.F. (1986): Long-distance running, bone density, and osteoarthritis. *J.A.M.A.*, 255:1147–1151.

45. Lanyon, L.E. (1980): Bone remodelling, mechanical stress, and osteoporosis. In: *Osteoporosis: Recent Advances in Pathogenesis and Treatment*, edited by H.F. DeLuca, H.M. Frost, W.S.S. Jee, C.C. Johnston, Jr., and A.M. Parfitt, pp. 129–138. University Park Press, Baltimore.

46. LaPorte, R.E., Adams, L.L., Savage, D.D., Brenes, G., Dearwater, S., and Cook, T. (1984): The spectrum of physical activity, cardiovascular disease and health: An epidemiologic perspective. *Am. J. Epidemiol.*, 120:507–517.

47. Lehmann, J.F., and De Lateur, B.J. (1982): Diathermy and superficial heat and cold therapy. In: *Krusen's Handbook of Physical Medicine and Rehabilitation*, edited by F.J. Kottke, G.K. Stillwell, and J.F. Lehmann, Third Edition, pp. 275–350. W.B. Saunders Company, Philadelphia.

48. Lucas, D.B. (1966): Spinal bracing. In: *Orthotics: Etcetera*, edited by S. Licht, pp. 274–305. Elizabeth Licht, Publisher, New Haven, Connecticut.

49. Mack, P.B., LaChance, P.A., Vose, G.P., and Vogt, F.B. (1967): Bone demineralization of foot and hand of Gemini-Titan IV, V and VII astronauts during orbital flight. *Am. J. Roentgenol.*, 100:503–511.

50. Margulies, J.Y., Simkin, A., Leichter, I., Bivas, A., Steinberg, R., Giladi, M., Stein, M., Kashtan, H., and Milgrom, C. (1986): Effect of intense physical activity on the bone-mineral content in the lower limbs of young adults. *J. Bone Joint Surg.*, 68-A:1090–1093.

51. Minaire, P., Meunier, P., Edouard, C., Bernard, J., Courpron, P., and Bourret, J. (1974): Quantitative histological data on disuse osteoporosis: Comparison with biological data. *Calcif. Tissue Res.*, 17:57–73.

52. Minaire, P., Berard, E., Meunier, P., Edouard, C., Goedert, G., and Pilonchery, G. (1981): Effects of disodium dichloromethylene diphosphonate on bone loss in paraplegic patients. *J. Clin. Invest.*, 68:1086–1092.

53. Minaire, P., Meunier, P.J., DePassio, J., Edouard, C., Pilonchery, G., Goedert, G., Argemi, B., Gueris, J., Kanis, J., Ulmann, A., and Caulin, F. (1984): The effect of calcitonin on the acute bone loss of paraplegic patients. *Proceedings of the Copenhagen International Symposium on Osteoporosis*, June 3-8, 1984, p. 136, (Abstr.)

54. Morris, J.M., Lucas, D.B., and Bresler, B. (1961): Role of the trunk in stability of the spine. *J. Bone Joint Surg.*, 43-A:327–351.

55. Murphy, S.B., Walker, P.S., and Schiller, A.L. (1984): Adaptive changes in the femur after implantation of an Austin Moore prosthesis. *J. Bone Joint Surg.*, 66-A:437–443.

56. Naftchi, N.E., Viau, A.T., Sell, G.H., and Lowman, E.W. (1980): Mineral metabolism in spinal cord injury. *Arch. Phys. Med. Rehabil.*, 61:139–142.

57. Nilsson, B.E., and Westlin, N.E. (1971): Bone density in athletes. *Clin. Orthop.*, 77:179–182.

58. Nilsson, B.E., Andersson, S.M., Havdrup, T., and Westlin, N.E. (1978): Ballet-dancing and weightlifting - effects on BMC, *A.J.R.*, 131:541–542, (Abstr.).

59. Nordin, B.E.C., Horsman, A., Crilly, R.G., Marshall, D.H., and Simpson, M. (1980): Treatment of spinal osteoporosis in postmenopausal women. *Br. Med. J.*, 280:451–454.

60. Osteoporosis and activity (1983): *Lancet*, 1:1365–1366.

61. Pocock, N.A., Eisman, J.A., Yeates, M.G., Sambrook, P.N., and Eberl, S. (1986): Physical fitness is a major determinant of femoral neck and lumbar spine bone mineral density. *J. Clin. Invest.*, 78:618–621.

62. Ragan, C., and Briscoe, A.M. (1964): Effect of exercise on the metabolism of ^{40}calcium and of ^{47}calcium in man. *J. Clin. Endocrinol. Metab.*, 24:385–392.

63. Rambaut, P.C., and Johnston, R.S. (1979): Prolonged weightlessness and calcium loss in man. *Acta. Astronaut.*, 6:1113–1122.

64. Rambaut, P.C., and Goode, A.W. (1985): Skeletal changes during space flight. *Lancet*, 2:1050–1052.

65. Riggs, B.L., and Melton, L.J. (1986): Medical progress: Involutional osteoporosis. *N. Engl. J. Med.*, 314:1676–1686.

66. Saville, P.D. (1973): The syndrome of spinal osteoporosis. *Clin. Endocrinol. Metab.*, 2:177–185.

67. Schneider, V.S., and McDonald, J. (1984): Skeletal calcium homeostasis and countermeasures to prevent disuse osteoporosis. *Calcif. Tissue Int.*, 36:S151–S154.

68. Sinaki, M. (1982): Postmenopausal spinal osteoporosis: physical therapy and rehabilitation principles. *Mayo Clin. Proc.*, 57:699–703.

69. Sinaki, M., and Mikkelsen, B.A. (1984): Postmenopausal spinal osteoporosis: flexion versus extension exercises. *Arch. Phys. Med. Rehabil.*, 65:593–596.

70. Sinaki, M., McPhee, M.C., Hodgson, S.F., Merritt, J.M., and Offord, K.P. (1986): Relationship between bone mineral density of spine and strength of back extensors in healthy postmenopausal women. *Mayo Clin. Proc.*, 61:116–122.

71. Smith, E.L., Jr., Reddan, W., and Smith, P.E. (1981): Physical activity and calcium modalities for bone mineral increase in aged women. *Med. Sci. Sports Ex.*, 13:60–64.

72. Smith, E.L., Jr., Smith, P.E., Ensign, C.J., and Shea, M.M. (1984): Bone involution decrease in exercising middle-aged women. *Calcif. Tissue Int.*, 36:S129–S138.

73. Snorrason, E. (1965): Exercise for healthy persons. In: *Therapeutic Exercise*, edited by S. Licht, Second

Edition, pp. 896–911. Elizabeth Licht, Publisher, New Haven, Connecticut.

74. Stamford, B.A. (1973): Effects of chronic institutionalization on the physical working capacity and trainability of geriatric men. *J. Gerontol.*, 28:441–446.

75. Stevenson, F.H. (1952): The osteoporosis of immobilisation in recumbency. *J. Bone Joint Surg.*, 34-B:256–265.

76. Stewart, A.F., Adler, M., Byers, C.M., Segre, G.V., and Broadus, A.E. (1982): Calcium homeostasis in immobilization: An example of resorptive hypercalciuria. *N. Engl. J. Med.*, 306:1136–1140.

77. Stillwell, G.K. (1973): The law of Laplace: some clinical applications. *Mayo Clin. Proc.*, 48:863–869.

78. Thomsen, K., Gotfredsen, A., and Christiansen, C. (1986): Is postmenopausal bone loss an age-related phenomenon? *Calcif. Tissue Int.*, 39:123–127.

79. Tilton, F.E., Degioanni, J.J.C., and Schneider, V.S. (1980): Long-term follow-up of Skylab bone demineralization. *Aviat. Space Environ. Med.*, 51:1209–1213.

80. Tonino, A.J., Davidson, C.L., Klopper, P.J., and Linclau, L.A. (1976): Protection from stress in bone and its effects: Experiments with stainless steel and plastic plates in dogs. *J. Bone Joint Surg.*, 58-B:107–113, 1976.

81. Unthoff, H.K., and Finnegan, M. (1983): The effects of metal plates on post-traumatic remodelling and bone mass. *J. Bone Joint Surg.*, 65-B:66–71.

82. Urist, M.R. (1973): Orthopaedic management of osteoporosis in postmenopausal women. *Clin. Endocrinol. Metab.*, 2:159–176.

83. Vogel, J.M. (1973): Bone mineral changes in the Apollo astronauts. In: *Proceedings of the International Conference on Bone Mineral Measurement*, edited by R.B. Mazess, pp. 352–361. U.S. Department of Health, Education, and Welfare, DHEW Publication No. (NIH)75-683, NIH, Bethesda, Maryland.

84. Watson, R.C. (1973): Bone growth and physical activity in young males. In: *Proceedings of the International Conference on Bone Mineral Measurement*, U.S. Department of Health, Education, and Welfare. DHEW Publication No. (NIH)75-683, pp. 380–386, NIH, Bethesda, Maryland.

85. Whedon, G.D., Deitrick, J.E., and Shorr, E. (1949): Modification of the effects of immobilization upon metabolic and physiologic functions of normal men by the use of an oscillating bed. *Am. J. Med.*, 6:684–711.

86. Whedon, G.D., and Shorr, E. (1957): Metabolic studies in paralytic acute anterior poliomyelitis. II. Alterations in calcium and phosphorus metabolism. *J. Clin. Invest.*, 36:966–981.

87. Whedon, G.D. (1984): Disuse osteoporosis: Physiological aspects. *Calcif. Tissue Int.*, 36:S146–S150.

88. White, M.K., Martin, R.B., Yeater, R.A., Butcher, R.L., and Radin, E.L. (1984): The effects of exercise on the bones of postmenopausal women. *Int. Orthop.*, 7:209–214.

89. Wolff, J., editor (1892): *Das Gesetz der Transformation der Knochen*. A. Hirschwald, Berlin.

90. Wyse, D.M., and Pattee, C.J. (1954): Effect of the oscillating bed and tilt table on calcium, phosphorus and nitrogen metabolism in paraplegia. *Am. J. Med.*, 17:645–661.

91. Yano, K., Wasnich, R.D., Vogel, J.M., and Heilbrun, L.K. (1984): Bone mineral measurements among middle-aged and elderly Japanese residents in Hawaii. *Am. J. Epidemiol.*, 119:751–764.

92. Yeater, R.A., and Martin, R.B. (1984): Senile osteoporosis: The effects of exercise. *Postgrad. Med.*, 75:147–163.

93. Zanzi, I., Ellis, K.J., Aloia, J., and Cohn, S.H. (1981): Effect of physical activity on body composition. In: *Osteoporosis: Recent Advances in Pathogenesis and Treatment*, edited by H.F. DeLuca, H.M. Frost, W.S.S. Jee, C.C. Johnston, Jr., and A.M. Parfitt, pp. 139–146, University Park Press, Baltimore.

Osteoporosis: Etiology, Diagnosis, and Management, edited by B. Lawrence Riggs and L. Joseph Melton, III. Raven Press, New York © 1988.

20

Practical Management of the Patient with Osteoporosis

B. Lawrence Riggs

Division of Endocrinology, Metabolism and Internal Medicine, Mayo Clinic and Mayo Foundation; Mayo Medical School; Rochester, Minnesota 55905

Previous chapters have covered various aspects of diagnosis and treatment in detail. These have provided an extensive review of experimental studies on the strengths and weaknesses of diagnostic procedures and the therapeutic value of drugs and their mechanisms of action in the osteoporotic patient. This chapter describes an approach to the practical management of the individual patient with osteoporosis. The general comments refer mainly to patients with type I (postmenopausal) osteoporosis associated with vertebral fractures, the main form of osteoporosis encountered in clinical practice. The latter portion of the chapter reviews management of the different osteoporosis syndromes.

The recommendations in this chapter are my own and may differ in some aspects from those of other workers. Nonetheless, they are similar to those used by my colleagues at the Mayo Clinic and are, I believe, well within the mainstream of informed opinion.

DIAGNOSIS

All patients presenting with osteoporosis should undergo a comprehensive medical evaluation to: (1) exclude secondary causes of osteoporosis (see Chapter 6, this volume), (2) assess the extent of bone loss and fractures, (3) provide baseline measurements against which one can evaluate the effectiveness of subsequent treatment, and (4) in selected instances, to determine whether bone turnover is high or low. Table 1 summarizes the components of a typical diagnostic evaluation for osteoporosis.

General Medical Examination

Careful history taking and physical examination should be performed in all patients. Historical points of particular importance include the chronology and location of fractures, the time course and characteristics of back pain, previous treatment, age at onset and type (natural or surgical) of menopause, family history of osteoporosis, use of tobacco or alcohol, level of physical activity, and presence of risk factors such as previous gastrointestinal surgery and corticosteroid use. The presence of systemic symptoms such as weakness and weight loss or of abnormal physical findings suggests that the osteoporosis may be caused by an underlying disease. Even patients with severe osteoporosis and multiple compression fractures seldom appear ill and do not report loss of weight.

Physical examination should include careful

TABLE 1. *Diagnostic evaluation for osteoporosis*

Routine

History and physical examination
Radiographs of chest, complete blood cell count, chemistry group, and urinalysis
Radiographs of lumbar and thoracic spinal column
Erythrocyte sedimentation rate
Serum protein electrophoresis

Optional

Lumbar spine bone density (dual photon absorptiometry or quantitative computed tomography)
Iliac crest biopsy (after tetracycline double labeling for bone histomorphometry)
Bone marrow examination (to exclude multiple myeloma and metastatic malignancy)

---

measurement of height (at maximal stretch) and a search for findings suggestive of systemic diseases. Blue sclerae, particularly when associated with a thinning of the skin and hyperelasticity of the joints, suggests osteogenesis imperfecta tarda or some related inborn error of collagen metabolism. Patients with osteogenesis imperfecta tarda usually have a "robin's egg blue" color which should not be confused with the bluish tint present in some patients with severe osteoporosis. Extreme thinning of the skin suggests osteogenesis imperfecta tarda or Cushing's syndrome, but some patients with severe osteoporosis also may have thin skin. Cushing's syndrome and hyperthyroidism have characteristic manifestations. The presence of hepatomegaly or splenomegaly is an ominous sign and suggests an underlying lymphoma or other malignancy.

All patients should have a complete blood cell count, multichannel serum chemistry group, determination of erythrocyte sedimentation rate, and urinalysis. Abnormalities in any of these studies suggest the presence of a secondary disease process. Increased serum alkaline phosphatase levels (in the absence of liver disease or fracture healing) suggest osteomalacia or a destructive skeletal process. Serum protein electrophoresis should be performed for all osteoporotic patients at the time of their initial evaluation. A normal serum protein electrophoresis pattern excludes the presence of multiple myeloma in 90% of patients.

Radiographic Assessment

Radiographs of the thoracic and lumbar spinal column should be obtained for all patients to evaluate severity, to relate symptoms of back pain to the underlying vertebral deformity, and to provide a baseline for assessing the effect of therapy on fracture occurrence. Quantitative assessment of vertebral compression fractures is discussed in Chapter 7, *this volume*. For clinical purposes, it is sufficient to note the number of vertebral deformities categorized on the basis of anterior wedge compressions, vertebral collapse fractures, and "ballooning" (biconcave compression of the end plates). A secondary reason for obtaining the radiographs is to detect secondary disease states that may have produced the osteoporosis. These are discussed in Chapter 7, *this volume*.

Densitometry

The development, during the past 5 years, of practical methods for measuring density of vertebral bones represents a major advance in patient care. Although these techniques were originally limited to research centers, their use is becoming widespread and, within the near future, they undoubtedly will be available in most medium-sized or large hospitals. Two techniques are generally available—dual photon absorptiometry (Chapter 9, *this volume*), and quantitative computed tomography (Chapter 8). Both have advantages and disadvantages, but they are roughly comparable in clinical utility. Bone density in the appendicular skeleton also can be measured by single-photon absorptiometry (Chapter 9). In the past, the main site of measurement has been the midradius, although recently there has been increased interest in measuring the ultradistal radius. Although bone density at these appendicular sites correlates moderately well ($r = 0.5$ to 0.8) with bone density of the vertebrae, the correlation is too weak to allow vertebral density to be predicted accurately for individual patients. Thus, appendicular density measurements cannot substitute for vertebral densitometry. However, they may provide supplementary information on the extent of cortical bone loss.

Bone Biopsy

Iliac crest biopsy is indicated in many patients with osteoporosis and, ideally, should be performed after tetracycline double labeling so rates of bone turnover and bone mineralization can be assessed (Chapter 11, *this volume*). Its major indications in osteoporosis are (1) to exclude occult or coexisting osteomalacia, (2) to characterize bone turnover quantitatively, (3) to detect subtle variants of osteogenesis imperfecta in young adults with idiopathic osteoporosis, and (4) to evaluate therapeutic response, particularly in a patient who is not responding well to established therapy. In addition to the dynamic skeletal parameters, the bone marrow in the biopsy sample can be examined to detect multiple myeloma or metastatic carcinoma. Because of the unique information that it provides, more and more patients are undergoing bone biopsy at the time of their initial evaluation. Conventional decalcified histologic specimens provide insufficient information, and the bone biospy specimen should be processed only in laboratories capable of cutting and processing thin, undecalcified sections. Quantitative measurements of the various histomorphometric parameters should be provided to the clinician, not just a subjective interpretation.

Other Studies

Skeletal remodeling activity can be assessed visually with a ^{99m}Tc-diphosphonate scan (Chapter 9). My experience is that this usually is not needed in evaluation of osteoporotic patients. Although a vertebral fracture can be judged as recent if it coincides with a local area of isotope uptake, this information usually is clear from the clinical history. Isotope scans also can be useful in detecting nonuniform skeletal uptake. In involutional osteoporosis, uptake is uniform (except for areas of recent fracture) whereas in certain conditions that may be confused with osteoporosis, such as osteomalacia, multiple myeloma, and diffuse mastocytosis, it may be nonuniform.

In osteoporotic patients who appear to be ill, who have normocytic anemia, or who show rapid progression on standard therapy, the bone marrow should be examined to exclude diffuse carcinoma or multiple myeloma. Although most patients with osteoporosis due to hyperthyroidism or Cushing's syndrome have clinical manifestations of the underlying endocrine disorder, exceptions occasionally occur. Thus, thyroid and adrenal function should be tested in atypical cases.

Serum 25-hydroxyvitamin D determination is indicated when osteoporosis is associated with gastrointestinal disease or when osteomalacia is suspected clinically. Serum 1,25-dihydroxyvitamin D determination has little, if any, value in the diagnosis of patients with osteoporosis. Although mean values for serum 1,25-dihydroxyvitamin D may be low in patients with type I osteoporosis, the decrease is small and there is a large overlap of individual patients with age- and sex-matched normals (4).

The serum immunoreactive parathyroid hormone level may be useful in detecting the small proportion of osteoporotic patients who have type III osteoporosis (Chapter 6), but whether it is cost-effective as a routine test for all osteoporotic patients is uncertain. Analysis for bone-specific markers soon may become part of the routine evaluation for osteoporosis (Chapter 10). We have found that the combination of serum bone alkaline phosphatase and osteocalcin (bone Gla-protein) determination provides a specific and relatively sensitive noninvasive way to estimate bone formation rate (unpublished data). These tests are not widely available now but soon will be. Very likely, these will become routine tests in evaluating all new osteoporotic patients in order to determine which of them should have iliac crest biopsies.

GENERAL THERAPEUTIC MEASURES

Both physicians and patients, at times, fail to understand that pain is relieved by general measures rather than by drug therapy. Acute pain from new vertebral fracture subsides in weeks or a few months even in the absence of drug therapy, whereas chronic pain due to spinal deformity may persist even if drug therapy has favorably altered the balance between resorption and formation of bone. Thus, adequate attention to general measures is a crucial part of management of osteoporotic patients. Many of these are described in detail in Chapter 19, *this volume.*

Acute back pain responds to analgesics, heat, and general massage to alleviate muscle spasm. If the pain is severe, stronger analgesics such as codeine sulfate or its derivatives may be required. Sometimes, a brief period of bed rest is necessary to control pain.

Chronic back pain often is caused by spinal deformity resulting from previous vertebral fractures and thus is difficult to relieve completely. Instructions in posture, gait training, and institution of regular back extension exercises to strengthen the flabby paravertebral muscles usually are beneficial.

Occasionally, an orthopedic back brace is required. All patients with osteoporosis should have a diet adequate in calcium, proteins, and vitamins, should be reasonably active physically, and should take precautions to prevent falls.

DRUG THERAPY

The drugs commonly used in the treatment of involutional osteoporosis are estrogen, calcitonin, calcium, and vitamin D. All of these act by inhibiting bone resorption. Thus, the best result that can be expected is to maintain bone mass or to slow the rate of bone loss. Estrogen and calcitonin have been approved by the United States Food and Drug Administration (FDA) for use in osteoporosis. Calcium and vitamin D have not been specifically approved for this indication but have a long tradition of use. The FDA has reviewed and specifically refused to approve the vitamin D metabolite 1,25-dihydroxyvitamin D for use in osteoporosis and has rescinded its approval for stanozolol and other anabolic steroids on the grounds that the therapeutic effect was not sufficient to justify the side effects. Sodium fluoride also has not been approved by the FDA for use in osteoporosis. This approval may be forthcoming soon, however, if two ongoing NIH-sup-

ported clinical trials confirm the positive findings of previous retrospective studies (14).

Estrogen

Although a number of estrogen preparations are available, the most common one used in the United States is conjugated estrogen. Equivalent dosages of various estrogen preparations commonly used in the treatment of osteoporosis are given in Table 2. Unfortunately, the major physiologic estrogen, estradiol acetate, has poor biologic availability when given orally. At effective dosages, estrogen will induce menometrorrhagia, mastodynia, and dependent edema in a significant minority of treated patients. These symptoms are more prevalent and more severe on higher dosages. When "break-through bleeding" (bleeding during estrogen administration) occurs, it is mandatory to obtain endometrial tissue, by either dilatation and curettage or Vabra-suction curettage, for pathologic examination to exclude malignant changes.

In addition, as discussed in (Chapters 12 and 15, *this volume,* there are two classes of diseases that can be produced or exacerbated by estrogen therapy. First, it has been clearly shown that postmenopausal estrogen therapy results in an increased incidence of carcinoma of the endometrium—about 0.5% to 1.0% per year of treatment (7). It still is controversial whether estrogen therapy causes carcinoma of the breast, but results of recent studies are somewhat reassuring (22). Concurrent administration of a progestin during the last 10 to 14 days of the cycle prevents endometrial hyperplasia and, presumably, thus prevents endome-

TABLE 2. *Equivalent dosages of estrogen preparations*

Preparation	Trade name	Dosage
Conjugated estrogen	Premarin (Ayerst)	0.625 mg/day
Estropipate	Ogen (Abbott)	0.75 mg/day
Ethanylestradiol	Estinyl (Schering)	0.025 mg/day
Transdermal estradiol	Estraderm (Ciba)	0.11 patch every 3.5 days

trial carcinoma (7). Also, it may decrease the risk of breast carcinoma (5). Giving a progestin has certain disadvantages, however. First, the large majority of women taking estrogen and progestin cyclically will have regular withdrawal bleeding, an event that some postmenopausal women are unwilling to accept. Also, there is some evidence that available progestins may be atherogenic by affecting serum lipid patterns unfavorably. This is much more true with the 19-nortestosterone derivatives (which is the class of progestins used in birth control pills) than with the 17-acetoxyprogesterone derivatives. Therefore, a drug in this latter class of progestins, such as medroxyprogesterone acetate (Provera®, Upjohn), is recommended for use in postmenopausal women (Table 3). Unfortunately, the physiologic progestin, progesterone acetate, has poor biologic availability when given orally.

The second group of induced diseases occur because of the nonphysiologic route of administration of estrogens. After oral administration, the liver is exposed to high blood concentrations during the first pass in the portal vein. This leads to increased hepatic production of certain estrogen-dependent proteins (including coagulation factors and renin substrate) and bile cholesterol (8). These increases probably account for the increased incidence, in estrogen-treated subjects, of venous thrombosis and pulmonary embolism, hypertension, and gallstones. Whether estrogen therapy increases the incidence of heart attacks and strokes is unclear; contradictory results have been reported (20,21). Tests are now underway to determine whether cyclic administration of estradiol acetate by transdermal patches will obviate the side effects resulting from excessive hepatic stimulation (1).

Estrogen should be given cyclically at the lowest effective dosage. For prevention of bone loss after menopause, this is 0.625 mg of conjugated estrogen, or its equivalent, daily (6). Recently, it has been shown that 0.3 mg daily will suffice if calcium supplements are given concurrently (3). My experience has been that dosages at about twice these levels

are needed to control bone loss in patients with established osteoporosis. In most patients, a progestin such as medroxyprogesterone acetate, 10 mg daily, should be given during the last 14 days of the cycle. Although some gynecologists believe that endometrial curettage should be performed routinely prior to estrogen therapy and at yearly intervals thereafter, this is impractical for most clinicians. Thus, if the bleeding at the time of cyclic estrogen withdrawal is normal in amount, it may be safely ignored. Metrorrhagia or menorrhagia, however, should be investigated promptly.

Alternative programs being studied include continuous administration of estrogen with the progestin given continuously (to induce endometrial atrophy) or sequentially for 2 weeks every 3 months (to induce endometrial bleeding). Until more information about safety and effectiveness of these alternative programs is available, the standard regimen should be used. Histories of breast cancer, endometrial cancer (but not squamous carcinoma of the cervix), deep venous thrombosis, or pulmonary emboli are contraindications to the use of estrogen. Significant varicose veins, moderate to severe hypertension, and a strong positive family history of breast cancer are relative contraindications. All women receiving estrogen therapy should have blood pressure measurements and breast and pelvic examinations yearly.

Calcitonin

This drug has the disadvantages of expense ($1,000 to $1,500 per year) and requirement for parenteral administration. It is usually well-tolerated, however. About 5 to 10% patients will experience nausea or flushing after the injection. These symptoms can be minimized by giving the dose at bedtime and by giving an antihistamine, such as 50 mg diphenhydramine (Benadryl®) 30 min before this. Occasionally, there may be local irritation at the site of injection.

A more common and serious complication is the development of resistance to the action of calcitonin. This occurs in 25 to 50% of patients after 6 to 24 months of continuous therapy. The usual dosage is 0.5 ml (100 U) daily by subcutaneous injection. The main preparation that has been used in the United States is salmon calcitonin (Calcimar®, USV Pharmaceutical). Recently, human calcitonin has become available (Cibacalcin®, Ciba Pharmaceutical). This has the potential advantages of sustained efficacy in long-term use, low risk of antigenicity, and decreased occurrence of drug resistance. The injection sites should be rotated in a manner analogous to that for daily insulin injection. Because of the possibility of inducing secondary hyperparathyroidism, calcium supplements should always be given in conjunction with calcitonin.

Calcium

The dosage of supplementary calcium should be 1,000 to 1,500 mg of elemental calcium daily plus a dietary intake of 1,000 mg of calcium daily.

A myriad of calcium preparations are available; the most commonly used are given in Table 3. Of the various calcium salts, calcium carbonate is the most widely used and has the advantage that elemental calcium represents 40% of its total weight. Thus, fewer tablets are required to reach a given dose of elemental calcium. It has two disadvantages, however. First, in some patients, the preparation is constipating or produces gaseousness and flatulence, or both. Second, in the absence of stomach acid, calcium carbonate is insoluble and is poorly absorbed. About 40% of postmenopausal women and elderly women have relative achlorhydria and generate free stomach acid only during meals. Recker (10) has shown that, in such patients, calcium is absorbed when calcium carbonate is taken with meals but not when taken on an empty stomach. Thus, if a patient has not been tested for achlorhydria, it is important to give the dose of calcium with meals. About 10% of this population, however, have absolute achlorhydria and at no time do they absorb calcium given as calcium carbonate. Calcium given as calcium phosphate or calcium citrate is more soluble and is better absorbed by achlorhydric patients, but these preparations contain only about 17 or 24% of elemental calcium, respectively. For reasons that are unclear, some patients who tolerate calcium carbonate treatment will not tolerate these latter preparations.

Vitamin D

This usually is given with calcium therapy in order to increase the fractional calcium absorption. It should not be used if there is a history of renal nephrolithiasis or if renal function is significantly impaired. The main side effects are hypercalciuria and hypercalcemia. Unfortunately, these may not occur until the drug has been used for months or even years. At times, severe hypercalcemia may occur abruptly and may be life-threatening. Thus, the smallest dosage that will increase calcium absorption

TABLE 3. *Calcium preparations in common use*

Trade name	Form of salt	Elemental calcium/tablet, mg	Cost, dollars for taking 1,500 mg/day
Os-Cal (Marion)	carbonate	250	0.30
Os-Cal 500 (Marion)	carbonate	500	0.30
Generic oyster shell calcium	carbonate	250	0.15
Tums (Norcliff Thayer)	carbonate	250	0.25
Posture (Ayerst)	phosphate	600	0.35
Calcitriol	citrate	200	0.70

should be used. This usually is 50,000 U every 7 to 10 days. The practice in the past of using higher dosages, such as 50,000 U daily, has been largely abandoned because of the high incidence of hypercalcemia and hypercalciuria. While the patient is receiving vitamin D therapy, serum and urine calcium determinations should be made every 2 or 3 months initially and no less than every 6 months subsequently.

TREATMENT OF SPECIFIC TYPES OF OSTEOPOROSIS

Type I (Postmenopausal) Osteoporosis

Patients with vertebral fractures, even mild nontraumatic wedge fractures, should be treated. Osteopenic patients without vertebral fractures but with bone density values below the age-adjusted normal range also should receive treatment. Those with Colles' fracture of the distal forearm should undergo vertebral densitometry to determine the need for drug therapy. All osteoporotic patients should have a total calcium intake of 2,000 to 2,500 mg/day. Although the role of calcium deficiency in the pathogenesis of osteoporosis is controversial (8), there is indirect evidence that high dosages of calcium supplements decrease bone turnover (12,17), perhaps by decreasing parathyroid hormone secretion (12), and may also decrease the fracture rate modestly (14).

In addition, patients with more extensive disease should receive estrogen therapy, particularly when they have a normal to increased rate of bone turnover. One-third of the osteoporotic patients with low turnover (Chapter 11) do not respond to estrogen or other antiresorptive drugs (11). At present, the only direct way of determining the state of bone turnover is by bone biopsy after tetracycline double labeling. In general, however, osteoporotic women within 10 years of menopause will have high rates of bone turnover, whereas those older than age 70 usually will not. Higher rates of bone turnover are also suggested by a high frequency of vertebral compressions [the average

rate is about one per year (14)] and by high normal values for serum phosphate and urinary calcium.

Estrogen therapy should be begun at a dosage of 0.625 mg of conjugated estrogen (or its equivalent in another estrogen preparation) per day. This should be given for 25 days each month and accompanied by a progestin (such as medroxyprogesterone acetate, 10 mg daily) for the last 10 days of the cycle. When there is evidence of significant impairment of calcium absorption, vitamin D in a dosage of 50,000 U once every 7 to 10 days should be added.

It is not practical clinically to assess calcium absorption (which requires the use of radiocalcium) but it can be estimated by using urinary calcium excretion in the published regression on calcium absorption (13). In general, when urinary calcium excretion is less than 75 mg/day in an osteoporotic patient consuming at least 800 mg of calcium daily, absorption is impaired.

When there is evidence of progression of bone loss or continued vertebral fractures after at least one year of therapy with low doses of estrogen, the dosage of estrogen should be doubled. Calcitonin appears to have no advantage over estrogen as an antiresorptive agent; it is indicated chiefly as an alternative antiresorptive agent when there are contraindications to the use of estrogen.

Type II (Senile) Osteoporosis

Regardless of whether they present with hip fracture or vertebral fractures, these elderly patients have already lost most of the bone they will lose. Their bone density differs little from that of their peers without fractures (16), and generally they do not have a high bone turnover rate. There is no evidence that estrogen or calcitonin therapy is beneficial in such patients. Moreover, because of their age and increased incidence of asymptomatic atherosclerosis, there may be increased risk associated with estrogen therapy. Treatment consists primarily of calcium supplementation (because of impaired calcium absorption) and instruction in measures that decrease the risk of falls. The latter includes use of shoes with flat heels, removal of loose floor rugs, avoidance of slippery surfaces (such as recently waxed floors or icy sidewalks), and use of a light if it is necessary to get up from bed during the night.

Idiopathic Osteoporosis in Premenopausal Women

Because these women are not estrogen-deficient, there is no reason to prescribe sex steroids. Some of the patients with this disorder have impaired calcium absorption, which can be corrected by administration of vitamin D. The mainstay of treatment, therefore, is calcium supplementation with or without pharmacologic dosages of vitamin D. When there is evidence of increased bone turnover, calcitonin can be added as an antiresorptive agent.

Osteoporosis in Men

A careful search should be made for secondary causes of osteoporosis which will be found in approximately 40% of these patients. Approximately 10 to 20% of men with osteoporosis will be found to have partial or complete hypogonadism of various causes (19). Those patients with documented low plasma testosterone levels should receive replacement therapy, such as testosterone enanthate, 200 to 400 mg intramuscularly every 4 weeks. Calcium supplementation, with or without pharmacologic dosages of vitamin D also is usually given.

Osteoporosis Associated with Glucocorticoid Excess

The most common cause of secondary osteoporosis is chronic use of glucocorticoids in pharmacologic dosages. The most important single treatment is reducing the dosage of the glucocorticoid or, if possible, discontinuing it. Administering glucocorticoids once daily or on alternate days may maintain a more favorable balance between the antiinflammatory or immunosuppressive effect and the osteopenic effect in some patients. All of these patients should receive calcium supplements and those who are postmenopausal women should also be given estrogens. Although glucocorticoids inhibit calcium absorption, the use of pharmacologic doses of vitamin D or its metabolites in this circumstance is controversial. There is increasing evidence that glucocorticoids do not induce major alterations in vitamin D metabolism (18).

ASSESSMENT OF THERAPEUTIC EFFECTS

All available regimens for the treatment of osteoporosis are only partially successful and are ineffective in some patients. The most sensitive way to determine the effectiveness of a given therapeutic regimen is measuring the rate of loss of bone from the lumbar spine by repeated densitometric studies using dual-photon absorptiometry or quantitative computed tomography. Unless the rate of bone loss is unusually high, repeat measurements made annually over to 2 to 3 years usually are required (15). If vertebral densitometry is not available, progression of the disease can be assessed by measuring the patient's standing height serially and by identifying the occurrence of new vertebral fractures on annual radiographs of the lumbar and thoracic spinal column. However, the absence of new fractures does not necessarily mean that bone loss has been prevented (because fractures occur sporadically) nor does their presence mean that treatment is ineffective (because patients whose bone loss has been arrested at a bone density value below the fracture threshold will continue to have fractures, albeit at a decreased rate).

PREVENTION OF OSTEOPOROSIS

Considering the magnitude of the problem of osteoporosis, prevention is the only cost-effective approach. As a result of an intensive public education program on the significance of osteoporosis, more and more individuals are consulting their physicians for advice on prevention. Certain measures may be recommended to the entire population, male and female. For adults, dietary calcium should be increased to at least 1,000 mg daily. This can be accomplished by ensuring that there are at least three exchange units of dairy products in the daily diet. An exchange unit would be one glass of whole or skim milk, one dish of ice cream, one can of yogurt, or one thick slice of cheese. Adolescents need at least 1,500 mg daily. Increased physical activity, especially of the weight-bearing type, should be encouraged. Bone toxins, such as cigarettes and heavy alcohol consumption, should be eliminated. Women who have premature menopause should receive estrogen replacement until age 50 years.

Because it would be impossible logistically to treat and follow the entire population at risk (all postmenopausal women and all elderly men!), it will be necessary to develop criteria for selecting those who are at greatest risk for future fractures. Prophylactic therapy with agents, such as estrogen, that are effective but have potential risks can be justified in high-risk patients.

There is no agreement, however, on how to identify such high-risk patients. Because there is a close relationship between bone density and the risk of fractures (12), measurement of bone density at the site of potential fracture would seem to be the best method currently available to predict the risk of fracture. Because measurements of bone density are expensive, it is doubtful that screening the millions of people who potentially are at risk is cost-effective (2,9).

A better approach might be to use historical risk factors to select those who are believed to be at sufficient risk of type I osteoporosis to warrant vertebral densitometry. Risk factors that might be discriminatory are given in Table 4. It is not yet possible to weight these factors according to their relative importance to establish a quantitative index. Nonetheless, the more of these that are present in a given person, the greater the likelihood that vertebral density values will be low. Persons found to

TABLE 4. *Possible discriminatory historical risk factors*

Postmenopausal (within 20 years after menopause)
White or Asian
Premature menopause
Positive family history
Short stature and small bones
Leanness
Low calcium intake
Inactivity
Nulliparity
Gastric or small-bowel resection
Long-term glucocorticoid therapy
Long-term use of anticonvulsants
Hyperparathyroidism
Thyrotoxicosis
Smoking
Heavy alcohol use

have low or relative low values should be counseled and started on prophylactic treatment consisting of supplementary calcium at 1,500 mg daily and, in women within 10 years of menopause, estrogen replacement therapy in a cyclic dosage equivalent to 0.625 mg of equine estrogen daily plus sequential progestin. For women over age 75, densitometry is less useful because the bones in most of these women are already below the fracture threshold and those with fractures differ only slightly in bone density from those who do not have fractures.

REFERENCES

1. Chetkowski, R.D., Meldrum, D.R., Steingold, K.A., Randle, D., Lu, J.K., Eggena, P., Hershman, J.M., Alkjaersig, N.K., Fletcher, A.P., and Judd, H.L. (1986): Biologic effects of transdermal estradiol. *N. Engl. J. Med.*, 314:1615–1620.
2. Cummings, S.R., and Black, D. (1986): Should perimenopausal women be screened for osteoporosis. *Ann. Int. Med.*, 104:817–823.
3. Ettinger, B., Genant, H.K., and Cann, C.E. (1987): Postmenopausal bone loss is prevented by treatment with low-dosage estrogen with calcium. *Ann. Int. Med.*, 106:40–45.
4. Gallagher, J.C., Riggs, B.L., Eisman, J., Hamstra, A., Arnaud, S.B., and DeLuca, H.F. (1979): Intestinal calcium absorption and serum vitamin D metabolites in normal subjects and osteoporotic patients: effect of age and dietary calcium. *J. Clin. Invest.*, 64:729–736.
5. Gambrell, R.D., Jr., Maier, R.C., and Sanders,

B.I. (1983): Decreased incidence of breast cancer in postmenopausal estrogen-progestogen users. *Obstet. Gynecol.*, 62:435–443.

6. Genant, H.K., Cann, C.E., Ettinger, B., and Gordan, G.S. (1982): Quantitative computed tomography of vertebral spongiosa: a sensitive method for detecting early bone loss after oophorectomy. *Ann. Int. Med.*, 97:699–705.

7. Judd, H.L., Meldrum, D.R., Deftos, L.J., and Henderson, B.E. (1983): Estrogen replacement therapy: indications and complications (UCLA Conference). *Ann. Int. Med.*, 98:195–205.

8. Kolata, G. (1986): How important is dietary calcium in preventing osteoporosis. *Science*, 233:519–520.

9. Ott, S. (1986): (Editorial) Should women get screening bone mass measurements? *Ann. Int. Med.*, 104:874–876.

10. Recker, R.R. (1985): Calcium absorption and achlorhydria. *N. Engl. J. Med.*, 313:70–73.

11. Riggs, B.L, Jowsey, J., Goldsmith, R.S., Kelly, P.J., Hoffman, D.L., and Arnaud, C.D. (1972): Short- and long-term effects of estrogen and synthetic anabolic hormone in postmenopausal osteoporosis. *J. Clin. Invest.*, 51:1659–1663.

12. Riggs, B.L, and Melton, L.J., III (1986): Involutional osteoporosis. *N. Engl. J. Med.*, 314:1676–1686.

13. Riggs, B.L., and Nelson, K.I. (1985): Effect of long-term treatment with calcitriol on calcium absorption and mineral metabolism in postmenopausal osteoporosis. *J. Clin. Endocrinol. Metab.*, 61:457–461.

14. Riggs, B.L., Seeman, E., Hodgson, S.F., Taves, D.R., and O'Fallon, W.M. (1982): Effect of the fluoride/calcium on vertebral fracture occurrence in postmenopausal osteoporosis. *N. Engl. J. Med.*, 306:446–450.

15. Riggs, B.L., Wahner, H.W., Melton, L.J., III, Richelson, L.S., Judd, H.L., and Offord, K.P. (1986): Rates of bone loss in the appendicular and axial skeletons of women: Evidence of substantial vertebral bone loss before menopause. *J. Clin. Invest.*, 77:1487–1491.

16. Riggs, B.L., Wahner, H.W., Seeman, E., Offord, K.P., Dunn, W.L., Mazess, R.B., Johnson, K.A., and Melton, L.J., III (1982): Changes in bone mineral density of the proximal femur and spine with aging. *J. Clin. Invest.*, 70:716–723.

17. Schwartz, E., Panariello, V.A., and Saeli, J. (1965): Radioactive calcium kinetics during high calcium intake in osteoporosis. *J. Clin. Invest.*, 44:1547.

18. Seeman, E., Kumar, R., Hunder, G.G., Scott, M., Heath, H., III, and Riggs, B.L. (1980): Production, degradation, and circulating levels of 1,25-dihydroxy vitamin D in health and in chronic glucocorticoid excess. *J. Clin. Invest.*, 66:664–669.

19. Seeman, E., Melton, L.J., III, O'Fallon, W.M., and Riggs, B.L. (1983): Risk factors for spinal osteoporosis in men. *Am. J. Med.*, 75:977–983.

20. Stampfer, M.J., Willett, W.C., Colditz, G.A., Rosner, B., Speizer, F.E., and Hennekens, C.H. (1985): A prospective study of postmenopausal estrogen therapy and coronary heart disease. *N. Engl. J. Med.*, 313:1044–1049.

21. Wilson, P.W.F., Garrison, R.J., and Castelli, W.P. (1985): Postmenopausal estrogen use, cigarette smoking, and cardiovascular morbidity in women over 50. *N. Engl. J. Med.*, 313:1038–1043.

22. Wingo, P.A., Layde, P.M., Lee, N.C., Rubin, G., and Ory, H.W. (1987): The risk of breast cancer in postmenopausal women who have used estrogen replacement therapy. *J. Am. Med. Assoc.*, 257:209–215.

Subject Index

A

Absorptiometry
  photon. *See* Photon absorptiometry
  X-ray, 265–270
Acid phosphatase, tartrate-resistant, 310–311
Acromegaly, osteoporosis in, 163–164
Adenosine, and bone cell function, 19
Adrenal function
  and androgen conversion to estrogen, 340
  and hypercorticolism with osteoporosis, 162–163
  and rate of bone loss, 336
Adrenalectomy, and osteoporosis, 170
Aging
  and androgen conversion to estrogen, 340
  and bone mass changes, 50–51
  and calcitonin levels, 382
  and fracture epidemiology, 134–138
  and histomorphometry of bone, 323
  and hydroxyproline excretion in urine, 308–309
  loss of bone in, 111–112, 334
    and mineral content analysis with computed tomography, 226–227
  and mean wall thickness of bone, 70, 72–73
  and osteocyte death, 79–80
  and parathyroid hormone levels, 374–375
  and vitamin D levels, 376–378
Albumin, serum, in bone, 102–103
Alcohol intake, and osteoporosis, 170, 349, 350
Alkaline phosphatase, 297–302, 483
  aging affecting, 375
  bone, 7, 299, 301–302
  estrogen therapy affecting, 343
  glucocorticoids affecting, 25
  intestinal, 298
  liver, 298
  and matrix mineralization, 8
  in menopause, 338
  in metabolic bone disease, 299
  in osteoporosis, 300–301
  placental, 298
  renal, 298
  structure and function of, 297–298
  vitamin D affecting, 24
Aluminum-containing antacids, and calcium in urine, 364, 369
Amenorrhea, exercise-induced, 163
  and bone mineral content, 232, 340–341
cAMP
  and calcitonin action, 23
  and parathyroid hormone action, 21
  urinary excretion of

estrogen therapy affecting, 343, 347
  parathyroid hormone affecting, 374
Analgesics in back pain, 461, 484
Androgens
  conversion to estrogen, aging affecting, 340
  and metabolism of bone, 26–27
  therapy with, 344–345
Anisotropy of bone, 112, 434
Ankle fractures, epidemiology of, 146
Anorexia nervosa, and osteoporosis, 163, 168
Anticonvulsant therapy, bone loss from, 167
Appendicular skeleton
  bone loss in, 334
  fractures of long bones in, 116–117
    epidemiology of, 133
  mineral content of
    compared to axial skeleton, 246, 251, 253–254
    computed tomography of, 234–238, 266–267
    dual-photon absorptiometry of, 262–263
    single-photon absorptiometry of, 254–257
Area moment of inertia, 114, 116, 436
  polar, 114, 116
Arrest lines in bone, 48–49
Arthritis, rheumatoid
  onset after estrogen therapy, 349
  osteoporosis in, 168–169
Axial skeleton. *See* Spine

B

Back strengthening exercises, 462–466, 484
Back supports or braces, 462, 466–469, 484
Barton's fracture, 118
Bending and torsion stresses, 115, 436
Biochemical markers of bone remodeling, 297–312
  acid phosphatase, tartrate-resistant, 310–311
  alkaline phosphatase, 297–302
  in formation of bone, 297–308
  hydroxylysine glycoside, urinary, 310
  hydroxyproline, urinary, 307–310
  osteocalcin, 302–307
  procollagen I carboxyterminal extension peptide, 307
  in resorption of bone, 308–311
Biochemistry of bone, 95–107
  collagen in, 95–99
  in disease, 106–107
  and molecular biology, 104–106
  noncollagenous proteins in, 99–103
Biomechanics of bone, 433–438
  in fractures, 111–126